Advances in Molecular and Cellular Microbiology 22

Antimicrobial Drug Discovery

Emerging Strategies

Edited by

George Tegos

University of New Mexico
Department of Pathology
Center for Molecular Discovery
University of New Mexico Health Sciences
Albuquerque
USA

and

Eleftherios Mylonakis

Harvard Medical School
Massachusetts General Hospital
Division of Infectious Diseases
Boston
USA

www.cabi.org

amcm **Advances in Molecular and Cellular Microbiology**

Through the application of molecular and cellular microbiology, we now recognize the diversity and dominance of microbial life forms on our planet, which exist in all environments. These microbes have many important planetary roles, but for us humans a major problem is their ability to colonize our tissues and cause disease. The same techniques of molecular and cellular microbiology have been applied to the problems of human and animal infection during the past two decades and have proved to be immensely powerful tools in elucidating how microorganisms cause human pathology. This series has the aim of providing information on the advances that have been made in the application of molecular and cellular microbiology to specific organisms and the diseases that they cause. The series is edited by researchers active in the application of molecular and cellular microbiology to human disease states. Each volume focuses on a particular aspect of infectious disease and will enable graduate students and researchers to keep up with the rapidly diversifying literature in current microbiological research.

Series Editor

Professor Michael Wilson
University College London

Titles Available from CABI

17. *Helicobacter pylori* in the 21st Century
Edited by Philip Sutton and Hazel Mitchell

18. Antimicrobial Peptides: Discovery, Design and Novel Therapeutic Strategies
Edited by Guangshun Wang

19. Stress Response in Pathogenic Bacteria
Edited by Stephen P. Kidd

20. Lyme Disease: an Evidence-based Approach
Edited by John Halperin

22. Antimicrobial Drug Discovery: Emerging Strategies
Edited by George Tegos and Eleftherios Mylonakis

Titles Forthcoming from CABI

Tuberculosis: Diagnosis and Treatment
Edited by Timothy McHugh

Microbial Metabolomics
Edited by Silas Villas-Bôas and Katya Ruggiero

Bacteriophages in Health and Disease
Edited by Paul Hyman and Stephen T. Abedon

The Human Microbiota and Microbiome
Edited by Julian Marchesi

Earlier titles in the series are available from Cambridge University Press (www.cup.cam.ac.uk).

CABI is a trading name of CAB International

CABI
Nosworthy Way
Wallingford
Oxfordshire OX10 8DE
UK

Tel: +44 (0)1491 832111
Fax: +44 (0)1491 833508
E-mail: info@cabi.org
Website: www.cabi.org

CABI
875 Massachusetts Avenue
7th Floor
Cambridge, MA 02139
USA

Tel: +1 800 552 3083 (toll free)
Tel: +1 (0)617 395 4051
E-mail: cabi-nao@cabi.org

A catalogue record for this book is available from the British Library, London, UK.

Library of Congress Cataloging-in-Publication Data

Antimicrobial drug discovery : emerging strategies / editors, George Tegos and Eleftherios Mylonakis.
p. ; cm. -- (Advances in molecular and cellular microbiology ; 22)
Includes bibliographical references and index.
ISBN 978-1-84593-943-4 (alk. paper)
I. Tegos, George. II. Mylonakis, Eleftherios. III. Series: Advances in molecular and cellular microbiology ; 22.
[DNLM: 1. Anti-Infective Agents--pharmacology. 2. Drug Design. 3. Disease Models, Animal. 4. High-Throughput Screening Assays--methods. 5. Photosensitizing Agents--pharmacology. QV 250]

615.7'92--dc23

2012001019

ISBN: 978 1 84593 943 4

Commissioning editor: Rachel Cutts
Editorial assistant: Alexandra Lainsbury
Production editor: Tracy Head

Typeset by SPi, Pondicherry, India.
Printed and bound in the UK by CPI Group (UK) Ltd, Croydon, CR0 4YY.

Contents

Contributors

Ahirrao, Pallavi, Rayat-Bahra Institute of Pharmacy, Saharaun, Kharar, Mohali District, Punjab, India, pahirrao11@gmail.com

Alex, Deepu, Department of Microbiology and Immunology, Georgetown University Medical Center, Washington, DC 20057, USA, Da82@georgetown.edu

Amaral, Leonard, Grupo de Micobactérias, Unidade de Microbiologia Médica, Instituto de Higiene e Medicina Tropical (IHMT), Universidade Nova de Lisboa, Rua da Junqueira 100, 1349-008 Lisbon, Portugal; UPMM (Unidade de Parasitologia e Microbiologia Médicas), Instituto de Higiene e Medicina Tropical (IHMT), Universidade Nova de Lisboa, Rua da Junqueira 100, 1349-008 Lisbon, Portugal; and Cost Action BM0701 (ATENS) of the European Commission/European Science Foundation, Brussels, Belgium, LAmaral@ihmt.unl.pt

Apidianakis, Yiorgos, Department of Surgery, Harvard Medical School and Massachusetts General Hospital, Boston, Massachusetts, USA; and Department of Biological Sciences, University of Cyprus, Nicosia, Cyprus, apidiana@ucy.ac.cy

Armstrong-James, Darius, Division of Infectious Diseases, Faculty of Medicine, Imperial College London, London SW7 2AZ, UK, d.armstrong@imperial.ac.uk

Ball, Anthony R., Department of Microbiology, Toxikon Corporation, Bedford, MA 01730, USA, aball@toxikon.com

Bignell, Elaine M., Division of Infectious Diseases, Faculty of Medicine, Imperial College London, London SW7 2AZ, UK, e.bignell@imperial.ac.uk

Bini, Davide, Department of Biotechnology and Biosciences, University of Milano-Bicocca, Piazza della Scienza 2, 20126 Milan, Italy, davidebini@hotmail.com

Boberek, Jaroslaw M., Department of Pathology and Infectious Diseases, The Royal Veterinary College, University of London, London, UK, jboberek@rvc.ac.uk

Bonvin, Alexandre M.J.J., Bijvoet Center for Biomolecular Research, Science Faculty, Utrecht University, 3584CH, Utrecht, The Netherlands, a.m.j.j.bonvin@uu.nl

Brackman, Gilles, Laboratory of Pharmaceutical Microbiology, Ghent University, Harelbekestraat 72, 9000 Ghent, Belgium, Gilles.Brackman@ugent.be

Calderone, Richard, Department of Microbiology and Immunology, Georgetown University Medical Center, Washington, DC 20057, USA, calderor@georgetown.edu

Cannon, Richard D., Sir John Walsh Research Institute, University of Otago, PO Box 647, Dunedin 9054, New Zealand, richard.cannon@otago.ac.nz

Cerca, Pedro, Grupo de Micobactérias, Unidade de Microbiologia Médica, Instituto de Higiene e Medicina Tropical (IHMT), Universidade Nova de Lisboa, Rua da Junqueira 100, 1349-008 Lisbon, Portugal, pcerca@ihmt.unl.pt

Chen, Hui, Department of Microbiology and Immunology, Georgetown University Medical Center, Washington, DC 20057, USA, chen@georgetown.edu

Chen, Yuan, School of Chemical and Biomedical Engineering, Nanyang Technological University, Singapore 637459, chenyuan@ntu.edu.sg

Cherkasov, Artem, Prostate Centre at the Vancouver General Hospital, University of British Columbia, 2640 Oak Street, British Columbia V6H 3Z6, Canada, acherkasov@prostatecentre.com

Cipolla, Laura, Department of Biotechnology and Biosciences, University of Milano-Bicocca, Piazza della Scienza 2, 20126 Milan, Italy, laura.cipolla@unimib.it

Coenye, Tom, Laboratory of Pharmaceutical Microbiology, Ghent University, Harelbekestraat 72, 9000 Ghent, Belgium, tom.coenye@UGent.be

Coleman, Jeffrey J., Division of Infectious Diseases, Massachusetts General Hospital, Harvard Medical School, 55 Fruit St, GRJ-504, Boston, MA 02114, USA, jjcoleman@partners.org

Cotter, Paul D., Teagasc Food Research Centre Moorepark, Fermoy, Cork, Ireland and Alimentary Pharmabiotic Centre, Cork, Ireland, paul.cotter@teagasc.ie

Couto, Isabel, Grupo de Micobactérias, Unidade de Microbiologia Médica, Instituto de Higiene e Medicina Tropical (IHMT), Universidade Nova de Lisboa, Rua da Junqueira 100, 1349-008 Lisbon, Portugal and Centro de Recursos Microbiológicos (CREM), Faculdade de Ciências e Tecnologia, UNL, 2829-516 Caparica, Portugal, icouto@ihmt.unl.pt

Dai, Tianhong, Wellman Center for Photomedicine, Massachusetts General Hospital, Boston, Massachusetts, USA; and Department of Dermatology, Harvard Medical School, Boston, MA 02114, USA, tdai@partners.org

Demain, Arnold L., Charles A. Dana Research Institute for Scientists Emeriti (RISE), Drew University, Madison, NJ 07940, USA, ademain@drew.edu

Fanning, Séamus, University College Dublin, School of Agriculture, Food Sciences and Veterinary Medicine, UCD Center Food Safety, Dublin 4, Ireland, sfanning@ucd.ie

Fjell, Christopher D., Centre for Microbial Diseases and Immunity Research, University of British Columbia, 2259 Lower Mall, Vancouver, British Columbia V6T 1Z4, Canada, cfjell@interchange.ubc.ca

Fonzi, William, Department of Microbiology and Immunology, Georgetown University Medical Center, Washington, DC 20057, USA, fonziw@georgetown.edu

Gabrielli, Luca, Department of Biotechnology and Biosciences, University of Milano-Bicocca, Piazza della Scienza 2, 20126 Milan, Italy, l.gabrielli2@campus.unimib.it

Gay-Andrieu, Francoise, Department of Microbiology and Immunology, Georgetown University Medical Center, Washington, DC 20057 USA, francoise.gayandrieu@free.fr

Gibbons, Simon, Centre for Pharmacognosy and Phytotherapy, The School of Pharmacy, University of London, London, UK, simon.gibbons@pharmacy.ac.uk

Goh, Shan, Department of Pathology and Infectious Diseases, The Royal Veterinary College, University of London, London, UK, sgoh@rvc.ac.uk

Good, Liam, Department of Pathology and Infectious Diseases, The Royal Veterinary College, University of London, London, UK, lgood@rvc.ac.uk

Groutas, William, Wichita State University, Department of Chemistry, Wichita, Kansas, USA, Bill.groutas@wsu.edu

Gupta, Shiv, Department of Natural Products, National Institute of Pharmaceutical Education and Research (NIPER), Sector 67, SAS Nagar, Punjab, India, shivgupta218@gmail.com

Hamblin, Michael R., Wellman Center for Photomedicine, Massachusetts General Hospital, Boston, Massachusetts, USA; Department of Dermatology, Harvard Medical School, Boston, MA 02114, USA; and Harvard-MIT Division of Health Sciences and Technology, Cambridge, Massachusetts, USA, hamblin@helix.mgh.harvard.edu

Hancock, Robert E.W., Centre for Microbial Diseases and Immunity Research, University of British Columbia, 2259 Lower Mall, Vancouver, British Columbia V6T 1Z4, Canada, bob@cmdr.ubc.ca

Hill, Colin, Microbiology Department, University College Cork, Cork, Ireland; and Alimentary Pharmabiotic Centre, Cork, Ireland, c.hill@ucc.ie

Holmes, Ann R., Sir John Walsh Research Institute, University of Otago, PO Box 647, Dunedin 9054, New Zealand, ann.holmes@otago.ac.nz

Jachak, Sanjay M., Department of Natural Products, National Institute of Pharmaceutical Education and Research (NIPER), Sector 67, SAS Nagar, Punjab, India, sanjayjachak@niper.ac.in

Jenssen, Håvard, Roskilde University, Dept. of Science, Systems and Models, Universitetsvej 1, Building 18.1, DK-4000 Roskilde, Denmark, jenssen@ruc.dk

Kastritis, Panagiotis L., Bijvoet Center for Biomolecular Research, Science Faculty, Utrecht University, 3584CH, Utrecht, The Netherlands, pkastrit@gmail.com

Kokai-Kun, John F., Biosynexus Incorporated, Gaithersburg, MD 20877, USA; current address: Lonza Walkersville, Inc., 8830 Biggs Ford Road, Walkersville, MD 21793, USA, john.kokai-kun@lonza.com

Kontoyiannis, Dimitrios P., Department of Infectious Diseases, Infection Control and Employee Health, The University of Texas MD Anderson Cancer Center, Houston, Texas, USA, dkontoyi@mdanderson.org

Kristiansen, Jette, Department of Chemistry, University of Copenhagen, Universitetsparken 5, DK-2100 Copenhagen, Denmark; and NRG, Sundgade 54, 6320 Egernsund, Denmark, malthe@dadlnet.dk

Lewis, Kim, Antimicrobial Discovery Center and the Department of Biology, Northeastern University, Boston, MA 02115, USA, k.lewis@neu.edu

Li, Dongmei, Department of Microbiology and Immunology, Georgetown University Medical Center, Washington, DC 20057, USA, dl33@georgetown.edu

Liu, Shaobin, School of Chemical and Biomedical Engineering, Nanyang Technological University, Singapore 637459, liushaobin@ntu.edu.sg

Machado, Lisa, Grupo de Micobactérias, Unidade de Microbiologia Médica, Instituto de Higiene e Medicina Tropical (IHMT), Universidade Nova de Lisboa, Rua da Junqueira 100, 1349-008 Lisbon, Portugal, lisa.machado@ihmt.unl.pt

Marsh, Alan J., Teagasc Food Research Centre, Moorepark, Fermoy, Cork, Ireland; and Microbiology Department, University College Cork, Cork, Ireland, Alan.Marsh@teagasc.ie

Martins, Ana, Institute of Pharmacognosy, Faculty of Pharmacy, University of Szeged, Eotvos u. 6, H-6720 Szeged, Hungary, martins.a@pharm.u-szeged.hu

McCusker, Matthew, University College Dublin, School of Agriculture, Food Sciences and Veterinary Medicine, UCD Centre Food Safety, Dublin, Ireland

Molnar, Joseph, Cost Action BM0701 (ATENS) of the European Commission/European Science Foundation, Brussels, Belgium; and Department of Medical Microbiology and Immunobiology, Faculty of Medicine, University of Szeged, Dóm tér 10, H-6720 Szeged, Hungary, molnarj@comser.szote.u-szeged.hu

Monk, Brian C., Sir John Walsh Research Institute, University of Otago, PO Box 647, Dunedin 9054, New Zealand, brian.monk@otago.ac.nz

Mylonakis, Eleftherios, Division of Infectious Diseases, Massachusetts General Hospital, Harvard Medical School, 55 Fruit St, GRJ-504, Boston, MA 02114, USA, emylonakis@partners.org

Nelis, Hans J., Laboratory of Pharmaceutical Microbiology, Ghent University, Harelbekestraat 72, 9000 Ghent, Belgium, Hans.Nelis@ugent.be

Niimi, Kyoko, Sir John Walsh Research Institute, University of Otago, PO Box 647, Dunedin 9054, New Zealand, niimi.kyoko@otago.ac.nz

Nosanchuk, Joshua D., Departments of Medicine (Division of Infectious Diseases) and Microbiology and Immunology, Albert Einstein College of Medicine, 1300 Morris Park Ave, New York, NY 10461, USA, josh.nosanchuk@einstein.yu.edu

Ntokou, Eleni, Short-Term Student Mission of the Cost Action BM0701 of the European Commission, European Science Foundation, Brussels, Belgium; and Department of Microbiology, Medical School, University of Thessaly, Viopolis, 41110 Larissa, Greece, elenintokou@gmail.com

Parra, Karlett J., Department of Biochemistry and Molecular Biology, University of New Mexico, School of Medicine, Albuquerque, NM 87131, USA, KJParra@salud.unm.edu

Rodrigues, Liliana, Grupo de Micobactérias, Unidade de Microbiologia Médica, Instituto de Higiene e Medicina Tropical (IHMT), Universidade Nova de Lisboa, Rua da Junqueira 100, 1349-008 Lisbon, Portugal; and UPMM (Unidade de Parasitologia e Microbiologia Médicas), Instituto de Higiene e Medicina Tropical (IHMT), Universidade Nova de Lisboa, Rua da Junqueira 100, 1349-008 Lisbon, Portugal, lrodrigues@ihmt.unl.pt

Ross, R. Paul, Teagasc Food Research Centre, Moorepark, Fermoy, Cork, Ireland; and Microbiology Department, University College Cork, Cork, Ireland, paul.ross@teagasc.ie

Roy, Somendu K., Department of Natural Products, National Institute of Pharmaceutical Education and Research (NIPER), Sector 67, SAS Nagar, Punjab, India, somenduroy@gmail.com

Russo, Laura, Department of Biotechnology and Biosciences, University of Milano-Bicocca, Piazza della Scienza 2, 20126 Milan, Italy, l.russo2@campus.unimib.it

Sharma, Sulbha K., Wellman Center for Photomedicine, Massachusetts General Hospital, Boston, Massachusetts, USA, and Department of Dermatology, Harvard Medical School, Boston, Massachusetts, USA, ssharma0@partners.org

Sklar, Larry A., University of New Mexico Center for Molecular Discovery (UNMCMD) and Department of Pathology, School of Medicine, Albuquerque, NM 87131, USA, lsklar@salud.unm.edu

Spengler, Gabriella, Department of Medical Microbiology and Immunobiology, Faculty of Medicine, University of Szeged, Dóm tér 10, H-6720 Szeged, Hungary, spengler.gabriella@med.u-szeged.hu

Spizek, Jaroslav, Institute of Microbiology, Academy of Sciences of the Czech Republic, Videnska 1083, 142 20 Prague 4, Czech Republic, spizek@biomed.cas.cz

Stach, Jem, School of Biology, University of Newcastle, Newcastle upon Tyne, UK, jem.stach@newcastle.ac.uk

Strouse, J. Jacob, University of New Mexico Center for Molecular Discovery (UNMCMD), Albuquerque, NM 87131, USA, jjstrouse@salud.unm.edu

Sun, Nuo, Department of Microbiology and Immunology, Georgetown University Medical Center, Washington, DC 20057, USA, nuosun@gmail.com

Tegos, George P., Center for Molecular Discovery and Department of Pathology, University of New Mexico, Albuquerque, NM 87131, USA; Wellman Center for Photomedicine, Massachusetts General Hospital, Boston, Massachusetts, USA; and Department of Dermatology, Harvard Medical School, Boston, Massachusetts, USA, gtegos@partners.org

Trofa, David, Departments of Medicine (Division of Infectious Diseases) and Microbiology and Immunology, Albert Einstein College of Medicine, 1300 Morris Park Ave, New York, NY 10461, USA, davidtrofa@gmail.com

Viveiros, Miguel, Grupo de Micobactérias, Unidade de Microbiologia Médica, Instituto de Higiene e Medicina Tropical (IHMT), Universidade Nova de Lisboa, Rua da Junqueira 100, 1349-008 Lisbon, Portugal; and Cost Action BM0701 (ATENS) of the European Commission/European Science Foundation, Brussels, Belgium, MViveiros@ihmt.unl.pt

Waldrop, Grover L., Division of Biochemistry and Molecular Biology, Department of Biological Sciences, Room 206, Life Sciences Building, Louisiana State University, Baton Rouge, LA 70803, USA, gwaldro@lsu.edu

To my family, students, colleagues and the memory of my advisor Costas Drainas

George Tegos

To my family, students and mentors

Eleftherios Mylonakis

Introduction

One of the scientific highlights of the 20th century was, without doubt, the development of successful prevention and control efforts for infectious diseases. After the development of penicillin and the subsequent development and synthesis of other antimicrobial agents, vaccines and antiseptics, victory against pathogens was declared (Sigerist, 1971). By the 1980s, pharmaceutical companies were convinced that there were already enough antimicrobial agents – the feeling at the time was that research should get ready to 'close the book on infectious diseases' and the emphasis was shifted to other clinical problems such as cancer, diabetes and heart disease.

However, the extensive and inappropriate use of antimicrobial agents gradually led to the development of pervasive resistance. Penicillin was first put into widespread use in the early 1940s, and by 1944, half of all clinical *Staphylococcus* spp. isolates were resistant to this proclaimed 'miracle drug' (Livermore, 2000). Today, infectious disease is the second most important killer in the world, third in developed nations and fourth in the USA behind heart disease, cancer and stroke (Vicente *et al.*, 2006; Kraus, 2008). Worldwide, 17 million people die each year from bacterial infections and numerous others from viral, fungal and parasitic diseases (Butler and Bush, 2006).

Pathogenic microorganisms have demonstrated an impressive ability to adapt and develop resistance to antimicrobial agents (Fig. I.1). Four classes of antimicrobial-resistant pathogens are emerging as major threats to public health: methicillin-resistant *Staphylococcus aureus* (MRSA), vancomycin-resistant *Enterococcus faecalis* (VRE), multidrug-resistant and extensively drug-resistant strains of *Mycobacterium tuberculosis* (MDR-TB and XDR-TB, respectively). These are a rising threat in the developing world, together with multidrug-resistant mycobacteria, Gram-negative pathogens and fungi (Dye, 2009; Jassal and Bishai, 2009; Nicolau, 2011). In addition to these established threats, we are confronting ever more challenging clinical scenarios including carbapenem-resistant *Klebsiella pneumoniae* encoding the New Delhi metallo-β-lactamase as well as other Enterobacteriaceae encoding this enzyme, and *Escherichia coli* outbreaks caused by previously unknown strains, all of which are responsible for significant morbidity and mortality (Norrby *et al.*, 2005; Cornaglia *et al.*, 2011; Turner, 2011).

There is a clear and emergent need for new strategies in antimicrobial drug discovery. The rapid emergence of resistance to essentially all broad-spectrum antimicrobial agents has been well established. For example, as noted above, resistance to penicillin was observed within 3–4 years, while the interval was 5 years for tetracycline and 1 year for methicillin (Palumbi, 2001). With the

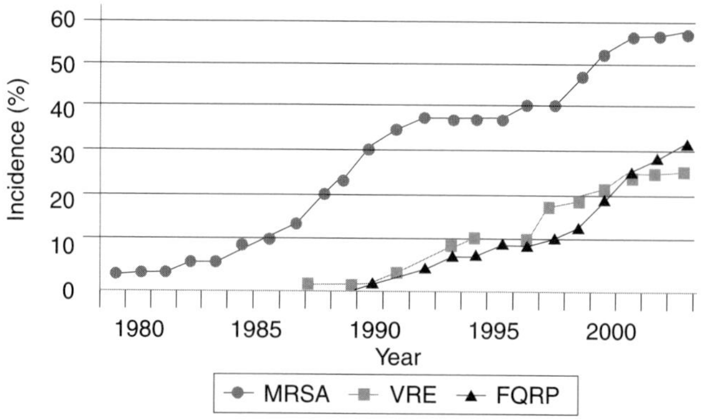

Fig. I.1. The incidence of resistant strains is increasing rapidly whereas the number of new antibacterial agents approved in the USA is decreasing (Dalovisio, 2005). MRSA, methicillin-resistant *Staphylococcus aureus*; VRE, vancomycin-resistant *Enterococcus*; FQRP, fluoroquinolone-resistant *Pseudomonas* spp.

possible exception of tigecycline and the narrow-spectrum agents linezolid and daptomycin, fluoroquinolones are the last class of truly broad-spectrum antimicrobial agents.

It is therefore necessary to develop strategies to address novel and unprecedented threats. At the present time, the field of antimicrobial drug discovery is being revitalized with new concepts and an array of technologies and platforms that are under investigation. However, as we expand our understanding of the mechanisms of multidrug resistance, there is a clear switch in conventional drug discovery ventures. There is also a consensus belief that the 'antibiotic era' should be radically conceptually enriched or amplified. Investing in revitalizing old targets as well as the quest for new ones, putting together more inclusionary approaches and multidisciplinary ventures in the interface of science and technology (translation) and exploring the special host–pathogen relationship are some of the most notable current efforts as we move towards a new era.

As an example, efflux mechanisms are broadly recognized as major components of resistance to many classes of chemotherapeutic agents as well as antimicrobial agents. Efflux occurs as a result of the activity of membrane transporter proteins widely known as multidrug efflux systems (Paulsen *et al.*, 2002). These are implicated in a variety of physiological roles other than efflux, and identifying natural substrates and inhibitors is an active and expanding research discipline (Piddock, 2006; Tegos, 2006). Multidrug efflux systems perform essential roles in cellular metabolism and activity. They differ in membrane topology, energy coupling mechanisms and, most importantly, substrate specificities. Based on their sequence similarity, they are classified into six superfamilies. The first five families are found in microorganisms (the MET family appears to be restricted to higher eukaryotes), but representatives of all groups are also expressed in mammalian cells. The most challenging clinical scenarios in a wide range of Gram-negative pathogens involve the resistant nodulation division (RND) systems.

At the University of New Mexico Center for Molecular Discovery, a comprehensive attempt to define the 'transporter–ligand interactome' is under development (Tegos *et al.*, 2011). This effort uses a hybrid chemogenomics–chemoinformatics discovery platform employing efflux systems from specific organisms, the National Institutes of Health Molecular Libraries Small Molecule Repository (MLSMR) chemical library and high-throughput screening (HTS) flow cytometry to map the chemical and biological space around efflux systems. This approach integrates data from genomic, proteomic and medicinal chemistry databases in concert with physical screening campaigns. It provides the rationale to chemically characterize substrates and subsequently accelerate the discovery of potent functional inducers or repressors as well as efflux pump inhibitors (EPIs). This project includes a multidisciplinary international consortium with investigators who are experts in specific transporter systems and translational research, and represents one of the first comprehensive efforts to employ the MLSMR in a selected group of organisms with efflux systems as targets. This effort aligns the discovery of lead chemotypes with secondary validation of lead probes as well as implementation of a translational plan to move forward lead EPIs to pre-clinical development based on prior art and collaborative ventures (Tegos *et al.*, 2002, 2006, 2008; Belofsky *et al.*, 2004, 2006; Dai *et al.*, 2010; Kishen *et al.*, 2010; Fiamegos *et al.*, 2011; Prates *et al.*, 2011).

On a slightly different note, there are potential ways and platforms to accelerate discovery. A variety of diverse model non-vertebrate hosts (e.g. the fly *Drosophila melanogaster*, the microscopic nematode *Caenorhabditis elegans* and the greater wax moth caterpillar *Galleria mellonella*), and fairly recently zebrafish, have been used to model microbial virulence and pathogenicity as well as the toxicity and efficacy of novel antimicrobial compounds (Fuchs and Mylonakis, 2006; Apidianakis and Rahme, 2009; Fuchs *et al.*, 2010; Adams *et al.*, 2011). These heterologous hosts fill an important niche in pathogenesis research and provide us with a unique opportunity to identify novel compounds and study basic, evolutionarily conserved aspects of virulence and the host response. However, model host systems have different strengths and weaknesses, and the selection of a model system depends on the virulence factors and host responses of interest (Mylonakis *et al.*, 2007; Mylonakis, 2011). Findings from these models can be validated and studied in mammalian systems. This approach is the basis for the 'multi-host' pathogenesis system that is based on cross-species studies among divergent model hosts and allows the discovery of fundamental virulence and host–response mechanisms that are independent of the host (Kerekov *et al.*, 2011; Zaborina *et al.*, 2011).

An example of an alternative transformation for a discovery platform is photodynamic therapy (PDT). PDT was initially established as (and remains) a promising modality against malignancies. More recently, photodynamic inactivation (PDI) has been investigated as a modality for antimicrobial discovery and development strategy. The concept of PDI is quite straightforward and requires microbial exposure to visible light energy, typically wavelengths in the visible region, which causes the excitation of photosensitizer molecules (either exogenous or endogenous), resulting in the production of singlet oxygen and other reactive oxygen species that react with intracellular components and consequently lead to cell inactivation. It is an area of increasing interest, as research is advancing both in understanding the photochemical, photophysical and biological mechanisms involved in inactivation and in developing potent and clinically compatible photosensitizers for novel delivery platforms in applications in the clinical setting and beyond, such as environmental disinfectants (St Denis *et al.*, 2011). The very nature of PDT makes it ideal for the treatment of skin, wound and burn infections, all of which are easily accessible for light therapies (Dai *et al.*, 2011). PDT may have prospective applications in the treatment of soft-tissue infections. Several new PDT clinical applications have been developed in recent years. Ondine Biomedical has a large clinical trial in progress using methylene blue PDT for nasal decontamination of MRSA before surgery (http://www.ondinebio.com/wp-content/uploads/2011/04/OBP-NR-041511-Final.pdf). The same company is planning a second clinical trial of photodisinfection for the *in situ* microbial disinfection of endotracheal tubes as a means of preventing ventilator-associated pneumonia (http://www.ondinebio.com/wp-content/uploads/2011/05/OBP-NR-051011-Final.pdf).

In this book, *Antimicrobial Drug Discovery: Emerging Strategies*, we attempt to shed light on these new approaches and outline some of the most exciting developments on the field, with a focus on bacterial and fungal pathogens. Chapters 1 and 2 outline the elements of drug resistance to provide a conceptual basis and highlight the requirement for and shaping of novel strategies. The next section (Chapters 3–6) emphasizes the efforts being made to modulate mechanisms of efflux. This section focuses on the AcrAB-TolC multidrug efflux systems of *Escherichia coli* and *Salmonella* (Chapter 3), provides an array of methodologies and approaches to identify natural inhibitors of efflux (Chapter 4), discusses tactic elements for fungal pump inhibitors (Chapter 5) and makes the case for the importance of the vacuolar ATPase in antifungal drug discovery (Chapter 6).

In the quest for new targets and approaches, the next chapters outline the impact of multidrug tolerance of biofilms and persister cells (Chapter 7), the strategy of bacterial quorum-sensing inhibition (Chapter 8), the attempt to exploit a protein essential for cell division in bacteria, filamentous temperature-sensitive mutant Z (FtsZ) (Chapter 9) for antibacterial therapy and the antistaphylococcal enzyme lysostaphin as a countermeasure for staphylococcal disease (Chapter 10).

The next section is devoted to discovery ventures with a heavy bio- or chemoinformatics component, such as strategies to identify modified ribosomally synthesized antimicrobials (Chapter 11) and quantitative structure–activity relationship-based discovery of antimicrobial peptides (Chapter 12). Bacterial acetyl-CoA carboxylase is discussed as an emerging target for antibiotic development (Chapter 13) as well as underexploited targets in lipopolysaccharide biogenesis for the design of antibacterial agents (Chapter 14). The last chapter in this section is devoted to prediction and dissection of biomolecular interactions by information-driven docking for discovery (Chapter 15).

The last section hosts a variety of approaches spanning a conceptual introduction to current trends for antifungal agents (Chapter 16) and pathosystematic 'systems biology' for the rational design of antifungal interventions (Chapter 17). Special emphasis is given to the use of non-vertebrate hosts for the development of *in vivo* HTS discovery utilizing *C. elegans* (Chapter 18) and *D. melanogaster* (Chapter 19) as versatile models for discovery. Finally, a set of chapters provides the highlights and discusses the potential of new antimicrobial technological platforms such as PDT (Chapter 19), nanoparticles (Chapter 20) and nanotubes (Chapter 21).

Editing this book would have been a mission impossible without the contribution of a diverse group of colleagues who offered their substantial reviewing efforts and suggestions: Jun Chen, Mark Haynes, Peter Simons and Jacob Strouse (University of New Mexico Center for Molecular Discovery, Albuquerque, New Mexico, USA), Michael La Fleur (Arietis Corp., Boston, Massachusetts, USA), Beth Fuchs (Division of Infectious Diseases, Harvard Medical School and Massachusetts General Hospital, Boston, Massachusetts, USA) and Nikos Karousis (Theoretical and Physical Chemistry Institute, National Hellenic Research Foundation, Athens, Greece).

George Tegos
Eleftherios Mylonakis

References

Adams, K.N., Takak, I.K., Connolly, L.E., Wiedenhoft, H., Winglee, K., Humbert, O., Edelstein, P.H., Cosma, C.L. and Ramakrishnan, L. (2011) Drug tolerance in replicating mycobacteria mediated by a macrophage-induced efflux mechanism. *Cell* 145, 39–53.

Apidianakis, Y. and Rahme, L.G. (2009) *Drosophila melanogaster* as a model host for studying *Pseudomonas aeruginosa* infection. *Nature Protocols* 4, 1285–1294.

Belofsky, G., Percivil, D., Lewis, K., Tegos, G.P. and Ekart, J. (2004) Phenolic metabolites of *Dalea versicolor* that enhance antibiotic activity against multi-drug resistant bacteria. *Journal of Natural Products* 67, 481–484.

Belofsky, G., Carreno, R., Lewis, K., Ball, A., Casadei, G. and Tegos, G.P. (2006) Metabolites of the "smoke tree", *Dalea spinosa*, potentiate antibiotic activity against multidrug-resistant *Staphylococcus aureus. Journal of Natural Products* 69, 261–264.

Butler, M.A. and Bush, A.D. (2006) Natural products – the future scaffolds for novel antibiotics? *Biochemical Pharmacology* 71, 919–929.

Cornaglia, G., Giamarellou, H. and Rossolini, G.M. (2011) Metallo-β-lactamases: a last frontier for β-lactams? *Lancet Infectious Diseases* 11, 381–393.

Dai, T., Tegos, G.P., Zhiyentayev, T., Mylonakis, E. and Hamblin, M.R. (2010) Photodynamic therapy for methicillin-resistant *Staphylococcus aureus* infection in a mouse skin abrasion model. *Lasers in Surgery and Medicine* 42, 38–44.

Dai, T., Kharkwal, G.B., Tanaka, M., Huang, Y.Y., Bil De Arce, V.J. and Hamblin, M.R. (2011) Animal models of external traumatic wound infections. *Virulence* 2, 296–315.

Dalovisio, J.R. (2005) IDSA: Infancy to adulthood in four decades. *Clinical Infectious Diseases* 40, 574–578.

Dye, C. (2009) Doomsday postponed? Preventing and reversing epidemics of drug-resistant tuberculosis. *Nature Reviews Microbiology* 7, 81–87.

Fiamegos, Y., Kastritis, P.L., Exarchou, V., Han, H., Bonvin, A.M.J.J., Vervoort, J., Lewis, K., Hamblin, M.R. and Tegos, G.P. (2011) Antimicrobial and efflux pump inhibitory activity of caffeoylquinic acids from *Artemisia absinthium* against Gram-positive pathogenic bacteria. *PLoS One* 6, e18127.

Fuchs, B. and Mylonakis, E. (2006) Using non-mammalian hosts to study fungal virulence and host defense. *Current Opinion in Microbiology* 9, 346–351.

Fuchs, B., O'Brien, E., Khoury, J. and Mylonakis, E. (2010) Methods for using *Galleria mellonella* as a model host to study fungal pathogenesis. *Virulence* 1, 475–482.

Jassal, M. and Bishai, W.R. (2009) Extensively drug-resistant tuberculosis. *Lancet Infectious Diseases* 9, 19–30.

Kerekov, N., Mihaylova, N., Prechl, J. and Tchorbanov, A. (2011) Humanized SCID mice models of SLE. *Current Pharmaceutical Design* 17, 1261–1266.

Kishen, A., Upadya, M., Tegos, G.P. and Hamblin, M.R. (2010) Efflux pump inhibitor potentiates antimicrobial photodynamic inactivation of *Enterococcus faecalis* biofilm. *Photochemistry and Photobiology* 86, 1343–1349.

Kraus, C. (2008) Low hanging fruit in infectious disease drug development. *Current Opinion in Microbiology* 11, 434–438.

Livermore, D.M. (2000) Antibiotic resistance in staphylococci. *International Journal of Antimicrobial Agents* 16 Suppl. 1, S3–10.

Mylonakis, E. (2011) The need to redefine antimicrobial drug discovery. *Current Pharmaceutical Design* 17, 1223–1224.

Mylonakis, E., Casadevall, A. and Ausubel, F.M. (2007) Exploiting amoeboid and non-vertebrate animal model systems to study the virulence of human pathogenic fungi. *PLoS Pathogens* 3, e101.

Nicolau, D. (2011) Current challenges in the management of the infected patient. *Current Opinion in Infectious Diseases* (Suppl. 1), S1–S10.

Norrby, S.R., Nord, C.E. and Finch, R. (2005) Lack of development of new antimicrobial drugs: a potential serious threat to public health. *Lancet Infectious Diseases* 5, 115–119.

Palumbi, S. (2001) Humans as the world's greatest evolutionary force. *Science* 293, 1786–1790.

Paulsen, I.T., Chen, J., Nelson, K.E. and Saier, M.H.J. (2002) Comparative genomics of microbial drug efflux systems. In: Lewis, K. (ed.) *Microbial Multidrug Efflux*. Horizon Press, Norfolk, UK, pp. 5–21.

Piddock, L. (2006) Multidrug-resistance efflux pumps – not just for resistance. *Nature Reviews Microbiology* 20, 629–636.

Prates, R., Kato, I.T., Ribeiro, M.S., Tegos, G.P. and Hamblin, M.R. (2011) Influence of multidrug efflux systems on methylene blue-mediated photodynamic inactivation of *Candida albicans. Journal of Antimicrobial Chemotherapy* 66, 1525–1532.

Sigerist, H. (1971) *The Great Doctors 372*. Dover Publications, New York.

St Denis, T., Dai, T., Izikson, L., Astrakas, C., Anderson, R.R., Hamblin, M.R. and Tegos, G.P. (2011) All you need is light: antimicrobial photoinactivation as an evolving and emerging discovery strategy against infectious disease. *Virulence* 2, 1–12.

Tegos, G. (2006) Substrates and inhibitors of microbial efflux pumps; redefine the role of plant antimicrobials. In: Rai, M. and Carpinella, C.M. (eds) *Naturally Occurring Bioactive Compounds: a New and Safe Alternative for Control of Pests and Microbial Diseases*. Cambridge University Press, Cambridge, UK.

Tegos, G., Stermitz, F.R., Lomovskaya, O. and Lewis, K. (2002) Multidrug pump inhibitors uncover remarkable activity of plant antimicrobials. *Antimicrobial Agents and Chemotherapy* 46, 3133–3141.

Tegos, G.P., Anbe, M., Yang, C., Demidova, T.N., Satti, M., Mroz, P., Janjua, S., Gad, F. and Hamblin, M.R. (2006) Protease-stable polycationic photosensitizer conjugates between polyethyleneimine and chlorin(e6) for broad-spectrum antimicrobial photoinactivation. *Antimicrobial Agents and Chemotherapy* 50, 1402–1410.

Tegos, G., Masago, K., Aziz, F., Higginbotham, A., Stermitz, F.R. and Hamblin, M.R. (2008) Inhibitors of bacterial multidrug efflux pumps potentiate antimicrobial photoinactivation. *Antimicrobial Agents and Chemotherapy* 52, 3202–3209.

Tegos, G., Haynes, M., Strouse, J.J., Khan, M.M.T., Bologa, C.G., Oprea, T.I. and Sklar, L.A. (2011) Microbial efflux pump inhibition: tactics and

strategies. *Current Pharmaceutical Design* 17, 1291–1302.
Turner, M. (2011) Microbe outbreak panics Europe. *Nature* 474, 137.
Vicente, M., Hodgson, J., Massidda, O., Tonjum, T., Henriques-Normark, B. and Ron, E.Z. (2006) The fallacies of hope: will we discover new antibiotics to combat pathogenic bacteria in time? *FEMS Microbiology Reviews* 30, 841–852.
Zaborina, O., Zaborin, A., Romanowski, K., Babrowski, T. and Alverdy, J. (2011) Host stress and virulence expression in intestinal pathogens: development of therapeutic strategies using mice and *C. elegans*. *Current Pharmaceutical Design* 17, 1254–1260.

1 Emerging Antimicrobial Drug-discovery Strategies: an Evolving Necessity

Anthony R. Ball[1] and George P. Tegos[2]
[1]*Department of Microbiology, Toxikon Corporation, Bedford, Massachusetts, USA;*
[2]*Center for Molecular Discovery and Department of Pathology, University of New Mexico School of Medicine, Albuquerque, New Mexico, USA*

1.1 Introduction

Antimicrobials may lose their efficacy immediately after their clinical use begins through the development of resistance by microbial pathogens, either by mutation or through acquisition of genes already present in the environment. The variety of these resistance mechanisms has led to the generation of an elite class of microorganisms, the so-called 'superbugs'. These are the causative agents of recalcitrant infections and have been involved in a series of clinically challenging conditions. The answer to these complex clinical problems is not trivial. The approval rate of new antimicrobials has been substantially reduced, but when they hit the pharmacy shelves, the path to resistance will occur sooner or later. This has often been described as the 'end of the antibiotic era'. The new era dictates a radical transformation and diversification of the antimicrobial drug-discovery platform. New concepts of enriching the available arsenal of antimicrobial agents through repurposing, synergies, substantial alterations and innovative explorations are under investigation. These are emerging as new strategies incorporating advancing knowledge in microbial physiology, chemical biology and translational research. This chapter provides an outline of the problem and the lessons learned from previous antimicrobial explorations, and highlights pivotal elements that will determine drug-discovery strategies in the near future.

1.2 The Infection Reality

The 20th century gave rise worldwide to a large array of often successful prevention and control efforts for infectious diseases. This fostered a mindset that the war against infectious microbes was over and research efforts were needed in more pressing matters such as cancer, diabetes and heart disease. Funding for infectious disease research and pathogens was de-emphasized. In the 1980s, consensus among pharmaceutical companies was that there were enough antibiotics, and these companies began redirecting their research accordingly (Binder *et al.*, 1999).

Optimism transformed into scepticism as a series of outbreaks and epidemics of new, re-emerging and antimicrobial-resistant infections arose. These microorganisms possessed effective and dynamic virulence and pathogenic capabilities, of both nosocomial and community-acquired origin, and emerged not only in the developing world but also in the developed world. These organisms soon dominated the scientific literature and gave rise to the term 'superbugs'. Infectious disease in the 21st century is again the epicentre of a global dialogue capturing the attention of academics, governments, public health officials and the general public alike. Demain and Spizek (Chapter 2, this volume) have provided an excellent overview of the past 40 years in antibiotic discovery, and the purpose of this chapter is to address the contribution of emergent multidrug-resistant (MDR) microorganisms, followed by highlighting some of the non-traditional approaches to treatment.

Every year, over 13 million deaths worldwide that are attributed to the emergence of new infectious diseases or to the re-emergence of diseases previously controlled can also be attributed to widespread multidrug resistance. Dynamic shifts in global socio-economic trends, environmental ecological factors and the microorganisms themselves have resulted in heightened public health concern with an emphasis on antimicrobial resistance. Controlling this challenge in the new millennium will require rational as well as unconventional antimicrobial drug-discovery efforts that are aligned with and help to foster public awareness, with an emphasis on combating the emerging problem (Binder *et al.*, 1999).

1.3 A New Generation of Resistant Pathogens

Four main classes of antibiotic-resistant pathogens are emerging as major threats to public health. These are:

1. Methicillin-resistant *Staphylococcus aureus* (MRSA).
2. MDR and pandrug-resistant (PDR) Gram-negative bacteria.
3. MDR and extensively drug-resistant (XDR) strains of *Mycobacterium tuberculosis* (MDR-TB and XDR-TB).
4. *Candida* species, the third leading cause of catheter-related infection.

MRSA is estimated to cause ~19,000 deaths per year in the USA alone (Deleo *et al.*, 2010), resulting in an estimated US$3–4 billion in additional healthcare costs. Alarmingly, the rising prevalence of MRSA increases the likelihood that vancomycin-resistant *S. aureus* (VRSA) (Gould, 2010) – just as deadly as MRSA but more challenging to treat – will become the new scourge of hospitals. In fact, vancomycin-resistant *Enterococcus faecalis* has been a common threat in hospitals for at least 15 years (Chavers *et al.*, 2003; Nordmann *et al.*, 2007).

Pathogens from the second class, comprising MDR and PDR Gram-negative bacteria, while far less prevalent than MRSA or Gram-positive pathogens, form a niche of opportunistic healthcare-associated infections in patients who are critically ill or immunocompromised. These infections pose the gravest threat because they are truly untreatable (McGowan, 2006; Dijkshoorn *et al.*, 2007; Nordmann *et al.*, 2007; Baldry, 2010; McKenna, 2011). Strains of *Acinetobacter baumannii*, *Escherichia coli*, *Klebsiella pneumoniae*, *Pseudomonas aeruginosa*, *Stenotrophomonas maltophilia* and *Burkholderia cepacia* are resistant to some (MDR) or all (PDR) of the antibiotic classes commonly used to treat Gram-negative bacteria: penicillins, cephalosporins, carbapenems, monobactams, quinolones, aminoglycosides and tetracyclines (Oteo *et al.*, 2008; Pitout and Laupland, 2008). Polymyxins are the only drug class with consistent activity against *P. aeruginosa*, *S. maltophilia* and *Acinetobacter* spp., but most *B. cepacia* isolates are resistant, and polymyxins carry the risk of nephrotoxicity, especially in the elderly (McGowan, 2006). *P. aeruginosa* and *B. cepacia* are important pathogens in patients with cystic fibrosis (Quinn, 1998; Saiman and Siegel, 2004). Resistance is achieved through a multipronged approach of enzyme product and target-site alteration, to which is coupled a loss of outer-membrane proteins (OMPs) and porins and the production of multidrug efflux pumps. The prospects of finding new antibiotics for Gram-negative pathogens are especially poor because of their outer membrane, which blocks the entry of some antibiotics in conjunction with specific and non-specific efflux pumps that expel many of the remainder (Lee *et al.*, 2000). Thus, Gram-negative microorganisms possess 'intrinsic resistance' because of the presence of an effective permeability barrier, a feature that limits penetration of hydrophilic solutes due to the narrow porin channels and low fluidity of the lipopolysaccharide leaflet that acts to reduce inward diffusion of lipophilic solutes (Plesiat and Nikaido, 1992). Taken together, it is not surprising that a survey published in 1993 (Vaara, 1993) revealed that

90% of natural-origin antibiotics lack activity in the model Gram-negative bacteria, *E. coli*. Moreover, of the 20 antibiotics that have been through some stage of clinical trial assessment since 1998, only tigecycline exhibits any activity against Gram-negative bacteria (Meyer, 2005).

The third class of antibiotic-resistant pathogens, MDR-TB and XDR-TB, is a rising threat in the developing world (Dye, 2009; Jassal and Bishai, 2009). MDR-TB is defined as *M. tuberculosis* resistant to isoniazid and rifampicin, whereas XDR-TB is also resistant to fluoroquinolone and at least one second-line injectable agent such as amikacin, kanamycin and/or capreomycin. MDR-TB treatment requires a 2-year course of antibiotics and carries serious side effects; XDR-TB is even more difficult to cure and often fatal (Keshavjee *et al.*, 2008; Koul *et al.*, 2011). Cases of MDR-TB and XDR-TB have been reported in the USA and other developed countries. According to the World Health Organization (WHO), MDR-TB is a growing problem specifically because incidents of MDR-TB, as opposed to simply tuberculosis (TB), are not always reported and it was estimated that, in 2008, a total of 440,000 cases of TB infection were due to MDR-TB or XDR-TB, with the top four countries being China, India, the Russian Federation and South Africa (WHO, 2010).

The fourth class comprises *Candida* spp., which are the third leading cause of catheter-related infections and are associated with the highest crude mortality of all catheter-related infections (Crump and Collignon, 2000). Candidaemia is the fourth most common cause of bloodstream infections in hospitals in the USA, and major risk factors include intravascular catheters, parenteral hyperalimentation and broad-spectrum antibiotic usage (Chi *et al.*, 2011). Diagnostically, traditional blood culture has a sensitivity of only 50% as a means of detecting invasive candidiasis, and antifungal therapy is limited by toxicity and the development of resistance. Although prevention of invasive candidiasis using azole prophylaxis can be effective in selected high-risk patient populations, selection for invasive infection by resistant non-*albicans Candida* spp. or moulds is a potentially devastating consequence. Despite improvements in antifungal therapy, the high mortality rate due to *Candida* infections has improved little over the last two decades. Even with appropriate therapy attributable mortality remains at 15–49% (Wey *et al.*, 1998; Gudlaugsson *et al.*, 2003), and an episode of candidaemia significantly increases the length of hospital stay and cost of care. In one analysis carried out in 1997, the estimated cost of an episode of care for candidaemia was US$34,123 per Medicare patient and US$44,536 per private insurance patient, with an overall economic impact of US$2 billion dollars annually in the USA (Rentz *et al.*, 1998).

In addition to the established threats posed by these microorganisms, even more challenging scenarios are emerging and include: carbapenem-resistant *K. pneumoniae* and the New Delhi metallo-β-lactamase-containing Enterobacteriaceae, as well as the German *E. coli* outbreak caused by a previously unknown strain (Norrby *et al.*, 2005; Heintz *et al.*, 2010; Cornaglia *et al.*, 2011; Haque *et al.*, 2011; Turner, 2011a,b). Antibiotic resistance is compounded by the inappropriate prescription of antibiotics for viral diseases, excessive use of antibiotics in agriculture and in feedstuffs for livestock, and the inability of patients to responsibly finish antibiotic regimens, all of which select for resistant bacterial strains. Moreover, antibiotics are incapable of eradicating bacterial spores, such as those of Gram-positive *Bacillus* spp., and are much less effective against bacterial biofilms (Russell, 1990; Prince, 2002).

1.4 Is There Still a Role for Target-based Antibiotic Discovery?

While the rate of resistant pathogens is on the rise, the number of new antibiotic/antimicrobial approvals is on the decline (Butler and Cooper, 2011; Cooper and Shlaes, 2011). Where will new antibiotics come from? In the past, this question has mostly been answered through synthetic tailoring of a small group of 'scaffolds': a fixed part of a molecule on which functional groups can be exchanged or substituted. Antimicrobial drug discovery and development have slowed considerably, as novel classes have not been discovered in decades and regulatory approval is tougher to obtain. Lead optimization to market approval has about a 10-year lag time, an incredibly long duration for a category of drug with an average lifespan of less than 10 years before widespread resistance emerges. Thus, microbes may already be drug resistant when the product reaches the pharmacy shelves (Palumbi, 2001; Norrby *et al.*, 2005; Quadri, 2007). Conventional techniques and newer genomic-mining approaches have yet to yield a novel class of antimicrobials. In retrospect, there has been an emphasis on developing analogues of existing antimicrobials by improving efficacy, minimizing resistance and alleviating toxicity. Undoubtedly, new compounds are waiting to be discovered – or perhaps synthesized – that may exhibit novel mechanisms of action on previously unexploited microbial targets or that use new strategies (pro-drugs and anti-infectives), which may pave the way for combating drug resistance and emerging pathogens in the years to come (Hamad, 2010; Ostrosky-Zeichner *et al.*, 2010; Hurdle *et al.*, 2011). Nevertheless, the use of microbial genomics to validate novel targets or yield new antibiotics, although exciting, has raised doubt regarding the utility of target-based discovery programmes (McDevitt and Rosenberg, 2001; Nagaraj and Singh, 2010; Lipkin, 2010). This has shifted the emphasis in validation of retooled discovery target-based strategies.

1.4.1 Revitalizing old targets

Most drugs that are used clinically function as inhibitors of enzymes from well-described pathways. This list includes peptidoglycan, ribosomal proteins, nucleic acids and folate synthesis, as well as topoisomerization (Simmons *et al.*, 2010). The next generation of existing scaffolds should continue to have success in the clinic, and these classical targets will thus remain useful. However, a complementary and perhaps more promising strategy will be to develop new scaffolds for these targets, thereby avoiding cross-resistance with existing drugs. For example, the recently introduced mutilin retapamulin targets the 50S subunit of the bacterial ribosome and is unaffected by resistance to other 50S-targeting classes such as macrolides (Hu and Zhou, 2009). Lipid II is another target that deserves renewed focus, and the success of glycopeptide antibiotics bodes well for other lipid II-binding molecules such as the mannopeptimycins (Breukink and De Kruijff, 2006) and lantibiotics (Piper *et al.*, 2009).

1.4.2 Grouping targets by inhibitor scaffold

To identify new targets, candidates are often grouped by functional criterion, such as membership of a validated pathway or as essential for growth in the laboratory. The attendant danger of single-target bias argues in favour of a strategy that begins with a wider funnel at its early stages. A different way of grouping targets – by a common inhibitor scaffold, rather than by pathway – may reveal not only new targets but also new clues about how to inhibit them. For example, ATP-binding enzymes are a group of targets that can be inhibited by ATP-mimetic scaffolds, and they deserve particular attention for two reasons. First, bacterial genomes encode hundreds of ATP-binding proteins. They include well-validated targets such as DNA gyrase, the target of the quinolones, as well as a host of new or underexplored targets, including: the chambered protease ClpP (Brotz-Oesterhelt *et al.*, 2005), ATP synthase (Hurdle *et al.*, 2011), aminoacyl-tRNA synthetases (Ataide and Ibba, 2006; Rock *et al.*, 2007), acyl-CoA carboxylase (Morens *et al.*, 2004) and the sensor kinase PhoQ that is essential for *Salmonella* virulence, as well as several widely conserved essential genes encoding proteins of unknown function that are predicted to bind ATP (Zhao *et al.*, 2008), suggesting that this class might include a particularly broad range of relevant targets. Insight from outside the antibiotic arena is also important for antibiotics; the observation that zinc-dependent hydrolases are efficiently inhibited by small molecules with zinc-chelating groups has led to the development of inhibitors that target a wide range of enzymes, including angiotensin-converting enzyme, histone deacetylases and matrix metalloproteases. Indeed, semi-synthetic derivatives of actinonin – a zinc-chelating natural product that inhibits the zinc-dependent bacterial enzyme peptide deformylase – have been considered as antibiotic candidates (Sharma *et al.*, 2009).

It is apparent that the pharmaceutical industry has a significant number of lead compounds to focus on. In retrospect, emerging pathogens may shift priorities towards the development of strategies and modalities that, until recently, have been seen as liabilities (e.g. antimicrobials with narrow activity spectra). The battle against MRSA is indicative of this approach, as focusing on agents with preferential activity against Gram-positive as opposed to Gram-negative bacteria is essential. One group used a repurposed series of eukaryotic cholesterol synthesis inhibitors to block the production of the golden pigment staphyloxanthin (Daum, 2008; Liu *et al.*, 2008), from which the species name *aureus* is derived. Another group identified inhibitors of the tubulin-like protein FtsZ to block cell division (Margolin, 2005; Vollmer, 2008). Such genus-selective agents may have the benefit of sparing more of the endogenous microflora than conventional antibiotics, thereby avoiding complications due to secondary *Clostridium difficile* infections.

1.5 Exploiting the Microbial 'Phenotype': a Quest for Novel Targets and Approaches

Advances in microbial physiology and translational research have shed light on a series of pathways, components and phenotypes that may serve as potential targets for antimicrobial drug discovery. Recent studies have dissected social interaction at the molecular level through analysis of both synthetic and natural microbial populations. These approaches have revealed novel molecular mechanisms that stabilize cooperation among cells and define new roles of population structure for the evolution of cooperative interactions. These new interactions are changing the view of microbial processes, with emphasis on pathogenesis and antibiotic resistance, and suggest new ways to fight infection by exploiting social interactions (Leeder *et al.*, 2011; Xavier, 2011). Evidently, bacteria have the ability to enter into a dormant (non-dividing) state known as persistence. The molecular mechanisms that underlie the formation of dormant persister cells are now being unravelled (Lewis, 2007). Accumulating evidence suggests that the seemingly disparate phenomena of latent bacterial infections, unculturable microorganisms and biofilm multidrug tolerance can all be defined as persistent states (Lewis, 2010).

Targeting bacterial virulence is a model approach under investigation for the development of new antimicrobials that can be used to disarm pathogens in the host (Finlay and Falkow, 1997; Lee *et al.*, 2003; Marra, 2004). Virulence in *S. aureus* is regulated by the action of many global gene regulators, the best studied being the four-gene operon *agr*. This operon is essential for virulence in numerous clinical isolates, including the community-acquired MRSA strains of the USA300 PFGE (pulsed field gel electrophoresis) type (Cassat *et al.*, 2006; Klingenberg *et al.*, 2007; Pang *et al.*, 2010). The only strategy for inhibiting *agr* signalling that has worked *in vivo* used a peptide antagonist based on the structure of the natural ligand for the agrC receptor (Lyon *et al.*, 2002). This approach has obvious limitations, as peptides are difficult to work with therapeutically and because the mechanism of action is limited to blocking pheromone binding. There is a wealth of lead small molecules that act as quorum sensing inhibitors in Gram-negative pathogenic systems (Rasmussen and Givskov, 2006) such as *P. aeruginosa* (Müh *et al.*, 2006; Lesic *et al.*, 2007; Borlee *et al.*, 2010) and enterohaemorrhagic *E. coli* (Gutierrez *et al.*, 2009). Unfortunately, there is no apparent molecular or functional similarity with *S. aureus*. These bacteria have completely different quorum-sensing systems that use lactones and furanones as pheromones, unlike the peptide pheromones used by Gram-positive bacteria, especially *S. aureus*.

One solution low on the radar would exploit weak points in the regulation or metabolism of pathogens through 'stealth antimicrobials' that exert a low selective pressure.

For example, most Gram-positive *Enterococcus* spp. are non-virulent and are commonly found in the gastrointestinal tract of humans and animals, yet some, like the nosocomial vancomycin-resistant V583 strain of *E. faecalis*, are clinically problematic worldwide (Fisher and Phillips, 2009). Interestingly, the V583 genome differs widely in size (20% difference compared with the commensal OG1RF strain) and one-quarter of the genome is comprised of mobile and foreign DNA as well as pathogenicity islands (Coburn *et al.*, 2004; Engelbert *et al.*, 2004; Lebreton *et al.*, 2009). Seemingly, expression of these virulence factors is not without consequence. Himes (2011) demonstrated that commensal *E. faecalis* is able to kill V583 in head-to-head growth studies through a proposed pheromonal-mediated response whereby V583 carrying plasmid pTEF2 will self-induce pore formation. Loss of pTEF2 by V583 would negate pheromonal killing at the cost of pTEF2, which is functionally similar to the conjugative plasmid pCF10 (Paulsen *et al.*, 2003; Hirt *et al.*, 2005).

Another story is told by siderophores such as iron chelators. Pathogens encounter iron-limiting environments when colonizing mammalian hosts (Brandon *et al.*, 2003). *In vivo* iron is present in limited quantities with a free serum iron concentration of about 10^{-24} M (Payne, 1993), and most important human pathogens are severely restricted in iron acquisition.

A pseudomonal 'Trojan horse', pyridine-2,6-dithiocarboxylic acid (PDTC) is a siderophore in *Pseudomonas* spp. (Ockels *et al.*, 1978) that facilitates solubilization and high-affinity uptake of ferric iron and inhibits non-PDTC producers (Hersman *et al.*, 2000; Sebat *et al.*, 2001; Cornelis and Matthijs, 2002) through sequestration. PDTC was shown to be active against *M. tuberculosis* at 0.13 μg/ml (Byrne *et al.*, 2007) and capable of completely inhibiting the growth of *E. coli*, *Arthrobacter* sp. and *Staphylococcus epidermidis* as well as non-PDTC-producing strains of *Pseudomonas* at concentrations between 10 and 25 μM. PDTC-producing strains are insensitive; however, the combination of PDTC with other antimicrobials could address this. The Trojan horse concept employs siderophores (such as PDTC) as mediators to facilitate the cellular uptake of antibiotic compounds (Miethke and Marahiel, 2007).

Another strategy worth considering utilizes the natural predator of bacteria, the bacteriophage. Bacteriophage lytic enzymes (lysins) are highly evolved molecules that digest the bacterial cell wall. Small quantities of purified recombinant lysin added to Gram-positive bacteria cause immediate and log-fold lysis of specific bacteria (Fischetti *et al.*, 2006). Following replication inside the bacterial host, the phage must exit to disseminate, and lytic enzymes have been refined over millions of years for exactly this purpose (Fischetti, 2005; Loeffler *et al.*, 2003). Lysins target and weaken the cell wall by attacking one of the four major bonds in peptidoglycan, and their activity can be as an endo-β-*N*-acetylglucosaminidase or *N*-acetylmuramidase, both acting on the sugar moiety of the bacterial wall, as an endopeptidase, which acts on the peptide moiety, or as an *N*-acetylmuramoyl-L-alanine amidase, which hydrolyses the amide bond connecting the glycan strand and peptide moieties (Fischetti, 2005). During their discovery, the potential for lysins was realized, but industrialization of antibiotics in the 1940s shifted the focus away. Now, with increasing incidence of multidrug-resistant pathogens, the potential of phage-based therapy is being re-examined (Thiel, 2004), and in Russia, phage-based therapies have been developed to treat a vast array of pathogenic microbes (Sulakvelidze *et al.*, 2001). In 2006, the US Food and Drug Administration (FDA) approved a cocktail of six individually purified phages as a treatment for *Listeria monocytogenes* contamination of ready-to-eat meat and poultry products. This is the first time the FDA has regulated the use of a phage preparation as a food additive (http://www.accessdata.fda.gov/scripts/fcn/fcnDetailNavigation.cfm?rpt=grasListing&id=198). In addition to whole phage, phage-derived lysins are also being examined for their potential therapeutic effect. Phage lysins have been used to control a wide range of pathogens including group A streptococci (Nelson *et al.*, 2001), *Streptococcus pneumoniae* (Loeffler and Fischetti, 2003), *Bacillus anthracis* (Schuch *et al.*, 2002), *E. faecalis*

(Yoong *et al.*, 2004) and *S. aureus* (O'Flaherty *et al.*, 2005).

In animal models, lysins have been effective in controlling pathogenic antibiotic-resistant bacteria on mucosal surfaces and in blood, often without eliciting an immune response (Fischetti, 2005). Moreover, no blood constituent has been found to inactivate lysins (V.A. Fischetti, personal communication). Key advantages over antibiotics include specificity for the pathogen without disturbing the normal flora, the low chance of resistance and the ability to kill colonizing pathogens on mucosal surfaces.

The lysin PlyC has been shown to kill exponential-phase cultures of *Streptococcus pyogenes*, reducing the number of colony-forming units by 6 logs at a concentration of 10 ng/ml (Nelson *et al.*, 2006). Cpl-1, another lysin, is a muramidase that binds to choline and has *in vivo* activity in a penicillin-resistant pneumococcal bacteraemia mouse model. A 2 mg dose, administered intravenously, reduced pneumococcal titres by 10 logs and led to 100% survival at 48 h compared with 20% survival of the buffer-treated control; however, it was mildly immunogenic (Fischetti, 2005).

1.6 A More Inclusionary Approach?

Multidrug efflux is a key target of these efforts. Efflux mechanisms are broadly recognized as major components of resistance to many classes of antimicrobials (Alekshun and Levy, 2007). Efflux occurs due to the activity of membrane transporter proteins widely known as multidrug efflux systems (MES) (Piddock, 2006a,b; Cannon *et al.*, 2009). They are implicated in a variety of physiological roles other than efflux, and identifying their natural substrates and inhibitors is an active and expanding research discipline (Finlay and Falkow, 1997; Stavri *et al.*, 2007; Tegos *et al.*, 2011). One plausible alternative is the combination of conventional antimicrobial agents/antibiotics with small molecules that block MES, known as multidrug efflux pump inhibitors (EPIs) or through the creation of hybrid-like molecules with dual-action moieties (Tegos *et al.*, 2011). An array of approaches in academic and industrial research settings, varying from high-throughput screening (HTS) ventures to bioassay-guided purification and determination, have yielded a number of promising EPIs in a series of pathogenic systems (Lomovskaya and Watkins, 2001; Lomovskaya and Bostian, 2006; Tegos, 2006; Fiamegos *et al.*, 2011). This synergistic discovery platform has been exploited in translational directions, as well as beyond the potentiation of conventional antimicrobial treatments (Ball *et al.*, 2006; Hamblin and Tegos, 2006; Tegos and Hamblin, 2006; Tegos *et al.*, 2008). Different tactical elements of this platform, as well as advances in assay development, genomics, proteomics and physiological information regarding MES, lights the trail for new, highly informative and comprehensive EPI-discovery strategies and inspired novel combinatorial ventures (Ejim *et al.*, 2011). Most infections are treated with a single antibiotic or antimicrobial (TB being a notable exception), ruling out the use of molecules with high intrinsic resistance rates. However, pairing these compounds into additive or synergistic combinations could rescue candidates formerly thought to be untenable for development. Although development of combination therapies carries the risk of unforeseen toxicity, precedents such as amoxicillin/clavulanate and isoniazid/rifampicin/pyrazinamide/ethambutol support the idea that antibacterial combination therapies can be quite successful, especially in suppressing the development of resistance (Bal *et al.*, 2010). Whether natural or synthetic, broad-spectrum or narrow, single agents or combinations, new scaffolds will be an essential component of a sustainable plan for combating resistance.

Natural sources, such as specific plants, have a distinct role to play in the effort to identify lead EPIs as well as potential antimicrobial agents. The natural antimicrobial discovery approach, a process ranging from identifying a hit to isolating a pure compound, has increased over the last decade and is thought of as more than promising (Lewis and Ausubel, 2006; Cegelski *et al.*, 2008; Gibbons, 2008; Ji *et al.*, 2009; Demain and Sanchez, 2009). Nevertheless, there are significant technical bottlenecks. There are a limited number of natural product extract libraries, and their analysis typically involves exacting isolation of different components of the extract and subsequent time-consuming spectroscopic identification of the separate compounds. Additionally, large-scale synthesis of natural products is often a daunting challenge.

A new and powerful platform that has recently gained ground by promising to bypass substantial drawbacks associated with new antimicrobial discovery is the development of facile whole-animal screens (Mylonakis, 2011). This utilizes an array of hosts including the well-studied nematode *Caenorhabditis elegans* (Sifri *et al.*, 2005; Tampakakis *et al.*, 2008), the great wax moth *Galleria mellonella* (Vilcinskas, 2011), the fruit fly *Drosophila melanogaster* (Apidianakis and Rahme, 2009, 2011; Chamilos *et al.*, 2011) and the zebrafish infection model (Mukhopadhyay and Peterson, 2006; Adams *et al.*, 2011; Meijer and Spaink, 2011; Stoop *et al.*, 2011). These model hosts have been used to simulate infection by pathogens (Aballay *et al.*, 2000; Labrousse *et al.*, 2000; Garsin *et al.*, 2003; Sifri *et al.*, 2003; Begun *et al.*, 2005; Maadani *et al.*, 2007; Peleg *et al.*, 2009), infectivity or immunomodulatory efficacy, while at the same time discriminating against toxicity (Fuchs and Mylonakis, 2006; Pukkila-Worley *et al.*, 2009). Antimicrobial discovery assays have been developed using a wide array of MDR pathogens. These assays have identified several small molecules not previously known to harbour anti-infective properties and will expedite drug development efforts.

In retrospect, target-based conventional discovery offers an array of promising approaches. This list includes:

1. The light-based photodynamic therapy platform (PDT), which has been transformed into a discovery and treatment alternative option for localized infections (Hamblin and Hasan, 2004; Dai *et al.*, 2009a) from its original aim as a cancer therapeutic modality (Dolmans *et al.*, 2003). PDT is under investigation on many different fronts including inactivation of MDR pathogens (Demidova and Hamblin, 2004; Tang *et al.*, 2007; Hajim *et al.*, 2010; Dovigo *et al.*, 2011; Maisch *et al.*, 2011; Xing *et al.*, 2011), inhibition of microbial biofilm formation (Garcez *et al.*, 2007; Arciola, 2009; Di Poto *et al.*, 2009; Fontana *et al.*, 2009; Biel, 2010; Collins *et al.*, 2010; Kishen *et al.*, 2010; Street *et al.*, 2010; Suci *et al.*, 2010; Soukos and Goodson, 2011) and its effect on efflux systems and virulence determinants (Zolfaghari *et al.*, 2009; Hamblin *et al.*, 2011; Sharma *et al.*, 2011), as well as exploring the efficacy of novel photoactive drugs and modalities employing animal models (Dai *et al.*, 2009b, 2010; Sharma *et al.*, 2011). All the reported studies have found that PDT can kill drug-resistant microbes as easily as their native counterparts (Wilson and Yianni, 1995; Soncin *et al.*, 2002). European and US-based companies employ PDT and light-based modalities for localized infections for endodontics, nasal decolonization and gingivitis.

2. Nanotechnology-based technologies (Hansen *et al.*, 2008) with an emphasis on the discovery of novel antimicrobial nanostructures (Mazzola, 2003) or employing nanoparticles for delivery purposes (Han *et al.*, 2009). Nanotechnology refers to the design, production and application of materials that are in the nanoscale range (< 100nm). The unique physical and chemical properties of nanoparticles, particularly their small size and high volume-to-surface ratio, allow this technology to surpass barriers and gain access to biological molecules and systems. As modern science permits the manipulation of nanosized materials, the size, shape and chemical characteristics may be altered to facilitate molecular interactions. As such, nanosized materials can be engineered as vehicles to carry various therapeutic or diagnostic agents and are potentially useful for medical applications (Kim *et al.*, 2010), including targeted drug delivery (Griffiths *et al.*, 2010), gene therapy (Sekhon and Kamboj, 2010) and cell labelling (Kell *et al.*, 2008).

An indicative core of new, promising chemotherapeutics is provided in Table 1.1.

1.7 Conclusions

The field of antimicrobial drug discovery is evolving rapidly as key elements of MDR

Table 1.1. Classes of alternative chemotherapeutics: efflux pump inhibitors (EPIs), siderophores, photodynamic therapy platform (PDT)-based combinations and dual-action antimicrobials.

Alternative chemotherapeutics	Synergist(s)	Microorganism(s)	Target(s)	Reference(s)
EPIs				
Gram-negative				
MC-207,110	Levofloxacin	*Pseudomonas aeruginosa*	MexAB–OprM, MexCD–OprJ, MexEF–OprN, MexXY–OprM	Lomovskaya *et al.* (2001)
Quinolone-pyridopyrimidine derivatives	β-Lactams, fluoroquinolones	*P. aeruginosa*	MexAB-OprM	Nakayama *et al.* (2003)
3-Arylpiperidines	Novobiocin, linezolid	*Escherichia coli*	AcrAB–TolC	Thorarensen *et al.* (2002)
Alkoxy- and alkylamino-quinolines	Chloramphenicol	*Enterobacter aerogenes*, *Klebsiella pneumoniae*	MarRAB, AcrAB-tolC and RamA	Chevalier *et al.* (2004)
Gram-positive				
3-Phenyl-1,4-benzothiazine derivatives	Fluoroquinolones	*Staphylococcus aureus*	NorA	Sabatini *et al.* (2008)
Reserpine	Ethidium bromide, fluoroquinolones, chloramphenicol	*S. aureus*, *Bacillus subtilis*, *Streptococcus pneumoniae*, *Streptomyces coelicolor*	NorA, Bmr, cmlR1, cmlR2	Markham *et al.* (1999); Vecchione *et al.* (2009); Neyfakh *et al.* (1991)
INF series	Ciprofloxacin, ethidium bromide	*S. aureus*	NorA	Markham *et al.* (1999)
Perperine series	Ethidium bromide	*S. aureus*	NorA	Sangwan *et al.* (2008)
Tariquidar	Ciprofloxacin	*S. aureus*	NorA	Leitner *et al.* (2011)
Thioridazine and chlorpromazine	Ethidium bromide, macrolides	*Mycobacterium avium*, *Mycobacterium smegmatis*		Rodrigues *et al.* (2008)
Siderophores				
Pyridine-2,6-dithiocarboxylic acid	Antimicrobial cations and metals	*P. aeruginosa*, *E. coli*, *Staphylococcus epidermidis*	Metal sequestration	Sebat *et al.* (2001)
Dihydropyridinone monosulfactam (BAL30072)	Meropenem	*Acinetobacter baumannii*	Permeabilizer, β-lactamase inhibitor	Russo *et al.* (2011)
PDT combinations				
Methylene blue	Visible light	*S. aureus*, *Helicobacter pylori*, *P. aeruginosa*, *E. coli*	Reactive oxygen species	Choi *et al.* (2010)
Methylene blue, toluidine blue	Visible light, EPIs	*S. aureus*, *P. aeruginosa*, *Candida albicans*	Reactive oxygen species	Tegos *et al.* (2008); Prates *et al.* (2011)

Continued

Table 1.1. Continued.

Alternative chemotherapeutics	Synergist(s)	Microorganism(s)	Target(s)	Reference(s)
Rose bengal	Visible light, EPIs	*Enterococcus faecalis*	Reactive oxygen species	Kishen *et al.* (2010)
Chlorin(e6)–polyethylenimine derivative	Visible light	*S. aureus*, *E. faecalis*, *E. coli*	Permeabilizer, reactive oxygen species	Huang *et al.* (2010)
Dual-action antimicrobials				
Berberine–indole derivatives	–	*S. aureus*, *E. faecalis*, *Enterococcus faecium*, *Bacillus anthracis*, *Bacillus cereus*	DNA, membrane	Ball *et al.* (2006)
Oxazolidinone–quinolone derivatives	–	*S. aureus*, *E. faecalis*, *E. faecium*, *E. coli*, *H. pylori*	DNA gyrase and topoisomerase IV	Hubschwerien *et al.* (2003)
Ketolide–quinolone derivatives	–	*S. aureus*, *S. pneumoniae*, *Streptococcus pyogenes*, *Moraxella catarrhalis*, *Haemophilus influenzae*	DNA gyrase and ribosome	Pavlovic *et al.* (2010)
Piperazine–quinolone derivative	Ethidium bromide	*S. aureus*	NorA, MepA	German *et al.* (2008)
Desferridanoxamine–lorabid, desferridan oxamine–ciprofloxacin and desferridanoxamine–triclosan derivatives	–	*B. subtilis*, *S. aureus*, *Micrococcus luteus*, *Mycobacterium vaccae*, *E. faecalis*, *Enterobacter cloacae*, *E. coli*, *P. aeruginosa*	Iron sequestration, various	Wencewicz *et al.* (2009)
Spermidine–carbacephalosporin derivatives	–	*E. coli*	Iron sequestration, peptidoglycan	Minnick *et al.* (1992)
Bisaryl urea–quinolone derivatives	–	*P. aeruginosa*	DNA gyrase, MexAB-OprM	German *et al.* (2008)

phenomena are resolved and elucidated. One could argue that the dogmas of the past will not fit into the new picture, and radical, unconventional approaches should be pursued exclusively to combat emerging pathogens. For example, although it was thought that combinatorial chemistry and HTS would yield many new hits and leads, the results were disappointing, despite the extraordinary amount of money spent (Horrobin, 2001). Developed in the early 1990s, speed and miniaturization were accomplished by HTS, but the discovery of new leads did not accelerate. HTS methods allowed 100,000–200,000 chemicals to be assayed per day, and combinatorial and other chemical libraries of 1 million compounds were commercially available. As use of the conventional 96-microwell format for HTS could cost US$1 million to screen 500,000 compounds against a single target, some companies went to 384-, 1536- and even 3456-well formats to cut expenses. However, the premise of 'the more compounds screened, the more leads found' did not prevail. No drugs were approved resulting from HTS by 1999 (Fox *et al.*, 1999) and not a single drug derived solely by combinatorial chemistry was introduced up to 2005.

The idea of enriching the available arsenal of antimicrobial agents through repurposing, synergies and substantial alterations is more realistic. The number of options is without doubt substantially larger, but the new challenges require tailoring particular solutions for a specific clinical problem. The often-described 'end of the antibiotic era' may be seen with optimism as a 'new opportunity era'. This concept requires alignment of all involved parts with emphasis on resources and funding but above all in mentality and multidisciplinary explorations.

Acknowledgements

G.P.T. is supported by the National Institutes of Health (NIH, Bethesda, MD) (grant 5U54MH084690-02). Research conducted in the Hamblin Laboratory was supported by the NIH (R01 AI050875 to Michael R. Hamblin) and the US Air Force MFEL Program (FA9550-04-1-0079). The authors would like to thank Mark Haynes and Peter Simons (University of New Mexico Center for Molecular Discovery, Albuquerque, New Mexico) for fruitful discussions.

References

Aballay, A., Yorgey, P. and Ausubel, F.M. (2000) *Salmonella typhimurium* proliferates and establishes a persistent infection in the intestine of *Caenorhabditis elegans*. *Current Biology* 10, 1539–1542.

Adams, K., Takaki, K., Connolly, L.E., Wiedenhoft, H., Winglee, K., Humbert, O., Edelstein, P.H., Cosma, C.L. and Ramakrishnan, L. (2011) Drug tolerance in replicating mycobacteria mediated by a macrophage-induced efflux mechanism. *Cell* 145, 39–53.

Alekshun, M. and Levy, S.B. (2007) Molecular mechanisms of antibacterial multidrug resistance. *Cell* 128, 1037–1050.

Apidianakis, Y. and Rahme, L.G. (2009) *Drosophila melanogaster* as a model host for studying *Pseudomonas aeruginosa* infection. *Nature Protocols* 4, 1285–1294.

Apidianakis, Y. and Rahme, L.G. (2011) *Drosophila melanogaster* as a model for human intestinal infection and pathology. *Disease Models and Mechanisms* 4, 21–30.

Arciola, C. (2009) New concepts and new weapons in implant infections. *International Journal of Artificial Organs* 32, 533–536.

Ataide, S. and Ibba, M. (2006) Small molecules: big players in the evolution of protein synthesis. *ACS Chemical Biology* 1, 285–297.

Bal, A.M., Kumar, A. and Gould, I.M. (2010) Antibiotic heterogeneity: from concept to practice. *Annals of the New York Academy of Sciences* 1213, 81–91.

Baldry, S. (2010) Attack of the clones. *Nature Reviews Microbiology* 8, 390.

Ball, A., Casadei, G., Samosorn, S., Bremner, J.B., Ausubel, F.F., Moy, T.I. and Lewis, K. (2006) Conjugating berberine to a multidrug efflux pump inhibitor creates an effective antimicrobial. *ACS Chemical Biology* 1, 594–600.

Begun, J., Sifri, C.D., Goldman, S., Calderwood, S.B. and Ausubel, F.M. (2005) *Staphylococcus aureus* virulence factors identified by using a high-throughput *Caenorhabditis elegans*-killing model. *Infection and Immunity* 73, 872–877.

Biel, M. (2010) Photodynamic therapy of bacterial and fungal biofilm infections. *Methods in Molecular Biology* 635, 175–194.

Binder, S., Levitt, A.M., Sacks, J.I. and Hughes, J.M. (1999) Emerging infectious diseases: public health issues for the 21st century. *Science* 284, 1311–1313.

Borlee, B., Geske, G.D., Blackwell, H.E. and Handelsman, J. (2010) Identification of synthetic inducers and inhibitors of the quorum-sensing regulator LasR in *Pseudomonas aeruginosa* by high-throughput screening. *Applied and Environmental Microbiology* 76, 8255–8258.

Brandon, M., Paszczynski, A., Korus, R. and Crawford, R. (2003) The determination of the stability constant for the iron(II) complex of the biochelator pyridine-2,6-bis(monothiocarboxylic acid). *Biodegradation* 14, 73–82.

Breukink, E. and De Kruijff, B. (2006) Lipid II as a target for antibiotics. *Nature Reviews Drug Discovery* 4, 321–332.

Brötz-Oesterhelt, H., Beyer, D., Kroll, H.P., Endermann, R., Ladel, C., Schroeder, W., Hinzen, B., Raddatz, S., Paulsen, H., Henninger, K., Bandow, J.E., Sahl, H.G. and Labischinski, H. (2005) Dysregulation of bacterial proteolytic machinery by a new class of antibiotics. *Nature Medicine* 10, 1082–1087.

Butler, M.S. and Cooper, M.A. (2011) Antibiotics in the clinical pipeline in 2011. *Journal of Antibiotics* 64, 413–425.

Byrne, S., Gu, P., Zhou, J., Denkin, S., Chong, C., Sullivan, D., Liu, J. and Zhang, Y. (2007) Pyrrolidine dithiocarbamate and diethyldithiocarbamate are active against growing and nongrowing persister *Mycobacterium tuberculosis. Antimicrobial Agents and Chemotherapy* 51, 4495–4497.

Cannon, R., Lamping, E., Holmes, A.R., Niimi, K., Baret, P.V., Keniya, M.V., Tanabe, K., Niimi, M., Goffeau, A. and Monk, B.C. (2009) Efflux-mediated antifungal drug resistance. *Clinical Microbiology Reviews* 2, 291–321.

Cassat, J., Dunman, P.M., Murphy, E., Projan, S.J., Beenken, K.E., Palm, K.I., Yang, S.I., Rice, K.C., Bayles, K.W. and Smeltzer, M.S. (2006) Transcriptional profiling of a *Staphylococcus aureus* clinical isolate and its isogenic *agr* and *sarA* mutants reveals global differences in comparison to the laboratory strain RN6390. *Microbiology* 152, 3075–3090.

Cegelski, L., Marshall, G.R., Eldridge, G.R. and Hultgren, S.J. (2008) The biology and future prospects of antivirulence therapies. *Nature Reviews Microbiology* 6, 17–27.

Chamilos, G., Samonis, G. and Kontoyiannis, D.P. (2011) *Drosophila melanogaster* as a model host for the study of microbial pathogenicity and the discovery of novel antimicrobial compounds. *Current Pharmaceutical Design* 17, 1246–1253.

Chavers, L., Moser, S.A., Benjamin, W.H., Banks, S.E., Steinhauer, J.R., Smith, A.M., Johnson, C.N., Funkhouser, E., Chavers, L.P., Stamm, A.M. and Waites, K.B. (2003) Vancomycin-resistant enterococci: 15 years and counting. *Journal of Hospital Infection* 53, 159–171.

Chevalier, J., Bredin, J., Mahamoud, A., Malléa, M., Barbe, J. and Pagès, J.M. (2004) Inhibitors of antibiotic efflux in resistant *Enterobacter aerogenes* and *Klebsiella pneumoniae* strains. *Antimicrobial Agents and Chemotherapy* 48, 1043–1046.

Chi, H., Yang, Y.S., Shang, S.T., Chen, K.H., Yeh, K.M., Chang, F.Y. and Lin, J.C. (2011) *Candida albicans* vs. non-*albicans* bloodstream infections: the comparison of risk factors and outcome. *Journal of Microbiology, Immunology and Infection* 44, 369–375.

Choi, S.S., Le, H.K. and Chae, H.S. (2010) *In vitro* photodynamic antimicrobial activity of methylene blue and endoscopic white light against *Helicobacter pylori* 26695. *Journal of Photochemistry and Photobiology B: Biology* 101, 206–209.

Coburn, P., Pillar, C.M., Jett, B.D., Haas, W. and Gilmore, M.S. (2004) *Enterococcus faecalis* senses target cells and in response expresses cytolysin. *Science* 306, 2270–2272.

Collins, T., Markus, E.A., Hassett, D.J. and Robinson, J.B. (2010) The effect of a cationic porphyrin on *Pseudomonas aeruginosa* biofilms. *Current Microbiology* 61, 411–416.

Cooper, M. and Shlaes, D. (2011) Fix the antibiotics pipeline. *Nature* 472, 32–32.

Cornaglia, G., Giamarellou, H. and Rossolini, G.M. (2011) Metallo-β-lactamases: a last frontier for β-lactams? *Lancet Infectious Disease* 11, 381–393.

Cornelis, P. and Matthijs, S. (2002) Diversity of siderophore mediated iron uptake systems in fluorescent pseudomonads: not only pyroverdine. *Environmental Microbiology* 3, 787–798.

Crump, J. and Collignon, P.I. (2000) Intravascular catheter-associated infections. *European Journal of Clinical Microbiology and Infectious Diseases* 19, 1–8.

Dai, T., Huang, Y.Y. and Hamblin, M.R. (2009a) Photodynamic therapy for localized infections – state of the art. *Photodiagnosis and Photodynamic Therapy* 6, 170–188.

Dai, T., Tegos, G.P., Lu, Z., Huang, L., Zhiyentayev, T., Franklin, M.J., Baer, D.G. and Hamblin, M.R. (2009b) Photodynamic therapy for *Acinetobacter baumannii* burn infections in mice. *Antimicrobial Agents and Chemotherapy* 53, 3929–3934.

Dai, T., Tegos, G.P., Zhiyentayev, T., Mylonakis, E. and Hamblin, M.R. (2010) Photodynamic therapy for methicillin-resistant *Staphylococcus aureus* infection in a mouse skin abrasion model. *Lasers in Surgery and Medicine* 42, 38–44.

Daum, R. (2008) Removing the golden coat of *Staphylococcus aureus. New England Journal of Medicine* 359, 85–87.

Deleo, F., Otto, M., Kreiswirth, B.N. and Chambers, H.F. (2010) Community-associated meticillin-resistant *Staphylococcus aureus. Lancet* 375, 1557–1568.

Demain, A.L. and Sanchez, S. (2009) Microbial drug discovery: 80 years of progress. *Journal of Antibiotics* 62, 5–16.

Demidova, T. and Hamblin, M.R. (2004) Photodynamic therapy targeted to pathogens. *International Journal of Immunopathology and Pharmacology* 17, 245–254.

Di Poto, A., Sbarra, M.S., Provenza, G., Visai, L. and Speziale, P. (2009) The effect of photodynamic treatment combined with antibiotic action or host defence mechanisms on *Staphylococcus aureus* biofilms. *Biomaterials* 18, 3158–3166.

Dijkshoorn, L., Nemec, A. and Seifert, H. (2007) An increasing threat in hospitals: multidrug-resistant *Acinetobacter baumannii. Nature Reviews Microbiology* 5, 939–951.

Dolmans, D., Fukumura, D. and Jain, R.K. (2003) Photodynamic therapy for cancer. *Nature Reviews Cancer* 3, 380–387.

Dovigo, L., Pavarina, A.C., Mima, E.G., Giampaolo, E.T., Vergani, C.E. and Bagnato, V.S. (2011) Fungicidal effect of photodynamic therapy against fluconazole-resistant *Candida albicans* and *Candida glabrata. Mycoses* 54, 123–130.

Dye, C. (2009) Doomsday postponed? Preventing and reversing epidemics of drug-resistant tuberculosis. *Nature Reviews Microbiology* 7, 81–87.

Ejim, L., Farha, M.A., Falconer, S.B., Wildenhain, J., Coombes, B.K., Tyers, M., Brown, E.D. and Wright, G.D. (2011) Combinations of antibiotics and nonantibiotic drugs enhance antimicrobial efficacy. *Nature Chemical Biology* 7, 348–350.

Engelbert, M., Mylonakis, E., Ausubel, F.M., Calderwood, S.B. and Gilmore, M.R. (2004) Contribution of gelatinase, serine protease, and *fsr* to the pathogenesis of *Enterococcus faecalis* endophthalmitis. *Infection and Immunity* 72, 3628–3633.

Fiamegos, Y., Kastritis, P.L., Exarchou, V., Han, H., Bonvin, A.M.J.J., Vervoort, J., Lewis, K., Hamblin, M.R. and Tegos, G.P. (2011) Antimicrobial and efflux pump inhibitory activity of caffeoylquinic acids from *Artemisia absinthium* against Gram-positive pathogenic bacteria *PLoS One* 6, e18127.

Finlay, B. and Falkow, S. (1997) Common themes in microbial pathogenicity revisited. *Microbiology and Molecular Biology Reviews* 61, 136–169.

Fischetti, V.A. (2005) Bacteriophage lytic enzymes: novel anti-infectives. *Trends in Microbiology* 13, 491–496.

Fischetti, V., Nelson, D. and Schuch, R. (2006) Reinventing phage therapy: are the parts greater than the sum? *Nature Biotechnology* 24, 1508–1511.

Fisher, K. and Phillips, C. (2009) The ecology, epidemiology and virulence of *Enterococcus. Microbiology* 155, 1749–1757.

Fontana, C., Abernethy, A.D., Som, S., Ruggiero, K., Doucette, S., Marcantonio, R.C., Boussios, C.I., Kent, R., Goodson, J.M., Tanner, A.C. and Soukos, N.S. (2009) The antibacterial effect of photodynamic therapy in dental plaque-derived biofilms. *Journal of Periodontal Research* 44, 751–759.

Fox, S., Farr-Jones, S. and Yund, M.A. (1999) High throughput screening for drug discovery: continually transitioning into new technology. *Journal of Biomolecular Screening* 4, 183–186.

Fuchs, B. and Mylonakis, E. (2006) Using non-mammalian hosts to study fungal virulence and host defense. *Current Opinion in Microbiology* 9, 346–351.

Garcez, A., Ribeiro, M.S., Tegos, G.P., Nunez, S.C., Jorge, A.O. and Hamblin, M.R. (2007) Antimicrobial photodynamic therapy combined with conventional endodontic treatment to eliminate root canal biofilm infection. *Lasers in Surgery and Medicine* 39, 59–66.

Garsin, D., Villanueva, J.M., Begun, J., Kim, D.H., Sifri, C.D., Calderwood, S.B., Ruvkun, G. and Ausubel, F.M. (2003) Long-lived *C. elegans daf-2* mutants are resistant to bacterial pathogens. *Science* 300, 1921.

German, N., Kaatz, G.W. and Kerns, R.J. (2008) Synthesis and evaluation of PSSRI-based inhibitors of *Staphylococcus aureus* multidrug efflux pumps. *Bioorganic and Medicinal Chemistry Letters* 18, 1368–1373.

Gibbons, S. (2008) Phytochemicals for bacterial resistance – strengths, weaknesses and opportunities. *Planta Medica* 74, 594–602.

Gould, I. (2010) VRSA – doomsday superbug or damp squib? *Lancet Infectious Disease* 10, 816–818.

Griffiths, G., Nyström, B., Sable, S.B. and Khuller, G.K. (2010) Nanobead-based interventions for the treatment and prevention of tuberculosis. *Nature Reviews Microbiology* 8, 827–834.

Gudlaugsson, O., Gillespie, S., Lee, K., Vande Berg, J., Hu J., Messer, S., Herwaldt, L., Pfaller, M. and Diekema, D. (2003) Attributable mortality of nosocomial candidemia, revisited. *Clinical Infectious Diseases* 37, 1172–1177.

Gutierrez, J., Crowder, T., Rinaldo-Matthis, A., Ho, M.C., Almo, S.C. and Schramm, V.L. (2009) Transition state analogs of 5 -methylthioadenosine nucleosidase disrupt quorum sensing. *Nature Chemical Biology* 5, 251–257.

Hajim, K., Salih, D.S. and Rassam, Y.R. (2010) Laser light combined with a photosensitizer may eliminate methicillin-resistant strains of *Staphylococcus aureus. Lasers in Medical Science* 25, 743–748.

Hamad, B. (2010) The antibiotics market. *Nature Reviews Drug Discovery* 9, 675–676.

Hamblin, M. and Hasan, T. (2004) Photodynamic therapy: a new antimicrobial approach to infectious disease? *Photochemical and Photobiological Sciences* 3, 436–450.

Hamblin, M. and Tegos, G. (2006) *Potentiation of Antimicrobial Photodynamic Therapy by Inhibitors of Microbial Multidrug Resistance*

Pumps. The General Hospital Corporation, Massachusetts General Hospital, Boston, Massachusetts.

Hamblin, M., Tegos, G.P., St Denis, T. and Huang, L. (2011) Antimicrobial photodynamic therapy: can resistance develop? *Photodiagnosis and Photodynamic Therapy* 8, 178.

Han, G., Martinez, L.R., Mihu, M.R., Friedman, A.J., Friedman, J.M. and Nosanchuk, J.D. (2009) Nitric oxide releasing nanoparticles are therapeutic for *Staphylococcus aureus* abscesses in a murine model of infection. *PLoS One* 4, e7804.

Hansen, S., Maynard, A., Baun, A., Joel, A. and Tickner, J.A. (2008) Late lessons from early warnings for nanotechnology. *Nature Nanotechnology* 3, 444–447.

Haque, N., Bari, M.S., Bilkis, L., Haque, S. and Sultana, S. (2011) Methicillin resistant *Staphylococcus aureus* – an overview. *Journal of Clinical Pharmacy and Therapeutics* 20, 159–164.

Heintz, B.H., Halilovic, J. and Christensen, C.L. (2010) Vancomycin-resistant enterococcal urinary tract infections. *Pharmacotherapy* 30, 1136–1149.

Hersman, L., Huang, A., Maurice, P.A. and Forsythe, J.H. (2000) Siderophore production and iron reduction by *Pseudomonas mendocina* in response to iron deprivation. *Geomicrobiology Journal* 17, 261–273.

Himes, P. (2011) Genetic basis for loss of fitness by vancomycin resistant *E. faecalis* strain V583. In: *Boston Bacterial Meeting*, 16–17 June, Cambridge, Massachusetts.

Hirt, H., Manias, D.A., Bryan, E.M., Klein, J.R., Marklund, J.K., Staddon, J.H., Paustian, M.L., Kapur, V. and Dunny, G.M. (2005) Characterization of the pheromone response of the *Enterococcus faecalis* conjugative plasmid pCF10: complete sequence and comparative analysis of the transcriptional and phenotypic responses of pCF10-containing cells to pheromone induction. *Journal of Bacteriology* 187, 1044–1054.

Horrobin, D. (2001) Realism in drug discovery – could Cassandra be right? *Nature Biotechnology* 19, 1099–1100.

Hu, C. and Zou, Y. (2009) Mutilins derivatives: from veterinary to human-used antibiotics. *Mini Reviews in Medicinal Chemistry* 12, 1397–1406.

Huang, L., Huang, Y.Y., Mroz, P., Tegos, G.P., Zhiyentayev, T., Sharma, S.K., Lu, Z., Balasubramanian, T., Krayer, M., Ruzié, C., Yang, E., Kee, H.L., Kirmaier, C., Diers, J.R., Bocian, D.F., Holten, D., Lindsey, J.S. and Hamblin, M.R. (2010) Stable synthetic cationic bacteriochlorins as selective antimicrobial photosensitizers. *Antimicrobial Agents and Chemotherapy* 54, 3834–3841.

Hubschwerien, C., Specklin, J., Baseschilin, D., Borer, Y., Haefeli, S., Sigwalt, C., Schroeder, S. and Locher, H.H. (2003) Structure–activity relationship in the oxazolidinone–quinolone hybrid series: influence of the central spacer on the antibacterial activity and the mode of action. *Bioorganic and Medicinal Chemistry Letters* 13, 4229–4233.

Hurdle, J., O'Neill, A.J., Chopra, I. and Lee, R.E. (2011) Targeting bacterial membrane function: an underexploited mechanism for treating persistent infections. *Nature Reviews Microbiology* 9, 62–75.

Jassal, M. and Bishai, W.R. (2009) Extensively drug-resistant tuberculosis. *Lancet Infectious Disease* 9, 19–30.

Ji, H., Li, X. and Zhang, H.Y. (2009) Natural products and drug discovery. *EMBO Reports* 10, 194–200.

Kell, A., Stewart, G., Ryan, S., Peytavi, R., Boissinot, M., Huletsky, A., Bergeron, M.G. and Simard, B. (2008) Vancomycin-modified nanoparticles for efficient targeting and preconcentration of Gram-positive and Gram-negative bacteria. *ACS Nano* 2, 1777–1788.

Keshavjee, S., Gelmanova, I.Y., Farmer, P.E., Mishustin, S.P., Strelis, A.K., Andreev, Y.G., Pasechnikov, A.D., Atwood, S., Mukherjee, J.N., Rich, M.L., Furin, J.J., Nardell, E.A., Kim, J.Y. and Shin, S.S. (2008) Treatment of extensively drug-resistant tuberculosis in Tomsk, Russia: a retrospective cohort study. *Lancet* 372, 1403–1409.

Kim, B.Y.S., Rutka, J.T. and Chan, W.C.W. (2010) Nanomedicine. *New England Journal of Medicine* 363, 2434–2443.

Kishen, A., Upadya, M., Tegos, G.P. and Hamblin, M.R. (2010) Efflux pump inhibitor potentiates antimicrobial photodynamic inactivation of *Enterococcus faecalis* biofilm. *Photochemistry and Photobiology* 86, 1343–1349.

Klingenberg, C., Rønnestad, A., Anderson, A.S., Abrahamsen, T.G., Zorman, J., Villaruz, A., Flaegstad, T., Otto, M. and Sollid, J.E. (2007) Persistent strains of coagulase-negative staphylococci in a neonatal intensive care unit: virulence factors and invasiveness. *Clinical Microbiology and Infection* 13, 1100–1111.

Koul, A., Arnoult, E., Lounis, N., Guillemont, J. and Andries, K. (2011) The challenge of new drug discovery for tuberculosis. *Nature* 469, 483–490.

Labrousse, A., Chauvet, S., Couillault, C., Kurz, C.L. and Ewbank, J.J. (2000) *Caenorhabditis*

elegans is a model host for *Salmonella typhimurium*. *Current Biology* 10, 1543–1545.
Lebreton, F., Riboulet-Bisson, E., Serror, P., Sanguinetti, M., Posteraro, B., Torelli, R., Hartke, A., Auffray, Y. and Giard, J.C. (2009) *ace*, which encodes an adhesin in *Enterococcus faecalis*, is regulated by Ers and is involved in virulence. *Infection and Immunity* 77, 2832–2839.
Lee, A., Mao, W., Warren, M.S., Mistry, A., Hoshino, K., Okumura, R., Ishida, H. and Lomovskaya, O. (2000) Interplay between efflux pumps may provide either additive or multiplicative effects on drug resistance. *Journal of Bacteriology* 182, 3142–3150.
Lee, Y., Almqvist, F. and Hultgren, S.I. (2003) Targeting virulence for antimicrobial chemotherapy. *Current Opinions in Pharmacology* 3, 513–519.
Leeder, A., Palma-Guerrero, J. and Glass, N.L. (2011) The social network: deciphering fungal language. *Nature Reviews Microbiology* 9, 440–451.
Leitner, I., Nemeth, J., Feurstein, T., Abrahim, A., Matzneller, P., Lagler, H., Erker, T., Langer, O. and Zeitlinger, M. (2011) The third-generation P-glycoprotein inhibitor tariquidar may overcome bacterial multidrug resistance by increasing intracellular drug concentration. *Journal of Antimicrobial Chemotherapy* 66, 834–839.
Lesic, B., Lépine, F., Déziel, E., Zhang, J., Zhang, Q., Padfield, K., Castonguay, M.H., Milot, S., Stachel, S., Tzika, A.A., Tompkins, R.G. and Rahme, L.G. (2007) Inhibitors of pathogen intercellular signals as selective anti-infective compounds. *PLoS Pathogens* 3, 1229–1239.
Lewis, K. (2007) Persister cells, dormancy and infectious disease. *Nature Reviews Microbiology* 5, 48–56.
Lewis, K. (2010) Persister cells. *Annual Reviews in Microbiology* 64, 357–372.
Lewis, K. and Ausubel, F.M. (2006) Prospects for plant-derived antibacterials. *Nature Biotechnology* 24, 1504–1507.
Lipkin, W. (2010) Microbe hunting. *Microbiology and Molecular Biology Reviews* 74, 363–377.
Liu, C., Liu, G.Y., Song, Y., Yin, F., Hensler, M.E., Jeng, W.Y., Nizet, V., Wang, A.H. and Oldfield, E. (2008) A cholesterol biosynthesis inhibitor blocks *Staphylococcus aureus* virulence. *Science* 319, 1391–1394.
Loeffler, J. and Fischetti, V.A. (2003) Synergistic lethal effect of a combination of phage lytic enzymes with different activities on penicillin-sensitive and -resistant *Streptococcus pneumoniae* strains. *Antimicrobial Agents and Chemotherapy* 47, 375–377.
Loeffler, J., Djurkovic, S. and Fischetti, V.A. (2003) Phage lytic enzyme Cpl-1 as a novel antimicrobial for pneumococcal bacteremia. *Infection and Immunity* 71, 6199–6204.
Lomovskaya, O. and Bostian, K.A. (2006) Practical applications and feasibility of efflux pump inhibitors in the clinic – a vision for applied use. *Biochemical Pharmacology* 71, 910–918.
Lomovskaya, O. and Watkins, W. (2001) Inhibition of efflux pumps as a novel approach to combat drug resistance in bacteria. *Journal of Molecular Microbiology and Biotechnology* 3, 225–236.
Lomovskaya, O., Warren, M.S., Lee, A., Galazzo, J., Fronko, R., Lee, M., Blais, J., Cho, D., Chamberland, S., Renau, T., Leger, R., Hecker, S., Watkins, W., Hoshino, K., Ishida, H,V. and Lee, V.I. (2001) Identification and characterization of inhibitors of multidrug resistance efflux pumps in *Pseudomonas aeruginosa*: novel agents for combination therapy. *Antimicrobial Agents and Chemotherapy* 45, 105–116.
Lyon, G., Wright, J.S., Muir, T.W. and Novick, R.P. (2002) Key determinants of receptor activation in the *agr* autoinducing peptides of *Staphylococcus aureus*. *Biochemistry* 41, 10095–10104.
Maadani, A., Fox, K.A., Mylonakis, E. and Garsin, D.A. (2007) *Enterococcus faecalis* mutations affecting virulence in the *Caenorhabditis elegans* model host. *Infection and Immunity* 75, 2634–2637.
Maisch, T., Hackbarth, S., Regensburger, J., Felgentrager, A., Baumler, W., Landthaler, M. and Röder, B. (2011) Photodynamic inactivation of multi-resistant bacteria (PIB) – a new approach to treat superficial infections in the 21st century. *Journal of the German Society of Dermatology* 9, 360–366.
Margolin, W. (2005) FtsZ and the division of prokaryotic cells and organelles. *Nature Reviews Molecular Cell Biology* 11, 862–871.
Markham, P., Westhaus, E., Klyachko, K., Johnson, M.E. and Neyfakh, A.A. (1999) Multiple novel inhibitors of the NorA multidrug transporter of *Staphylococcus aureus*. *Antimicrobial Agents and Chemotherapy* 43, 2404–2408.
Marra, A. (2004) Can virulence factors be viable antibacterial targets? *Expert Review of Anti-infective Therapy* 2, 61–72.
Mazzola, L. (2003) Commercializing nanotechnology. *Nature Biotechnology* 21, 1137–1143.
McDevitt, D. and Rosenberg, M. (2001) Exploiting genomics to discover new antibiotics. *Trends in Microbiology* 9, 611–617.
McGowan, J.E. Jr (2006) Resistance in nonfermenting Gram-negative bacteria: multidrug resistance to the maximum. *American Journal of Medicine* 119, S29–S36.

McKenna, M. (2011) The enemy within. *Scientific American* 304, 46–53.
Meijer, A. and Spaink, H.P. (2011) Host–pathogen interactions made transparent with the zebrafish model. *Current Drug Targets* 12, 1000–1017.
Meyer, A. (2005) Prospects and challenges of developing new agents for tough Gram-negatives. *Current Opinion in Pharmacology* 5, 1–5.
Miethke, M. and Marahiel, M. (2007) Siderophore-based iron acquisition and pathogen control. *Microbiology and Molecular Biology Reviews* 71, 413–451.
Minnick, A.A., McKee, J.A., Dolence, E.K. and Miller, M.J. (1992) Iron transport-mediated antibacterial activity of and development of resistance to hydroxamate and catechol siderophore–carbacephalosporin conjugates. *Antimicrobial Agents and Chemotherapy* 36, 840–850.
Morens, D., Folkers, G.K. and Fauci, A.S. (2004) The challenge of emerging and re-emerging infectious diseases. *Nature* 430, 242–249.
Müh, U., Schuster, M., Heim, R., Singh, A., Olson, E.R. and Greenberg, E.P. (2006) Novel *Pseudomonas aeruginosa* quorum-sensing inhibitors identified in an ultra-high-throughput screen. *Antimicrobial Agents and Chemotherapy* 50, 3674–3679.
Mukhopadhyay, A. and Peterson, R.T. (2006) Fishing for new antimicrobials. *Current Opinion in Chemical Biology* 10, 327–333.
Mylonakis, E. (2011) The need to redefine antimicrobial drug discovery. *Current Pharmaceutical Design* 17, 1223–1224.
Nagaraj, N. and Singh, O.V. (2010) Using genomics to develop novel antibacterial therapeutics. *Critical Reviews in Microbiology* 36, 340–348.
Nakayama, K., Ishida, Y., Ohtsuka, M., Kawato, H., Yoshida, K., Yokomizo, Y., Ohta, T., Hoshino, K., Otani, T., Kurosaka, Y., Yoshida, K., Ishida, H., Lee, V.I., Renau, T.E. and Watkins, W.J. (2003) MexAB-OprM specific efflux pump inhibitors in *Pseudomonas aeruginosa*. Part 2: achieving activity *in vivo* through the use of alternative scaffolds. *Bioorganic and Medicinal Chemistry Letters* 13, 4205–4208.
Nelson, D., Loomis, L. and Fischetti, V.A. (2001) Prevention and elimination of upper respiratory colonization of mice by group A streptococci by using a bacteriophage lytic enzyme. *Proceedings of the National Academy of Sciences USA* 98, 4107–4112.
Nelson, D., Schuch, R., Chahales, P., Zhu, S. and Fischetti, V.A. (2006) PlyC: a multimeric bacteriophage lysin. *Proceedings of the National Academy of Sciences USA* 103, 10765–10770.
Neyfakh, A., Bidnenko, V. and Chen, L. (1991) Efflux-mediated multidrug resistance in *Bacillus subtilis* – similarities and dissimilarities with the mammalian system. *Proceedings of the National Academy of Sciences USA* 88, 4781–4785.
Nordmann, P., Naas, T., Fortineau, N. and Poirel, L. (2007) Superbugs in the coming new decade; multidrug resistance and prospects for treatment of *Staphylococcus aureus, Enterococcus* spp. and *Pseudomonas aeruginosa* in 2010. *Current Opinion in Microbiology* 10, 436–440.
Norrby, S., Nord, C.E. and Finch, R. (2005) Lack of development of new antimicrobial drugs: a potential serious threat to public health. *Lancet Infectious Disease* 5, 115–119.
Ockels, W., Romer, A., Budzikiewicz, H. (1978) An Fe(II) complex of pyridine-2, 6-di(monothiocarboxylic acid) – a novel bacterial metabolic product. *Tetrahedron Letters* 36, 3341–3342.
O'Flaherty, S., Coffey, A., Meaney, W., Fitzgerald, G.F. and Ross, R.P. (2005) The recombinant phage lysin LysK has a broad spectrum of lytic activity against clinically relevant staphylococci, including methicillin-resistant *Staphylococcus aureus. Journal of Bacteriology* 187, 7161–7164.
Ostrosky-Zeichner, L., Casadevall, A., Galgiani, J.N., Odds, F.C. and Rex, J.H. (2010) An insight into the antifungal pipeline: selected new molecules and beyond. *Nature Reviews Drug Discovery* 9, 719–727.
Oteo, J., Pérez-Vázquez, M. and Campos, J. (2008) Extended-spectrum β-lactamase producing *Escherichia coli*: changing epidemiology and clinical impact. *Current Opinion in Infectious Disease* 23, 320–326.
Palumbi, S. (2001) Humans as the world's greatest evolutionary force. *Science* 293, 1786–1790.
Pang, Y., Schwartz, J., Thoendel, M., Ackermann, L.W., Horswill, A.R. and Nauseef, W.M. (2010) *agr*-dependent interactions of *Staphylococcus aureus* USA300 with human polymorphonuclear neutrophils. *Journal of Innate Immunity* 2, 546–559.
Paulsen, I., Banerjei, L., Myers, G.S.A., Nelson, K.E.R., Seshadri, R., Read, T.D., Fouts, D.E., Eisen, J.A., Gill, S.R., Heidelberg, J.F., Tettelin, H., Dodson, R.J., Umayam, L., Brinkac, L., Beanan, M., Daugherty, S., Deboy, R.T., Durkin, S., Kolonay, J., Madupu, R., Nelson, W., Vamathevan, J., Tran, B., Upton, J., Hansen, T., Shetty, J., Khouri, H., Utterback, T., Radune, D., Ketchum, K.A., Dougherty, B.A. and Fraser, C.M. (2003) Role of mobile DNA in the evolution of vancomycin-resistant *Enterococcus faecalis. Science* 28, 2071–2074.
Pavlovic, D., Fajdetic, A. and Mutak, S. (2010) Novel hybrids of 15-membered 8a- and

9a-azahomoerythromycin A ketolides and quinolones as potent antibacterials. *Bioorganic and Medicinal Chemistry* 18, 8566–8582.
Payne, S.M. (1993) Iron acquisition in microbial pathogenesis. *Trends in Microbiology* 1, 66–69.
Peleg, A., Jara, S., Monga, D., Eliopoulos, G.M., Moellering, R.C. Jr and Mylonakis, E. (2009) *Galleria mellonella* as a model system to study *Acinetobacter baumannii* pathogenesis and therapeutics. *Antimicrobial Agents and Chemotherapy* 53, 2605–2609.
Piddock, L. (2006a) Clinically relevant chromosomally encoded multidrug resistance efflux pumps in bacteria. *Clinical Microbiology Reviews* 19, 382–402.
Piddock, L. (2006b) Multidrug-resistance efflux pumps – not just for resistance. *Nature Reviews Microbiology* 20, 629–636.
Piper, C., Cotter, P.D., Ross, R.P. and Hill, C. (2009) Discovery of medically significant antibiotics. *Current Drug Discovery Technology* 6, 1–18.
Pitout, J. and Laupland, K.B. (2008) Extended-spectrum β-lactamase-producing Enterobacteriaceae: an emerging public-health concern. *Lancet Infectious Disease* 8, 159–166.
Plesiat, P. and Nikaido, H. (1992) Outer membranes of Gram-negative bacteria are permeable to steroid probes. *Molecular Microbiology* 6, 1323–1333.
Prates, R., Kato, I.T., Ribeiro, M.S., Tegos, G.P. and Hamblin, M.R. (2011) Influence of multidrug efflux systems on methylene blue-mediated photodynamic inactivation of Candida albicans. *Journal of Antimicrobial Chemotherapy* 66, 1525–1532.
Prince, A.S. (2002) Biofilms, antimicrobial resistance, and airway infection. *New England Journal of Medicine* 347, 1110–1111.
Pukkila-Worley, R., Holson, E., Wagner, F. and Mylonakis, E. (2009) Antifungal drug discovery through the study of invertebrate model hosts. *Current Medicinal Chemistry* 16, 1588–1595.
Quadri, L. (2007) Strategic paradigm shifts in the antimicrobial drug discovery process of the 21st century. *Infectious Disorders – Drug Targets* 7, 230–237.
Quinn, J. (1998) Clinical problems posed by multiresistant nonfermenting Gram-negative pathogens. *Clinical Infectious Diseases* 27, S117–S124.
Rasmussen, T. and Givskov, M. (2006) Quorum-sensing inhibitors as anti-pathogenic drugs. *International Journal of Medical Microbiology* 296, 149–161.
Rentz, A., Halpern, M.T. and Bowden, R. (1998) The impact of candidemia on length of hospital stay, outcome, and overall cost of illness. *Clinical Infectious Diseases* 27, 781–788.
Rock, F., Mao, W., Yaremchuk, A., Tukalo, M., Crépin, T., Zhou, H., Zhang, Y.K., Hernandez, V., Akama, T., Baker, S.I., Plattner, J.I., Shapiro, L., Martinis, S., Benkovic, S.I., Cusack, S. and Alley, M.R. (2007) An antifungal agent inhibits an aminoacyl-tRNA synthetase by trapping tRNA in the editing site. *Science* 316, 1759–1761.
Rodrigues, L., Wagner, D., Viveiros, M., Sampaio, D., Couto, I., Vavra, M., Kern, W.V. and Amaral, L. (2008) Thioridazine and chlorpromazine inhibition of ethidium bromide efflux in *Mycobacterium avium* and *Mycobacterium smegmatis*. *Journal of Antimicrobial Chemotherapy* 61, 1076–1082.
Russell, A.D. (1990) Bacterial spores and chemical sporicidal agents. *Clinical Microbiology Reviews* 3, 99–119.
Russo, T., Page, M., Beanan, J., Olson, R., Hujer, A., Hujer, K., Jacobs, M., Bajaksouzian, S., Endimiani, A. and Bonomo, R.A. (2011) *In vivo* and *in vitro* activity of the siderophore monosulfactam BAL30072 against *Acinetobacter baumannii*. *Journal of Antimicrobial Chemotherapy* 66, 867–873.
Sabatini, S., Kaatz, G.W., Rossolini, G.M., Brandini, D. and Fravolini, A. (2008) From phenothiazine to 3-phenyl-1,4-benzothiazine derivatives as inhibitors of the *Staphylococcus aureus* NorA multidrug efflux pump. *Journal of Medicinal Chemistry* 51, 4321–4330.
Saiman, L. and Siegel, J. (2004) Infection control in cystic fibrosis. *Clinical Microbiology Reviews* 17, 57–71.
Sangwan, P., Koul, J.L., Koul, S., Reddy, M.V., Thota, N., Khan, I.A., Kumar, A., Kalia, N.P. and Qazi, G.N. (2008) Piperine analogs as potent *Staphylococcus aureus* NorA efflux pump inhibitors. *Bioorganic and Medicinal Chemistry* 16, 9847–9857.
Schuch, R., Nelson, D. and Fischetti, V.A. (2002) A bacteriolytic agent that detects and kills *Bacillus anthracis*. *Nature* 418, 884–889.
Sebat, J., Paszczynski, J., Cortese, M.S. and Crawford, R.L. (2001) Antimicrobial properties of pyridine-2,6-dithiocarboxylic acid, a metal chelator produced by *Pseudomonas* spp. *Applied and Environmental Microbiology* 67, 3934–3942.
Sekhon, B.S. and Kamboj, S. (2010) Inorganic nanomedicine – part 1. *Nanomedicine: Nanotechnology, Biology and Medicine* 6, 516–522.
Sharma, A., Khuller, G.K. and Sharma, S. (2009) Peptide deformylase – a promising therapeutic target for tuberculosis and antibacterial drug discovery. *Expert Opinion on Therapeutic Targets* 13, 753–765.
Sharma, S., Dai, T., Kharkwal, G.B., Huang, Y.Y., Huang, L., De Arce, V.J., Tegos, G.P.

and Hamblin, M.R. (2011) Drug discovery of antimicrobial photosensitizers using animal models. *Current Pharmaceutical Design* 17, 1303–1319.

Sifri, C., Begun, J., Ausubel, F.M. and Calderwood, S.B. (2003) *Caenorhabditis elegans* as a model host for *Staphylococcus aureus* pathogenesis. *Infection and Immunity* 71, 2208–2217.

Sifri, C., Begun, J. and Ausubel, F.M. (2005) The worm has turned – microbial virulence modeled in *Caenorhabditis elegans. Trends in Microbiology* 13, 119–127.

Simmons, K., Chopra, I. and Fishwick, C.W. (2010) Structure-based discovery of antibacterial drugs. *Nature Reviews Microbiology* 8, 501–510.

Soncin, M., Fabris, C., Busetti, A., Dei, D., Nistri, D., Roncucci, G. and Jori, G. (2002) Approaches to selectivity in the Zn(II)-phthalocyanine-photosensitized inactivation of wild-type and antibiotic-resistant *Staphylococcus aureus. Photochemical and Photobiological Sciences* 1, 815–819.

Soukos, N. and Goodson, J.M. (2011) Photodynamic therapy in the control of oral biofilms. *Periodontology 2000* 55, 143–166.

Stavri, M., Piddock, L.J.V. and Gibbons, S. (2007) Bacterial efflux pump inhibitors from natural sources. *Journal of Antimicrobial Chemotherapy* 59, 1247–1260.

Stoop, E., Schipper, T., Rosendahl Huber, S.K., Nezhinsky, A.E., Verbeek, F.I., Gurcha, S.S., Besra, G.S., Vandenbroucke-Grauls, C.M., Bitter, W. and Van Der Sar, A.M. (2011) Zebrafish embryo screen for mycobacterial genes involved in the initiation of granuloma formation reveals a newly identified ESX-1 component. *Disease Models and Mechanisms* 4, 526–536.

Street, C., Pedigo, L.A. and Loebel, N.G. (2010) Energy dose parameters affect antimicrobial photodynamic therapy-mediated eradication of periopathogenic biofilm and planktonic cultures. *Photomedicine and Laser Surgery* (Suppl. 1), S61–S66.

Suci, P., Kang, S., Gmür, R., Douglas, T. and Young, M. (2010) Targeted delivery of a photosensitizer to *Aggregatibacter actinomycetemcomitans* biofilm. *Antimicrobial Agents and Chemotherapy* 54, 2489–2496.

Sulakvelidze, A., Alavidze, A. and Morris, J.G. Jr (2001) Bacteriophage therapy. *Antimicrobial Agents and Chemotherapy* 45, 649–659.

Tampakakis, E., Okoli, I. and Mylonakis, E. (2008) A *C. elegans*-based, whole animal, *in vivo* screen for the identification of antifungal compounds. *Nature Protocols* 3, 1925–1931.

Tang, H., Hamblin, M.R. and Yow, C.M. (2007) A comparative *in vitro* photoinactivation study of clinical isolates of multidrug-resistant pathogens. *Journal of Infection and Chemotherapy* 13, 87–91.

Tegos, G. (2006) Substrates and inhibitors of microbial efflux pumps; redefine the role of plant antimicrobials. In: Rai, M. and Carpinella, M.C. (ed.) *Naturally Occurring Bioactive Compounds: a New and Safe Alternative for Control of Pests and Microbial Diseases.* Cambridge University Press, Cambridge, UK.

Tegos, G. and Hamblin, M.R. (2006) Phenothiazinium antimicrobial photosensitizers are substrates of bacterial multidrug resistance pumps. *Antimicrobial Agents and Chemotherapy* 50, 196–203.

Tegos, G., Masago, K., Aziz, F., Higginbotham, A., Stermitz, F.R. and Hamblin, M.R. (2008) Inhibitors of bacterial multidrug efflux pumps potentiate antimicrobial photoinactivation. *Antimicrobial Agents and Chemotherapy* 52, 3202–3209.

Tegos, G., Haynes, M., Strouse, J.J., Khan, M.M.T., Bologa, C.G., Oprea, T.I. and Sklar, L.A. (2011) Microbial efflux pump inhibition: tactics and strategies. *Current Pharmaceutical Design* 17, 1291–1302.

Thiel, K. (2004) Old dogma, new tricks – 21st century phage therapy. *Nature Biotechnology* 22, 31–36.

Thorarensen, A., Presley-Bodnar, A.L. Marotti, K.R., Boyle, T.P., Heckaman, C.L., Bohanon, M.I., Tomich, P.K., Zurenko, G.E., Sweeney, M.T. and Yagi, B.H. (2002) 3-Arylpiperidines as potentiators of existing antibacterial agents. *Bioorganic and Medicinal Chemistry Letters* 11, 1903–1906.

Turner, M. (2011a) German *E. coli* outbreak caused by previously unknown strain. *Nature* doi:10.1038/news.2011.345.

Turner, M. (2011b) Microbe outbreak panics Europe. *Nature* 474, 137.

Vaara, M. (1993) Antibiotic-supersusceptible mutants of *Escherichia coli* and *Salmonella typhimurium. Antimicrobial Agents and Chemotherapy* 37, 2255–2260.

Vecchione, J., Blair, A. and Sello, J. (2009) Two distinct major facilitator superfamily drug efflux pumps mediate chloramphenicol resistance in *Streptomyces coelicolor. Antimicrobial Agents and Chemotherapy* 53, 4673–4677.

Vilcinskas, A. (2011) Anti-infective therapeutics from the lepidopteran model host *Galleria mellonella. Current Pharmaceutical Design* 17, 1240–1245.

Vollmer, W. (2008) Targeting the bacterial Z-ring. *Chemistry and Biology* 2, 93–94.

Wencewicz, T.A., Möllmann, U., Long, T.E. and Miller, M.J. (2009) Is drug release necessary for antimicrobial activity of siderophore-drug conjugates? Syntheses and biological studies of the naturally occurring salmycin "Trojan Horse" antibiotics and synthetic desferridanoxamine-antibiotic conjugates. *Biometals* 22, 633–648.

Wey, S., Mori, M., Pfaller, M.A., Woolson, R.F. and Wenzel, R.P. (1998) Hospital-acquired candidemia. The attributable mortality and excess length of stay. *Archives of Internal Medicine* 148, 2642–2645.

WHO (2010) *Global Tuberculosis Control*. World Health Organization Press, Geneva.

Wilson, M. and Yianni, C. (1995) Killing of methicillin-resistant *Staphylococcus aureus* by low-power laser light. *Journal of Medical Microbiology* 42, 62–66.

Xavier, J. (2011) Social interaction in synthetic and natural microbial communities. *Molecular Systems Biology* 7, 483.

Xing, B., Jiang, T., Bi, W., Yang, Y., Li, L., Ma, M., Chang, C.-K., Xu, B. and Yeow, E.K.L. (2011) Multifunctional divalent vancomycin: the fluorescent imaging and photodynamic antimicrobial properties for drug resistant bacteria. *Chemical Communications (Cambridge)* 47, 1601–1603.

Yoong, P., Schuch, R., Nelson, D. and Fischetti, V.A. (2004) Identification of a broadly active phage lytic enzyme with lethal activity against antibiotic-resistant *Enterococcus faecalis* and *Enterococcus faecium*. *Journal of Bacteriology* 186, 4808–4812.

Zhao, G., Weatherspoon, N., Kong, W., Curtiss, R. III and Shi, Y. (2008) A dual-signal regulatory circuit activates transcription of a set of divergent operons in *Salmonella typhimurium*. *Proceedings of the National Academy of Sciences USA* 105, 20924–20929.

Zolfaghari, P., Packer, S., Singer, M., Nair, S.P., Bennett, J., Street, C. and Wilson, M. (2009) *In vivo* killing of *Staphylococcus aureus* using a light-activated antimicrobial agent. *BMC Microbiology* 9, 27.

2 The Antibiotic Crisis

Arnold L. Demain[1] and Jaroslav Spizek[2]
[1]*Charles A. Dana Research Institute for Scientists Emeriti (RISE), Drew University, Madison, New Jersey, USA;* [2]*Institute of Microbiology, Academy of Sciences of the Czech Republic, Videnska, Prague, Czech Republic*

2.1 The Problem

The golden era of antibiotic discovery occurred from 1950 until 1970. Unfortunately in 1969, the US Surgeon General stated to Congress: 'The time has come to close the book on infectious disease.' Microbiologists knew at that time that technology had not yet won the war against infectious micro-organisms due to resistance development in pathogenic microbes and other problems. Resistance of bacteria to antibiotics continues to increase. The human population is ageing, and many patients undergo surgeries or have implanted joint replacements or are subjected to immunosuppressive therapy, making them possible victims of resistant bacteria. Some bacteria produce biofilms that make them extremely antibiotic resistant and thus very dangerous for such patients. Biofilm infections of some medical devices by common pathogens such as staphylococci are not only associated with increased morbidity and mortality but also significantly contribute to the emergence and dissemination of antibiotic resistance in the nosocomial setting (Lynch and Robertson, 2008). Microbial pathogens are thus extremely dangerous for these patients. Bacterial sepsis has already become one of the main causes of death in the elderly. The extensive use of antibiotics has selected antibiotic-resistant strains, some of them resistant to more than one antibiotic. Resistant bacteria were originally detected in hospitals; however, their occurrence is now more widely distributed. The large amounts of antibiotics used in human therapy, as well as those used for farm animals and even for fish in aquaculture, have resulted in the selection of pathogenic bacteria resistant to multiple drugs (Nikaido, 2009). Indeed, as taught by Joshua Lederberg, we know that technology will never win this war permanently and we must be satisfied merely to stay one step ahead of the pathogens for a long time to come; thus, the search for new drugs must not be stopped. In hospitals, resistant bacteria can survive for a prolonged time and can cause epidemics, for example in intensive care units. The risk of infection increases with the amount of time spent in the hospital. Vancomycin had long been considered the last hope for an antibiotic against methicillin-resistant *Staphylococcus aureus* (MRSA). However, strains resistant even to vancomycin have developed and the occurrence of antibiotic-resistant strains is apparently inevitable. Some pathogenic bacteria in intensive care units, such as *Acinetobacter baumannii*, have been described as 'pan-resistant'. The increasing resistance of these bacteria raises fears of failure of antibiotic treatment (Spizek *et al.*, 2010).

The antibiotic crisis is evidenced by the following facts:

1. Infectious disease was the leading cause of death in 1900, and today it is the second most important killer in the world, number three in developed nations and fourth in the USA (Kraus, 2008). It is the third leading cause of death in Europe, mostly in elderly and debilitated populations, and, despite existing antibiotic therapies and vaccines, infectious diseases remain the leading cause of mortality and morbidity (Vicente *et al.*, 2006). Worldwide, 17 million people die each year from bacterial infections (Butler and Buss, 2006). Americans are infected with bacteria at a rate of over 2.5 million people per year, resulting in 100,000 deaths. MRSA kills 19,000 people in the USA each year (Scott, 2009; Walsh and Fischbach, 2009).
2. It has been stated that 'hospitals are dangerous places to be – especially if you are sick, but even if not'. 15 million people are admitted to US hospitals annually, and 5–15% of these patients develop hospital-acquired infections, also known as nosocomial infections; 90,000–100,000 of them die (Overbye and Barrett, 2005; Brickner *et al.*, 2008; Carlson, 2009). People in modern society generally feel that pathogenic bacteria are unlikely to infect them and, if they occasionally do, there will always be an antibiotic to cure them. As stated by Kollef (2003), if we base our future health on the hope that new antibiotics to combat infectious diseases will be available within a short time, we, as a society, and certainly as individuals, may eventually be confronted by a catastrophic event.
3. *S. aureus* is responsible for half of nosocomial infections (Balaban and Dell'Acqua, 2005). MRSA incidence in US intensive care units among *S. aureus* isolates was 2% in 1974, 22% in 1995 and 64% in 2004.
4. *Streptococcus pneumoniae* causes bacterial pneumonia resulting in 40,000 deaths in the USA each year. By 1999, 25% of US isolates of this organism were penicillin resistant. Small children and the elderly are at higher risk. This is important, as the elderly are becoming a larger segment of the population as a consequence of improved living standards in developed societies (Vicente *et al.*, 2006).
5. A major problem today is tuberculosis (TB) caused by *Mycobacterium tuberculosis*, which currently infects 2 billion people. TB was once considered to be disappearing; however, it has come back recently. There are two main reasons for this: the association of this bacterium with AIDS and the fact that *M. tuberculosis* strains resistant to several of the drugs used to treat the disease now predominate. Multiple drug resistance has developed against two of the most important TB drugs, rifampicin and isoniazid. Each year, 9 million new cases are diagnosed and 2.6 million people die. No new drug has been commercialized against TB since 1964 (Koppal, 2004). TB is the second most important infectious killer; only AIDS (3 million deaths per year) is more dangerous. Multidrug-resistant mycobacteria arise for a complex set of reasons, an important one being the high failure rates for completion of therapeutic courses, which are often associated with a lack of resources required to observe compliance to relatively long-term therapeutic regimens. The emergence of multidrug-resistant *M. tuberculosis* resulted in the use of drugs that are much more expensive than those used previously. It is alarming that highly resistant strains continue to evolve and we face the risk of losing control, even in the industrialized world (Russell *et al.*, 2010).
6. The opportunistic pathogen *Pseudomonas aeruginosa* causes fatal wound infections, burn infections, and chronic and fatal infections of lungs in cystic fibrosis patients. Very few antibiotics can inhibit this pathogen. The bacterium almost never infects uncompromised tissues; however, it can infect practically any tissue of patients compromised in some manner. In addition to the above-mentioned infections, it causes urinary tract infections, respiratory system infections, dermatitis, soft tissue infection, bacteraemia, bone and joint infections, gastrointestinal infections and a variety of systemic infections, particularly in patients with severe burns and in cancer and AIDS patients who are immunosuppressed. Other pathogens such as *Pseudomonas cepacia* and *Enterococcus faecium* are not inhibited by any currently used antibiotic (Breiman *et al.*, 1994;

Goldman *et al.*, 1996; Tenover and Hughes, 1996; Stephens and Shapiro, 1997).

2.2 The Need for New Antibiotics

There are a number of reasons why new antibiotics are continually needed. One is the existence of naturally resistant bacteria, such as *P. aeruginosa*, *Stenotrophomonas maltophilia*, *E. faecium*, *Burkholderia cepacia* and *A. baumannii* (Tenover and Hughes, 1996).

Secondly, resistant pathogens continue to develop, such as enterococci resistant to all antibiotics (Chu *et al.*, 1996), and the organisms causing TB and malaria. Resistance is due to inactivation by enzymes such as β-lactamase, increased efflux of the antibiotic out of cells, decreased uptake of the antibiotic, modification of the target to decrease binding of the antibiotic, amplification of the target, bypassing the essentiality of the target, sequestration of the antibiotic, protection of the target, intracellular localization and biofilm formation (Singh and Barrett, 2006; Davies, 2007). Bacteria that form biofilms, including staphylococci, are very resistant to antibiotics and grow on wounds, scar tissue, medical implants such as joint prostheses, spinal instruments, vascular prosthetic grafts and heart valves. It is worth mentioning that some antibiotics can even induce biofilm formation (Hoffman *et al.*, 2005). All of the above modifications occur by mutation and/or by gene acquisition. The antibiotic resistance problem was examined thoroughly in the report of the colloquium sponsored by the American Academy of Microbiology entitled *Antibiotic Resistance: an Ecological Perspective on an Old Problem* (American Academy of Microbiology, 2009). In a worst-case scenario, the emergence of resistance towards a variety of antibiotics may lead to treatment failure in all patient classes, not only the elderly and the immunocompromised. As it takes a long time to develop a new antibiotic for clinical use, in the future we may be faced with bacterial infections that are resistant to all available drugs and find that it is too late to react.

In contrast to other drugs, antibiotics can start to lose their efficacy immediately after their clinical use begins through the development of antibiotic resistance by bacterial pathogens. Pathogens can become resistant to antibiotics through the acquisition of resistance genes from other bacteria or by modification of some of their own genes. In the case of acquisition of resistance genes by pathogens, antibiotic-producing organisms can be envisaged as a potential source of antibiotic resistance genes (Davies, 1994). This hypothesis was developed further by D'Costa *et al.* (2006), who demonstrated that soil-dwelling bacteria produce and encounter a myriad of antibiotics, evolving corresponding sensing and evading strategies. They are a reservoir of resistance determinants that can be mobilized into the microbial community. The authors of this important finding concluded that the study of this reservoir could provide an early warning system for future clinically relevant antibiotic resistance mechanisms. More recently, Wright (2010) showed that environmental microbes are highly drug resistant, that the genes that form the environmental resistome have the potential to be transferred to pathogens and that there is some evidence that some clinically relevant resistance genes originated in environmental microbes.

Bacterial pathogens mutate frequently, even during the course of a single treatment, and therefore their target can be modified to confer resistance in a very short time after the introduction of a new drug. In the most puzzling cases (as was the case for penicillin and more recently for linezolid, an oxazolidinone that interacts with the peptidyl-tRNA-binding P site on the 50S subunit), the emergence of resistant microorganisms has even preceded the clinical use of some antibiotics (Bush, 2004). The introduction of different classes of new antibiotics into medical use has been met by further developments in antibiotic resistance such that multidrug-resistant bacterial pathogens are now increasingly common.

A third reason has been the emergence of new disease agents, such as human immunodeficiency virus (HIV) causing AIDS, Hanta virus, Ebola virus, *Cryptospiridium*, Legionnaire's disease, Lyme disease, *Escherichia coli* O157:H7 and severe acute respiratory syndrome coronavirus (SARS-CoV). The World Health Organization concluded that at least 30 new diseases emerged in the 1980s and 1990s (DaSilva and Iaccarino, 1999). Antibiotic discovery is vital when considering the threat posed by the emergence of previously unknown or uncommon infectious diseases (Morens *et al.*, 2004). A contemporary example is provided by the frequent outbreaks of *Legionella* spp., an organism that only became a serious health threat when the extensive use of large air-conditioning systems created a favourable environment both for the multiplication of the pathogen and for its delivery as aerosols to the human respiratory system. Also important are emerging and re-emerging diseases such as influenza, hepatitis B, West Nile fever, hepatitis C, hantavirus pulmonary syndrome, children's diarrhoea caused by rotavirus, dengue fever and mad cow disease. The cost of combating these diseases is more than US$120 billion per year.

The increase in emerging and re-emerging diseases is a result of a number of factors: (i) increased international travel; (ii) increased human population density; (iii) increasing population age; (iv) global movement of wild, exotic animals; (v) destruction of animal habitats; (vi) inadequate public health in underdeveloped countries leading to poor preventive vaccine campaigns and ineffective monitoring of water and food cleanliness; and (vii) a decrease in new antibiotic discovery and development. An example of the global movement of wild animals is the use of exotic cats in China for meat, which has led to the host transition of SARS-CoV from animals to humans. With regard to inadequate public health, water pollution causes 14,000 deaths per day in developing countries. Nearly 2 million people die of diarrhoeal diseases every year, mainly due to contaminated water and poor sanitation.

Fourthly, food contamination is a major problem, with 9000 Americans dying each year as a result. The contamination is mainly due to microbes, the most serious of which are *E. coli*, *Listeria monocytogenes*, *Campylobacter jejuni* and *Salmonella* spp. The medical expenses of people and losses in productivity amount to US$7–35 billion per year in the USA from meat and poultry contamination by just seven bacteria.

Lastly, diseases caused by a known pathogen but attacking new populations, and the toxicity of some of the current compounds (Strohl, 1997), mean there is a continued need for new antibiotics.

2.3 Evidence for the Decrease in Discovery of New Antibiotics

The number of new antibiotics discovered has steadily decreased, as evidenced by the following:

1. There were 120 drug approvals by the US Food and Drug Administration (FDA) in 1996 and 1997 (Ryan, 2003). Due to the movement of the pharmaceutical industry away from natural products, especially antibiotics, the number of drug approvals dropped to 36 in 2004 and then to 20 in 2005 (Mullin, 2006a). Although 86 new drugs were approved by the FDA in 2003, the actual number of new chemical structures hit a 9-year low.
2. During 1978–1980, the average number of the FDA category of new molecular entities (NMEs), i.e. drugs with novel molecular structures, launched by the pharmaceutical industry was 43. By 1998–2000, the average number had dropped to 33. Evidence of the drop-off can be seen in the following data: 1996 = 53, 1997 = 39, 1998 = 30, 1999 = 35, 2000 = 27, 2001 = 24, 2002 = 17, 2003 = 21 and 2005 = 18 (Warner, 2004; Kostel, 2004).
3. Whereas FDA drug applications peaked at 131 in 1996, the number dropped steadily to 78 by 2002 (Warner, 2003). Launches of new drugs have dropped from an average of 44 per year during 1995–2000 to 33 during 2001–2006, and to 27 in 2007 (Malik, 2008).
4. The number of drugs classified by the FDA as new chemical entities (NCEs) developed by the top 20 pharmaceutical organizations continued to drop over the 15-year period between 1987 and 2002 (Handen, 2002). The number launched in 2003 was 30, the lowest in over 20 years (Class, 2004). Furthermore, fewer than half of the NCEs approved by the FDA in 2002 were really new (Willis, 2004).

The rest were protein-based products, off-patent generics and derivatives of existing drugs.
5. Another FDA category is new active substances (NASs). In 2001, there was a 20-year low in the number of these approved by the FDA (Jacobs, 2002). The number was 37 and was part of a continuous drop since 1997.
6. The drop-off in new drug approvals has been even more significant when one considers antibiotics (Genilloud *et al.*, 2010). Since 1983, the rate of antibacterial commercialization has become vanishingly low (Table 2.1). In 2002, there were 89 new drugs approved by the FDA but none was an antibiotic. Of the 74 new therapeutic agents approved by the FDA in 2007, only two were antibiotics. Of 2700 compounds in development in 2008, only 50 were antibacterials and, of these, only ten were from large pharmaceutical companies (Carlson, 2009). Possible reasons for the lack of discovery of new antibiotics were put forth by Baltz (2008) as follows: (i) enzymes essential to the viability of pathogens may not be readily 'druggable' (i.e. they may not have binding sites for inhibitors, the compounds cannot get into the cell or the compounds have poor pharmacological properties); (ii) targets are not accessible to *in vitro* screening (e.g. if they are ribosomal or part of a nascent peptidoglycan); and (iii) chemical libraries lack the molecular complexity of natural antibiotics. According to Baltz (2008), we can no longer depend on pharmaceutical companies alone to come up with new antibiotics. The effort will have to come from medical research by academia in collaboration with small firms including biotechnology companies and pharmaceutical corporations.

Table 2.1. New antibacterials that have been commercialized.

Years	Number
1983–1987	16
1988–1992	14
1993–1997	10
1998–2002	7
2003–2007	5
2008–2010	2

2.4 Reasons for the Drop-off in Discovery

A significant number of pharmaceutical companies have abandoned their anti-infective research programmes in recent years (Demain, 2002). This trend can be highlighted by the observation that it is quicker to name the few that still retain a programme, even if it is not prioritized, than to enumerate those who have abandoned their anti-infective research.

There are some trivial reasons that have usually not been considered at all. Vicente *et al.* (2006) were probably the first who mentioned the generally known phenomenon that many clinicians are satisfied with the available antibiotics. The authors referred to an informal enquiry of medical professionals working in hospitals in Madrid, Spain, and Cagliari, Italy, indicating that only about one-third of them thought that the discovery of new antibiotics was urgently required, whereas the rest were satisfied that most 'normal' cases can be treated with one or a few available drugs, despite their estimates that antibiotic therapy failure in compromised patients could be as high as 15%. We have also noted that this assumption is rather frequent among clinicians, who are usually convinced that infectious diseases can be successfully treated with the currently available antibiotics and that the treatment of diseases other than infectious diseases is more important.

Another reason is 'merger-mania' in the pharmaceutical industry. Mergers have markedly decreased the number of groups searching for new antibiotics. As recently as 2009, major companies had undergone mergers, such as Wyeth with Pfizer and Schering-Plough with Merck. The problem is that these large merged companies appear to be less productive than the original ones and that company size has no relationship to the frequency of discovery of new and useful drugs. Even many drug executives now realize that mergers can actually have a negative impact on research R&D productivity. Almost 40 major mergers in the pharmaceutical industry took place between 1985 and 2005 (Daemmrich and Bowden, 2005).

A third reason involves the nature of natural products. Among medicines used up to 1996, 80% were natural products or inspired by natural products (Harvey, 2007). Of the 868 NCEs approved between 1981 and 2002, 52% were natural or created around natural product structure. It is quite difficult to discover new natural products with antibacterial activity when those more prevalent in nature have already been discovered. As a result, there has been a misguided loss of interest by companies in natural products, especially those with antibiotic activity. The industry has opted to save funds by eliminating natural product departments or decreasing their relevance in the hunt for new drugs. Large pharmaceutical companies that dropped or significantly reduced research on antibiotic discovery include Merck, Wyeth (now part of Pfizer), Aventis, Eli Lilly, Bristol-Myers Squibb, Schering-Plough (now part of Merck), Abbott Laboratories, and Proctor and Gamble (Barrett, 2005). It is of some hope that small companies, including biotech firms, will continue to attempt antibiotic discovery. For example, in 1995, the large pharmaceutical companies had only three antibacterials in clinical development compared with 17 compounds being developed by the biotechnology industry (Bush, 2004; Carlson, 2009).

A fourth reason is the increased development time required for clinical trials. Clinical development time doubled between 1982 and 2002 to 6 years. This included 1 year of Phase I (involving 20–30 healthy volunteers for safety and dosage determination), 1.5 years for Phase II (100–300 patient volunteers for efficacy and side effects assessment) and 3.5 years for Phase III (1000–5000 patient volunteers monitoring the effects of long-term use). Added to this could be 2–10 years for discovery, 4 years for pre-clinical testing, 1 year of FDA review and approval, and 1 year of post-marketing testing. Although some estimate that the total time to get a drug on the market is 12–15 years (Burrill, 2002), the above breakdown indicates that it could be as long as 14–22 years.

The increased development time has markedly increased the cost of getting a drug to market; this rose from US$500–600 million in 1999 to US$900 million–US$1 billion in 2002 (Kettler, 1999; Agres, 2003). By 2003, the cost had risen to US$1.7 billion (Thayer, 2004), and by 2009, to US$1.8 billion (Morrow, 2010). Two-thirds of the cost was due to leads that failed in the clinic. One-half of all potential drugs failed because of adsorption, distribution, metabolism, excretion or toxicity problems. Approximately 70% of compounds get through Phase I of clinical trials, 33% of these get through Phase II and 25–30% of these get through Phase III. Overall, only about 8% of compounds entering trials become commercialized.

Because of the increased costs, the pharmaceutical industry's discovery efforts in the 1990s moved away from natural products to combinatorial chemistry followed by high-throughput screening (HTS). This was done because it was considered that natural product extracts were not amenable to HTS (Fox *et al.*, 1999). Although it was thought that combinatorial chemistry and HTS would yield many new hits and leads, the results were disappointing, despite the extraordinary amount of money spent (Horrobin, 2001). Developed in the early 1990s, speed and miniaturization were accomplished by HTS, but discovery of new leads did not accelerate. HTS methods allowed 100,000–200,000 chemicals to be assayed per day (Firn and Jones, 2000; Hefti and Bolten, 2003), and combinatorial and other chemical libraries of 1 million compounds were available commercially. As use of the conventional 96-microwell format for HTS could cost US$1 million to screen 500,000 compounds against a single target, some companies went to 384-, 1536- and even 3456-well formats to cut expenses. However, the premise of 'the more compounds screened, the more leads found' did not work. No drugs were approved resulting from HTS by 1999 (Fox *et al.*, 1999) and not a single drug derived solely by combinatorial chemistry was introduced up to 2005. The US pharmaceutical industry invested US$32 billion in 2002, triple the amount invested 10 years earlier, but the number of resulting NCEs dropped. Finally, one NCE of synthetic origin produced by combinatorial chemistry was approved by the FDA. It was the antitumour drug sorafenib (Nexavar) from Bayer, a kinase inhibitor, approved in 2006 for renal carcinoma (Newman and Cragg, 2007).

The problems were that HTS had not been applied to natural product libraries and that combinatorial chemistry had not utilized natural products as scaffolds (Demain, 1999; Kingston and Newman, 2002; Waldmann and Breinbauer, 2002). This made no sense, as the role of combinatorial chemistry, like those of structure–function drug design and recombinant DNA technology two and three decades ago, was that of complementing and assisting natural product discovery and development, not replacing them. Combinatorial chemistry is great for improving leads but not for the discovery of new leads. However, when combinatorial chemistry is applied to natural products, it works. For example, workers at Vicuron (Clough *et al.*, 2003) produced 500 combinatorial analogues of the natural but poorly soluble thiazole peptide antibiotic GE2270A. Of these, eight had both good solubility and good activity. A number of other examples were cited by Ganesan (2004). The chemist Waldmann (2003) stated that 'biological investigation of the million compound speculative combinational libraries of the first generation yielded disappointingly low hit rates'. He urged the use of biologically validated compounds as scaffolds for library generation. He further stated that 'biologically active natural products can be regarded as chemical entities that were evolutionarily selected and validated for binding to particular protein domains'. It is encouraging that natural products are finally being used by chemists as combinatorial chemistry scaffolds for synthesis of potential drugs. It is hoped that new products will result from such efforts (Newman, 2008).

Despite the great costs of genomics research, the use of genomics has not had a major effect on drug discovery. After 10 years of bacterial genomics, there were still no promising antibacterial agents on the market or even in clinical testing resulting from genomic studies (Shlaes *et al.*, 2004; Coates and Hu, 2007).

It is clear that the advent of combinatorial chemistry, HTS, genomics and proteomics has not yet done the job predicted for them. Indeed, investment in genomics and HTS has had no effect on the number of products in preclinical development or Phase I clinical trials. However, instead of downgrading natural product screening, there is real opportunity in incorporating it with HTS, combinatorial chemistry, genomics, proteomics and new discoveries being made in biodiversity.

The pharmaceutical industry increased spending on R&D from US$2 billion in 1980 to US$30 billion in 2001, but further increases stopped at that time (Tralau-Stewart *et al.*, 2009). One reason was the drop-off in discovery of new small molecules. Data from 48 drug companies showed that R&D spending increased by 80% from 1992 to 2002, whereas new drug launches dropped by 35% (Thayer, 2003). Similarly, from 1998 to 2001, the annual spending on R&D of the top 20 pharmaceutical companies increased from US$26 billion in 1998 to US$31 billion in 1999, to US$35 billion in 2000 and to US$37 billion in 2001, but the number of new drug applications decreased from 34 to 23 to 21 to 16 in those same years. Another study showed that the R&D dollars spent per entity launched was US$44 million in 1978–1980 but this increased to US$878 million in 1998–2000 (Centre for Medicines Research International, 2000). It is obvious that the incorrect approaches described above have contributed to this problem.

The drop-off in rate of discovery is not due to a decrease in total investment by the pharmaceutical industry but more likely to an over-emphasis on promotion. The amount spent by the pharmaceutical industry to market, promote and advertise their products in 1991 was US$9.2 billion. By 2004, the amount was US$25 billion, mainly due to direct advertising to consumers, free drug samples and salaries for drug representatives. Apparently, there is one drug representative for every nine Managing Directors, each representative earning over US$100,000 per year (Hilleman, 2006). One major corporation spent 33% of sales on promotion but only 19% on R&D in 2004.

2.5 Why Natural Products are More Likely to Become Drugs than Synthetic Compounds

In total, 877 pharmaceuticals were commercialized from 1988 to 2008. Of these, 60% were from natural sources or derived from them (Lefevre *et al.*, 2008). Quality appears to be more important than quantity when it comes to new drug discovery. Whereas only 0.001% of the total synthetic compounds have become drugs, 0.2–0.3% of microbial metabolites have become drugs and another 0.2–0.3% have become lead compounds for chemical modification. This is more than two orders of magnitude difference. Natural product collections have a much higher hit rate in high-throughput screens than combinatorial libraries. Breinbauer *et al.* (2002) pointed out that the number of compounds in a chemical library is not the important point; it is the biological relevance, design and diversity of the library, and that a scaffold from nature provides viable, biologically validated starting points for the design of chemical libraries. Products from nature are unsurpassed in their ability to provide novelty and complexity (Bull *et al.*, 2000). With respect to the number of chirality centres, rings, bridges and functional groups in the molecule, natural products are spatially more complex than synthetic compounds (Henkel *et al.*, 1999).

Synthetic compounds highlighted via combinatorial chemistry and *in vitro* high-throughput assays are based on small chemical changes to existing drugs, and of the thousands, perhaps millions, of chemical 'shapes' available to pharmaceutical researchers, only a few hundred are being explored. Many compounds are probably being missed. Natural products differ from synthetic compounds by having more oxygen atoms and stereochemical elements such as chiral centres and polycyclic (often bridged) carbon skeletons (Ganesan, 2004). Most drugs in use today are chiral. In a survey comparing approximately 670,000 chemical combinatorial compounds, about 11,000 drugs and over 3000 natural products, it was found that 82% of natural products were chiral and 55% of drugs were chiral, but only 29% of combinatorial products were chiral (Feher and Schmidt, 2003).

According to Sam Danishefsky, the prominent chemist at the Memorial Sloan-Kettering Cancer Center in New York, it is appropriate 'to critically examine the prevailing supposition that synthesizing zillions of compounds at a time is necessarily going to cut the costs of drug discovery or fill pharma pipelines with new drugs any time soon' (Borman, 2002). Danishefsky continued:

> At the risk of sounding Neanderthal, I would even put in a pitch for industry getting back to the screening of natural products. Some of the most valuable products and promising leads in oncology are naturally derived or naturally inspired. For instance, paclitaxel, a chemically established drug, came from natural product sources, as did doxorubicin, the etoposides and the latter-day camptothecins. In fact, even tamoxifen arose from natural product leads, steroid hormones. Moreover, several of today's most promising pipeline candidates in oncology, such as ecteinascidin, halichondrin, bryostatin, and of course, the epothilones, all arose from natural product screening followed by synthetic modifications. A small collection of smart compounds may be more valuable than a much larger hodgepodge collection mindlessly assembled. Thus, the decision on the part of several pharma companies to get out of the natural products business is gross foolishness. There are major teachings in these natural products that we would do well to consider. They may be reflecting eons of wisdom and refinement. The much maligned natural product collections did, after all, bring us statin, β-lactam, aminoglycoside, and macrolide blockbuster drugs. In fact, one of the most promising approaches in diversity chemistry is to produce diversity-chemistry-derived collections that benefit from or partake of the 'wisdom' of natural products.

One also has to be wary of chemical rules established for the characteristics of successful drugs. A letter to the Editor by Frank R. Stermitz (2002) reads as follows: 'I see from your cover story on computers in chemistry that a good drug molecule should have a molecular weight of under 500. I'm sure that many people are glad that "computational screening" was not available before the development of avermectin (molecular weight 886), paclitaxel (molecular weight 854) or vancomycin (molecular weight 1,449).'

2.6 What Can Be Done to Correct the Situation?

One reason for companies abandoning the antibiotic area is that these compounds are taken for only a short time by the patient compared with: (i) drugs for heart disease, which are taken for the length of one's life; and (ii) those enhancing male sexual performance. Despite this dismal situation, there is hope. After all, antimicrobial pharmaceuticals are still big business. In 2002, the anti-infective market amounted to US$45 billion, made up of 62% antibacterials; 13% sera, immunoglobulins and vaccines; 12% anti-HIV antivirals; 7% antifungals; and 6% non-HIV antivirals (Bush, 2004). What is needed is a move back by the large companies to rational drug design and the use of more focused, more drug-like, compound libraries. Baltz (2008) argued that the lack of new antibiotics can be changed markedly by using high-throughput fermentations, isolating marine actinomycetes, mining genomes to find cryptic pathways and employing combinatorial biosynthesis.

New targets are available for screening natural products. Inhibitors of peptide deformylase and fatty acid biosynthesis, new targets not based on genomics, are in clinical trials. Other targets include lipid A biosynthesis and tRNA synthetases. Eighteen antibacterial drugs were in clinical trials in 2004 (Bush *et al.*, 2004). They included carbapenems, cephalosporins, glycopeptides, quinolones, a glycolipodepsipeptide, a dihydrofolate reductase inhibitor, an oxazolidinone, two peptides and a peptide deformylase inhibitor. Furthermore, major improvements have been made in detection, characterization and purification of small molecules.

New screening technologies are also very important. For example, a new means of discovering antifungal drugs uses an assay based on the application of the nematode *Caenorhabditis elegans* as host for *Candida albicans* and other pathogenic *Candida* spp. (Breger *et al.*, 2007). The yeast is ingested by the worm, which causes an infection in the intestinal tract of the worm and kills it. Known antifungal agents such as amphotericin B and caspofungin prolong the worm's survival. The test is done in liquid medium contained in 96-well plates and appears to be a valuable discovery tool. Of 1266 compounds tested, 1.2% (15 compounds) were active. The most active were caffeic acid phenethyl ester and the fluoroquinolone enoxacin. Another novel method to discover new antimicrobial agents employs the laboratory nematode *C. elegans* infected with *Enterococcus faecalis* (Moy *et al.*, 2006). Antibiotics rescue the infected nematode in an assay done in 96-well microtitre plates. Some of the new targets for antimicrobials were recently reviewed by Aminov (2010).

Additional targets for new antibiotics have been proposed by Devasahayam *et al.* (2010). They include the following: (i) proteins carrying out bactericidal functions, which could include the essential enoyl-ACP reductase Fab-I of fatty acid synthesis; (ii) virulence factors such as CrtM from *S. aureus*, which is used to produce staphyloxanthin, an antioxidant allowing *S. aureus* to evade the reactive oxygen species response of the host; (iii) multidrug-resistant efflux pumps of fungi and the type III secretion system of Gram-negative pathogens; (iv) proteins involved in formation of the lipopolysaccharide outer membrane of the Gram-negative organisms, such as RfaE; (v) proteins such as DltA involved in D-alanylation of lipoteichoic acid in Gram-positive pathogens; (vi) signalling proteins such as the QseC histidine kinase involved in virulence gene activation in *Salmonella typhimurium* and *Francisella tularensis*; (vii) inhibitors of ATP synthesis or agents disrupting proton motive force in *M. tuberculosis*; (viii) activators of host response pathways such as activators of the Toll-like receptor; and (ix) antitumour necrosis factor-α agents for patients with sepsis.

The production of antibiotics in heterologous hosts, known as combinatorial biosynthesis, is capable of yielding new antibiotics (Baltz, 2006; Zhang *et al.*, 2008). Recombinant DNA methods are used to introduce genes encoding natural product synthetases into producers of other natural products or into non-producing strains to obtain modified or hybrid antibiotics. Galm and Shen (2006) have described such production of over 50 secondary metabolites. The first demonstration of combinatorial biosynthesis involved gene transfer from a streptomycete strain producing the isochromanequinone antibiotic actinorhodin into strains producing granaticin, dihydrogranaticin and mederomycin (which are also isochromanequinones). This led to the discovery of two new antibiotic derivatives, mederrhodin A and dihydrogranatirhodin. Since this breakthrough paper by Hopwood *et al.* (1985), many hybrid antibiotics have been produced by recombinant DNA technology. Many of these have been obtained after the biosynthetic paths were elucidated and the biosynthetic genes isolated (Mendez and Salas, 2003). Techniques used are: (i) targeted gene disruption in which single genes are inactivated; (ii) tailoring by introducing a single gene or a few genes from another pathway; and (iii) a combination of (i) and (ii). New antibiotics can also be created by changing the order of the genes of an individual pathway in its native host (Hershberger, 1996). Antibiotics produced by combinatorial biosynthesis include novel erythromycins (Donadio *et al.*, 1993), other novel polyketides that contain sugars at normally unglycosylated positions (Trefzer *et al.*, 2002), macrolides with new sugar moieties (Zhao *et al.*, 1999) and new peptide antibiotics (Stachelhaus *et al.*, 1995). Over 200 new polyketides have been made by combining polyketide biosynthetic genes, such as polyketide synthases (PKSs), from different producers (Hutchinson and Fujii, 1995; Rodriguez and McDaniel, 2001).

A new enzymatic technique called glycorandomization is being used to prepare glycoside libraries and to make optimized or novel glycoside antibiotics. Sugars in natural products such as antibiotics are usually members of the 6-deoxyhexose family. Over 70 different variants have been found in products of bacteria, fungi and plants. Engineering the formation of new secondary metabolites in actinomycetes by glycosylation was reviewed by Salas and Mendez (2007). Novel deoxysugars can be placed on macrolide antibiotics by combinatorial biosynthesis (Oh *et al.*, 2007). The presence of glycosidic residues in antibiotics is very important for their activity (Kren and Rezanka, 2008).

The marine environment is an intriguing source for the discovery of new drugs (Hopwood, 2007; Gulder and Moore, 2009). Marine cyanobacteria are a rich source of novel secondary metabolites (Tan, 2007). They produce more than 300 nitrogenous secondary metabolites. Most are bioactive non-ribosomal peptides (NRPs) or mixed polyketide/NRPs. This source provides a much higher discovery rate of novel secondary metabolites (>75%) than other sources of microbes. Marine actinomycetes (Bull *et al.*, 2005; Jensen *et al.*, 2005) and marine fungi (Bhadury *et al.*, 2006) are other promising sources of new antibiotics.

Although the practice of genomics has not yielded commercial antibiotics, as described above, it still has potential for the discovery of new antibacterials (Mills, 2006). Genome sequencing has revealed many more gene clusters for biosynthesis of secondary metabolites than the number of metabolites known. These 'orphan' biosynthetic pathways (Gross, 2007) are now being activated by determination of optimum conditions for production. *Streptomyces coelicolor* was known to produce four secondary metabolites at the time that the genome sequence revealed 18 additional biosynthetic pathways. Genome sequencing of the marine organism *Salinispora tropica* revealed a circular genome of 5,183,331 bp (Udwary *et al.*, 2007). A large portion (9.9%) is devoted to secondary metabolism, greater than ever before seen. It contained genes encoding PKS systems of every known family, non-ribosomal peptide synthases and hybrid clusters. Genome mining involves powerful techniques for the discovery of new natural products (Zerikly and Challis, 2009). In recent years, a number of additional 'silent' secondary metabolites have been found by genome mining. These include coelichelin (Lautru *et al.*, 2005) from *S. coelicolor*, geosmin (Cane *et al.*, 2006) from *Streptomyces avermitilis*, and epi-isozizaene (Lin *et al.*, 2006), germicidins (Song *et al.*, 2006) and mycothiol (Park *et al.*, 2006) from *S. coelicolor*. Coelichelin is a peptide that appears to be a siderophore involved in iron uptake, and the germicidins are a group of five related compounds. Germicidin A was previously known to be an inhibitor of spore germination in *Streptomyces viridochromogenes*. Three of the germicidins were new compounds (Song *et al.*, 2006). Many new compounds have been isolated from other mined microbes (Gross, 2007). As hundreds of microbial genomes have been sequenced, genome mining has great importance for the future of drug discovery. Multiple gene clusters encoding secondary metabolite production are common in species of *Streptomyces*, other filamentous actinomycetes and mycobacteria (Busti *et al.*, 2006). *S. coelicolor* and *S. avermitilis* contain 20–30 of these clusters. In contrast, most other bacterial genomes lack them. The use of actinomycetes, traditionally the most successful sources of natural products, in novel drug discovery has recently been discussed by Genilloud *et al.* (2010), who suggested that novel molecules with potential therapeutic applications are still waiting to be discovered from these natural sources, especially from actinomycetes. According to the authors, *Streptomyces* continues to be one of the best factories among actinomycetes and can deliver novel scaffolds if appropriate tools are put in a place in a cost-effective manner. They also proposed that: 'the challenge today is to be able to translate current developments into industrial-scale processes, and this remains the major hurdle that will have to be overcome if we want to revitalize natural products discovery'.

Specific strains of streptomycetes (i.e. *Streptomyces albus*, *S. coelicolor*, *Streptomyces lividans*, *Streptomyces griseofuscus*, *Streptomyces ambofaciens*, *S. avermitilis*, *Streptomyces fradiae*, *Streptomyces roseosporus*, *Streptomyces toyocaensis* and *Saccharopolyspora erythrea*, formerly *Streptomyces erythreus*) can also serve as hosts for heterologous expression of secondary metabolite gene clusters to address the expression of different cryptic secondary metabolite pathways in well-defined hosts (Baltz, 2010). In Baltz's review, the heterologous hosts are divided into two general groups: hosts derived from industrial polyketide producers and hosts derived from NRP producers. The author proposed that 'the information should provide an experimental basis to help researchers choose hosts for current application and future development to express heterologous secondary metabolite pathways in yields sufficient for rapid scale-up, biological testing and commercial production'.

Like the bacteria, fungi have many extra clusters of secondary metabolite biosynthesis genes (Sanchez *et al.*, 2008). Genome sequencing of eight species of *Aspergillus* (*A. clavatus*, *A. flavus*, *A. fumigatus*, *A. nidulans*, *A. niger*, *A. oryzae*, *A. terreus* and *A. fischeri*) showed many more clusters, including PKS and NRP synthetase (NRPS) sequences, than those of secondary metabolites known to be produced by these species. Sequencing of the *A. nidulans* genome revealed 27 PKSs and 14 NRPSs, whereas previously fewer than ten biosynthetic gene clusters were known (Chiang *et al.*, 2008). Production of 'silent' secondary metabolites by fungi can be brought about by addition of inhibitors of DNA methyltransferase and histone deacetylase (Williams *et al.*, 2008), or by disrupting the activities of such enzymes (Schwab *et al.*, 2007).

Uncultured microbes are a new source of antibiotics. Existing bacterial species in nature are estimated to number somewhere between 10^7 and 10^9 (Schloss and Handelsman, 2004). Less than 0.3% of soil bacteria and less than 0.00001% of water-associated bacteria are estimated to have been grown in common laboratory media (Amann *et al.*, 1995).

One gram of soil has been estimated to contain up to 10 billion microorganisms of thousands of different species (Rosello-Mora and Amann, 2001). Another estimate is that 30 g of soil contains >500,000 species (Doolittle, 1999). These numbers are much higher than the 5000–6000 individual prokaryotic microbes available in culture collections or described in the literature (Daniel, 2004). Another piece of data is that in 1 g of soil, 10^7 cells could be counted but only 10^4 (0.1%) could be cultivated (Kellenberger, 2001). Using a new synthetic statistical approach to measure biodiversity, Hong *et al.* (2006) estimated that a 5 g sample of marine sediment contained 2000–3000 bacterial species. Estimates of the number of prokaryotic cells are 4×10^7/g in forest soil and 2×10^9/g in cultivated soils and grasslands (Daniel, 2004). It is obvious that the vast majority of microbes in nature have never been cultured in a laboratory. Some uncultured microbes have finally been grown by: (i) the use of low-nutrient oligotrophic growth media, which prevent overgrowth by rapidly growing species; (ii) using signalling molecules; (iii) using inhibitors of undesirable organisms; (iv) using very long periods of incubation, sometimes in the natural environment; (v) protection of cells from exogenous peroxides; (vi) inclusion of humic acid; (vii) use of hypoxic (1–2% oxygen) and anoxic atmospheres; (viii) use of a high concentration (5%) of carbon dioxide along with high-throughput PCR methodology; (ix) construction of a diffusion chamber containing a simulated natural environment; and (x) encapsulating cells in gel microdroplets under low-nutrient flux conditions and detecting microcolonies by flow cytometry (Zengler *et al.* 2002, 2005; Connon and Giovannoni, 2002; Kaeberlein *et al.*, 2002; Wery *et al.*, 2003; Stevenson *et al.*, 2004).

To discover new drugs from natural sources, a metagenomic approach is also recommended (Lorenz and Eck, 2005; Lefevre *et al.*, 2008). This involves cultivation-independent approaches such as extraction of nucleic acids ('environmental DNA') from the soil, insertion into vectors (plasmids, cosmids or bacterial artificial chromosomes (BACs)) and propagation in bacteria such as *E. coli* (Martinez *et al.*, 2005). Metagenomics can be defined as the genomic analysis of assemblages of organisms, and deals mainly with the genomes of unculturable microbes (Handelsman, 2004). It has yielded new antibiotics and enzymes. DNA is isolated from soil or water and cloned into *E. coli* or *S. lividans* by the use of BACs. BACs can carry large DNA inserts up to 350 kb in size. Clones containing environmental (= metagenomic) DNA are then screened for activity. The size of metagenomic DNA can be as large as 40 kb from aquatic environments and 70 kb from soil (Handelsman *et al.*, 1998; Rondon *et al.*, 2000; Stokes *et al.*, 2001). These new compounds included 13 long-chain *N*-acyl tyrosine antibiotics (Brady and Clardy, 2000) and a new turbomycin (Gillespie *et al.*, 2002) with broad spectrum activity and no haemolytic activity; these are triaryl cation antibiotics. Siderophores, terragines, indole derivatives, indirubins, fatty acid dienic alcohol isomers and triaryl cations have also been produced (Pelzer *et al.*, 2005).

In a recent review, Donadio *et al.* (2010) proposed that, in addition to retrieving microbial strains from underexplored environments, genome mining, increased sensitivity assays and HTS and even chemical derivatization of known microbial products could be applied with the aid of so-called 'click' chemistry. To be useful, the click reaction must be of wide scope, give consistently high yields with various starting materials, be easy to perform, be insensitive to oxygen or water and use only readily available reagents, and, finally, the reaction work-up and product isolation must be simple, without the need for chromatographic purification (Kolb and Sharpless, 2003).

In addition to the application of new technologies to solve the antibiotic crisis, there are additional possible remedies. One could involve more government support of small companies and academic institutions attempting to discover new antibiotics. Most of the antibacterials in clinical trials are from small pharmaceutical companies and the biotechnology industry. Whereas the major pharmaceutical companies had only three antibacterial products in clinical development in 2005, the biotechnology companies and small pharmaceutical organizations had 17. In general, about one-half to two-thirds of new products of the pharmaceutical industry are being licensed in from such companies. In 2006, small companies provided 50–60% of pharmaceutical revenues (Mullin, 2006b).

Another approach involves measures by which the government might encourage large pharmaceutical companies to return to antibiotic discovery. The Infectious Diseases Society of America has suggested the following: (i) a shorter approval process for new antibiotics; (ii) patent extensions; (iii) orphan drug status; (iv) tax credits; (v) limitation of liability; and (vi) advanced purchasing commitment by governments. We have a further suggestion. We believe governments throughout the world should establish institutes devoted solely to the discovery of new antibiotics. In the USA, the National Institutes of Health has recently announced the establishment of the National Center for Advancing Translational Sciences (NCATS) (Reed, 2011; Weissmann, 2011), which we hope will be devoted to the use of genome mining, combinatorial biosynthesis, metagenomics, glycorandomization and new methods of HTS for inhibitors of novel targets. This would demonstrate that the US government is interested in solving the terrible problems that we in the world are facing as potential victims of antibiotic-resistant pathogenic microorganisms. It may be that the ensuing scientific discoveries might not provide the platform for the discovery of broad-spectrum antibacterials with sufficient blockbuster potential to attract large pharmaceutical companies. However, a greater scientific understanding could be expected to provide a sound basis for the discovery and development of 'targeted' antibiotics with commercial returns attractive enough for small pharmaceutical and biotechnology companies. Certainly, a failure to fund microbiological research means that we may fail to yield vital new drugs in time, and society will face a return to the pre-antibiotic era for infections caused both by drug-resistant pathogens and by new ones that may produce a disease as a result of environmental or social changes. The final issue to be examined is whether the research needed to find new antibacterials will have sufficient continuity within the pharmaceutical and biotechnological industries. If this should prove not to be the case, strategic reasons should perhaps motivate the public sector to devote a more sustained effort, at least in the initial stages of discovery, to obtain new antimicrobials.

Acknowledgements

We thank Maria Falzone for assistance in the preparation of the manuscript. The work of J.S. was supported by Research Project 2B08064 of the Ministry of Education, Youth and Sport of the Czech Republic.

References

Agres, T. (2003) Alliances eye early-stage drugs. *Drug Discovery and Development* 6, 17–18.

Amann, R.I., Ludwig, W. and Schleifer, K.H. (1995) Phylogenetic identification and *in situ* detection of individual microbial cells without cultivation. *Microbiological Reviews* 59, 143–169.

American Academy of Microbiology (2009) *Antibiotic Resistance: an Ecological Perspective on an Old Problem.* American Society for Microbiology, Washington, DC.

Aminov, R.I. (2010) A brief history of the antibiotic era: lessons learned and challenges for the future. *Frontiers in Microbiology* 1, 1–7.

Balaban, N. and Dell'Acqua, G. (2005) Barriers on the road to new antibiotics. *Scientist* 19 42–43.

Baltz, R. (2006) Molecular engineering approaches to peptide, polyketide and other antibiotics. *Nature Biotechnology* 24, 1533–1540.

Baltz, R.H. (2008) Renaissance in antibacterial discovery from actinomycetes. *Current Opinion in Pharmacology* 8, 557–563.

Baltz, R.H. (2010) *Streptomyces* and *Saccharopolyspora* hosts for heterologous expression of secondary metabolite gene clusters. *Journal of Industrial Microbiology and Biotechnology* 37, 759–772.

Barrett, J.F. (2005) Can biotech deliver new antibiotics? *Current Opinion in Microbiology* 8, 498–503.

Bhadury, P., Mohammad, B.T. and Wright, P.C. (2006) The current status of natural products from marine fungi and their potential as anti-infective agents. *Journal of Industrial Microbiology and Biotechnology* 33, 325–337.

Borman, S. (2002) Organic lab sparks drug discovery. *Chemical and Engineering News* 80, 23–24.

Brady, S.F. and Clardy, J. (2000) Long-chain *N*-acyl amino acid antibiotics isolated from heterologously expressed environmental DNA. *Journal of the American Chemical Society* 122, 12903–12904.

Breger, J., Fuchs, B.B., Aperis, G., Moy, T.I., Ausubel, F.M. and Mylonakis, E. (2007) Antifungal chemical compounds identified using a *C. elegans* pathogenicity assay. *PLoS Pathogens* 3, e18.

Breiman, R., Butler, J., Tenover, F., Elliot, J. and Facklam, R. (1994) Emergence of drug-resistant pneumocoocal infections in the United States. *Journal of the American Medical Association* 271, 1831–1835.

Breinbauer, R., Manger, M., Scheck, M. and Waldmann, H. (2002) Natural product guided compound library development. *Current Medicinal Chemistry* 9, 2129–2145.

Brickner, S.J., Barbachyn, M.R., Hutchinson, D.K. and Manninen, P.R. (2008) Linezolid (ZYVOX), the first member of a completely new class of antibacterial agents for treatment of serious Gram-positive infections. *Journal of Medicinal Chemistry* 1, 1981–1990.

Bull, A.T., Ward, A.C. and Goodfellow, M. (2000) Search and discovery strategies for biotechnology. *Microbiology and Molecular Biology Reviews* 64, 573–606.

Bull, A.T., Stach, J.E.M., Ward, A.C. and Goodfellow, M. (2005) Marine actinobacteria: perspectives, challenges, future directions. *Antonie van Leeuwenhoek* 87, 65–79.

Burrill, G.S. (2002) Personalized medicine or blockbusterology? *BioPharm* 15, 46–50.

Bush, K. (2004) Why it is important to continue antibacterial drug discovery. *ASM News* 70, 282–287.
Bush, K., Macielag, M. and Weidner-Wells, M. (2004) Taking inventory: antibacterial agents currently at or beyond phase 1. *Current Opinion in Microbiology* 7, 466–476.
Busti, E., Monciardini, P., Cavaletti, L., Bamonte, R., Lazzarini, A., Sosio, M. and Donadio, S. (2006) Antibiotic-producing ability by representatives of a newly discovered lineage of actinomycetes. *Microbiology* 152, 675–683.
Butler, M.S. and Buss, A.D. (2006) Natural products – the future scaffolds for novel antibiotics? *Biochemical Pharmacology* 71, 919–929.
Cane, D.E., He, X., Kobayashi, S., Omura, S. and Ikeda, H. (2006) Geosmin biosynthesis in *Streptomyces avermitilis*. Molecular cloning, expression and mechanistic study of the germacradienol/geosmin synthase. *Journal of Antibiotics* 59, 471–479.
Carlson, B. (2009) Combating hospital-acquired infections. *Genetic Engineering Biotechnology News* 29, 18.
Centre for Medicines Research International (2000) *The Pharmaceutical R&D Compendium.* Surrey, UK.
Chiang, Y.-M., Szewczyk, E., Nayak, T., Davidson, A.D., Sanchez, J.F., Lo, H.-C., Ho, W.-Y. *et al.* (2008) Molecular genetic mining of the *Aspergillus* secondary metabolome: discovery of the emericellamide biosynthetic pathway. *Chemistry and Biology* 15, 527–532.
Chu, D.T.W., Plattner, J.J. and Katz, L. (1996) New directions in antibacterial research. *Journal of Medicinal Chemistry* 39, 3853–3874.
Class, S. (2004) Health care in focus. *Chemical and Engineering News* 82, 18–29.
Clough, J., Chen, S., Gordon, E.M., Hackbarth, C., Lam, S., Trias, J., White, R.J., Candiani, G., Donadio, S., Romanò, G., Ciabatti, R. and Jacobs, J.W. (2003) Combinatorial modification of natural products: synthesis and *in vitro* analysis of derivatives of thiazole peptide antibiotic GE2270 A: A-ring modifications. *Bioorganic & Medicinal Chemistry Letters* 13, 3409–3414.
Coates, A.R.M. and Hu, Y. (2007) Novel approaches to developing new antibiotics for bacterial infections. *British Journal of Pharmacology* 152, 1147–1154.
Connon, S.A. and Giovannoni, S.J. (2002) High-throughput methods for culturing microorganisms in very-low-nutrient media yield diverse new marine isolates. *Applied and Environmental Microbiology* 68, 3878–3885.
Daemmrich, A.A. and Bowden, M.E. (2005) A rising drug industry. *Chemical and Engineering News* 83, 28–42.
Daniel, R (2004) The soil metagenome – a rich resource for the discovery of novel natural products. *Current Opinion in Biotechnology* 15, 199–204.
DaSilva, E. and Iaccarino, M. (1999) Emerging diseases: a global threat. *Biotechnology Advances* 17, 363–384.
Davies, J. (1994) Inactivation of antibiotics and the dissemination of resistance genes. *Science* 264, 375–382.
Davies, J. (2007) Resistance redux. *EMBO Reports* 8, 616–621.
D'Costa, V.M., McGrann, K.M., Hughes, D.W. and Wright, D.G. (2006) Sampling the antibiotic resistome. *Science* 311, 374–377.
Demain, A.L. (1999) Pharmaceutically active secondary metabolites of microorganisms. *Applied Microbiology and Biotechnology* 52, 455–463.
Demain, A.L. (2002) Prescription for an ailing pharmaceutical industry. *Nature Biotechnology* 20, 331.
Devasahayam, G., Scheld, W.M. and Hoffman, P.S. (2010) Newer antibacterial drugs for a new century. *Expert Opinion on Investigational Drugs* 19, 215–235.
Donadio, S., McAlpine, J.B., Shelden, P.J., Jackson, M. and Katz, L. (1993) An erythromycin analog produced by reprogramming polyketide synthesis. *Proceedings of the National Academy of Sciences USA* 90, 7119–7123.
Donadio, S., Maffioli, S., Monciardini, P., Sosio, M. and Jabes, D. (2010) Antibiotic discovery in the twenty-first century: current trends and future perspectives. *Journal of Antibiotics* 63, 423–430.
Doolittle, W. (1999) Phylogenetic classification and the universal tree. *Science* 284, 2124–2128.
Feher, M. and Schmidt, J.M. (2003) Property distributions: differences between drugs, natural products, and molecules from combinatorial chemistry. *Journal of Chemical Information and Computer Science* 43, 218–227.
Firn, R.D. and Jones, C.G. (2000) The evolution of secondary metabolism – a unifying model. *Molecular Microbiology* 37, 989–994.
Fox, S., Farr-Jones, S. and Yund, M.A. (1999) New directions in drug discovery. *Genetic and Engineering News* 19, 10, 36, 56, 66, 80.
Galm, U. and Shen, B. (2006) Expression of biosynthetic gene clusters in heterologous hosts for natural product production and combinatorial biosynthesis. *Expert Opinion in Drug Discovery* 1, 409–437.
Ganesan, A. (2004) Natural products as a hunting ground for combinatorial chemistry. *Current Opinion in Biotechnology* 15, 584–590.
Genilloud, O., Gonzáles, I., Salazar, O., Martín, J., Tormo, J.S. and Vicente, F. (2010) Current

approaches to exploit actinomycetes as a source of novel natural products. *Journal of Industrial Microbiology and Biotechnology* 38, 375–389.

Gillespie, D.E., Brady, S.F., Bettermann, A.D., Cianciotto, N.P., Liles, M.R., Rondon, M.R., Clardy, J., Goodman, R.M. and Handelsman, J. (2002) Isolation of antibiotics turbomycin A and B from a metagenomic library of soil microbial DNA. *Applied and Environmental Microbiology* 68, 4301–4306.

Goldman, D.A., Weinstein, R.A., Wenzel, R.P., Tablan, O.C., Duma, R.J., Gaynes, R.P., Schlosser, J. and Martone, W.J. (1996) Strategies to prevent and control the emergence and spread of antimicrobial-resistant microorganisms in hospitals. *Journal of the American Medical Association* 275, 234–240.

Gross, H. (2007) Strategies to unravel the function of orphan biosynthesis pathways: recent examples and future prospects. *Applied Microbiology and Biotechnology* 75, 267–277.

Gulder, T.A.M. and Moore, B.S. (2009) Chasing the treasures of the sea – bacterial marine natural products. *Current Opinion in Microbiology* 12, 252–260.

Handelsman, J. (2004) Metagenomics: application of genomics to uncultured microorganisms. *Microbiology and Molecular Biology Reviews* 68, 669–685.

Handelsman, J., Rondon, M.R., Brady, S.F., Clardy, J. and Goodman, R.M. (1998) Molecular biological access to the chemistry of unknown soil microbes: a new frontier for natural products. *Chemistry and Biology* 5, R245–R249.

Handen, J.S. (2002) The industrialization of drug discovery. *Drug Discovery Today* 7, 83–85.

Harvey, A.L. (2007) Natural products as a screening resource. *Current Opinion in Chemical Biology* 11, 480–484.

Hefti, E. and Bolten, B.M. (2003) Advances in high-throughput screening advances – do they lead to new drugs? *Genetic Engineering News* 23, 7–10.

Henkel, T., Brunne, R.M., Mueller, H. and Reichel, F. (1999) Statistical investigation into the structural complementarity of natural products and synthetic compounds. *Angewandte Chemie International Edition* 38, 643–647.

Hershberger, C.L. (1996) Metabolic engineering of polyketide biosynthesis. *Current Opinion in Biotechnology* 7, 560–562.

Hilleman, B. (2006) Regulatory trends. *Chemical and Engineering News* 84, 80–99.

Hoffman, L.R., D'Argenio, D.A., MacCoss, M.J., Zhang, Z., Jones, R.A. and Miller, S.I. (2005) Aminoglycoside antibiotics induce biofilm formation. *Nature* 436, 1171–1175.

Hong, S.-H., Bunge, J., Jeon, S.O. and Epstein, S.S. (2006) Predicting microbial species richness. *Proceedings of the National Academy of Sciences USA* 103, 117–122.

Hopwood, D.A. (2007) Therapeutic treasures from the deep. *Nature Chemical Biology* 3, 457–458.

Hopwood, D.A., Malpartida, F., Kieser, H.M., Ikeda, H., Duncan, J., Fujii, I., Rudd, B.A.M., Floss, H.G. and Omura, S. (1985) Production of 'hybrid' antibiotics by genetic engineering. *Nature* 314, 642–644.

Horrobin, D.F. (2001) Realism in drug discovery – could Cassandra be right? *Nature Biotechnology* 19, 1099–1100.

Hutchinson, R. and Fujii, J. (1995) Polyketide synthase gene manipulation: a structure–function approach in engineering novel antibiotics. *Annual Reviews in Microbiology* 49, 201–238.

Jacobs, M. (2002) Pharmaceutical balancing act. *Chemical and Engineering News* 80, 5.

Jensen, P.R., Mincer, T.J., Williams, P.G. and Fenical, W. (2005) Marine actinomycete diversity and natural product discovery. *Antonie van Leeuwenhoek* 87, 43–48.

Kaeberlein, T., Lewis, K. and Epstein, S.S. (2002) Isolating 'uncultivable' microorganisms in pure culture in a simulated natural environment. *Science* 296, 1127–1129.

Kellenberger, E. (2001) Exploring the unknown: the silent revolution of microbiology. *EMBO Reports* 2, 5–7.

Kettler, H.E. (1999) Updating the cost of a new chemical entity. Office of Health Economics, London.

Kingston, D.G.I. and Newman, D.J. (2002) Mother nature's combinatorial libraries; their influence on the synthesis of drugs. *Current Opinion in Drug Discovery and Development* 5, 304–316.

Kolb, H.C. and Sharpless, B.K. (2003) The growing impact of click chemistry on drug discovery. *Drug Discovery Today* 8, 1128–1137.

Kollef, M.H. (2003) The importance of appropriate initial antibiotic therapy for hospital-acquired infections. *American Journal of Medicine* 115, 582–584.

Koppal, T. (2004) Global teams battle. *Drug Discovery and Development* 4, 28–32.

Kostel, K. (2004) Industry snapshot. *The Scientist* 18, 45.

Kraus, C.N. (2008) Low hanging fruit in infectious disease drug development. *Current Opinion in Microbiology* 11, 434–438.

Kren, V. and Rezanka, T. (2008) Sweet antibiotics – the role of glycosidic residues in antibiotic and antitumor activity and their randomization. *FEMS Microbiology Reviews* 32, 858–889.

Lautru, S., Deeth, R.J., Bailey, L.M. and Challi, G.L. (2005) Discovery of a new peptide natural product from *Streptomyces coelicolor* genome mining. *Nature Chemical Biology* 1, 265–269.

Lefevre, F., Robe, P., Jarrin, C., Ginolhac, A., Zago, C., Auriol D., Vogel, T.M., Simonet, P. and Nalin, R. (2008) Drugs from hidden bugs: their discovery via untapped resources. *Research in Microbiology* 159, 153–161.

Lin, X., Hopson, R. and Cane, D.E. (2006) Genome mining in *Streptomyces coelicolor*: molecular cloning and characterization of a new sesquiterpene synthase from *S. coelicolor*. *Journal of the American Chemical Society* 128, 6022–6023.

Lorenz, P. and Eck, J. (2005) Metagenomics and industrial applications. *Nature Reviews Microbiology* 3, 510–516.

Lynch, A.S. and Robertson, G.T. (2008) Bacterial and fungal biofilm infections. *Annual Reviews of Medicine* 59, 415–428.

Malik, N.N. (2008) Drug discovery: past, present and future. *Drug Discovery Today* 13, 909–912.

Martinez, A., Hopke, J., MacNeil, I.A. and Osburne, M.S. (2005) Accessing the genomes of uncultivated microbes for novel natural products. In: Zhang, L. and Demain, A.L. (eds) *Natural Products, Drug Discovery and Therapeutic Medicine*. Humana Press, Totowa, New Jersey, pp. 295–312.

Mendez, C. and Salas, J.A. (2003) On the generation of novel anticancer drugs by recombinant DNA technology: the use of combinatorial biosynthesis to produce novel drugs. *Combinatorial Chemistry and High Throughput Screening* 6, 513–526.

Mills, S.D. (2006) When will the genomics investment pay off for antibacterial discovery? *Biochemical Pharmacology* 71, 1096–1102.

Morens, D.M., Folkers, G.K. and Fauci, A.S. (2004) The challenge of emerging and re-emerging infectious diseases. *Nature* 430, 242–249.

Morrow, K.J. (2010) Using selection to advance drug discovery. *American Biotechnology Laboratory Magazine* 28, 24–25.

Moy, T.I., Ball, A.R., Anklesaria, G., Lewis, K. and Ausubel, F.M. (2006) Identification of novel antimicrobials using a live-animal infection model. *Proceedings of the National Academy of Sciences USA* 103, 10414–10419.

Mullin, R. (2006a) Pharma in flux. *Chemical and Engineering News* 84, 30–35.

Mullin, R. (2006b) Tufts report anticipates upturn. Cites drugmakers' actions to accelerate drug development. *Chemical and Engineering News* 84, 9.

Newman, D.J. (2008) Natural products as leads to potential drugs: an old process or the new hope for drug discovery? *Journal of Medicinal Chemistry* 51, 2589–2599.

Newman, D.J. and Cragg, G.M. (2007) Natural products as sources of new drugs over the last 25 years. *Journal of Natural Products* 70, 461–477.

Nikaido, H. (2009) Multidrug resistance in bacteria. *Annual Reviews of Biochemistry* 78, 119–146.

Oh, T.-J., Mo, S.J., Yoon, Y.J. and Sohng, J.K. (2007) Discovery and molecular engineering of sugar-containing natural product biosynthetic pathways in actinomycetes. *Journal of Microbiology and Biotechnology* 17, 1909–1921.

Overbye, K.M. and Barrett, J.F. (2005) Antibiotics: where did we go wrong? *Drug Discovery Today* 10, 45–52.

Park, J.H., Cha, C.J. and Roe, J.H. (2006) Identification of genes for mycothiol biosynthesis in *Streptomyces coelicolor* A3. *Journal of Microbiology* 44, 121–125.

Pelzer, S., Vente, A. and Bechthold, A. (2005) Novel natural compounds obtained by genome-based screening and genetic engineering. *Current Opinion in Drug Discovery and Development* 8, 228–238.

Reed, J.C. (2011) NCATS could mitigate pharma valley of death. National Center for Advancing Translational Sciences essential to capitalize on basic research. *Genetic Engineering and Biotechnology News* 31, 6–8.

Rodriguez, E. and McDaniel, R. (2001) Combinatorial synthesis of antimicrobials and other natural products. *Current Opinion in Microbiology* 4, 526–534.

Rondon, M.R., August, P.R., Bettermann, A.D., Brady, S.F., Grossman, T.H., Liles, M.R., Loiacono, K.A., Lynch, B.A., MacNeil, I.A., Minor, C., Tiong, C.L., Gilman, M., Osburne, M.S., Clardy, J., Handelsman, J. and Goodman, R.M. (2000) Cloning the soil metagenome: a strategy for assessing the genetic and functional diversity of uncultured microorganisms. *Applied and Environmental Microbiology* 66, 2541–2547.

Rosello-Mora, R. and Amann, R. (2001) The species concept for prokaryotes. *FEMS Microbiology Reviews* 25, 39–67.

Russell, D.G., Barry, C.E. III and Flynn, J.A.L. (2010) Tuberculosis: what we don't know can, and does hurt us. *Science* 328, 852–855.

Ryan, J.F. (2003) Tough times. *Today's Chemist at Work* 12, 7.

Salas, J.A. and Mendez, C. (2007) Engineering the glycosylation of natural products in actinomycetes. *Trends in Microbiology* 15, 219–232.

Sanchez, J.F., Chiang, Y.-M. and Wang, C.C.C. (2008) Bacterial hosts for natural product formation. *Molecular Pharmaceutics* 5, 226–233.

Schloss, P.D. and Handelsman, J. (2004) Status of the microbial census. *Molecular Biology Reviews* 68, 686–691.

Schwab, E.K., Bok, J.W., Tribus, M., Galehr, J., Graessle, S. and Keller, N.P. (2007) Histone

deacetylase activity regulates chemical diversity in *Aspergillus. Eukaryotic Cell* 6, 1656–1664.
Scott, R.W. (2009) Defensin mimetics: nature knows best. *American Biotechnology Laboratory* 27, 16–19.
Shlaes, D.M., Projan, S.J. and Edwards, J.E. Jr (2004) Antibiotic discovery: state of the state. *ASM News* 70, 275–281.
Singh, S.B. and Barrett, J.F. (2006) Empirical antibacterial drug discovery – foundation in natural products. *Biochemical Pharmacology* 71, 1006–1015.
Song, L., Barona-Gomez, F., Corre, C., Xiang, C.L., Udwary, D.W., Austin, M.B., Noel, J.P., Moore, B.S. and Challis, G.L. (2006) Type III polyketide synthase β-ketoacyl-ACP starter unit and ethylmalonyl-CoA extender unit selectivity discovered by *Streptomyces coelicolor* genome mining. *Journal of the American Chemical Society* 128, 14754–14755.
Spizek, J., Novotna, J., Rezanka, T. and Demain, A.L. (2010) Do we need new antibiotics? The search for new targets and new compounds. *Journal of Industrial Microbiology and Biotechnology* 37, 1241–1248.
Stachelhaus, T., Schneider, A. and Marahiel, M.A. (1995) Rational design of peptide antibiotics by targeted replacement of bacterial and fungal domains. *Science* 269, 69–72.
Stephens, J.S. and Shapiro, L. (1997) Bacterial protein secretion – a target for new antibiotics? *Chemistry and Biology* 4, 637–641.
Stermitz, F.R. (2002) Letter to the Editor. *Chemical and Engineering News* 80, 51.
Stevenson, B.S., Eichorst, S.A., Wertz, J.T., Schmidt, T.M. and Breznak, J.T. (2004) New strategies for cultivation of previously uncultured microbes. *Applied and Environmental Microbiology* 70, 4748–4755.
Stokes, H.W., Holmes, A.J., Nield, B.S., Holley, M.P., Nevalainen, K.M.H., Mabbutt, B.C. and Gillings, M.R. (2001) Gene cassette PCR: sequence-independent recovery of entire genes from environmental DNA. *Applied and Environmental Microbiology* 67, 5240–5246.
Strohl, W.R. (1997) Industrial antibiotics: today and the future. In: Strohl, W.R. (ed.) *Biotechnology of Antibiotics.* Marcel Dekker, New York, pp. 1–47.
Tan, L.T. (2007) Bioactive natural products from marine cyanobacteria for drug discovery. *Phytochemistry* 68, 954–979.
Tenover, F.C. and Hughes, J.M. (1996) The challenges of emerging infectious diseases. *Journal of the American Medical Association* 275, 300–304.
Thayer, A.M. (2003) Biomarkers emerge. *Chemical and Engineering News* 81, 33–37.
Thayer, A.M. (2004) Blockbuster model breaking down. *Modern Drug Discovery* 7, 23–24.
Tralau-Stewart, C.L., Wyatt, C.A., Kleyn, D.E. and Ayad, A. (2009) Drug discovery: new models for industry–academic partnerships. *Drug Discovery Today* 14, 95–101.
Trefzer, A., Pelzer, S., Schimana, J., Stockert, S., Bihlmaier, C., Fiedler, H.-P., Welzel, K., Vente, A. and Bechthold, A. (2002) Biosynthetic gene cluster of simocyclinone, a natural multihybrid antibiotic. *Antimicrobial Agents and Chemotherapy* 46, 1174–1182.
Udwary, D.W., Zeigler, L., Asokar, R.N., Singan, V., Lapidas, A., Fenical, W., Jensen, P.R. and Moore, B.S. (2007) Genome sequencing reveals complex secondary metabolome in the marine actinomycete *Salinospora tropica. Proceedings of the National Academy of Sciences USA* 104, 10376–10381.
Vicente, M., Hodgson, J., Massidda, O., Tonjum, T., Henriques-Normark, B. and Ron, E.Z. (2006) The fallacies of hope: will we discover new antibiotics to combat pathogenic bacteria in time? *FEMS Microbiology Reviews* 30, 841–852.
Waldmann, H. (2003) At the crossroads of chemistry and biology. *Bioorganic and Medicinal Chemistry* 11, 3045–3051.
Waldmann, H. and Breinbauer, R. (2002) Nature provides the answer. *Screening* 6, 46–48.
Walsh, C.T. and Fischbach, M.A. (2009) Squashing superbugs – the race for new antibiotics. *Scientific American* 301, 44–51.
Warner, S. (2003) Pipeline anxiety: scientists pumped into new roles. *The Scientist* 17, 46.
Warner, S. (2004) High-priced biotech drugs: are they worth it? *The Scientist* 18, 20–24.
Weissmann, G. (2011) Is drug development too slow? NIH to the rescue! *FASEB Journal* 25, 1110–1122.
Wery, N., Gerike, U., Sharman, A., Chaudhuri, J.B., Hough, D.W. and Danson, M.J. (2003) Use of a packed-cell bioreactor for isolation of diverse protease-producing bacteria from Antarctic soil. *Applied and Environmental Microbiology* 69, 1457–1464.
Williams, R.B., Henrikson, J.C., Hoover, A.R., Lee, A.E. and Cichewicz, H. (2008) Epigenetic remodeling of fungal secondary metabolome. *Organic and Biomolecular Chemistry* 6, 1895–1897.
Willis, R.C. (2004) The discovery doldrums: NCEs are coming slowly; Juergen Drews explains why. *Modern Drug Discovery* 4, 23–24.
Wright, G.D. (2010) Antibiotic resistance in the environment: a link to the clinic? *Current Opinion in Microbiology* 13, 589–594.
Zengler, K., Toledo, G., Rappe, M., Elkins, J., Mathur, E.J., Short, J.M. and Keller, M. (2002) Cultivating the uncultured. *Proceedings of the National Academy of Sciences USA* 99, 15681–15686.

Zengler, K., Paradkar, A. and Keller, M. (2005) New methods to access microbial diversity for small molecule discovery. In: Zhang, L. and Demain, A.L. (eds) *Natural Products: Drug Discovery and Therapeutic Medicine*. Humana Press, Totowa, New Jersey, pp. 275–293.

Zerikly, M. and Challis, G.L. (2009) Strategies for the discovery of new natural products by genome mining. *ChemBioChem* 10, 625–633.

Zhang, H., Wang, Y. and Pfeifer, B.A. (2008) Bacterial hosts for natural product formation. *Molecular Pharmaceutics* 5, 212–225.

Zhao, L., Ahlert, J., Xue, Y., Thorson, J.S., Sherman, D.H. and Liu, H.-W. (1999) Engineering a methymycin/pikromycin–calicheamicin hybrid: construction of two new macrolides carrying a designed sugar moiety. *Organic Letters* 15, 133–136.

3 Structure, Genetic Regulation, Physiology and Function of the AcrAB–TolC Efflux Pump of *Escherichia coli* and *Salmonella*

Leonard Amaral,[1] Ana Martins,[2] Gabriella Spengler,[3] Marta Martins,[1] Liliana Rodrigues,[1] Matthew McCusker,[4] Eleni Ntokou,[5] Pedro Cerca,[1] Lisa Machado,[1] Miguel Viveiros,[1] Isabel Couto,[1] Séamus Fanning,[4] Jette Kristiansen[6] and Joseph Molnar[7]

[1]*Grupo de Micobactérias, Unidade de Microbiologia Médica, Instituto de Higiene e Medicina Tropical, Universidade Nova de Lisboa, Lisbon, Portugal;* [2]*Institute of Pharmacognosy, Faculty of Pharmacy, University of Szeged, Szeged, Hungary;* [3]*Department of Medical Microbiology and Immunobiology, Faculty of Medicine, University of Szeged, Szeged, Hungary;* [4]*University College Dublin, School of Agriculture, Food Sciences and Veterinary Medicine, UCD Centre Food Safety, Dublin, Ireland;* [5]*Short-Term Student Mission of the Cost Action BM0701 of the European Commission/European Science Foundation, Brussels, Belgium;* [6]*Department of Chemistry, University of Copenhagen, Universitetsparken 5, Copenhagen, Denmark;* [7]*Cost Action BM0701 (ATENS) of the European Commission/European Science Foundation, Brussels, Belgium*

3.1 Introduction

Gram-negative bacteria that live in the wild are equipped with two mechanisms that allow them to survive in an environment that contains a noxious agent, provided that the concentration of this agent is below that which kills the organism. When a given Gram-negative bacterium infects a human and that human is treated ineffectively with an antibiotic or antimicrobial agent, the bacterium can rapidly invoke the two mechanisms that render it resistant to the therapeutic agent as well as to other non-related therapeutic agents. The two mechanisms that render the bacterium multidrug resistant (MDR) are the downregulation of porins (Viveiros *et al.*, 2007; Davin-Regli *et al.*, 2008) and upregulation of efflux pumps (Viveiros *et al.*, 2007; Gootz, 2010). Porins are tribarrel structures that traverse the cell envelope and permit the penetration of hydrophilic compounds (nutrients) as well as hydrophilic antibiotics and antimicrobial agents from the environment to the cytoplasm (Bolla *et al.*, 2004; Kumar *et al.*, 2010). Efflux pumps are structures that traverse the cell envelope and recognize structurally unrelated noxious compounds, including antibiotics or antimicrobial agents, that have penetrated into the periplasm or cytoplasm, and extrude these agents to the outside of the cell before they reach their intended targets (Blair and Piddock, 2009; Husain and Nikaido, 2010). In this chapter, porins will not be further discussed. Instead, we will focus on AcrAB–TolC, the main efflux pump of the pathogenic Gram-negative bacteria *Escherichia coli*, *Salmonella* sp. and *Enterobacter aerogenes* (Bolla *et al.*, 2004), describing its structure and function and the effects that phenothiazines have on the genes that regulate and code for the AcrAB–TolC efflux pump and on the activity of the pump itself.

3.2 The AcrAB–TolC Efflux Pump

The AcrAB efflux pump is a member of the resistance nodulation division (RND) family of transporters. Although Gram-negative bacteria have more than one and as many as 20 or more efflux pumps that can extrude noxious agents (Viveiros *et al.*, 2005), AcrAB–TolC is considered to be the main efflux pump of *E. coli*, *Salmonella* sp. and *E. aerogenes* (Pagès and Amaral, 2009; Amaral *et al.*, 2011b). This redundancy of efflux pumps affords survival of the organism when its main efflux pump, AcrAB, is deleted (Viveiros *et al.*, 2005). As an example, deletion of the AcrAB efflux pump is accompanied by overexpression of other efflux pumps, such as the AcrEF pump (Viveiros *et al.*, 2005). Nevertheless, the efficiency of the latter is far less than that of the main efflux pump, AcrAB (Viveiros *et al.*, 2005).

The structure of the AcrAB–TolC efflux pump as it exists in the bacterium is not known precisely. However, the structures of the components that make up the pump have been determined and are schematically presented in Fig. 3.1. Briefly, the transporter AcrB is a trimeric structure that is attached at the plasma membrane by the flanking fusion protein AcrA and is contiguous with TolC, which ends at the surface of the cell. Noxious agents that penetrate the periplasm or cytoplasm find their way into the cavity of the transporter by means that are not yet understood. These agents are substrates of the pump and bind to a specific internal site of the transporter (Eicher *et al.*, 2009; Pos, 2009; Husain and Nikaido, 2010; Schulz *et al.*, 2010) and are extruded to the TolC conduit by mechanisms that are not yet fully understood. However, studies by Su and Yu (2007) have shown that, whereas binding of the AcrAB substrate to purified AcrB takes place rapidly at low pH, the dissociation of the substrate is pH dependent: at low pH, the dissociation constant, K_d, is high, and with increasing pH, K_d decreases to a point such that at neutral pH dissociation is very slow (Fig. 3.2). The very slow dissociation of the substrate from the transporter when the pH is at or near neutral would result in a marked reduction in the effectiveness of the pump. This does not take place, and the reason that extrusion continues in a pH that denies dissociation of the substrate has been postulated to be due to the mobilization of hydronium ions from the surface of the cell to the periplasm/cytoplasm through aquaporins (Amaral *et al.*, 2011a). Movement of hydronium ions from the surface of the cell is due to events that depend on and use the proton motive force (PMF) as an energy source for activity, such as a PMF-dependent efflux pump of the RND family of transporters (Thanassi *et al.*, 1997; Zgurskaya and Nikaido, 2000; Levy, 2002; Martins *et al.*, 2009b). The movement of hydronium ions from the periplasm/cytoplasm through the internal cavity of the transporter reduces the pH to a point that permits the dissociation of the substrate (Amaral *et al.*, 2011a). Extrusion of the substrate is probably due to the movement of water through the transporter and the conduit provided by TolC to the outside of the cell. Movement of water is believed to be assisted by the fusion proteins via peristaltic action (Seeger *et al.*, 2008; Pos, 2009; Schulz *et al.*, 2010). Furthermore, the movement of hydronium ions through the AcrB–TolC conduit provides the means by which toxic agents are extruded from the cell (Amaral *et al.*, 2011a). Figure 3.3 summarizes the sequence of events believed to take place for functioning of the AcrAB–TolC pump.

The role and source of energy for the activity of the efflux pump has not received sufficient attention. It is generally thought that the PMF is the source of energy required for efflux activity (Thanassi *et al.*, 1997; Zgurskaya and Nikaido, 2000; Levy, 2002; Martins *et al.*, 2009b). The PMF results from metabolic

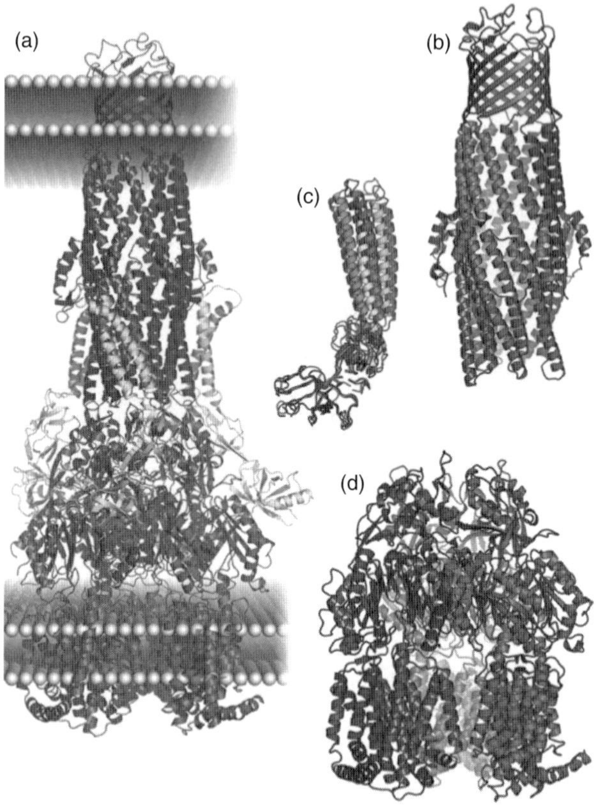

Fig. 3.1. Structure of TolC, fusion protein AcrA and transporter AcrB, and a model of the AcrAB–TolC pump and its relationship to the components of the cell envelope. (a) Outer membrane of the Gram-negative bacterium. (b) TolC component of the AcrAB–TolC efflux pump. (c) Fusion protein of the AcrAB–TolC efflux pump. (d) Theoretical assembly of the AcrAB–TolC efflux pump.

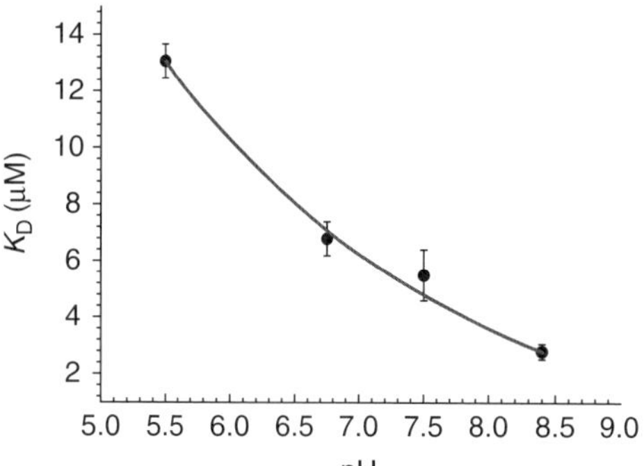

Fig. 3.2. Effect of pH on dissociation of substrate from purified AcrB. Note that dissociation of substrate takes place at low pH and that at high pH dissociation is very low. (From Su and Yu, 2007.)

activities of the bacterium that result in the production of protons. Protons do not exist as free entities; rather, when generated, they are rapidly bound to water, forming a temporary hydronium ion (Boyer, 1988; von Ballmoos, 2007). Hydronium ions are postulated to translocate to the surface of the cell (Mulkidjanian *et al.*, 2005, 2006; Mulkidjanian, 2009), where they are bound to components of the lipopolysaccharide layer or to the basic amino acids of adsorbed proteins (Mulkidjanian *et al.*, 2005; Mulkidjanian, 2009). The binding of these hydronium ions results in a pH at the surface of the cell that is two to three units lower than that of the bulk milieu (Mulkidjanian *et al.*, 2006; Mulkidjanian, 2009). The concentration of hydronium ions at the surface is considerably

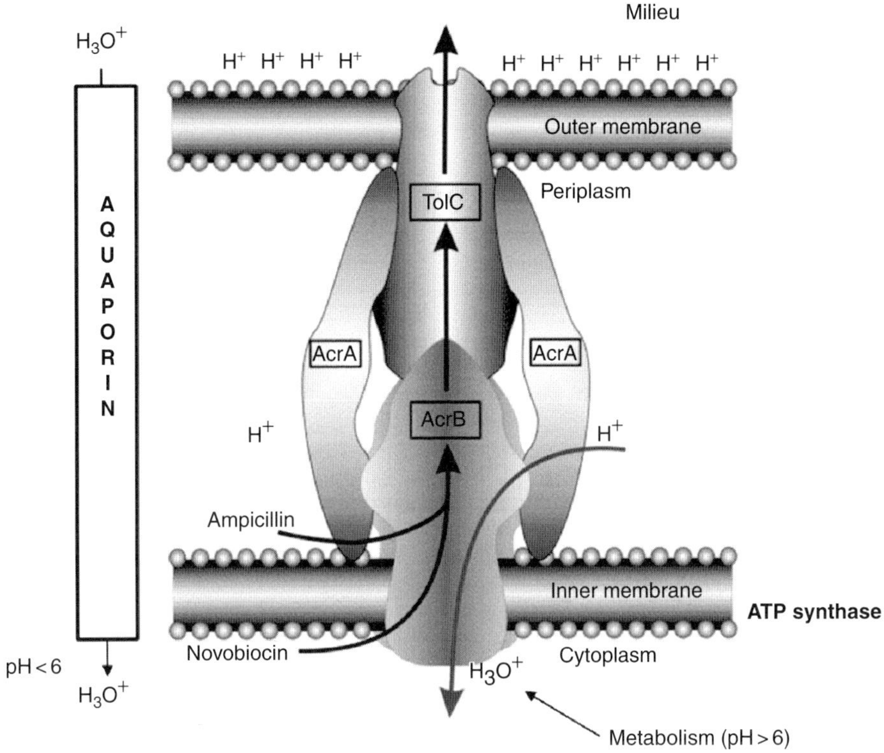

Fig. 3.3. Model showing the hypothetical events associated with efflux. At near neutral pH, hydronium ions from hydrolysis of ATP by ATP synthase pass through the AcrB transporter, reducing the pH to a point that causes release of the substrate. When the hydronium ions reach the surface of the cell, they are distributed over the surface and bind to lipopolysaccharides and basic amino acids. When there is a need for hydronium ions for activity of the efflux pump and the pH is lower than neutral, and the hydrolysis of ATP is not favoured, hydronium ions from the surface of the cell via the proton motive force mobilize through the aquaporins and reach the transporter where they are pushed through the transporter by the peristaltic action caused by the fusion proteins. Substrates bound to the transporter dissociate when the pH is reduced by the flow of hydronium ions and are carried out by the flow of water. (Modified from Pos, 2009.)

greater than that at the periplasm of the cell. The difference in hydronium ion concentration between the surface and the periplasm results in an electrochemical gradient that creates the PMF. The generation of hydronium ions is primarily the result of ATP synthase activity (Dimroth *et al.*, 2000; Turina *et al.*, 2006; Nakamoto *et al.*, 2008; Mulkidjanian, 2009). At a pH < 6 or so, ATP synthase activity favours synthesis of ATP, whereas at a higher pH, it favours hydrolysis of ATP (Feniouk and Yoshida, 2008; Bald and Koul, 2010; Maeda, 2010). Consequently, at pH > 6 or so, the generation of hydronium ions takes place, and their translocation to the surface of the cell is postulated to take place via the channel provided by AcrB–TolC (Martins *et al.*, 2009b; Amaral *et al.*, 2011a). The translocated hydronium ions are bound to the surface of the cell and therefore contribute to the PMF (Mulkidjanian *et al.*, 2005, 2006; Mulkidjanian, 2009). When Gram-negative bacteria are challenged with a noxious agent such as ethidium bromide in an environment of pH > 7, efflux is totally dependent on a metabolic source of energy (Martins *et al.*, 2009b; Amaral *et al.*, 2011a,b). In contrast, at a pH < 6, because efflux is independent of metabolic energy (Martins *et al.*, 2009b; Amaral *et al.*, 2011a,b), the hydronium ions of the milieu are the source for repletion of hydronium ions that have been mobilized to the periplasm by the PMF (Martins *et al.*, 2009b; Amaral *et al.*, 2011a).

3.3 The Role of Efflux Pumps in MDR Phenotypes of Clinical Gram-negative Isolates

Most Gram-negative clinical isolates that present with an MDR phenotype when studied overexpress their main efflux pump (Soto *et al.*, 2003; Chang *et al.*, 2007; Pagès and Amaral, 2009). However, the degree of resistance to given antibiotics is not completely due to the activity of an efflux pump. Consequently, efflux pump inhibitors (EPIs) rarely reduce resistance to a given antibiotic to a level compatible to that of a wild-type reference strain denoted as susceptible. The reason for this is due to the presence of mutations that have accumulated during prolonged therapy of the patient with a given antibiotic (Martins *et al.*, 2009a). As an example, *E. coli* can be induced to high-level resistance to tetracycline by serial exposure to increasing concentration of the antibiotic (Viveiros *et al.*, 2005, 2007). In addition, the organism assumes an MDR phenotype (Viveiros *et al.*, 2005). Induced resistance can be totally reversed by an EPI or by transfer to a drug-free medium (Viveiros *et al.*, 2005, 2007). Induced resistance results from increased activity of genes that regulate and code for the AcrB transporter; the latter gene continues to increase its activity with each serial exposure to increasing concentrations of the antibiotic. However, when the organism is then maintained at the same high concentration over many serial passages, the resistance to tetracycline escalates, whereas the activity of the gene encoding the AcrB component of the pump decreases (Martins *et al.*, 2009a). At this point, reversal of resistance to tetracycline is not possible, although a reduction in resistance by an EPI is still noted. Examination by phenotypic array of the progeny strains during culture in medium containing a constant high concentration of tetracycline reveals the accumulation of mutations with time. As the extent of mutations increases, there is a reduction in the activity of the *acrB* gene (Martins *et al.*, 2009a). These results are relevant to the process by which MDR develops in the patient who is treated with a constant dose of antibiotic and results in increasing resistance of the infecting Gram-negative bacterium, sometimes 1000 times greater than that of the reference strain. Moreover, the contributions made by efflux versus mutations to the MDR phenotype of a Gram-negative MDR clinical isolate will reflect the duration of therapy. During early therapy, efflux pumps would be overexpressed. With prolongation of therapy, overexpressed efflux pumps and mutations are expected, and with further prolongation of therapy, efflux pumps are no longer overexpressed and the MDR phenotype may be exclusively the result of mutations (Martins *et al.*, 2009a). The process of prolonged exposure to a constant concentration of an antibiotic may activate a master mutator gene that results in mutations of essential targets (Chopra *et al.*, 2003; Martins *et al.*, 2009a).

3.4 Phenothiazines

Phenothiazines are heterocyclic compounds whose origins lie in the first phenothiazine, methylene blue (Fig. 3.4). The biological properties of methylene blue were studied by the German physician-chemist Paul Ehrlich during the late 1880s and shown to exhibit a variety of antimicrobial properties (Guttmann and Ehrlich, 1891). Among these properties was the ability to inhibit microbial growth, as well as microbial mobility. Because of the ability of methylene blue to inhibit microbial mobility, the dye was administered to humans to see if it could also retard movement, which it promptly did soon after oral administration (Bodoni, 1899; Kristiansen and Amaral, 1997). Subjects who received the dye became lethargic and calm, albeit with a blue tinge that took a long time to disappear. Because of the success of salvarsan, an antimicrobial agent created by Ehrlich, interest in methylene blue was limited to its neuroleptic properties. It took more than 50 years and a highly convoluted path for the

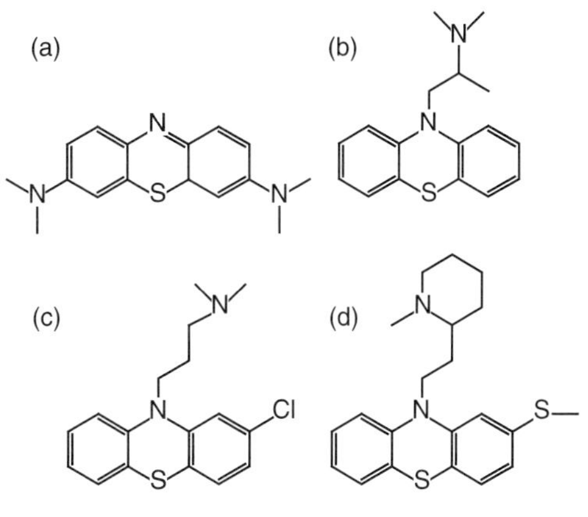

Fig. 3.4. Structure of phenothiazines known to affect the activity of bacterial efflux pumps: (a) methylene blue; (b) promethazine; (c) chlorpromazine; (d) thioridazine.

synthesis of the first colourless phenothiazine, promethazine, which, by serendipity, was eventually used as a lead compound for the synthesis of the first commercial neuroleptic chlorpromazine (CPZ) (Charpentier *et al.*, 1952). Global use of CPZ soon led to observations that it had a wide gamut of antimicrobial (Kristiansen and Amaral, 1997; Amaral *et al.*, 2001) and antimycobacterial (Amaral *et al.*, 1996) properties. CPZ was shown to inhibit the replication of bacteria (Amaral *et al.*, 1992) and mycobacteria (Amaral *et al.*, 1996), cause the elimination of plasmids from Gram-negative bacteria (Amaral *et al.*, 2010b) and reduce resistance to antibiotics (Amaral *et al.*, 1992). However, these properties were produced with concentrations of CPZ that were hundreds of times greater than those that could be achieved safely in humans (maximum of 0.5 mg/l of plasma). Moreover, because CPZ produced serious and frequent side effects, interest in the development of derivatives with desirable antimicrobial properties did not materialize. However, due to the emergence of MDR tuberculosis (MDR-TB), interest in CPZ was revived, and by 1992, Crowle and his group demonstrated that a concentration of CPZ in the medium that was within clinical range could promote the killing of intracellular *Mycobacterium tuberculosis* (Crowle *et al.*, 1992). Soon after, Amaral and his group demonstrated that thioridazine (TZ) was equal to CPZ with respect to its *in vitro* antibacterial properties (Amaral *et al.*, 1996), and because TZ produced fewer serious side effects than its parental CPZ, studies by this group soon showed that, as was the case for CPZ, TZ also promoted the killing of intracellular antibiotic-susceptible and antibiotic-resistant strains of *M. tuberculosis* (Ordway *et al.*, 2003; Amaral *et al.*, 2004; Martins *et al.*, 2007) at concentrations that were lower than those used for chronic treatment of the psychotic patient. The use of TZ for therapy of non-antibiotic-responsive MDR and extensively drug-resistant TB soon followed on the basis of compassionate therapy (Amaral *et al.*, 2010a, 2011c).

Phenothiazines such as CPZ, promethazine and TZ inhibit the binding of calcium to calcium-binding proteins and enzymes (Hidaka and Shikano, 1983; Klee *et al.*, 1986; Osawa *et al.*, 1998; Mayur *et al.*, 2006). Inhibition of calcium binding results in the elimination of calcium signalling, a mechanism that is central to most biological processes (Ren *et al.*, 2009). Among the enzymes that are known to be inhibited by a phenothiazine such as CPZ are enzymes involved in the generation of hydronium ions that are shunted to the surface of the cell, as noted above. Consequently, it was not surprising that CPZ as well as TZ could reverse resistance that was mediated by the induced PMF-dependent efflux pump, AcrAB, of *E. coli* (Viveiros *et al.*, 2005), as well as that of other PMF-dependent efflux pumps of Gram-negative (Bailey *et al.*, 2008) and Gram-positive (Kristiansen *et al.*, 2007, Klitgaard *et al.*, 2008; Costa *et al.*, 2010; Rahbar *et al.*, 2010) bacteria. These demonstrations were soon followed by the development of new methods for the real-time assessment of efflux pump activity along physiological lines (Viveiros *et al.*, 2008, 2010). As shown in Fig. 3.5, the presence of a phenothiazine such as CPZ or TZ can promote accumulation of the universal efflux pump substrate ethidium bromide by *E. coli*, which results from inhibition of the efflux pump system. The effects of the phenothiazine can be removed by the addition of calcium (Fig. 3.6). The phenothiazine effects can be qualitatively reproduced by the divalent cation chelator

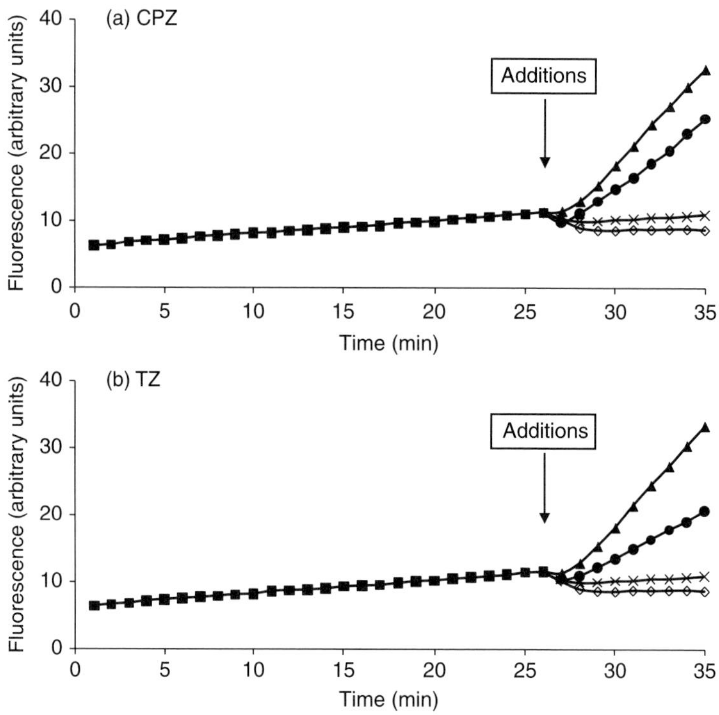

Fig. 3.5. Effect of phenothiazines on efflux of the AcrAB–TolC substrate ethidium bromide. Accumulation of ethidium bromide by *E. coli* AG100 cells was measured at pH 7 without glucose for 25 min (■). Additions for efflux evaluation in PBS (pH 7) were as follows: 15 mg/l phenothiazine (▲); 15 mg/l phenothiazine and 0.4% glucose (●); PBS control (x); PBS and 0.4% glucose control (◇). Note that accumulation of ethidium bromide during the first 25–27 min was due to the absence of metabolic energy: the addition of glucose stopped accumulation, while the addition of the phenothiazines with glucose rapidly resulted in accumulation of ethidium bromide.

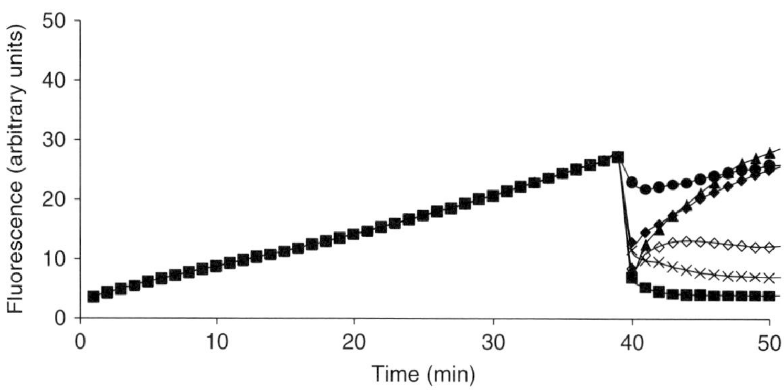

Fig. 3.6. Modulation of the effect of the phenothiazine chlorpromazine (CPZ) on efflux by calcium. Accumulation of ethidium bromide by *E. coli* AG100 cells took place at pH 7 without glucose for 40 min (■). Additions for efflux evaluation were made in PBS (pH 7) as follows: control without glucose (●); control with 0.4% glucose (■); 25 mg/l CPZ and 0.4% glucose (▲); 25 mg/l CPZ, 5 mM Ca^{2+} and 0.4% glucose (x); 30 mg/l CPZ and 0.4% glucose (◆); 30 mg/l CPZ, 5 mM Ca^{2+} and 0.4% glucose (◇). The addition of calcium eliminated the inhibitory effects of the phenothiazine on efflux of ethidium bromide. (From Martins, A. *et al.*, 2011.)

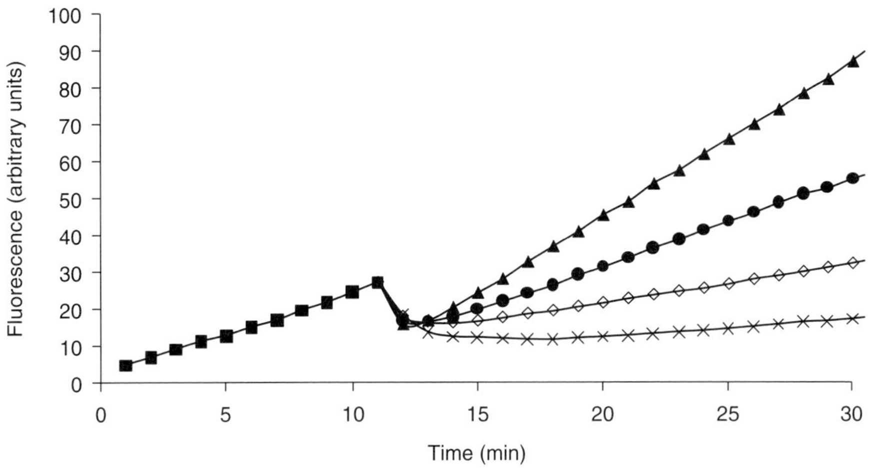

Fig. 3.7. Qualitative reproduction of the effects of phenothiazine on the efflux of ethidium bromide using the divalent cation chelator EDTA alone. Accumulation of ethidium bromide by *E. coli* AG100 cells took place at pH 7 without glucose for 10 min (■). Additions for efflux evaluation were made in PBS (pH 7) as follows: 5 mM EDTA (▲); 5 mM EDTA and 5 mM Ca^{2+} (●); 5 mM Ca^{2+} (×); PBS control (◇). (From Martins, A. *et al.*, 2011.)

EDTA alone, and the effect can be eliminated by the addition of Ca^{2+} to the assay (Fig. 3.7). The effects of the phenothiazine on the efflux pump system of *E. coli* are therefore mediated by its well-known property of inhibiting calcium binding to calcium-dependent systems. Therefore, the phenothiazine cannot be assigned an EPI role as its effects are indirect and are not mediated towards the efflux pump itself.

The effect of TZ on the accumulation of ethidium bromide by *Salmonella* sp. strains is very different from that of *E. coli*. As evident from Fig. 3.8, increasing concentrations of TZ at first promote the accumulation of ethidium bromide during the first 10 min, after which efflux follows. Efflux takes place whether or not the assay system contains glucose or any intermediates of glycolysis or the Krebs cycle. However, the addition of increasing concentrations of the fatty acid palmitic acid inhibits accumulation by TZ (Fig. 3.8). These results suggest that TZ inhibits enzymes involved in the generation of energy from glycolytic and Krebs cycle sources and does not affect the generation of energy from sources such as fatty acids. Furthermore, because the TZ-promoted efflux takes place in the absence of metabolic energy, the organism must have the ability to shunt its energy sources for efflux from glycolytic and Krebs sources to the metabolism of its own fat. The ability of *Salmonella* sp. to use its fat storage source when placed under stress has recently been shown by others (Dubois-Brissonnet *et al.*, 2011). The effect of TZ on accumulation that is followed by efflux has been noted only for *Salmonella* sp.

3.5 Effects of TZ on *Salmonella* sp. Genes that Regulate and Code for the AcrAB Efflux Pump

The effects of TZ on accumulation of ethidium bromide and subsequent efflux by *Salmonella* sp. suggest that the organism responds early to the presence of the noxious agent. Because other studies have indicated that the growth of *Salmonella* sp. is initially inhibited by CPZ during the first 6–8 h of culture, after which time the organism becomes increasingly resistant to the agent, the effects of TZ on the growth of *Salmonella* sp. were studied. As shown in Fig. 3.9, during the first 6–8 h of exposure to TZ, the growth of the organism is inhibited

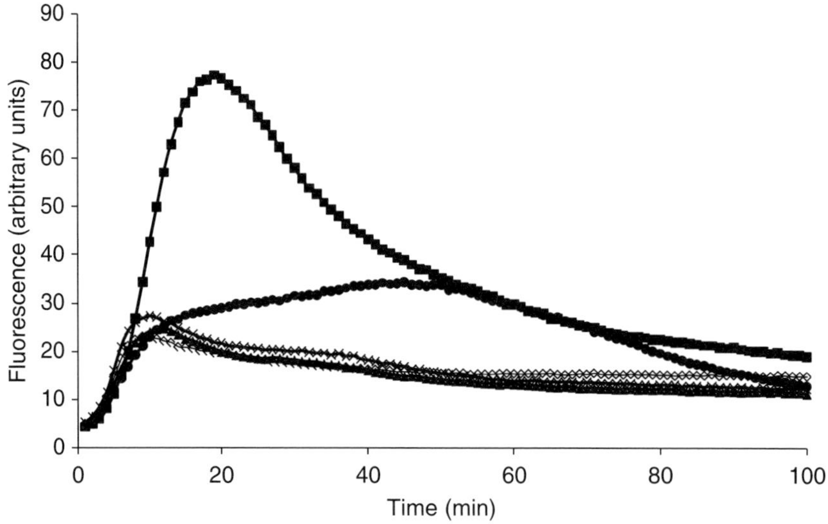

Fig. 3.8. Effect of palmitic acid on the phenothiazine thioridazine (TZ) is to promote accumulation of ethidium bromide. Accumulation of ethidium bromide by *Salmonella* Enteritidis 104 cells was measured at pH 8 with 50 mg/l TZ in medium containing 0.6% glucose (■) and increasing concentrations of: 1 mg/l palmitic acid (●); 5 mg/l palmitic acid (×); 10 mg/l palmitic acid (▲); 15 mg/l palmitic acid (◇). Note that only a single concentration of TZ is shown. This concentration produced accumulation of ethidium bromide, which peaked after approximately 20 min, after which efflux of ethidium bromide occurred. The efflux was independent of glucose and other glycolytic intermediates as well as ethanol. The presence of increasing concentrations of palmitic acid negated the effects of the TZ on accumulation of ethidium bromide and its subsequent efflux (Spengler *et al.*, 2012).

by a concentration of the agent that is below the minimum inhibitory concentration of 230 mg/l. After this period, the organism grows at a rate that is similar to that of the control. An assessment of the activity of the genes that regulate and code for the AcrAB efflux pump at intervals in cultures with or without TZ at 100 mg/l is summarized in Fig. 3.10. During the period when the organism is not growing, the stress gene *soxS* is first activated, followed by activation of the global regulator *ramA*, then by the local regulator *marA* and lastly by the gene encoding the transporter *acrB*. By the end of 8 h of exposure to TZ, the organism is able to extrude the noxious agent and achieve growth at its normal rate. It should be noted, as shown in Fig. 3.10, that exposure to TZ activates the two-component regulon PmrA/B. The PmrA/B regulon is activated by pH, as is the case when the organism has been phagocytosed by neutrophils (Gunn, 2008). Activation of this regulon first involves a sensor function for PmrB, which is activated to undergo self-phosphorylation. The phosphorylated PmrB transfers the phosphate group to PmrA, which then activates a major operon consisting of nine genes, resulting in the synthesis of lipid A, which is introduced into the nascent lipopolysaccharide layer of the outer membrane. When this takes place, the organism is resistant to almost everything (see Gunn, 2008, for a comprehensive review of the PmrA/B two-component regulon). Because TZ activates *pmrB* first followed later by activation of *pmrA*, in all probability, activation of *pmrD* takes place, resulting in the activation of *ramA*, and the sequence of activated genes that results in the overexpression of the transporter *acrB* takes place (Gunn, 2008). Consequently, one may suppose that the increased resistance to TZ involves the cascade of genes that regulate and code for the transporter of the AcrAB pump as well as the cascade of genes that are initiated by the activation of the PmrA/B two-component regulon.

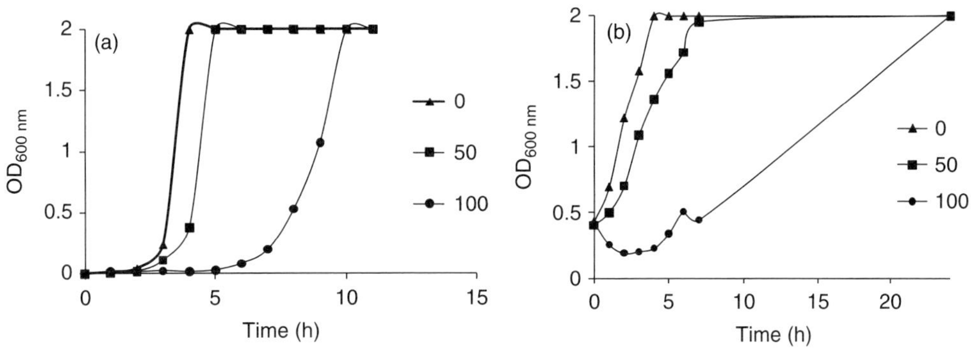

Fig. 3.9. Effect of phenothiazine thioridazine (TZ) concentrations on the growth of *Salmonella* sp. Growth curves of *Salmonella* Enteritidis 104 in Mueller–Hinton broth at pH 7 in the absence of TZ (▲) and in the presence of 50 mg/l TZ (■) and 100 mg/l TZ (●). (a) Minimum inhibitory concentration (MIC) inoculum; (b) inoculum from a mid-point logarithmic growth of fresh culture. Spectrophotometric evaluation of growth was carried out by measuring optical density (OD) at 600 nm. The dip in OD of the fresh culture was due to a TZ-sensitive component of the population. This component was also present with the MIC inoculums but was beyond the sensitivity of the spectrophotometer. Note that the presence of increasing concentrations of TZ inhibited growth for up to 8 h. Growth then proceeded such that by the end of the culture period of 24 h, the organism was resistant to the phenothiazine (MIC of TZ in excess of 230 mg/l) (Spengler *et al*., 2012).

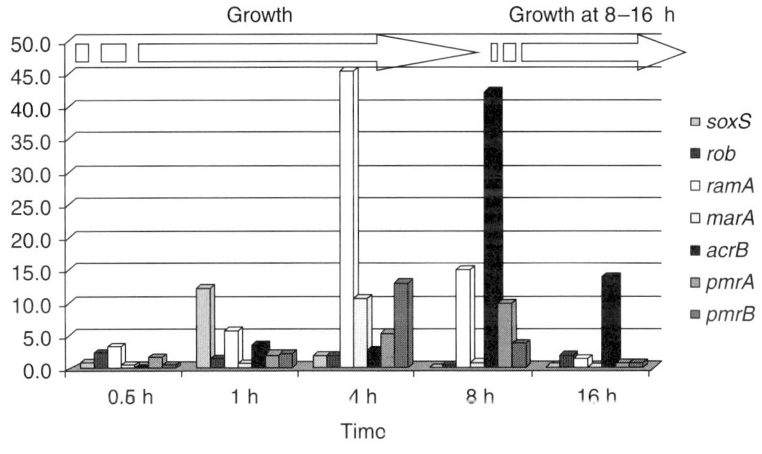

Fig. 3.10. Assessment of the activity of genes that regulate and code for the AcrAB efflux pump of *Salmonella*. Note that during the first 8 h, the organism was not growing. However, during this period of no growth, the genes that regulate and code for the AcrB transporter were sequentially activated; first *soxS*, followed 3 h later by *ramA*, *marA* and *pmrB*. After 8 h of culture, *ramA* decreased its activity, *marA* returned to baseline activity, *acrB* was maximally increased in activity and *pmrA* was now active. By the end of the 16 h culture period, only *acrB* remained elevated in activity (Spengler *et al*., 2012).

3.6 Does TZ Induce Similar Gene Responses when the Stress Gene *soxS* or the Global Regulator *ramA* is Deleted?

The effect of TZ on genes that regulate and code for the AcrAB efflux pump of *Salmonella* sp. raises the question of what happens when *Salmonella* sp. whose *soxS* stress gene is deleted is exposed to concentrations of TZ. First, as was evident with the genetically intact *Salmonella* sp. strain, a latent growth period of about 7–8 h takes place. However, growth is then followed by

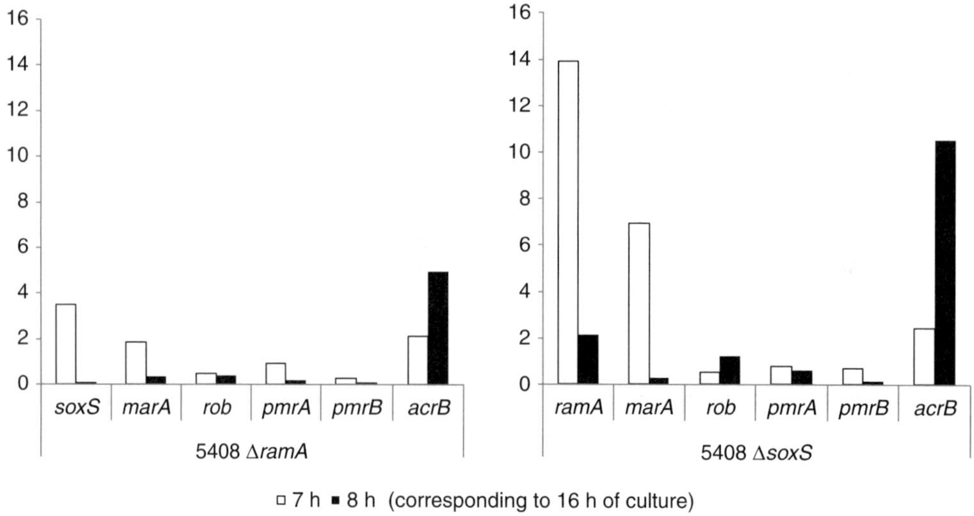

Fig. 3.11. Effect of phenothiazine thioridazine (TZ) on genes that regulate and code for the AcrB transporter of *Salmonella* Enteritidis 5408 whose *soxS* or *ramA* gene has been deleted. Note that, regardless of deletion of either the *ramA* or *soxS* gene, activation of transporter *acrB* took place. During the first 7 h, the organism was not growing in the culture containing 50 mg/l TZ. The activation of genes in the presence of TZ (50 mg/l) took place after 7 h. The values on the *y*-axis represent the level of gene expression of the treated cells compared with the untreated control (Spengler *et al.*, 2012).

less-than-normal rates of growth. The effect of TZ on the genes that regulate and code for AcrB is summarized in Fig. 3.11; the presence of a subinhibitory concentration of TZ promotes overexpression of the *acrB* gene, even though the stress gene *soxS* has been deleted. Similarly, TZ promotes the overexpression of the *acrB* gene of *Salmonella* whose global regulator gene *ramA* has been deleted. For both gene-deleted strains, overexpression of the local regulator *marA* gene results. As the PmrA/B two-component regulator genes are not significantly affected, there must be another genetic activating pathway that is invoked by TZ, even though the two main genes involved in a stress-related response are absent.

3.7 Methods Developed for the Assessment of Efflux Pumps in Bacteria

Methods for screening MDR clinical isolates for overexpressed efflux pumps have been developed (Martins, M. *et al.*, 2006, 2010, 2011). These methods employ agar containing increasing concentrations of ethidium bromide, and reference strains and MDR clinical isolates are streaked on the surface of the agar. The principle of the method is based on the assumption that isolates that overexpress their efflux pumps require higher concentrations of ethidium bromide for the production of fluorescence associated with the streak than do their wild-type counterpart strains. As noted by the example provided in Fig. 3.12, the strains that overexpress their efflux pumps do not fluoresce at concentrations of ethidium bromide in the agar that produce fluorescence in the strains that do not overexpress their efflux pumps. The method is useful for evaluating physiological conditions such as pH that impact on the efflux activity of the strain, as noted in Fig. 3.13. This method has recently been used for the identification of strains of *Staphylococcus aureus* that contain plasmids carrying the Qac efflux pump gene (Costa *et al.*, 2010).

The second method works on a real-time basis to assess the accumulation and efflux of the universal substrate ethidium

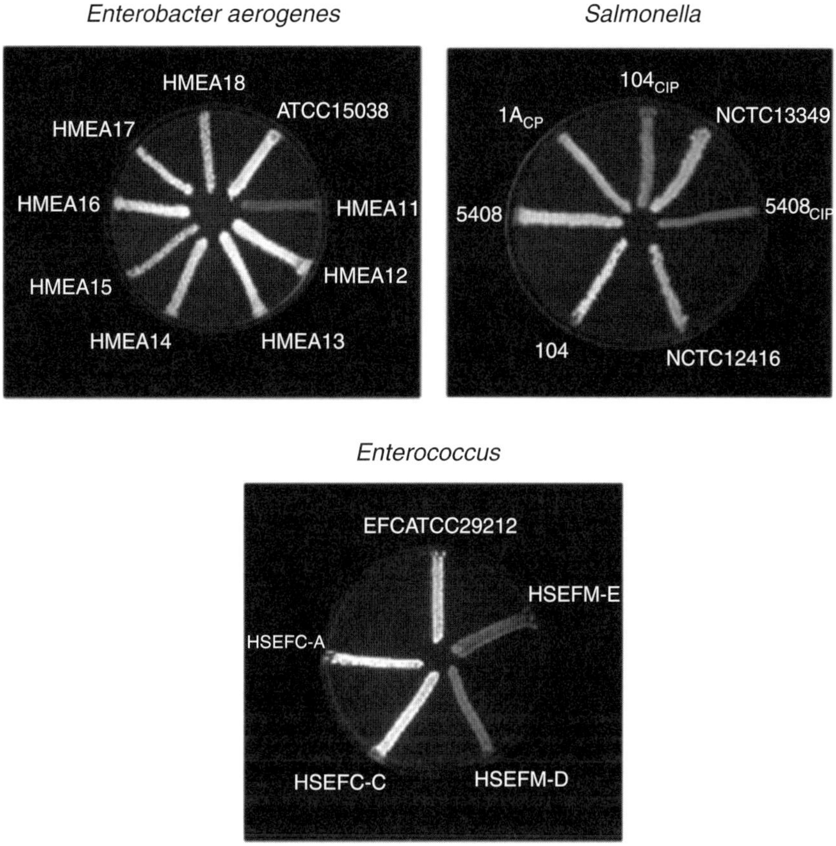

Fig. 3.12. Results of an ethidium bromide agar method to identify strains that overexpress their efflux pump systems. In the examples provided, only one concentration of ethidium bromide is shown. For *Enterobacter aerogenes*, the agar plate contains 1.5 mg/l ethidium bromide, while for the *Enterococcus* and *Salmonella* strains, the concentration shown is 2.5 mg/l. Note that lines of cultures that fluoresce are indicative of strains whose efflux pumps are expressed at a significantly lower level than that of the lines of cullture that do not fluoresce or have lower degrees of fluorescence (Spengler *et al.*, 2012).

bromide (Viveiros *et al.* 2008, 2010). Whereas the ethidium bromide method provides an overall understanding of efflux during an 18–20 h period, the semi-automated ethidium bromide method assesses efflux during an initial period of culture under minimal nutrient conditions. This means that physiological parameters can be manipulated from the onset or during the period of incubation. Among these physiological parameters are pH, metabolic energy, ions and agents that are to be studied for effect on accumulation/efflux of the universal substrate ethidium bromide. Figures 3.14–3.17 provide examples of the assay with respect to the presence of glucose and alternative sources of metabolic energy (Fig. 3.14), effect of pH on accumulation and efflux (Fig. 3.15) and the effects of EPIs (Fig. 3.16). The assay is sufficiently reproducible to yield Michaelis–Menton constants (K_m), as shown in Fig. 3.17 for competitive substrates relative to ethidium bromide (Martins *et al.*, 2009b).

The combined use of both methods provides a substantial understanding of the efflux pump system of a given bacterial strain. It is anticipated that, with extensive use of these methods, they will become standardized.

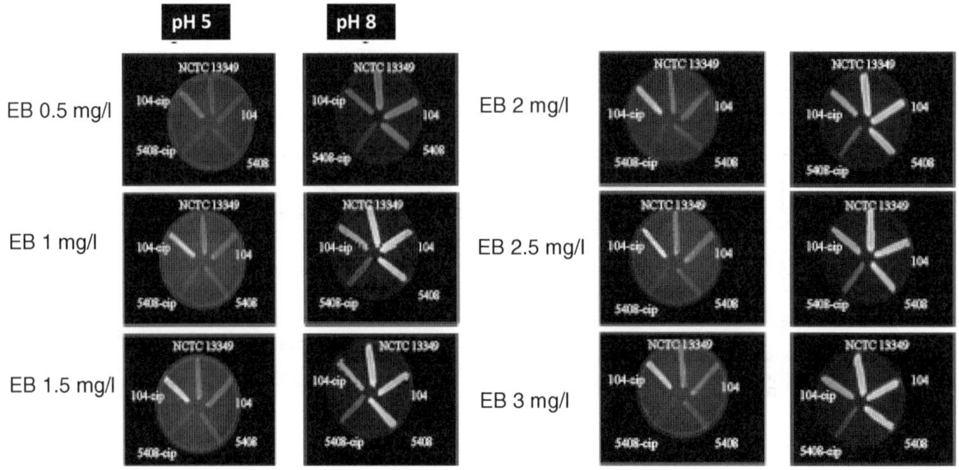

Fig. 3.13. Effect of pH on the accumulation of ethidium bromide by *Salmonella* by their AcrAB–TolC efflux pumps. Strains indicated by 'cip' overexpress their efflux pumps (O'Regan *et al.*, 2009). Note that strains 104-cip and 5408-cip were derived from their respective parents, 104 and 5408, by sequential exposure to increasing concentrations of ciprofloxacin. With the exception of the 104-cip strain that overexpressed its efflux pump sixfold compared with its parental strain (O'Regan *et al.*, 2009), the degree of fluorescence of the other strains conformed to the expectation of the assay at pH 5 and 8; namely, that at pH 5, there was less fluorescence associated with the line of culture than at pH 8, and that the degree of fluorescence was associated with the level of expression of the AcrAB–TolC efflux pump. The reason for the unexpected result yielded by the 104-cip strain is not yet known (Spengler *et al.*, 2012).

3.8 Future Perspectives

It is the general consensus that finding drugs that inhibit the overexpressed efflux pump of Gram-negative bacterial pathogens is a worthwhile goal (Pagès *et al.*, 2011). However, achieving this goal may not be possible given the following facts:

1. The redundancy of efflux pumps ensures that deletion of one or more of these efflux pumps will result in the overexpression of others (Viveiros *et al.*, 2005, 2007). Although the efficiency of the non-main efflux pumps is far less than that of the main one, they are still effective in rendering the bacterium resistant to the agent that induced resistance (Viveiros *et al.*, 2005).
2. Exposure to an EPI promotes a response from the bacterium similar to the initial response to an antibiotic (Martins *et al.*, 2009a), namely, overexpression of efflux pumps, as described in this chapter.

So how can an adjuvant be designed that will by-pass the above and effectively inhibit any efflux pump of a given Gram-negative bacterium? The answer may well be in the development of agents that block the outer-membrane protein of the RND efflux pump (e.g. TolC). TolC is present in all of the RND efflux pumps of a given bacterium (Piddock, 2006). Some agents have been identified that cause constriction of the part of the TolC conduit that connects to the outer cell membrane (B.F. Luisi, 2010, personal communication). However, these negatively charged polypeptides are extremely toxic. Nevertheless, they may serve as lead compounds that are reduced in toxicity or may even be non-toxic to humans.

Another more promising approach is the use of nano-antibodies that recognize antigenic determinants on the surface component of TolC. However, to our knowledge, this idea has not yet been developed at the level of experimentation.

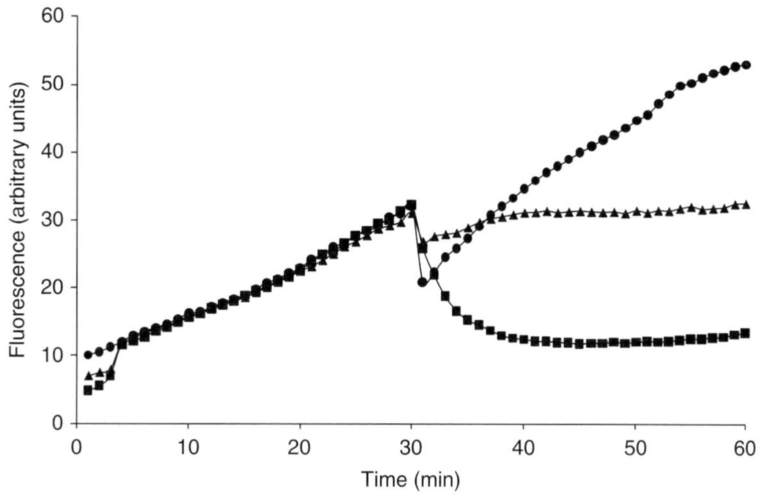

Fig. 3.14. Example of the method for assessment of accumulation and efflux of the AcrAB–TolC substrate ethidium bromide in deionized water. In this example, the assay was conducted in deionized water at pH 5.5. Accumulation of ethidium bromide by *Salmonella* Enteritidis cells without glucose (●) was measured, and at the end of 30 min accumulation, the following additions were made: 0.4% glucose (■) and 2% ethanol (▲). Note that ethanol was able to replace glucose as the sole source of metabolic energy. (From Amaral *et al.*, 2011b.)

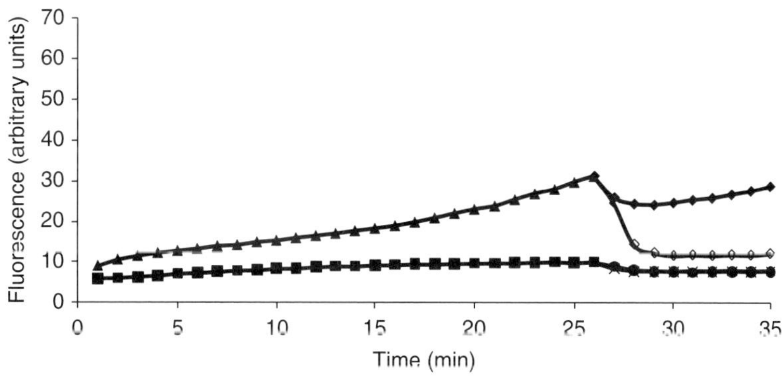

Fig. 3.15. Example of an assay for accumulation of ethidium bromide in PBS at pH 5 and 8. Accumulation of ethidium bromide was measured in *E. coli* AG100 cells in PBS at pH 5 (■) and pH 8 (▲) without glucose for 25 min. Additions for efflux evaluation were made in PBS at pH 5 or 8 as follows: pH 5 without glucose (x); pH 5 with 0.4% glucose (●); pH 8 without glucose (◆); pH 8 with 0.4% glucose (◇). (From Martins *et al.*, 2009b.)

In conclusion, we have presented a wide-ranging review of efflux pumps, the energetics of efflux, the genetics of regulation, the role that the environment plays in their function and their physiological workings. It is hoped that this review will attract the attention of scientists who are not currently in the field of bacterial efflux pumps, who, because of their distinct backgrounds, expertise and knowledge, may contribute in ways not yet known towards the control of efflux pumps of major MDR bacteria pathogens, thereby making effective therapy possible.

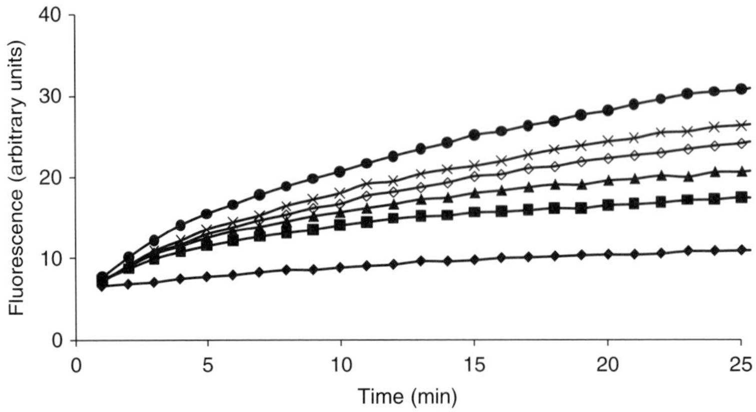

Fig. 3.16. Measurement of accumulation of ethidium bromide and competition with Phe-Arg β-naphthylamide (PAN). Accumulation of ethidium bromide was measured in *E. coli* AG100 cells at pH 5 with glucose and increasing concentrations of PAN as follows: control without PAN (◆); 2.5 mg/l PAN (■); 5 mg/l PAN (▲); 10 mg/l PAN (◇); 20 mg/l PAN (×); 40 mg/l PAN (●). (From Martins *et al.*, 2009b.)

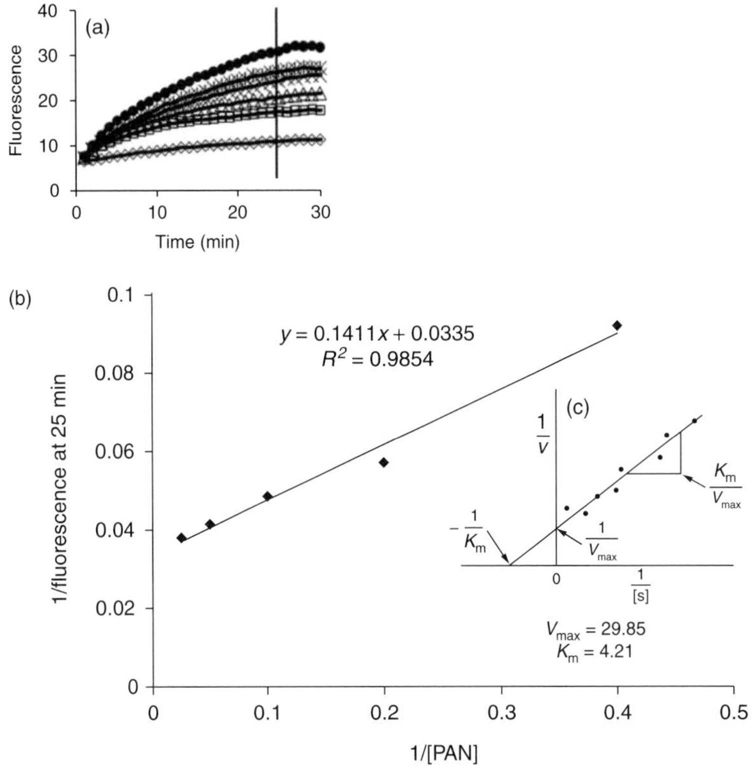

Fig. 3.17. Calculation of K_m from the competitive data between PAN and ethidium bromide. Increasing concentrations of PAN from 1 to 40 mg/l caused an increase in fluorescence (a). This data was then used for the derivation of the PAN K_m initially plotted in (b) and data employed in the Michaelis–Menten kinetics (c). (From Martins *et al.*, 2009b.)

References

Amaral, L., Kristiansen, J. and Lorian, V.S. (1992) Synergic effect of chlorpromazine on the activity of some antibiotics. *Journal of Antimicrobial Chemotherapy* 30, 556–558.

Amaral, L., Kristiansen, J.E., Abebe, L.S. and Millett, W. (1996) Inhibition of the respiration of multi-drug resistant clinical isolates of *Mycobacterium tuberculosis* by thioridazine: potential use for initial therapy of freshly diagnosed tuberculosis. *Journal of Antimicrobial Chemotherapy* 38, 1049–1053.

Amaral, L., Viveiros, M. and Kristiansen, J.E. (2001) Phenothiazines: potential alternatives for the management of antibiotic resistant infections of tuberculosis and malaria in developing countries. *Tropical Medicine and International Health* 6, 1016–1022.

Amaral, L., Viveiros, M. and Molnar, J. (2004) Antimicrobial activity of phenothiazines. *In Vivo* 18, 725–731.

Amaral, L., Boeree, M.J., Gillespie, S.H., Udwadia, Z.F. and van Soolingen, D. (2010a) Thioridazine cures extensively drug-resistant tuberculosis (XDR-TB) and the need for global trials is now! *International Journal of Antimicrobial Agents* 35, 524–526.

Amaral, L., Martins, A., Molnar, J., Kristiansen, J.E., Martins, M., Viveiros, M., Rodrigues, L., Spengler, G., Couto, I., Ramos, J., Dastidar, S., Fanning, S., McCusker, M. and Pages, J.M. (2010b) Phenothiazines, bacterial efflux pumps and targeting the macrophage for enhanced killing of intracellular XDRTB. *In Vivo* 24, 409–424.

Amaral, L., Cerca, P., Spengler, G., Machado, L., Martins, A., Couto, I., Viveiros, M., Fanning, S. and Pagès, J.M. (2011a) Ethidium bromide efflux by *Salmonella*: modulation by metabolic energy, pH, ions and phenothiazines. *International Journal of Antimicrobial Agents* 38, 140–145.

Amaral, L., Pages, J.M. and Fanning, S. (2011b) RND efflux pumps of Gram-negative bacteria. *Advances in Enzymology* 77, 61–108.

Amaral, L., Viveiros, M., Molnar, J. and Kristiansen, J.E. (2011c) Effective therapy with the neuroleptic thioridazine as an adjunct to second line of defence drugs, and the potential that thioridazine offers for new patents that cover a variety of “new uses”. *Recent Patents on Anti-infective Drug Discovery* 6, 84–87.

Bailey, A.M., Paulsen, I.T. and Piddock, L.J. (2008) RamA confers multidrug resistance in *Salmonella enterica* via increased expression of *acrB*, which is inhibited by chlorpromazine. *Antimicrobial Agents and Chemotherapy* 52, 3604–3611.

Bald, D. and Koul, A. (2010) Respiratory ATP synthesis: the new generation of mycobacterial drug targets? *FEMS Microbiology Letters* 308, 1–7.

Blair, J.M. and Piddock, L.J. (2009) Structure, function and inhibition of RND efflux pumps in Gram-negative bacteria: an update. *Current Opinion in Microbiology* 12, 512–519.

Bodoni, P. (1899) Dell’azione sedativa del bleu di metilene in vaire forme di psicosi. *Clinica Medica Italiana* 24, 217–222.

Bolla, J.M., Saint, N., Labesse, G., Pagès, J.M. and Dumas, C. (2004) Crystallization and preliminary crystallographic studies of MOMP (major outer membrane protein) from *Campylobacter jejuni. Acta Crystallographica Section D – Biological Crystallography* 60, 2349–2351.

Boyer, P.D. (1988) Bioenergetic coupling to proton-motive force: should we be considering hydronium ion coordination and not group protonation? *Trends in Biochemical Sciences* 13, 5–7.

Chang, T.M., Lu, P.L., Li, H.H., Chang, C.Y., Chen, T.C. and Chang, L.L. (2007) Characterization of fluoroquinolone resistance mechanisms and their correlation with the degree of resistance to clinically used fluoroquinolones among *Escherichia coli* isolates. *Journal of Chemotherapy* 19, 488–494.

Charpentier, P., Gaillot, P., Jacob, R., Gaudechon, J. and Buisson, P. (1952) Recherches sur les dimethylaminopropyl N-phenothiazines. *Comptes Rendus de l’Académie des Sciences* 35, 59–60.

Chopra, I., O’Neill, A.J. and Miller, K. (2003) The role of mutators in the emergence of antibiotic-resistant bacteria. *Drug Resistance Updates* 6, 137–145.

Costa, S.S., Ntokou, E., Martins, A., Viveiros, M., Pournaras, S., Couto, I. and Amaral, L. (2010) Identification of the plasmid-encoded *qacA* efflux pump gene in meticillin-resistant *Staphylococcus aureus* (MRSA) strain HPV107, a representative of the MRSA Iberian clone. *International Journal of Antimicrobial Agents* 36, 557–561.

Crowle, A.J., Douvas, G.S. and May, M.H. (1992) Chlorpromazine: a drug potentially useful for treating mycobacterial infections. *Chemotherapy* 38, 410–419.

Davin-Regli, A., Bolla, J.M., James, C.E., Lavigne, J.P., Chevalier, J., Garnotel, E., Molitor, A. and Pagès, J.M. (2008) Membrane permeability and regulation of drug “influx and efflux” in enterobacterial pathogens. *Current Drug Targets* 9, 750–759.

Dimroth, P., Kaim, G. and Matthey, U. (2000) Crucial role of the membrane potential for ATP synthesis by F_1F_o ATP synthases. *Journal of Experimental Biology* 203, 51–59.

Dubois-Brissonnet, F., Naïtali, M., Mafu, A.A. and Briandet, R. (2011) Induction of fatty acid composition modifications and tolerance to biocides in *Salmonella enterica* serovar Typhimurium by plant-derived terpenes. *Applied and Environmental Microbiology* 77, 906–910.

Eicher, T., Brandstätter, L. and Pos, K.M. (2009) Structural and functional aspects of the multidrug efflux pump AcrB. *Biological Chemistry* 390, 693–699.

Feniouk, B.A. and Yoshida, M. (2008) Regulatory mechanisms of proton-translocating F_OF_1-ATP synthase. *Results and Problems in Cell Differentiation* 45, 279–308.

Gootz, T.D. (2010) The global problem of antibiotic resistance. *Critical Reviews in Immunology* 30, 79–93.

Gunn, J.S. (2008) The *Salmonella* PmrAB regulon: lipopolysaccharide modifications, antimicrobial peptide resistance and more. *Trends in Microbiology* 16, 284–290.

Guttmann, P. and Ehrlich, P. (1891) Über die Wirkung des Methylenblau bei Malaria. *Berliner Klinische Wochenschrift* 39, 953–956.

Hidaka, H. and Shikano, K. (1983) [Overview on the research on calmodulin and its inhibitors]. *Nippon Rinsho* 41, 2138–2150 (in Japanese).

Husain, F. and Nikaido, H. (2010) Substrate path in the AcrB multidrug efflux pump of *Escherichia coli*. *Molecular Microbiology* 78, 320–330.

Klee, C.B., Ni, W.C., Draetta, G.F. and Newton, D.L. (1986) Different modes of interaction of calmodulin with its target enzymes. *Journal of Cardiovascular Pharmacology* 8, S52–S56.

Klitgaard, J.K., Skov, M.N., Kallipolitis, B.H. and Kolmos, H.J. (2008) Reversal of methicillin resistance in *Staphylococcus aureus* by thioridazine. *Journal of Antimicrobial Chemotherapy* 62, 1215–1221.

Kristiansen, J.E. and Amaral, L. (1997) The potential management of resistant infections with non-antibiotics. *Journal of Antimicrobial Chemotherapy* 40, 319–327.

Kristiansen, J.E., Hendricks, O., Delvin, T., Butterworth, T.S., Aagaard, L., Christensen, J.B., Flores, V.C. and Keyzer, H. (2007) Reversal of resistance in microorganisms by help of non-antibiotics. *Journal of Antimicrobial Chemotherapy* 59, 1271–1279.

Kumar, A., Hajjar, E., Ruggerone, P. and Ceccarelli, M. (2010) Structural and dynamical properties of the porins OmpF and OmpC: insights from molecular simulations. *Journal of Physics: Condensed Matter* 22, 454125.

Levy, S.B. (2002) Active efflux, a common mechanism for biocide and antibiotic resistance. *Symposium Series Society for Applied Microbiology* S65–S71.

Maeda, M. (2010) [H^+-transporting ATP synthases: insights into how their electrochemically driven motor might serve as a drug target]. *Yakugaku Zasshi* 130, 191–197 (in Japanese).

Martins, A., Iversen, C., Rodrigues, L., Spengler, G., Ramos, J., Kern, W.V., Couto, I., Viveiros, M., Fanning, S., Pages, J.M. and Amaral, L. (2009a) An AcrAB-mediated multidrug-resistant phenotype is maintained following restoration of wild-type activities by efflux pump genes and their regulators. *International Journal of Antimicrobial Agents* 34, 602–604.

Martins, A., Spengler, G., Rodrigues, L., Viveiros, M., Ramos, J., Martins, M., Couto, I., Fanning, S., Pagès, J.M., Bolla, J.M., Molnar, J. and Amaral, L. (2009b) pH modulation of efflux pump activity of multi-drug resistant *Escherichia coli*: protection during its passage and eventual colonization of the colon. *PLoS One* 4, e6656.

Martins, A., Machado, L., Costa, S., Cerca, P., Spengler, G., Viveiros, M. and Amaral, L. (2011) Role of calcium in the efflux system of *Escherichia coli*. *International Journal of Antimicrobial Agents* 37, 410–414.

Martins, M., Santos, B., Martins, A., Viveiros, M., Couto, I., Cruz, A., Pagès, J.M., Molnar, J., Fanning, S., Amaral, L. and Management Committee Members of Cost B16 European Commission/European Science Foundation (2006) An instrument-free method for the demonstration of efflux pump activity of bacteria. *In Vivo* 20, 657–664.

Martins, M., Schelz, Z., Martins, A., Molnar, J., Hajös, G., Riedl, Z., Viveiros, M., Yalcin, I., Aki-Sener, E. and Amaral, L. (2007) *In vitro* and *ex vivo* activity of thioridazine derivatives against *Mycobacterium tuberculosis*. *International Journal of Antimicrobial Agents* 29, 338–340.

Martins, M., Couto, I., Viveiros, M. and Amaral, L. (2010) Identification of efflux-mediated multi-drug resistance in bacterial clinical isolates by two simple methods. *Methods in Molecular Biology* 642, 143–157.

Martins, M., Viveiros, M., Couto, I., Costa, S.S., Pacheco, T., Fanning, S., Pagès, J.M. and Amaral, L. (2011) Identification of efflux pump-mediated multidrug-resistant bacteria by the ethidium bromide–agar cartwheel method. *In Vivo* 25, 171–178.

Mayur, Y.C., Jagadeesh, S. and Thimmaiah, K.N. (2006) Targeting calmodulin in reversing multi drug resistance in cancer cells. *Mini Reviews in Medicinal Chemistry* 6, 1383–1389.

Mulkidjanian, A.Y. (2009) Proton in the well and through the desolvation barrier. *Biochimica et Biophysica Acta* 1757, 415–427.

Mulkidjanian, A.Y., Cherepanov, D.A., Heberle, J. and Junge, W. (2005) Proton transfer dynamics at membrane/water interface and mechanism of biological energy conversion. *Biochemistry* (Moscow) 70, 251–256.

Mulkidjanian, A.Y., Heberle, J. and Cherepanov, D.A. (2006) Protons @ interfaces: implications for biological energy conversion. *Biochimica et Biophysica Acta* 1757, 913–930.

Nakamoto, R.K., Scanlon, J.A.B. and Al-Shawi, M.K. (2008) The rotary mechanism of the ATP synthase. *Archives of Biochemistry and Biophysics* 476, 43–50.

Ordway, D., Viveiros, M., Leandro, C., Bettencourt, R., Almeida, J., Martins, M., Kristiansen, J.E., Molnar, J. and Amaral, L. (2003) Clinical concentrations of thioridazine kill intracellular multidrug-resistant *Mycobacterium tuberculosis. Antimicrobial Agents and Chemotherapy* 47, 917–922.

O'Regan, E., Quinn, T., Pagès, J.M., McCusker, M., Piddock, L. and Fanning, S. (2009) Multiple regulatory pathways associated with high-level ciprofloxacin and multidrug resistance in *Salmonella enterica* serovar Enteritidis: involvement of RamA and other global regulators. *Antimicrobial Agents and Chemotherapy* 53, 1080–1087.

Osawa, M., Tomomori, C. and Ikura, M. (1998) [Calmodulin: the progress in three-dimensional structure analysis]. *Tanpakushitsu Kakusan Koso* 43(Suppl.), 1939–1944 (in Japanese).

Pagès, J.M. and Amaral, L. (2009) Mechanisms of drug efflux and strategies to combat them: challenging the efflux pump of Gram-negative bacteria. *Biochimica et Biophysica Acta* 1794, 826–833.

Pagès, J.M., Amaral, L. and Fanning, S. (2011) An original deal for new molecule: reversal of efflux pump activity, a rational strategy to combat Gram-negative resistant bacteria. *Current Medicinal Chemistry* 18, 2969–2980.

Piddock, L.J.V. (2006) Clinically relevant chromosomally encoded multidrug resistance efflux pumps in bacteria. *Clinical Microbiology Reviews* 19, 382–402.

Pos, K.M. (2009) Drug transport mechanism of the AcrB efflux pump. *Biochimica et Biophysica Acta* 1794, 782–793.

Rahbar, M., Mehrgan, H. and Hadji-nejad, S. (2010) Enhancement of vancomycin activity by phenothiazines against vancomycin-resistant *Enterococcus faecium in vitro. Basic and Clinical Pharmacology and Toxicology* 107, 676–679.

Ren, X., Wang, S., Wen, Y. and Yang, K. (2009) [An update of calcium signaling in bacteria a review]. *Wei Sheng Wu Xue Bao* 49, 1564–1570 (in Chinese).

Schulz, R., Vargiu, A.V., Collu, F., Kleinekathöfer, U. and Ruggerone, P. (2010) Functional rotation of the transporter AcrB: insights into drug extrusion from simulations. *PLoS Computational Biology* 6, e1000806.

Seeger, M.A., Diederichs, K., Eicher, T., Brandstätter, L., Schiefner, A., Verrey, F. and Pos, K.M. (2008) The AcrB efflux pump: conformational cycling and peristalsis lead to multidrug resistance. *Current Drug Targets* 9, 729–749.

Soto, S.M., Ruíz, J., Mendoza, M.C. and Vila, J. (2003) *In vitro* fluoroquinolone-resistant mutants of *Salmonella enterica* serotype Enteritidis: analysis of mechanisms involved in resistance. *International Journal of Antimicrobial Agents* 22, 537–540.

Spengler, G., Rodrigues, L., Martins, A., Martins, M., Mc Cusker, M., Cerca, P., Machado, L., Costa, S.S., Ntokou, E., Couto, I., Viveiros, M., Fanning, S., Molnar, J. and Amaral, L. (2012) Genetic response of *Salmonella enterica* serotype Enteritidis to thioridazine rendering the organism resistant to the agent. *International Journal of Antimicrobial Agents* 39, 16–21.

Su, C.C. and Yu, E.W. (2007) Ligand-transporter interaction in the AcrB multidrug efflux pump determined by fluorescence polarization assay. *FEBS Letters* 581, 4972–4976.

Thanassi, D.G., Cheng, L.W. and Nikaido, H. (1997) Active efflux of bile salts by *Escherichia coli. Journal of Bacteriology* 179, 2512–2518.

Turina, P., Rebecchi, A., D'Alessandro, M., Anefors, S. and Melandri, B.A. (2006) Modulation of proton pumping efficiency in bacterial ATP synthases. *Biochimica et Biophysica Acta* 1757, 320–325.

Viveiros, M., Jesus, A., Brito, M., Leandro, C., Martins, M., Ordway, D., Molnar, A.M., Molnar, J. and Amaral, L. (2005) Inducement and reversal of tetracycline resistance in *Escherichia coli* K-12 and expression of proton gradient-dependent multidrug efflux pump genes. *Antimicrobial Agents and Chemotherapy* 49, 3578–3582.

Viveiros, M., Dupont, M., Rodrigues, L., Couto, I., Davin-Regli, A., Martins, M., Pagès, J.M. and Amaral, L. (2007) Antibiotic stress, genetic response and altered permeability of *E. coli. PLoS One* 2, e365.

Viveiros, M., Martins, M., Couto, I., Rodrigues, L., Spengler, G., Martins, A., Kristiansen, J.E., Molnar, J. and Amaral, L. (2008) New methods for the identification of efflux mediated MDR bacteria, genetic assessment of regulators and efflux pump constituents, characterization of efflux systems and screening for inhibitors of efflux pumps. *Current Drug Targets* 9, 760–778.

Viveiros, M., Rodrigues, L., Martins, M., Couto, I., Spengler, G., Martins, A. and Amaral, L. (2010) Evaluation of efflux activity of bacteria by a semi-automated fluorometric system. *Methods in Molecular Biology* 642, 159–172.

von Ballmoos, C. (2007) Alternative proton binding mode in ATP synthases. *Journal of Bioenergetics and Biomembranes* 39, 441–445.

Zgurskaya, H.I. and Nikaido, H. (2000) Cross-linked complex between oligomeric periplasmic lipoprotein AcrA and the inner-membrane-associated multidrug efflux pump AcrB from *Escherichia coli. Journal of Bacteriology* 182, 4264–4267.

4 Small-molecule Efflux Pump Inhibitors from Natural Products as a Potential Source of Antimicrobial Agents

Sanjay M. Jachak,[1] Somendu K. Roy,[1] Shiv Gupta,[1] Pallavi Ahirrao[2] and Simon Gibbons[3]

[1]Department of Natural Products, National Institute of Pharmaceutical Education and Research (NIPER), SAS Nagar, Punjab, India; [2]Rayat-Bahra Institute of Pharmacy, Saharaun, Kharar, Punjab, India; [3]Centre for Pharmacognosy and Phytotherapy, The School of Pharmacy, University of London, London, UK

4.1 Introduction

Staphylococcus aureus (Gram-positive) and *Pseudomonas aeruginosa* (Gram-negative) are common nosocomial human pathogens. *S. aureus* is common in wound-related infections and has virulent effects including endocarditis, osteomyelitis, pneumonia, toxic-shock syndrome, food poisoning, carbuncles and boils (Miller *et al.*, 2005), whereas *P. aeruginosa* is a frequent cause of infections such as pneumonia, urinary tract infections (UTIs) and bacteraemia (Medscap Reference, 2009). Tuberculosis (TB) caused by the acid-fast bacterium *Mycobacterium tuberculosis* and *Candida* infections are other causes of death worldwide, especially in human immunodeficiency virus (HIV)-infected patients. There are a number of antibiotics (β-lactam, macrolides, fluoroquinolones, vancomycin and aminoglycosides) for the treatment of infectious diseases caused by Gram-positive and Gram-negative bacteria, but a major drawback is the rapid occurrence of resistance against these antibiotics as a result of mutations of the target protein, enzymatic inactivation of the antibiotic or inhibition of accumulation of the antibiotics by overexpression of efflux systems within the bacterial cell (Alekshun and Levy, 2007). Therefore, continuous discovery and development of new antibiotics from natural products is required, and these should be effective alone or in combination with new targets in microorganisms.

In the early 1990s, it was shown that efflux pumps (EPs) represent a potential target in microorganisms. The presence of EPs was first reported in *Escherichia coli*, encoded by various genes that cause resistance towards tetracyclines (McMurry *et al.*, 1980). Numerous EPs have since been discovered in microorganisms and are categorized into five main superfamilies: (i) ATP-binding cassette (ABC) transporters; (ii) major facilitators; (iii) resistance nodulation division (RND); (iv) small multidrug resistance (SMR); and (v) multidrug and toxic-compound extrusion (MATE) (Fig. 4.1) (Li and Nikaido, 2004, 2009; Zechini and Versace, 2009). Some of the EPs belonging to these superfamilies in bacteria are shown in Table 4.1.

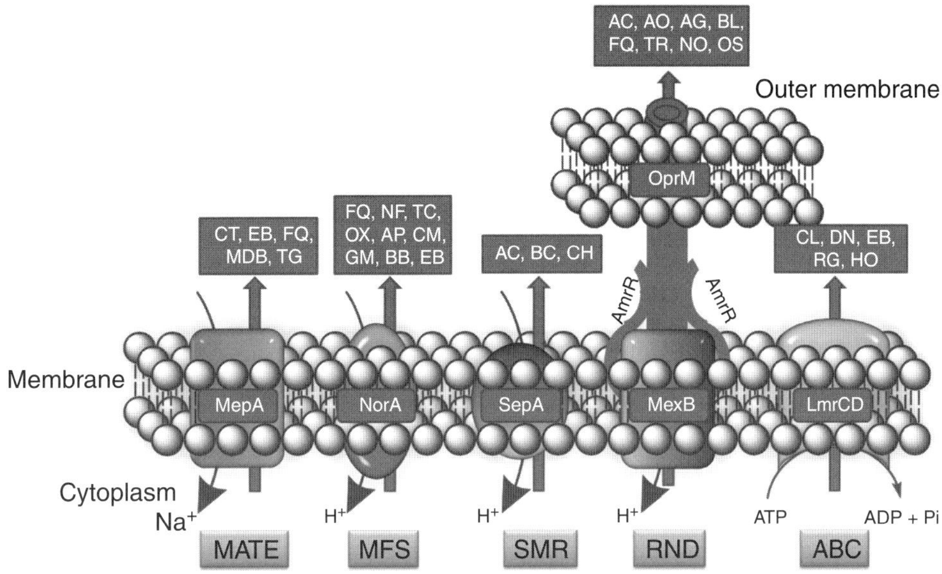

Fig. 4.1. Some examples of EPs and their substrates that are pumped through the bacterial cell membrane. ABC, ATP-binding cassette; MATE, multidrug and toxic-compound extrusion; MFS, major facilitator superfamily; RND, resistance nodulation division; SMR, small multidrug resistance; CT, ceftazidine; EB, ethidium bromide; FQ, fluoroquinolones; MDB, monovalent and divalent biocides; TG, tigecycline; NF, norfloxacine; TC, tetracyclines; OX, oxacillin; AP, ampicillin; CM, chloramphenicol; GM, gentamicin; BB, berberine; AC, acriflavin; BC, benzalkonium chloride; CH, chlorhexidine; AO, acridine orange; AG, aminoglycoside; BL, β-lactam; TR, triclosan; NO, novobiocine; OS, organic solvents; CL, cholate; DN, daunomycin; RG, rhodamine; HO, Hoechst 33342.

4.2 Screening for Efflux Pump Inhibitors

A number of pathogenic Gram-positive and Gram-negative bacteria and fungi, including *S. aureus*, *Mycobacterium* spp. and *Candida albicans*, remove antibiotics from their cells using EPs, enabling them to develop resistance. Thus, EP inhibitors (EPIs), in combination with a novel or conventional antibiotic, would set a new improved standard of therapy for bacterial infections. A number of *in vitro* assays are used for the determination of EPIs, as described below.

4.2.1 Accumulation assay (ethidium bromide or berberine)

Fluorescent molecules such as ethidium bromide and berberine have been characterized as substrates in a variety of microorganisms. In the presence of an active EPI, these substrates accumulate in the cells. The inhibitory activity of EPIs can thus be measured fluorometrically, as a reduction in fluorescence over time (Paixão *et al.*, 2009).

4.2.2 Susceptibility testing

The next step is susceptibility testing of any compound shown to prevent efflux, to eliminate synergy due to antibacterial activity. Growth inhibition of test compounds is determined using subinhibitory concentrations of berberine for Gram-positive bacteria and of erythromycin for Gram-negative bacteria. According to the Clinical and Laboratory Standards Institute (CLSI) recommendations, an EPI is defined as a compound that completely prevents cell growth in the presence

Table 4.1. Some of the efflux pumps present in bacteria.

Efflux pump(s)	Substrates	Organism(s)	Reference(s)
MF superfamily			
MdfA	CM, DR, FQ, NF, TC	*Salmonella typhimurium, Escherichia coli*	Bohn and Bouloc (1998); Nishino *et al.* (2006)
MdeA	BC, DQ, EB, FU, HO, LA, ML, MU, NO, QAC, type-A SG, TPP, VM	*Staphyloccoccus aureus, Staphylococcus haemolyticus, Bacillus cereus, Bacillus subtilis*	Huang *et al.* (2004); Yamada *et al.* (2006)
EmeA	AC, CL, EB, EM, FQ, NO	*Enterococcus faecalis*	Jonas *et al.* (2001)
QacAa	AC, CH, CV, DD, EB, QAC	*S. aureus*	Littlejohn *et al.* (1992)
RND superfamily			
MexB	AC, AG, AO, BB, BC, BL, CM, CV, DA, EB, EM, FU, ML, NO, OS, RG, SDS, SF, TC, TM, TR, TPP	*Pseudomonas aeruginosa, Pseudomonas syringae*	Cao *et al.* (2004); Daigle *et al.* (2007); Li *et al.* (1995); Poole *et al.* (1996); Sobel *et al.* (2005); Stoitsova *et al.* (2008)
CmeE	AO, AP, CAB, EB, PM, SDS, TR	*Campylobacter jejuni*	Akiba *et al.* (2006); Pumbwe *et al.* (2005)
SdeY	AC, BAC, EM, NF, RG, TC	*Serratia marcescens*	Chen *et al.* (2003)
VexF	BC, BS, DC, EB, EM, NF, NO, SDS,TC, TM	*Vibrio cholerae*	Rahman *et al.* (2007)
ABC superfamily			
DrrAB	DA, DR, EB, TC, NOR	*Mycobacterium tuberculosis*	Choudhuri *et al.* (2002); De Rossi *et al.* (2006)
Bcg0231	AP, CM, SM, VC	*Mycobacterium bovis BCG*	Danilchanka *et al.* (2008)
Rv0194	AP, EM, NO, VC	*M. tuberculosis*	Danilchanka *et al.* (2008)
SmdAB	DP, HO, NF, TC	*S. marcescens*	Matsuo *et al.* (2008)
VcaM	DN, DP, DR, FQ, HO, TC	*V. cholerae*	Huda *et al.* (2003)
MATE superfamily			
AbeM	AC, AG, DN, DR, FQ, HO, RG	*Acinetobacter baumannii*	Su *et al.* (2005)
NorMI	AC, BB, FQ, GM, TPP	*Brucella melitensis*	Braibant *et al.* (2002)
HmrM	AC, BB, DC, DN, DP, DR, EB, HO, TPP, FQ	*Haemophilus influenzae*	Piddock (2006); Xu *et al.* (2003)
PmpM	AC, BC, EB, TPP, FQ	*P. aeruginosa*	He *et al.* (2004)
DinF	AC, AP, BB, EB, TPP	*Ralstonia solanacearum*	Brown *et al.* (2007)
MepA	CI, EB, FQ, MDB, TG	*S. aureus*	Kaatz *et al.* (2005); Kaatz *et al.* (2006); McAleese *et al.* (2005)
SMR superfamily			
EmrE	AC, EB, MV, QAC, AG	*E. coli, P. aeruginosa*	Li *et al.* (2003); Yerushalmi *et al.* (1995)
TehAB	DL, EB, KT, MV, PF	*E. coli*	Turner *et al.* (1997)
Mmr	AC, CIP, EB, EM, NOR, TPP	*M. tuberculosis, Mycobacterium smegmatis*	De Rossi *et al.* (1998)

Continued

Table 4.1. Continued.

Efflux pump(s)	Substrates	Organism(s)	Reference(s)
MdtJI	DC, SDS, SD	*E. coli*	Higashi *et al.* (2008)
SsmE	AC, EB, NF	*S. marcescens*	Minato *et al.* (2008)
SepA	AC, BC, CH	*S. aureus*	Narui *et al.* (2002)

AC, acriflavine; AG, aminoglycosides; AO, acridine orange; AP, ampicillin; BB, berberine; BC, benzalkonium chloride; BL, β-lactams; BS, bile salts; CAB, cetyltrimethylammonium bromide; CH, chlorhexidine; CL, cholate; CM, chloramphenicol; CI, cetrimide; CV, crystal violet; DA, daunorubicin, DD, diamidines; DC, deoxycholate; DL, dequalinium; DN, daunomycin; DP, 4′,6-diamidino-2-phenylindole; DQ, dequalinium chloride; DR, doxorubicin; EB, ethidium bromide; EM, erythromycin; FQ, fluoroquinolones; FU, fusidic acid; GM, gentamicin; HO, Hoechst 33342; KT, potassium tellurite; LA, lincosamides; MDB, monovalent and divalent biocides; ML, macrolides; MU, mupirocin; MV, methyl viologen; NF, norfloxacin; NO, novobiocin; OS, organic solvents; PF, proflavine; PH, phloretin; PM, polymyxin B; QAC, quaternary ammonium compounds; RG, rhodamine 6G; SDS, sodium dodecyl sulfate; SD, spermidine; SF, sulfonamides; SM, streptomycin; TC, tetracyclines; TG, tigecycline; TM, trimethoprim; TPP, tetraphenylphosphonium; TR, triclosan; VC, vancomycin; VM, virginiamycin.

of subinhibitory concentrations of an antibiotic following an 18h incubation at 37°C for *S. aureus*, measured by determining the absorption at 600nm (Belofsky *et al.*, 2004; Paixão *et al.*, 2009).

4.2.3 Checkerboard assay

Compounds possessing minimum inhibitory concentrations (MICs) of > 125 μM are considered to be inactive antimicrobials. The MIC is further tested for synergy with a range of concentrations of antibiotics against a single concentration of tested compounds in strains containing active EPs. If the test compound possesses EPI activity, then it will potentiate the antibiotic given at a subinhibitory concentration. This is defined as the modulating factor (MF) (Eliopoulos and Moellering, 1991; Kamicker *et al.*, 2008):

$$\text{MF} = \frac{\text{MIC (Antibiotic)}}{\text{MIC(Antibiotic + Modulator)}}$$

4.2.4 Fractional inhibitory testing

Any compound exhibiting an MF of ≥ 8 in combination with a single concentration of EPI is further tested by the more robust fractional inhibitory concentration (FIC) method. This method can distinguish whether two compounds together have an additive, synergistic or antagonistic effect on the bacteria. FIC indices (FICI) are interpreted as synergistic for values ≤ 0.5 and as antagonistic for values ≥ 4. The results in between synergy and antagonism are defined as additive or indifferent (Odds, 2003; Kamicker *et al.*, 2008). FICI is calculated as:

$$\text{FIC(A)} = \frac{\text{MIC(A in presence of B)}}{\text{MIC (A alone)}}$$

$$\text{FIC(B)} = \frac{\text{MIC (B in presence of A)}}{\text{MIC (B alone)}}$$

$$\text{FICI} = \text{FIC(A)} + \text{FIC(B)}$$

4.2.5 Protonophore assay

Determination of FIC is followed by the protonophore assay, which uses an *E. coli* strain that allows radiolabelled lactose to accumulate in the cell via the proton motive force (i.e. the membrane potential and the pH gradient). Any potential EPI that also disrupts the proton motive force is not working through EP mechanisms and is excluded as a potential EPI (Kamicker *et al.*, 2008).

4.2.6 Time–kill studies

A time–kill test is the final *in vitro* step in the search for a successful EPI. It is a basic microbiology method for assessment of antimicrobial activity. The time–kill test is carried out to evaluate the microbial reduction by antimicrobials against selected organisms such as *S. aureus*, *P. aeruginosa*, *E. coli* and *Aspergillus niger* (Ackerman *et al.*, 1992; Accugen Laboratories, 2012).

4.3 Natural Product EPIs

Natural products have always played a major role in providing bioactive molecules with various scaffolds and showing numerous activities against infectious and non-infectious diseases. These molecules are biosynthesized by enzymatic transformation, and are highly regio-, enantio- and diastereospecific.

Some EPs have been shown to selectively extrude specific antibiotics, while others expel various antibiotics and are referred to as multidrug resistant (MDR). EPIs can restore the clinical utility of some older antibiotics, to increase their potency and avoid the development of resistance. Several natural products have been described as EPIs against various EPs present in the bacterial cell membrane (reviewed Tegos, 2006; Stavri *et al.*, 2007; Gibbons, 2008). In this chapter, we will describe some EPIs of plant origin against *Mycobacterium* EPs, the NorA pump in *S. aureus* and EPIs specific for *Candida albicans* EPs.

4.3.1 Mycobacterial EPIs

There are numerous antibiotics for the treatment of TB, which are categorized as first- and second-line drugs and act through different mechanisms. However, the development of resistance in *Mycobacterium* makes many anti-TB drugs ineffective. According to the World Health Organization (WHO), more than 110,000 deaths, approximately 490,000 cases of MDR to first-line TB drugs and 40,000 cases of extensive drug resistance to both first- and second-line TB drugs emerge every year (WHO, 2008). There are several natural products that have been tested against various resistant *Mycobacterium* strains, which act as EPIs and have shown promising results, reducing the MIC of some of the drugs used clinically in TB treatment (Fig. 4.2).

Plant flavonoids (see Fig. 4.2, compounds 1–3) and resveratrol (4) have been tested for their synergistic effect with ethidium bromide against the mc^2 155 strain of *Mycobacterium smegmatis*. Baicalein (1) could modulate the MIC of ethidium bromide at least to a small extent, whereas biochanin A (2) was shown to be the best modulator and could decrease the MIC of ethidium bromide four- to eightfold at 10 mg/l and 16- to 32-fold at 32 mg/l. Similarly genistein (3) at 32 mg/l and resveratrol (4) at 16 mg/l decreased the MIC of ethidium bromide twofold (Lechner *et al.*, 2008a).

A few other flavonoids such as (–)-epicatechin (5), kaempferol (6), isorhamnetin (7), taxifolin (8), rutin (9) at 32 mg/l, and myricetin (10) and quercetin (11) at 16 µg/ml in combination with isoniazid, decreased the MICs of isoniazid against various *Mycobacterium* strains (Lechner *et al.*, 2008b).

Totarol (12), ferruginol (13), sandaracopimeric acid (14), and 4-epiabetol (15) isolated from the leaves and bark of *Juniperus procera*, plumbagin (16) isolated from aerial parts of *Plumbago zeylanica*, and ferulenol (17) isolated from the rhizomes of *Ferula communis* decreased the MIC of isoniazid, two- to eightfold against the resistant *M. tuberculosis* H37Rv strain (Mossa *et al.*, 2004).

Synergy assays have indicated that farnesol (18) decreased the MIC of ethidium bromide eightfold against *M. smegmatis* mc^2 155 ATCC 700084 when incorporated at a concentration of 32 µg/ml and decreased the MIC fourfold at 16 µg/ml (Jin *et al.*, 2010).

Curcumin (19) and demethoxycurcumin (20) modulated the MIC of isoniazid by four- and 16-fold, respectively, against *M. smegmatis* mc^2 155 ATCC 700084 when co-administered at 32 µg/ml (Lechner *et al.*, 2008c).

4.3.2 *S. aureus* NorA multidrug EPIs

The NorA multidrug transporter is the most explored example of MF superfamily, contributing to the resistance of *S. aureus* by overexpressing the efflux system. The NorA pump can efflux berberine and fluoroquinolones such as ciprofloxacin and norfloxacin (Yoshida *et al.*, 1990). The natural products that showed good EPI activity against NorA EP in *S. aureus* are shown in Fig. 4.3.

Polyphenols

2-ARYLBENZOFURAN. Spinosan A (21) isolated from *Dalea spinosa*, when used at 48 µM, decreased the MIC of berberine approximately eight- and 62-fold, respectively, against wild-type *S. aureus*, whereas pterocarpan (22) at 56 µM reduced the MIC of berberine by fourfold (Belofsky *et al.*, 2006).

N-CAFFEOYLPHENALKYLAMIDES. *N-trans*-feruloyl 4′-*O*-methyldopamine (23) isolated from *Mirabilis jalapa* showed moderate activity as an EPI against MDR *S. aureus* overexpressing the multidrug efflux transporter NorA, causing an eightfold reduction in the norfloxacin MIC at 100 µg/ml (Michalet *et al.*, 2007).

CHALCONES. A chalcone (24) isolated from *Dalea versicolor* at 10 µg/ml concentration enhanced the activity of berberine fourfold against MDR *S. aureus* (Belofsky *et al.*, 2004).

COUMARINS. The coumarins 4-(((*E*)-5-(3,3-dimethyl-2-oxiranyl)-3-methyl-2-pentenyl) oxy)-7*H*-furo(3,2-g)chromen-7-one (25) and 7-(((E)-5-(3,3-dimethyl-2-oxiranyl)-3-methyl-2-pentenyl)oxy)-2H-2-chromenone (26) isolated from grape fruit oil exhibited the potential to decrease the MIC of norfloxacin

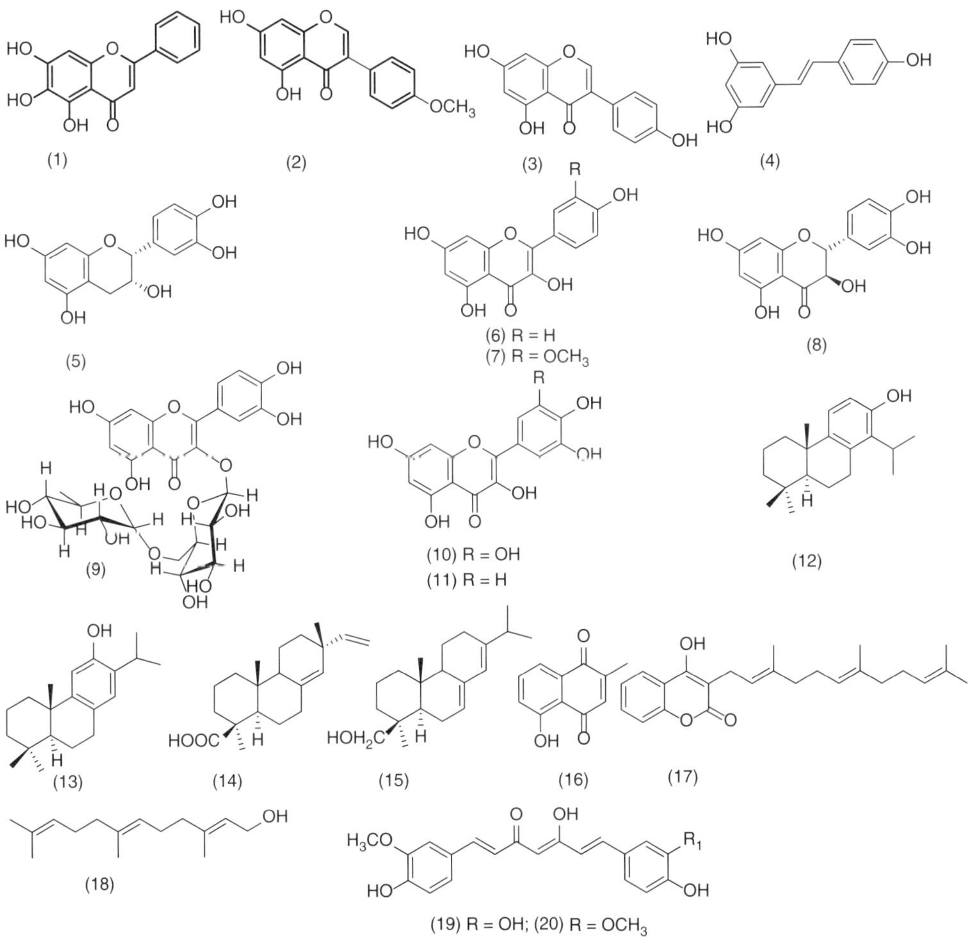

Fig. 4.2. *Mycobacterium* sp. efflux pump inhibitors from natural products (see text for details).

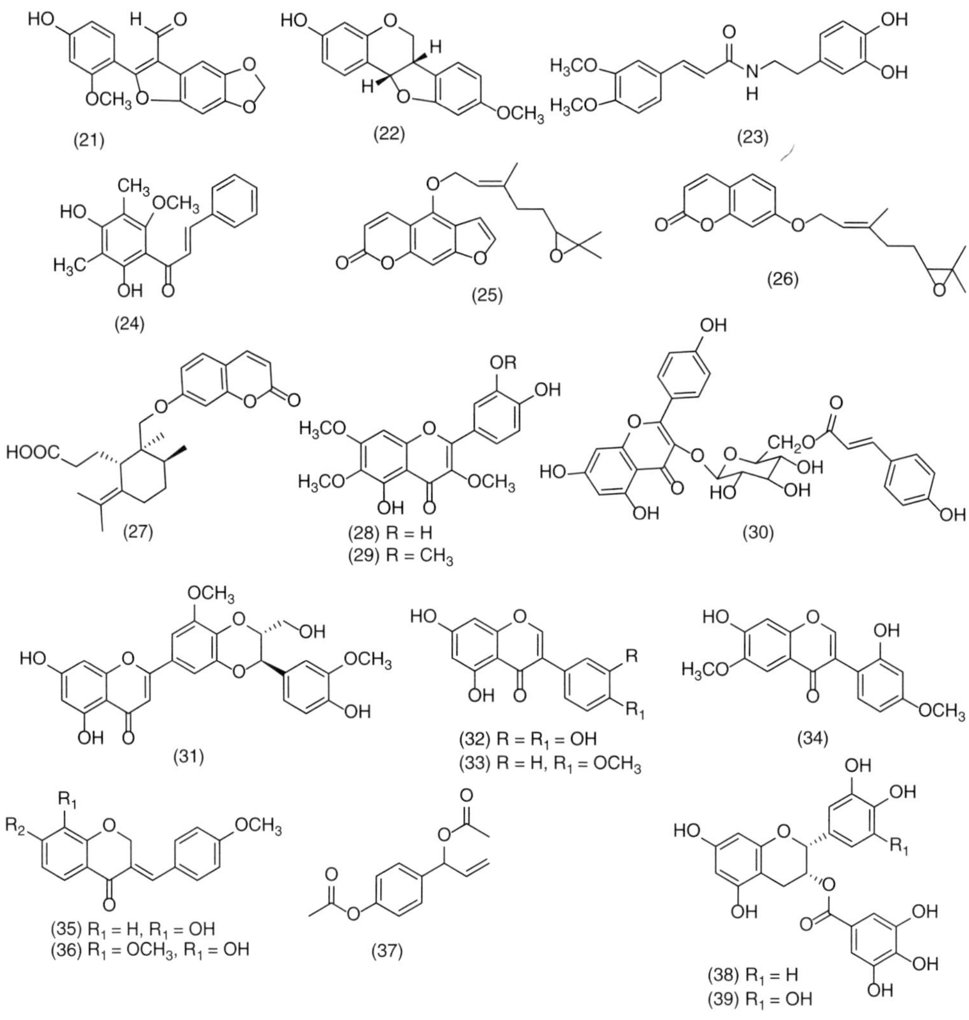

Fig. 4.3. *Staphylococcus aureus* NorA efflux pump inhibitors from natural products (see text for details).

by 20-fold in resistant *S. aureus* at a concentration of 35.7 mg/l and 30 mg/l, respectively (Abulrob *et al.*, 2004).

Galbanic acid (27), a sesquiterpene coumarin isolated from the roots of *Ferula szowitsiana*, at 300 μg/ml reduced the MIC of ciprofloxacin from 10–80 to ≤2.5–5 μg/ml and of ethidium bromide from 4–16 0.5–2 μg/ml against various resistant clinical isolates of *S. aureus* (Bazzaz *et al.*, 2010).

FLAVONOLS. Chrysosplenol-D (28) and chrysoplenetin (29), isolated from *Artemisia annua*, inhibited the growth of *S. aureus* in the presence of a subinhibitory concentration of berberine (30 μg/ml) with MICs of 25 mg/l and 6.25 mg/l, respectively (Stermitz *et al.*, 2002). Tiliroside (30), isolated from aerial parts of *Herissantia tiubae*, showed no antibacterial activity at 128 μg/ml against *S. aureus* (MIC of 256 μg/ml). However, when it was incorporated in the growth medium at 64 μg/ml (0.25 MIC) or 32 μg/ml (0.125 MIC), a reduction in the MIC of ciprofloxacin was observed up to 16- and eightfold, respectively (Falcão-Silva *et al.*, 2009).

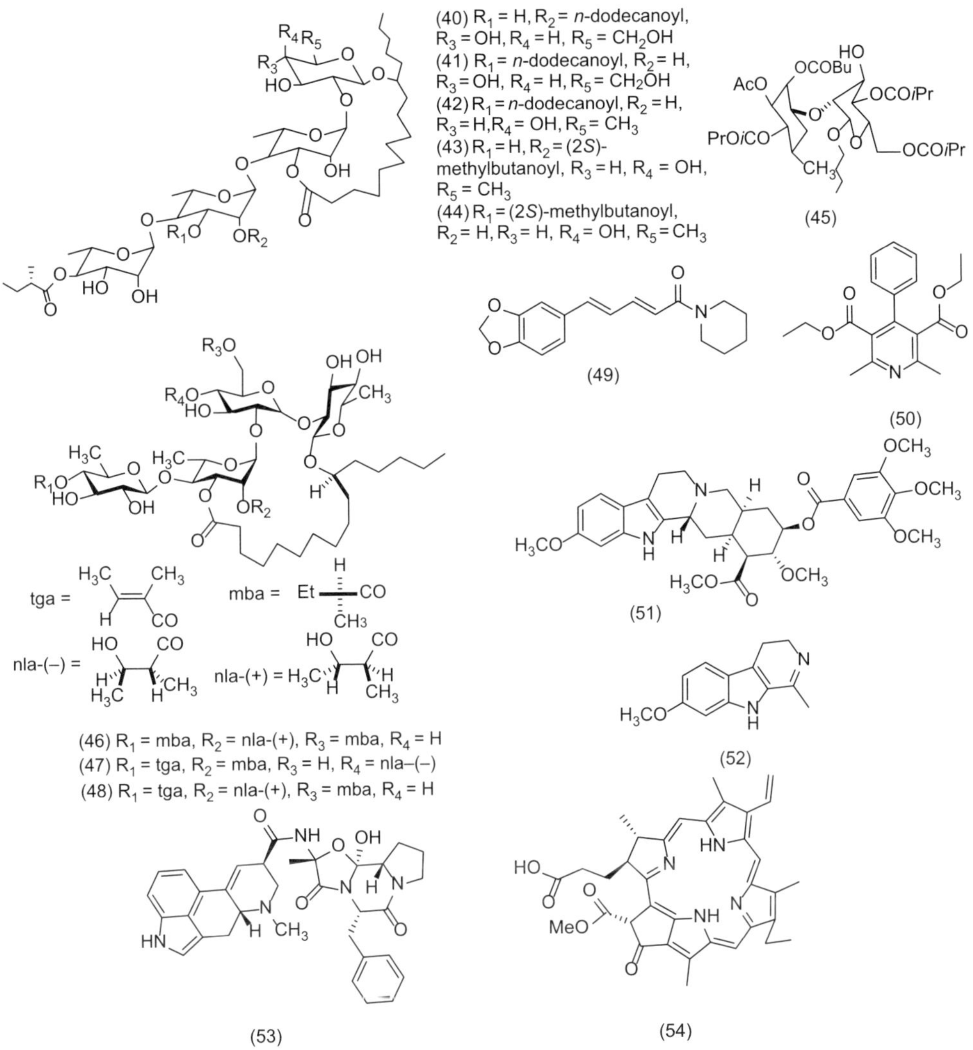

Fig. 4.3. Continued.

FLAVONOLIGNANS. The flavonolignan 5′-methoxyhydnocarpin-D (31) isolated from the leaves of *Berberis aetnensis*, at 10 μg/ml reduced the MIC of norfloxacin to 0.25 μg/ml against wild-type *S. aureus*, indicating complete inhibition of efflux of this antibiotic by the compound (Stermitz *et al.*, 2000).

ISOFLAVONES. The isoflavones genistein (3), orobol (32) and biochanin A (33) isolated from *Lupinus argenteus* decreased the MIC of norfloxacin two- to fourfold against a mutant strain of *S. aureus* when added at a concentration of 10 μg/ml (Morel *et al.*, 2003), whereas 6,4′-dimethoxy-7,2′-dihydroxyisoflavone (34), an isoflavone isolated from *D. spinosa*, at a concentration of 48 μM, showed a fourfold decrease in the MIC of berberine (89 μM) against wild-type *S. aureus* (Belofsky *et al.*, 2006).

HOMOISOFLAVONOIDS. The two homoisoflavonoids bonducellin (35) and 8-methoxybonducellin (36), isolated from *Caesalpinia digyna*, were found to potentiate berberine activity (unpublished data).

PHENYLPROPANOIDS. Acetoxycavicolacetate (37), isolated from the rhizomes of *Alpinia galangal*, was found to enhance ethidium bromide activity when incorporated at a concentration 50 μg/ml (unpublished data).

TANNINS. Epicatechin gallate (38) and epigallocatechin gallate (39) enhanced the activity of norfloxacin fourfold against a wild-type and a NorA-overexpressing *S. aureus* strain at a concentration of 20 μg/ml (Gibbons *et al.*, 2004).

Diterpenes

Ferruginol (13) isolated from *Chamaecyparis lawsoniana*, showed NorA pump inhibitory activity against resistant *S. aureus* bacteria. When used at a subinhibitory concentration (2 μg/ml), ferruginol resulted in twofold potentiation of norfloxacin activity against *S. aureus* strain SA-1199B (Smith *et al.*, 2007).

Oligosaccharides

Five murucoidins (XII–XVI) (40–44) were isolated from *Ipomoea murucoides*. Murucoidins XII, XIII, XV and XVI potentiated the activity of norfloxacin fourfold at concentrations of 25 μg/ml, while murucoidin XIV exerted the same potentiation effect at a concentration of 5 μg/ml against strains of *S. aureus* (Chérigo *et al.*, 2009).

A penta-ester compound (45) isolated from *Geranium caespitosum* reduced the MIC of berberine up to 40-fold at a concentration of 10 μg/ml against *S. aureus* SA-1199B (Stermitz *et al.*, 2003).

A phytochemical investigation of Mexican morning glory led to the isolation of orizabin XIX (46), orizabin IX (47) and orizabin XV (48), which showed a potentiation effect of norfloxacin against the NorA-overexpressing *S. aureus* SA-1199B. The amphipathic orizabin XIX increased the activity of norfloxacin fourfold (from 32 to 8 mg/l) at a concentration of 25 mg/l, while orizabin IX enhanced norfloxacin activity 16-fold at a concentration of 1 mg/l. Orizabin XV showed nearly equipotent activity with respect to orizabin IX in an ethidium bromide EPI assay (Pereda-Miranda *et al.*, 2006).

Alkaloids

Piperine (49), isolated from *Piper nigrum*, when co-administered at a concentration of 50 μg/ml with ciprofloxacin, inhibited growth of a mutant *S. aureus*, even at the 1 μg/ml concentration of ciprofloxacin (Khan *et al.*, 2006).

2,6-Dimethyl-4-phenylpyridine-3,5-dicarboxylic acid diethyl ester (50) isolated from *Jatropha elliptica*, reduced the MIC of ciprofloxacin at a concentration of 2 mg/l against NorA-overexpressing *S. aureus* SA-1199B (Marquez *et al.*, 2005).

Reserpine (51), isolated from *Rauwolfia vomitoria*, increased the activity of tetracycline (fourfold reduction in MIC) in two clinical isolates of methicillin-resistant *S. aureus*, IS-58 and XU212, which possessed the Tet(K) efflux protein. Reserpine also reversed the NorA pump and enhanced the activity of norfloxacin against *S. aureus* fourfold (Gibbons and Udo, 2000). Harmaline (52), isolated from *Perganum harmala*, reduced the MIC of ethidium bromide fourfold against *S. aureus* U949 (Mohtar *et al.*, 2009). Ergotamine (53), an indole alkaloid from *Claviceps purpurea*, displayed no direct antibacterial activity but, in combination, with norfloxacin at 20 μg/ml, caused a fourfold reduction in norfloxacin MIC against a norfloxacin-resistant strain of *S. aureus* (Gibbons, 2008).

Pheophorbide *a* (54) isolated from *B. aetnensis* enhanced the activity of ciprofloxacin 16-fold when co-administrated at a concentration of 0.5 μg/ml (Musumeci *et al.*, 2003).

4.4 Fungal EPIs

Analysis of the *C. albicans* genome has identified several EPs (CDR1, CDR2, CDR3, CDR4, CDR5, SNQ2 and YOR1) belonging to the ABC superfamily, responsible for the development of resistance to various azole antibiotics (itraconazole, fluconazole, ketoconazole and meconazole) on prolonged use. Tacrolimus (FK-506) (55), unnaramicin A (56), unnaramicin C (57),

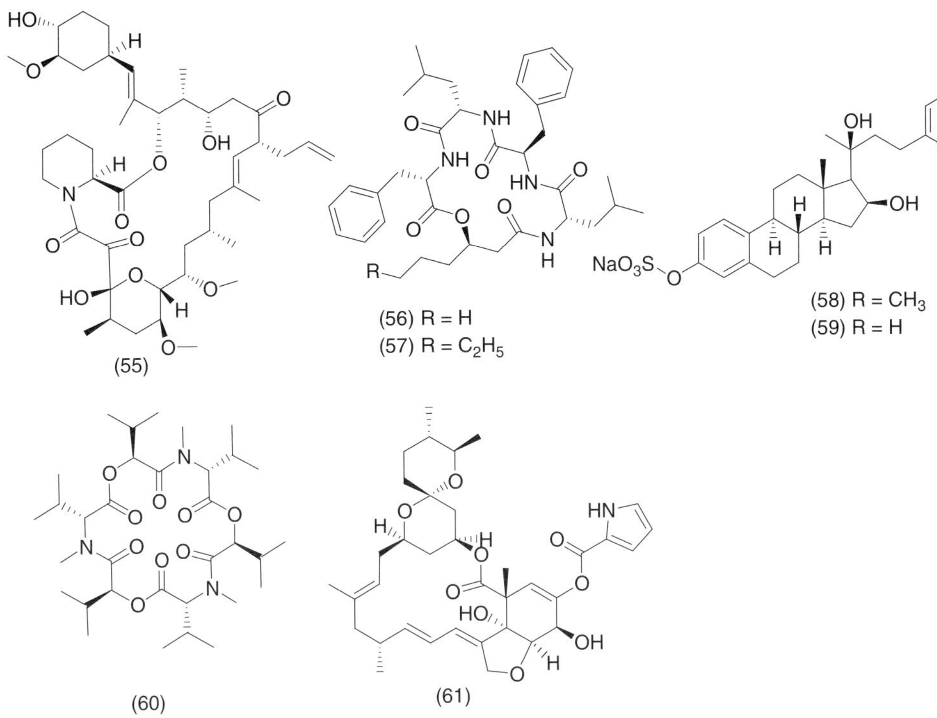

Fig. 4.4. *Candida albicans* efflux pump inhibitors from natural products (see text for details).

geodisterol-3-*O*-sulfite (58), 29-demethylgeodisterol-3-*O*-sulfite (59), enniatin B (60) and milbemycin α_9 (61) are examples of EPIs in the ABC superfamily (Cannon *et al.*, 2009, Tegos *et al.*, 2011) (Fig. 4.4).

Tacrolimus, isolated from the fermentation broth of *Streptomyces tsukubaensis* No. 9993, added at a subinhibitory concentration (10^{-5} to 10^{-3} mM) reduced the itraconazole MIC against azole-resistant *C. albicans* C26 (CDR1-expressing resistant strain) from 8 to 0.5 mg/l (Kino *et al.*, 1987, Maesaki *et al.*, 1998). The MIC of itraconazole against *C. albicans* resistant strain C40 (MDR strain) decreased from 0.5 to 0.06 mg/l in the presence of tacrolimus (Maesaki *et al.*, 1998). The cyclodepsipeptides unnaramicin A and unnaramicin C were isolated from the extracts of the marine bacterium *Photobacterium* sp. MBIC06485 (Oku *et al.*, 2008). Unnaramicin A and unnaramicin C reduced the MIC of fluconazole by 64-fold (from 320 to 5 μg/ml) against azole-resistant *C. albicans* at a concentration of 5 and 1.25 μM, respectively (Tanabe *et al.*, 2007). Geodisterol-3-*O*-sulfite and 29-demethylgeodisterol-3-*O*-sulfite, isolated from marine sponge *Topsentia* sp., enhanced the activity of fluconazole against an overexpressed MDR1 clinical isolate of *C. albicans* (DiGirolamo *et al.*, 2009). Enniatin B at concentration of 6.0 μM reduced the 50% inhibitory concentration of cycloheximide by eightfold (from 0.13 to 0.016 μg/ml) against a Pdr5p-overexpressing strain of *Saccharomyces cerevisiae* (Hiraga *et al.*, 2005). Milbemycin α_9 was found to enhance the activity of fluconazole and SCH-56592 against clinical isolates of *C. albicans* (Lee *et al.*, 2001).

4.5 Conclusion

Clinical reports signify that emergence of resistance to antibiotics in bacteria is increasing rapidly. So, there is an urgent need to develop an alternative source that reduces the bacterial resistance and potentiates the existing antibiotics. At present there is not a single antibiotic combined with an EPI on the market. Although drug discovery from natural products is time consuming and expensive, it can play a significant role in the discovery of new or novel lead molecules as EPIs. The EPIs discussed herein are in the preliminary stage of drug discovery. These EPIs require further detailed studies to ensure safety and efficacy before they will be drug candidates. Reserpine is one example that exhibited potential EPI activity, but has not been investigated further because it causes neurotoxicity (Markham and Neyfakh, 1996).

A majority of the EPIs discussed are active against Gram-positive bacteria (*S. aureus*). A few of them showed activity against acid-fast Gram-positive bacteria (*Mycobacteria*). Fewer studies have been published regarding activity against Gram-negative bacteria (*Pseudomonas, Escherichia*) because of the thick, lipophilic outer membrane that provides these organisms with a permeability barrier against hydrophilic compounds. Thus, detailed studies are necessary in the investigation of potential EPIs derived from natural products as lead molecules to combat resistant microorganisms.

References

Abulrob, A.N., Suller, M.T.E., Gumbleton, M., Simons, C. and Russell, A. (2004) Identification and biological evaluation of grapefruit oil components as potential novel efflux pump modulators in methicillin-resistant *Staphylococcus aureus* bacterial strains. *Phytochemistry* 65, 3021–3027.

Accugen Laboratories (2012) Time kill test. Available at: http://www.accugenlabs.com/killtimestudy.html (accessed 6 March 2012).

Ackerman, B.H., Vannier, A.M. and Eudy, E.B. (1992) Analysis of vancomycin time-kill studies with *Staphylococcus* species by using a curve stripping program to describe the relationship between concentration and pharmacodynamic response. *Antimicrobial Agents and Chemotherapy* 36, 1766–1769.

Akiba, M., Lin, J., Barton, Y.W. and Zhang, Q. (2006) Interaction of CmeABC and CmeDEF in conferring antimicrobial resistance and maintaining cell viability in *Campylobacter jejuni. Journal of Antimicrobial Chemotherapy* 57, 52–60.

Alekshun, M.N. and Levy, S.B. (2007) Molecular mechanisms of antibacterial multidrug resistance. *Cell* 128, 1037–1050.

Bazzaz, B.S.F., Memariani, Z., Khashiarmanesh, Z., Iranshahi, M. and Naderinasab, M. (2010) Effect of galbanic acid, a sesquiterpene coumarin from *Ferula szowitsiana*, as an inhibitor of efflux mechanism in resistant clinical isolates of *Staphylococcus aureus. Brazilian Journal of Microbiology* 41, 574–580.

Belofsky, G., Percivill, D., Lewis, K., Tegos, G.P. and Ekart, J. (2004) Phenolic metabolites of *Dalea versicolor* that enhance antibiotic activity against model pathogenic bacteria. *Journal of Natural Products* 67, 481–484.

Belofsky, G., Carreno, R., Lewis, K., Ball, A., Casadei, G. and Tegos, G.P. (2006) Metabolites of the "Smoke Tree", *Dalea spinosa*, potentiate antibiotic activity against multidrug-resistant *Staphylococcus aureus. Journal of Natural Products* 69, 261–264.

Bohn, C. and Bouloc, P. (1998) The *Escherichia coli cmlA* gene encodes the multidrug efflux pump Cmr/MdfA and is responsible for isopropyl-β-D-thiogalactopyranoside exclusion and spectinomycin sensitivity. *Journal of Bacteriology* 180, 6072–6075.

Braibant, M., Guilloteau, L. and Zygmunt, M.S. (2002) Functional characterization of *Brucella melitensis* NorMI, an efflux pump belonging to the multidrug and toxic compound extrusion family. *Antimicrobial Agents and Chemotherapy* 46, 3050–3053.

Brown, D.G., Swanson, J.K. and Allen, C. (2007) Two host-induced *Ralstonia solanacearum* genes, *acrA* and *dinF*, encode multidrug efflux pumps and contribute to bacterial wilt virulence. *Applied and Environmental Microbiology* 73, 2777–2786.

Cannon, R.D., Lamping, E., Holmes, A.R., Niimi, K., Baret, P.V., Keniya, M.V., Tanabe, K., Niimi, M., Goffeau, A. and Monk, B.C. (2009) Efflux-mediated antifungal drug resistance. *Clinical Microbiology Reviews* 22, 291–321.

Cao, L., Srikumar, R. and Poole, K. (2004) MexAB-OprM hyperexpression in NalC-type multidrug-resistant *Pseudomonas aeruginosa*: identification and characterization of the *nalC* gene encoding a repressor of PA3720-PA3719. *Molecular Microbiology* 53, 1423–1436.

Chérigo, L., Pereda-Miranda, R. and Gibbons, S. (2009) Bacterial resistance modifying tetrasaccharide agents from *Ipomoea murucoides. Phytochemistry* 70, 222–227.

Chen, J., Kuroda, T., Huda, M.N., Mizushima, T. and Tsuchiya, T. (2003) An RND-type multidrug efflux pump SdeXY from *Serratia marcescens. Journal of Antimicrobial Chemotherapy* 52, 176–179.

Choudhuri, B.S., Bhakta, S., Barik, R., Basu, J., Kundu, M. and Chakrabarti, P. (2002) Overexpression and functional characterization of an ABC (ATP-binding cassette) transporter encoded by the genes *drrA* and *drrB* of *Mycobacterium tuberculosis. Biochemical Journal* 367, 279–285.

Daigle, D.M., Cao, L., Fraud, S., Wilke, M.S., Pacey, A., Klinoski, R., Strynadka, N.C., Dean, C.R. and Poole, K. (2007) Protein modulator of multidrug efflux gene expression in *Pseudomonas aeruginosa. Journal of Bacteriology* 189, 5441–5451.

Danilchanka, O., Mailaender, C. and Niederweis, M. (2008) Identification of a novel multidrug efflux pump of *Mycobacterium tuberculosis. Antimicrobial Agents and Chemotherapy* 52, 2503–2511.

De Rossi, E., Branzoni, M., Cantoni, R., Milano, A., Riccardi, G. and Ciferri, O. (1998) *mmr*, a *Mycobacterium tuberculosis* gene conferring resistance to small cationic dyes and inhibitors. *Journal of Bacteriology* 180, 6068–6071.

De Rossi, E., Aínsa, J.A. and Riccardi, G. (2006) Role of mycobacterial efflux transporters in drug resistance: an unresolved question. *FEMS Microbiology Reviews* 30, 36–52.

DiGirolamo, J.A., Li, X.C., Jacob, M.R., Clark, A.M. and Ferreira, D. (2009) Reversal of fluconazole resistance by sulfated sterols from the marine sponge *Topsentia* sp. *Journal of Natural Products* 72, 1524–1528.

Eliopoulos, G.M. and Moellering, R.C. (1991) *Antibiotics In Laboratory Medicine*, 3rd edn. Williams and Wilkins, Baltimore, Maryland.

Falcão-Silva, V.S., Silva, D.A., Souza, M.F.V. and Siqueira, J.P. Jr (2009) Modulation of drug resistance in *Staphylococcus aureus* by a kaempferol glycoside from *Herissantia tiubae* (Malvaceae). *Phytotherapy Research* 23, 1367–1370.

Gibbons, S. (2008) Phytochemicals for bacterial resistance – strengths, weaknesses and opportunities. *Planta Medica* 74, 594–602.

Gibbons, S. and Udo, E.E. (2000) The effect of reserpine, a modulator of multidrug efflux pumps, on the *in vitro* activity of tetracycline against clinical isolates of methicillin resistant *Staphylococcus aureus* (MRSA) possessing the *tet*(K) determinant. *Phytotherapy Research* 14, 139–140.

Gibbons, S., Moser, E. and Kaatz, G.W. (2004) Catechin gallates inhibit multidrug resistance (MDR) in *Staphylococcus aureus. Planta Medica* 70, 1240–1242.

He, G.X., Kuroda, T., Mima, T., Morita, Y., Mizushima, T. and Tsuchiya, T. (2004) An H^+-coupled multidrug efflux pump, PmpM, a member of the MATE family of transporters, from *Pseudomonas aeruginosa. Journal of Bacteriology* 186, 262–265.

Higashi, K., Ishigure, H., Demizu, R., Uemura, T., Nishino, K., Yamaguchi, A., Kashiwagi, K. and Igarashi, K. (2008) Identification of a spermidine excretion protein complex (MdtJI) in *Escherichia coli. Journal of Bacteriology* 190, 872–878.

Hiraga, K., Yamamoto, S., Fukuda, H., Hamanaka, N. and Oda, K. (2005) Enniatin has a new function as an inhibitor of Pdr5p, one of the ABC transporters in *Saccharomyces cerevisiae. Biochemical and Biophysical Research Communications* 328, 1119–1125.

Huang, J., O'Toole, P.W., Shen, W., Amrine-Madsen, H., Jiang, X., Lobo, N., Palmer, L.M., Voelker, L.R., Fan, F., Gwynn, M.N. and McDevitt, D. (2004) Novel chromosomally encoded multidrug efflux transporter MdeA in *Staphylococcus aureus. Antimicrobial Agents and Chemotherapy* 48, 909–917.

Huda, N., Lee, E.W., Chen, J., Morita, Y., Kuroda, T., Mizushima, T. and Tsuchiya, T. (2003) Molecular cloning and characterization of an ABC multidrug efflux pump, VcaM, in non-O1 *Vibrio cholerae. Antimicrobial Agents and Chemotherapy* 47, 2413–2417.

Jin, J., Zhang, J.Y., Guo, N., Sheng, H., Li, L., Liang, J.C., Wang, X.L., Li, Y., Liu, M.Y. and Wu, X.P. (2010) Farnesol, a potential efflux pump inhibitor in *Mycobacterium smegmatis. Molecules* 15, 7750–7762.

Jonas, B.M., Murray, B.E. and Weinstock, G.M. (2001) Characterization of *emeA*, a *norA* homolog and multidrug resistance efflux pump, in *Enterococcus faecalis. Antimicrobial Agents and Chemotherapy* 45, 3574–3579.

Kaatz, G.W., McAleese, F. and Seo, S.M. (2005) Multidrug resistance in *Staphylococcus aureus* due to overexpression of a novel multidrug and toxin extrusion (MATE) transport protein. *Antimicrobial Agents and Chemotherapy* 49, 1857–1864.

Kaatz, G.W., Demarco, C.E. and Seo, S.M. (2006) MepR, a repressor of the *Staphylococcus aureus* MATE family multidrug efflux pump MepA, is a substrate-responsive regulatory protein. *Antimicrobial Agents and Chemotherapy* 50, 1276–1281.

Kamicker, B.J., Sweeney, M.T., Kaczmarek, F., Dib-Hajj, F., Shang, W., Crimin, K., Duignan, J. and Gootz, T.D. (2008) Bacterial efflux pump inhibitors. In: Champney, W.S. (ed.) *Methods in Molecular Medicine*. Humana Press, Totowa, New Jersey, pp. 187–204.

Khan, I.A., Mirza, Z.M., Kumar, A., Verma, V. and Qazi, G.N. (2006) Piperine, a phytochemical potentiator of ciprofloxacin against *Staphylococcus aureus. Antimicrobial Agents and Chemotherapy* 50, 810–812.

Kino, T., Hatanaka, H., Hashimoto, M., Nishiyama, M., Goto, T., Okuhara, M., Kohsaka, M., Aoki, H. and Imanaka, H. (1987) FK-506, a novel immunosuppressant isolated from a *Streptomyces.* I. Fermentation, isolation, and physico-chemical and biological characteristics. *Journal of Antibiotics* 40, 1249–1255.

Lechner, D., Gibbons, S. and Bucar, F. (2008a) Plant phenolic compounds as ethidium bromide efflux inhibitors in *Mycobacterium smegmatis. Journal of Antimicrobial Chemotherapy* 62, 345–348.

Lechner, D., Gibbons, S. and Bucar, F. (2008b) Modulation of isoniazid susceptibility by flavonoids in *Mycobacterium. Phytochemistry Letters* 1, 71–75.

Lechner, D., Gibbons, S., Jachak, S., Srivastava, A. and Bucar, F. (2008c) Curcuminoids as efflux pump inhibitors (EPIs) in *Mycobacterium smegmatis* mc^2 155. In: Skaltsounis, L. and Magiatis, P. (eds) *Book of Abstracts. 7th Joint Meeting of GA, AFERP, ASP, PSI and SIF*, Athens, Greece, p. 12.

Lee, M.D., Galazzo, J.L., Staley, A.L., Lee, J.C., Warren, M.S., Fuernkranz, H., Chamberland, S., Lomovskaya, O. and Miller, G.H. (2001) Microbial fermentation-derived inhibitors of efflux-pump-mediated drug resistance. *Il Farmaco* 56, 81–85.

Li, X.Z. and Nikaido, H. (2004) Efflux-mediated drug resistance in bacteria. *Drugs* 64, 159–204.

Li, X.Z. and Nikaido, H. (2009) Efflux-mediated drug resistance in bacteria: an update. *Drugs* 69, 1555–1623.

Li, X.Z., Nikaido, H. and Poole, K. (1995) Role of MexA-MexB-OprM in antibiotic efflux in *Pseudomonas aeruginosa. Antimicrobial Agents and Chemotherapy* 39, 1948–1953.

Li, X.Z., Poole, K. and Nikaido, H. (2003) Contributions of MexAB-OprM and an EmrE homolog to intrinsic resistance of *Pseudomonas aeruginosa* to aminoglycosides and dyes. *Antimicrobial Agents and Chemotherapy* 47, 27–33.

Littlejohn, T.G., Paulsen, I.T., Gillespie, M.T., Tennent, J.M., Midgley, M., Jones, I.G., Purewal, A.S. and Skurray, R.A. (1992) Substrate specificity and energetics of antiseptic and disinfectant resistance in *Staphylococcus aureus. FEMS Microbiology Letters* 95, 259–265.

Maesaki, S., Marichal, P., Hossain, M.A., Sanglard, D., Vanden-Bossche, H. and Kohno, S. (1998) Synergic effects of tactolimus and azole antifungal agents against azole-resistant *Candida albicans* strains. *Journal of Antimicrobial Chemotherapy* 42, 747–753.

Markham, P.N. and Neyfakh, A.A. (1996) Inhibition of the multi-drug transporter NorA prevents emergence of norfloxacin resistance in *Staphylococcus aureus. Journal of Antimicrobial Chemotherapy* 40, 2673–2674.

Marquez, B., Neuville, L., Moreau, N.J., Genet, J.P., Dos Santos, A.F., Caño De Andrade, M.C. and Goulart, S.A. (2005) Multidrug resistance reversal agent from *Jatropha elliptica. Phytochemistry* 66, 1804–1811.

Matsuo, T., Chen, J., Minato, Y., Ogawa, W., Mizushima, T., Kuroda, T. and Tsuchiya, T. (2008) SmdAB, a heterodimeric ABC-type multidrug efflux pump, in *Serratia marcescens. Journal of Bacteriology* 190, 648–654.

McAleese, F., Petersen, P., Ruzin, A., Dunman, P.M., Murphy, E., Projan, S.J. and Bradford, P.A. (2005) A novel MATE family efflux pump contributes to the reduced susceptibility of laboratory-derived *Staphylococcus aureus* mutants to tigecycline. *Antimicrobial Agents and Chemotherapy* 49, 1865–1871.

McMurry, L., Petrucci, R.E. and Levy, S.B. (1980) Active efflux of tetracycline encoded by four genetically different tetracycline resistance determinants in *Escherichia coli. Proceedings of the National Academy of Sciences USA* 77, 3974–3977.

Medscap Reference (2009) Pseudomonas aeruginosa *infections.* Available at: http://emedicine.medscape.com/article/226748-overview (accessed 6 March 2012).

Michalet, S., Cartier, G., David, B., Mariotte, A.M., Dijoux-Franca, M.G., Kaatz, G.W., Stavri, M. and Gibbons, S. (2007) *N*-Caffeoylphenalkylamide derivatives as bacterial efflux pump inhibitors. *Bioorganic and Medicinal Chemistry Letters* 17, 1755–1758.

Miller, L.G., Perdreau-Remington, F., Rieg, G., Mehdi, S., Perlroth, J., Bayer, A.S., Tang, A.W., Phung, T.O. and Spellberg, B. (2005) Necrotizing fasciitis caused by community-associated methicillin-resistant *Staphylococcus aureus* in Los Angeles. *New England Journal of Medicine* 352, 1445–1453.

Minato, Y., Shahcheraghi, F., Ogawa, W., Kuroda, T. and Tsuchiya, T. (2008) Functional gene cloning and characterization of the SsmE multidrug efflux pump from *Serratia marcescens. Biological and Pharmaceutical Bulletin* 31, 516–519.

Mohtar, M., Johari, S.A., Li, A.R., Isa, M.M., Mustafa, S., Ali, A.M. and Basri, D.F. (2009) Inhibitory and resistance-modifying potential of plant-based alkaloids against methicillin-resistant *Staphylococcus aureus* (MRSA). *Current Microbiology* 59, 181–186.

Morel, C., Stermitz, F.R., Tegos, G. and Lewis, K. (2003) Isoflavones as potentiators of antibacterial activity. *Journal of Agriculture and Food Chemistry* 51, 5677–5679.

Mossa, J.S., El Feraly, F.S. and Muhammad, I. (2004) Antimycobacterial constituents from *Juniperus procera*, *Ferula communis* and *Plumbago zeylanica* and their *in vitro* synergistic activity with isonicotinic acid hydrazide. *Phytotherapy Research* 18, 934–937.

Musumeci, R., Speciale, A., Costanzo, R., Annino, A., Ragusa, S., Rapisarda, A., Pappalardo, M.S. and Iauk, L. (2003) *Berberis aetnensis* C. Presl. extracts: antimicrobial properties and interaction with ciprofloxacin. *International Journal of Antimicrobial Agents* 22, 48–53.

Narui, K., Noguchi, N., Wakasugi, K. and Sasatsu, M. (2002) Cloning and characterization of a novel chromosomal drug efflux gene in *Staphylococcus aureus*. *Biological and Pharmaceutical Bulletin* 25, 1533–1536.

Nishino, K., Latifi, T. and Groisman, E.A. (2006) Virulence and drug resistance roles of multidrug efflux systems of *Salmonella enterica* serovar Typhimurium. *Molecular Microbiology* 59, 126–141.

Odds, F.C. (2003) Synergy, antagonism, and what the chequerboard puts between them. *Journal of Antimicrobial Chemotherapy* 52, 1.

Oku, N., Kawabata, K., Adachi, K., Katsuta, A. and Shizuri, Y. (2008) Unnarmicins A and C, new antibacterial depsipeptides produced by marine bacterium *Photobacterium* sp. MBIC06485. *Journal of Antibiotics* 61, 11–17.

Paixão, L., Rodrigues, L., Couto, I., Martins, M., Fernandes, P., De Carvalho, C.C.C.R., Monteiro, G.A., Sansonetty, F., Amaral, L. and Viveiros, M. (2009) Fluorometric determination of ethidium bromide efflux kinetics in *Escherichia coli*. *Journal of Biological Engineering* 3, 18–30.

Pereda-Miranda, R., Kaatz, G.W. and Gibbons, S. (2006) Polyacylated oligosaccharides from medicinal Mexican morning glory species as antibacterials and inhibitors of multidrug resistance in *Staphylococcus aureus*. *Journal of Natural Products* 69, 406–409.

Piddock, L.J.V. (2006) Clinically relevant chromosomally encoded multidrug resistance efflux pumps in bacteria. *Clinical Microbiology Reviews* 19, 382–402.

Poole, K., Tetro, K., Zhao, Q., Neshat, S., Heinrichs, D.E. and Bianco, N. (1996) Expression of the multidrug resistance operon *mexA-mexB-oprM* in *Pseudomonas aeruginosa*: *mexR* encodes a regulator of operon expression. *Antimicrobial Agents and Chemotherapy* 40, 2021–2028.

Pumbwe, L., Randall, L.P., Woodward, M.J. and Piddock, L.J.V. (2005) Evidence for multiple-antibiotic resistance in *Campylobacter jejuni* not mediated by CmeB or CmeF. *Antimicrobial Agents and Chemotherapy* 49, 1289–1293.

Rahman, M.M., Matsuo, T., Ogawa, W., Koterasawa, M., Kuroda, T. and Tsuchiya, T. (2007) Molecular cloning and characterization of all RND-type efflux transporters in *Vibrio cholerae* non-O1. *Microbiology and Immunology* 51, 1061–1070.

Smith, E.C.J., Williamson, E.M., Wareham, N., Kaatz, G.W. and Gibbons, S. (2007) Antibacterials and modulators of bacterial resistance from the immature cones of *Chamaecyparis lawsoniana*. *Phytochemistry* 68, 210–217.

Sobel, M.L., Hocquet, D., Cao, L., Plesiat, P. and Poole, K. (2005) Mutations in PA3574 (*nalD*) lead to increased MexAB-OprM expression and multidrug resistance in laboratory and clinical isolates of *Pseudomonas aeruginosa*. *Antimicrobial Agents and Chemotherapy* 49, 1782–1786.

Stavri, M., Piddock, L.J. V. and Gibbons, S. (2007) Bacterial efflux pump inhibitors from natural sources. *Journal of Antimicrobial Chemotherapy* 59, 1247–1260.

Stermitz, F.R., Lorenz, P., Tawara, J.N., Zenewicz, L.A. and Lewis, K. (2000) Synergy in a medicinal plant: antimicrobial action of berberine potentiated by 5-methoxyhydnocarpin, a multidrug pump inhibitor. *Proceedings of the National Academy of Sciences USA* 97, 1433–1437.

Stermitz, F.R., Scriven, L.N., Tegos, G. and Lewis, K. (2002) Two flavonols from *Artemisa annua* which potentiate the activity of berberine and norfloxacin against a resistant strain of *Staphylococcus aureus*. *Planta Medica* 68, 1140–1141.

Stermitz, F.R., Cashman, K.K., Halligan, K.M., Morel, C., Tegos, G.P. and Lewis, K. (2003) Polyacylated neohesperidosides from *Geranium caespitosum*: bacterial multidrug resistance pump inhibitors. *Bioorganic and Medicinal Chemistry Letters* 13, 1915–1918.

Stoitsova, S.O., Braun, Y., Ullrich, M.S. and Weingart, H. (2008) Characterization of the RND-type multidrug efflux pump MexAB-OprM of the plant pathogen *Pseudomonas syringae*. *Applied and Environmental Microbiology* 74, 3387–3393.

Su, X.Z., Chen, J., Mizushima, T., Kuroda, T. and Tsuchiya, T. (2005) AbeM, an H^+-coupled *Acinetobacter baumannii* multidrug efflux pump belonging to the MATE family of transporters.

Antimicrobial Agents and Chemotherapy 49, 4362–4364.

Tanabe, K., Lamping, E., Adachi, K., Takano, Y., Kawabata, K., Shizuri, Y., Niimi, M. and Uehara, Y. (2007) Inhibition of fungal ABC transporters by unnarmicin A and unnarmicin C, novel cyclic peptides from marine bacterium. *Biochemical and Biophysical Research Communications* 364, 990–995.

Tegos, G.P. (2006) Natural substrates and inhibitors of multidrug resistant pumps (MDRs) redefine the plant antimicrobials. In: Rai, M. and Carpinella, M.C. (eds) *Naturally Occurring Bioactive Compounds.* Elsevier Publication, Amsterdam, pp. 45–59.

Tegos, P., Haynes, M., Jacob-Strouse, J., Khan, M.T., Bologa, G., Oprea, I. and Sklar, A. (2011) Microbial efflux pump inhibition: tactics and strategies. *Current Pharmaceutical Design* 17, 1291–1302.

Turner, R.J., Taylor, D.E. and Weiner, J.H. (1997) Expression of *Escherichia coli* TehA gives resistance to antiseptics and disinfectants similar to that conferred by multidrug resistance efflux pumps. *Antimicrobial Agents and Chemotherapy* 41, 440–444.

WHO (2008) World Health Organization reports highest rates of drug-resistant tuberculosis to date. Available at: http://www.who.int/tb/features_archive/drs_factsheet.pdf (accessed 6 March 2012).

Xu, X.J., Su, X.Z., Morita, Y., Kuroda, T., Mizushima, T. and Tsuchiya, T. (2003) Molecular cloning and characterization of the HmrM multidrug efflux pump from *Haemophilus influenzae* Rd. *Microbiology and Immunology* 47, 937–943.

Yamada, Y., Shiota, S., Mizushima, T., Kuroda, T. and Tsuchiya, T. (2006) Functional gene cloning and characterization of MdeA, a multidrug efflux pump from *Staphylococcus aureus. Biological and Pharmaceutical Bulletin* 29, 801–804.

Yerushalmi, H., Lebendyker, M. and Schuldiner, S. (1995) EmrE, an *Escherichia coli* 12-kDa multidrug transporter, exchanges toxic cations and H^+ and is soluble in organic solvents. *Journal of Biological Chemistry* 270, 6856–6863.

Yoshida, H., Bogaki, M., Nakamura, S., Ubukata, K. and Konno, M. (1990) Nucleotide sequence and characterization of the *Staphylococcus aureus norA* gene, which confers resistance to quinolones. *Journal of Bacteriology* 172, 6942–6949.

Zechini, B. and Versace, I. (2009) Inhibitors of multidrug resistant efflux systems in bacteria. *Recent Patents on Anti-infective Drug Discovery* 4, 37–50.

5 Fungal Efflux-mediated Resistance: from Targets to Inhibitors

Brian C. Monk,[1] Kyoko Niimi,[1] Ann R. Holmes,[1] J. Jacob Strouse,[2] Larry A. Sklar[2] and Richard D. Cannon[1]
[1] *Sir John Walsh Research Institute, University of Otago, Dunedin, New Zealand;* [2] *University of New Mexico Center for Molecular Discovery, Albuquerque, New Mexico, USA*

5.1 Introduction

Fungi are responsible for significant infections of plants and animals. Fungi and their toxins cause considerable damage to agriculturally important cereal and fruit crops. Farmers often use large amounts of fungicides to prevent crop damage and this can lead to the emergence of fungicide resistance. In humans, fungi often cause relatively mild superficial infections, such as athlete's foot or vaginal thrush, in a large proportion of the healthy population. In the immunocompromised, however, they can cause life-threatening disseminated disease that is exacerbated by antifungal resistance. There are relatively few classes of antifungal agents (Sanglard and Bille, 2002; Monk and Goffeau, 2008). The pyrimidine analogues, such as 5-fluorocytosine, inhibit RNA and DNA synthesis. The polyene antifungals, such as nystatin and amphotericin B, insert in the fungal plasma membrane and associate with ergosterol, and this leads to the formation of annuli that disrupt membrane integrity. The azoles, such as the well-tolerated and widely used fluconazole (FLC), target synthesis of the major fungal membrane sterol, ergosterol, by inhibiting lanosterol 14α-demethylase. The echinocandin derivatives, including caspofungin, micafungin and anidulafungin, non-competitively inhibit the enzyme that synthesizes the essential cell-wall component β-1,3-glucan (Odds *et al.*, 2003). It is important to note that the targets of the pyrimidine analogues and azoles are intracellular, while the polyenes insert in the plasma membrane. It is not known whether the echinocandins interact with plasma membrane enzyme β-1,3-glucan synthase from the cytoplasm or periplasm.

Indiscriminate use of antifungals at sub-optimum dosages has led to the development of resistance by both phytopathogens and human pathogens. Resistance to azole antifungals is most prominent. The azoles are fungistatic and their stress response to azole exposure enables fungi to acquire resistance (Cannon *et al.*, 2007). While there are several mechanisms of resistance, including increased expression of the drug target and point mutations in the target, high-level azole resistance in clinical isolates of human pathogens such as *Candida albicans* correlates with overexpression of efflux pumps located in the plasma membrane (Sanglard and Bille, 2002; Cannon *et al.*, 2009). The pumps reduce intracellular azole concentrations to levels at which the intracellular target is no longer inhibited. Although fungal genomes contain numerous genes encoding efflux pumps, in *C. albicans* the ATP-binding cassette (ABC) transporter Cdr1p contributes most to the azole resistance of clinical isolates (Holmes *et al.*, 2008;

Tsao *et al.*, 2009). This was a significant discovery in our extensive search for pump inhibitors that could be used in combination with azoles to overcome efflux-mediated resistance – an approach analogous to the use of augmentin for bacterial infections where the β-lactamase inhibitor clavulanic acid is combined with the β-lactam amoxicillin.

In this chapter, we will describe our use of heterologous expression of fungal efflux pumps in *Saccharomyces cerevisiae* for medium- and high-throughput screening to identify pump inhibitors. We will also discuss strategies for overcoming some of the limitations of current antifungal drugs and for identifying novel drug targets not subject to efflux-mediated resistance.

5.2 Fungal Efflux Pumps as a Drug Target

There are two main types of fungal drug efflux pump (Cannon *et al.*, 2009). Major facilitator superfamily (MFS) transporters use the electrochemical gradient across the plasma membrane to expel drugs from cells (Fig. 5.1). ABC transporters, in contrast, use ATP binding and hydrolysis to efflux drugs. Although fungal cells contain many genes for both types of pump, clinical azole resistance is most often associated with overexpression of ABC transporters (Holmes *et al.*, 2008; Cannon *et al.*, 2009). Therefore, ABC pumps represent a prime target for overcoming efflux-mediated azole resistance. MFS pumps are valuable, none the less, as a counter-screen to ensure that pump inhibitors identified in screens of compounds are ABC pump-specific (Fig. 5.1).

There are several classes of fungal ABC transporter, and the pleiotropic drug resistance (PDR) family is often responsible for fungal drug resistance (Lamping *et al.*, 2010). Clinically important PDR transporters include *C. albicans* Cdr1p (CaCdr1p) and CaCdr2p, which are orthologues of *S. cerevisiae* Pdr5p (ScPdr5p), and mammalian G-type ABC transporters. CaCdr2p appears to be the product of recent gene duplication, with the induced expression of CaCdr2p providing a detectable, but less important, contribution to triazole resistance than CaCdr1p (Holmes *et al.*, 2006; Holmes *et al.*, 2008; Cannon *et al.*, 2009). Fungal PDR efflux pumps have relatively promiscuous substrate specificities that are thought to be defined primarily by their transmembrane domains. These specificities often partially overlap among family members in a particular organism and thus provide broad-spectrum protection against xenobiotic threat, including that posed by the widely used and well-tolerated imidazole and triazole drugs.

Typical PDR ABC pumps consist of two homologous halves. Each half contains a transmembrane domain (TMD) with six transmembrane spans and a cytosolic nucleotide-binding domain (NBD) (Fig. 5.1). PDR transporters have a 'reverse' topology to the $(TMD–NBD)_2$ of most full-sized eukaryotic ABC transporters (Dean, 2005; Lamping *et al.*, 2010). In addition to this distinctive topology, the NBDs of most fungal PDR transporters appear less symmetrical than their mammalian ABC transporter counterparts (Lamping *et al.*, 2010). This is partly due to the presence in PDR transporters of a Walker A motif in the N-terminal NBD that has a conserved lysine replaced with a cysteine. Interestingly, the mammalian homologues (e.g. ABCG2) of the fungal PDR group are all half-sized and thus symmetrical when they assemble into homotetrameric functional units. Single particle analysis of ScPdr5p suggests that the functional unit for full-sized family members is also a dimer comprising two full-sized subunits in total (Ferreira-Pereira *et al.*, 2003).

Fungal PDR transporters, like many other ABC pumps, are truly pleiotropic, and several hundred substrates have been reported (Kolaczkowski *et al.*, 1998). Many substrates appear to be chemically unrelated, but most are hydrophobic and sufficiently charged to facilitate oriented binding at a large hydrophobic binding site. This site is thought to be capable of attracting multiple substrates from the inner leaflet of the plasma membrane or from the cytoplasm. Golin and colleagues have demonstrated that ScPdr5p binds the substrates rhodamine 6G (R6G), cycloheximide and triazole drugs via sites that, at best, partially overlap, and that substrate size may be a key characteristic (Golin *et al.*, 2003, 2007). The presence of separate non-interacting binding

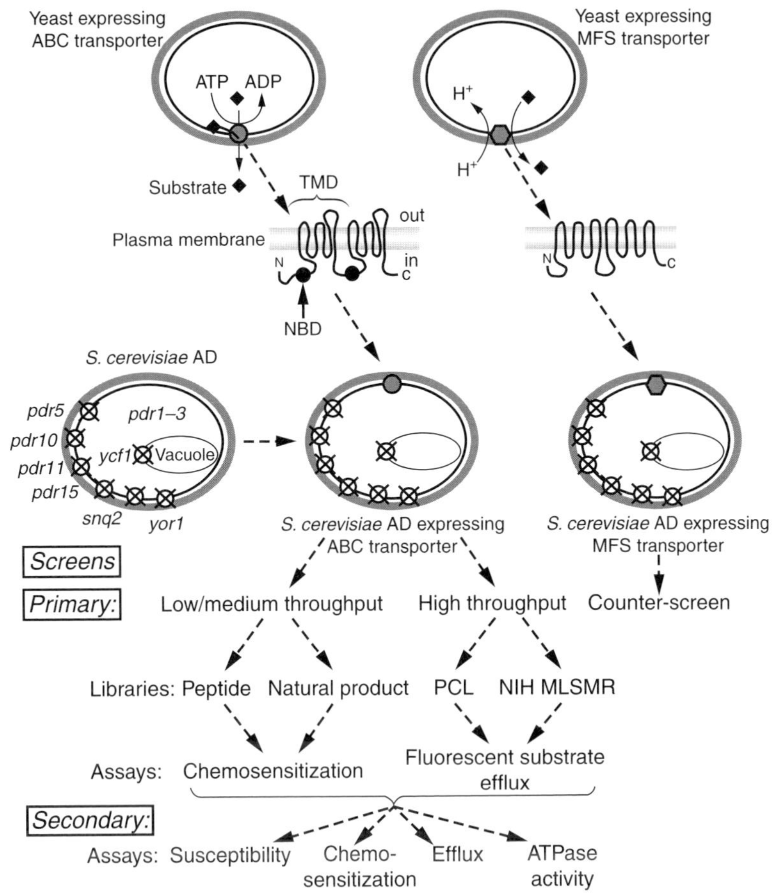

Fig. 5.1. Strategy for identifying inhibitors of fungal ABC efflux pumps. TMD, transmembrane domain; NBD, nucleotide-binding domain; PCL, Prestwick Chemical Library; NIH MLSMR, National Institutes of Health Molecular Libraries Small Molecule Repository.

sites and/or multiple efflux pump-mediated pathways across the lipid bilayer is consistent with the finding that efflux of ScPdr5p substrate R6G is not inhibited in the presence of the triazole substrate FLC. The ATPase activity of Pdr5p is not activated (or inhibited) by FLC, unlike certain mammalian ABC transporters, which are activated by substrates such as verapamil. This may indicate that the natural substrates of ScPdr5p and other PDR transporters are actually endogenous compounds, such as phospholipids, that permanently stimulate the efflux pumps.

There are several ways in which PDR pump inhibitors could act. They might be pump substrates that affect either ATP hydrolysis or transport competitively. They could be non-competitive inhibitors that 'lock' the pump partway through its reaction cycle by binding a substrate exit site, the NBD(s) or other sequences that modulate intersubunit interactions or affect conformation changes required for the reaction cycle. Inhibitors that bind to the NBDs (e.g. nucleotide analogues) might lack specificity, as NBDs are highly conserved between ABC transporters. We have developed a screening platform in which functional fungal PDR pumps are heterologously hyperexpressed in *S. cerevisiae*. This has allowed us to use whole-cell screens to identify PDR pump inhibitors that act from the outside of the cell and thus will not bind the NBD and will not suffer themselves from efflux-mediated resistance.

5.3 Heterologous Expression of PDR Transporters in *S. cerevisiae* for Drug Screening

The heterologous expression screening platform we have developed has several advantages for the identification of fungal PDR pump inhibitors. The high level of target expression in an *S. cerevisiae* strain depleted in endogenous pumps yields whole cell and *in vitro* screens with a high signal:noise ratio. The system is amenable to low-, intermediate- and high-throughput primary screens with growth inhibition and fluorescence read-outs. A comprehensive panel of secondary assays simplifies hit validation.

5.3.1 Hyperexpression of the pump target

A strong drug resistance and efflux phenotype is achieved by hyperexpression of the heterologous pump in a yeast strain with depleted pump activity. Decottignies and co-workers developed an *S. cerevisiae* mutant (AD12345678, denoted AD in Fig. 5.1) in which seven ABC pump genes were deleted in order to reduce background drug transport activity (Decottignies *et al.*, 1998). The expression of PDR genes in *S. cerevisiae* is controlled by transcription factors encoded by *PDR1* and *PDR3*. Strain AD is deleted in *PDR3* and has a gain-of-function mutation (*pdr1-3*) in *PDR1*. These mutations lead to the constitutive upregulation of the *PDR5* promoter and the coordinated overexpression of other members of the PDR gene network (Carvajal *et al.*, 1997).

We have further developed the host strain and plasmid vectors (Nakamura *et al.*, 2001; Lamping *et al.*, 2007) and patented the yeast system for the expression of heterologous membrane proteins (Monk *et al.*, 2002). The PDR pump to be studied is directionally cloned into plasmid pABC3 (GenBank accession number DQ903883.1), or derivatives allowing C-terminal fusions (green fluorescent protein (GFP) or monomeric red fluorescent protein (mRFP)) or tags (His, Cys, FLAG/His or His/Cys), downstream of the cloned open reading frame. The cloned PDR gene is then excised from the plasmid in a cassette, containing a *URA3* marker, flanked by *PDR5* upstream and downstream sequences. Upon transformation of AD to Ura$^+$, these sequences direct the integration of the cassette at the *PDR5* locus (Lamping *et al.*, 2007). Deletion of chromosomal *URA3* in AD prevents integration of the cassette at this locus. This cloning system ensures constant PDR gene copy number and stable strain phenotypes. The heterologous PDR gene is constitutively hyperexpressed from the *PDR5* promoter due to the *pdr1-3* mutation, which also induces the expression of several genes required for membrane protein synthesis and correct protein trafficking within the yeast cell (Balzi and Goffeau, 1995). The deletion of endogenous ABC pumps in AD makes it hypersensitive to antifungals and other xenobiotics. When CaCdr1p was hyperexpressed in AD, it comprised 29% plasma membrane protein and increased the resistance of AD to azole antifungals by 400–1000-fold (Lamping *et al.*, 2007). We have used this system to express PDR pumps from *C. albicans*, *Candida glabrata*, *Candida krusei* and *Cryptococcus neoformans*, the *C. albicans* MFS pump Mdr1p and human ABC pump ABCB1 (P-glycoprotein) (Lamping *et al.*, 2007, 2009). *S. cerevisiae* strains expressing the non-PDR pumps are useful for secondary screens to measure the specificity of pump inhibitors. Heterologous expression of efflux pumps ranged from 29% of plasma membrane protein for CaCdr1p to 3.2% for ABCB1. This highlights a limitation of the system. In general, the further the genetic distance of the source of the pump from *S. cerevisiae*, the lower the level of expression obtained. We are currently investigating ways of overcoming this limitation.

5.3.2 Primary screening assays to identify PDR inhibitors

We have developed a range of assays that measure pump function and can be used to identify pump inhibitors. Fungal PDR transporters are not essential for growth; the deletion of one or more PDR genes, or the transcriptional regulators *PDR1* and *PDR3*, is not lethal, so pump inhibition does not give a growth defect phenotype. However, an *S. cerevisiae* strain expressing a fungal PDR pump can grow on medium containing antifungal pump substrates. If the pump is inhibited, these cells are chemosensitized to the antifungal in the medium and the cells will not grow. This is the basis of the chemosensitization assay (Fig. 5.1), which we have used in low- and intermediate-throughput screens. We can also measure the efflux of fluorescent substrates, such as R6G, rhodamine-123 (R123) or Nile red (Holmes *et al.*, 2006; Ivnitski-Steele *et al.*, 2009) catalysed by PDR transporters. We have used the glucose- and time-dependent efflux of R6G in medium-throughput assays of pump inhibitors employing a microtitre plate spectrofluorimeter. We have also adapted the cell-associated fluorescence of energized cells to high-throughput screening (HTS) assays. Cells with active PDR pumps have low fluorescence, whereas if the pump is inhibited the cells have high fluorescence. This is detected by flow cytometric analysis of cells serially aspirated from wells of microtitre plates where each well contains a different test compound.

Having identified putative PDR pump inhibitors from library screens, it is important to confirm that they do, in fact, target the pump directly and specifically. For example a fluorescence-based HTS will identify antifungal inhibitors that indirectly affect efflux pumps, as well as specific pump inhibitors. Secondary assays can distinguish competitive pump inhibitors that share efflux pump substrate binding sites from inhibitors that block the reaction cycle (i.e. that inhibit ATPase activity).

5.3.3 Secondary assays

We employ a range of secondary assays that use either whole *S. cerevisiae* cells or membrane fractions for *in vitro* assays. Three types of whole-cell assays are applied in the analysis of hits from the screening assays:

1. Whole-cell susceptibility assays, involving either liquid minimum inhibitory concentration (MIC) assays or agar-based diffusion assays, confirm that potential pump inhibitors alone do not affect growth.
2. Chemosensitization assays (using solid or liquid media) are employed to demonstrate that compounds that inhibit the efflux of surrogate fluorescent substrates also reverse resistance to clinically important substrates such as FLC. Checkerboard chemosensitization assays – essentially liquid MIC assays in which the concentrations of both a pump inhibitor and an antifungal substrate are varied – are used to calculate the fractional inhibitory concentration index, which quantifies the degree of synergism between the two compounds (Holmes *et al.*, 2008). Defining the chemosensitization to a range of antifungal substrates by pump inhibitors helps elucidate the nature of the pump inhibition, and chemosensitization to *S. cerevisiae* strains expressing other efflux pumps to azoles reveals the specificity of the pump inhibition. Inclusion of strains expressing MFS pumps or mammalian ABC pumps as counter-screens indicates whether target specificity is acceptable. If it is not, use of these inhibitors might result in side-effects.
3. In order to determine that an inhibitor has a direct effect on efflux function, we measure the effect of the identified inhibitor on energy-dependent efflux of a fluorescent substrate, such as R6G, into the culture supernatant using a microtitre filter plate method (Holmes *et al.*, 2008). This is particularly important where the screen employs flow cytometry-based identification of putative inhibitors, as changes in whole-cell fluorescence may not be energy dependent and may reflect cell death or intracellular sequestration rather than inhibition of efflux.

In addition to whole-cell assays, *in vitro* secondary assays are also critical. Putative inhibitors are tested for their effects on the ATPase activities of membrane preparations from *S. cerevisiae* strains expressing the efflux pump. With a few exceptions (e.g. CaCdr2p), the ATPase activity of ABC transporters is vanadate- and oligomycin-sensitive and can be distinguished from the oligomycin-resistant ATPase activity of the dominant plasma membrane protein, H^+ATPase. It is important to demonstrate that efflux pump 'hits' inhibit the efflux of multiple substrates plus the ATPase activity of the transporter. For example, the immunosuppressant FK506 inhibits FLC and rhodamine transport by ScPdr5p and the ATPase activity of the enzyme. The *in vitro* ATPase assay is also used to indicate whether inhibitors act competitively or non-competitively in relation to nucleotide binding.

We have used the heterologous expression system with various primary and secondary screens to identify pump inhibitors from a range of compound libraries (Fig. 5.1).

5.4 Low-/Medium-throughput Screening of Inhibitors of Drug Efflux

We initially developed a low-/medium-throughput approach to antifungal discovery that sought to overcome the problem of antifungal resistance in key pathogenic fungi. We aimed to discover non-competitive inhibitors of ScPdr5p that targeted the extracellular surfaces of this molecule. This required the development of a biologically stable, surface-targeting resource of chemical and conformational diversity. This was provided using a D-octapeptide library that contained an N-terminal combinatorial D-pentapeptide component. The surface-targeting feature of the D-octapeptides built on the observation that a TRITC-tagged model D-peptide containing a C-terminal amidated tri-arginine motif was excluded from yeast cells and appeared to associate with cell wall phosphomannan. We therefore manually synthesized a 1.85×10^6 member D-octapeptide combinatorial library of the form D-NH_2-A-B-X_1-X_2-X_3-R-R-R-$CONH_2$ (where the amino acids A and B are known for each pool, X_1, X_2 and X_3 may be any of 18 amino acids except glycine and cysteine, and R is arginine). The combinatorial library comprised an 18×18 array of 324 peptide pools, with each pool theoretically containing 5832 (18^3) peptides (Niimi *et al.*, 2004; Monk *et al.*, 2005). A medium-throughput screen of these pools, depending on the number and complexity of the primary and secondary screens, took between 2 weeks and 1 month. The peptide pool that best met the screening criteria was selected for deconvolution to identify the active principal. This involved synthesizing and screening 18 derivatives at each position to sequentially identify X_1, X_2 and X_3. The manual peptide resynthesis required at each position took about 1 month and the subsequent primary and secondary screens required about 1 week per position. Once the primary sequence of the active principal was identified by deconvolution, the peptide was manually resynthesized, purified by HPLC and its activity confirmed. This process generally took another 2 months and included more comprehensive mode of action and toxicity studies.

We identified a chemosensitizer of *S. cerevisiae* Pdr5p by screening the D-octapeptide combinatorial library, in a 96-well microtitre plate format, using an *S. cerevisiae* strain deleted of five other ABC transporters plus the *pdr1-3* mutation (Niimi *et al.*, 2004). This strain is distinct from AD (represented in Fig. 5.1) as it retains the *PDR5* gene and Pdr5p is hyperexpressed in the plasma membrane. We screened for peptide pools, which, at a set D-octapeptide concentration (~50 μg/ml), did not affect growth yield in the absence of FLC, but in the presence of FLC (0.25 MIC: 50 μg/ml) blocked yeast growth. The chemosensitizing pools were titrated to identify the most potent pools and assayed for inhibition of ScPdr5p using the vanadate- and oligomycin-sensitive ATPase activity at pH 7.0 of a plasma membrane preparation obtained from the *S. cerevisiae* strain overexpressing Pdr5p. Deconvolution of the combinatorial library, including HPLC-purified candidate polypeptides, identified a D-octapeptide derivative, KN20 (D-NH_2-NWWKVRRR-$CONH_2$ + Mtr) as a non-competitive inhibitor (at 4 μM) of *in vitro* Pdr5p ATPase activity and a potential chemosensitizer (at 40 μM) of FLC efflux by Pdr5p. Mtr (4-methoxy-2,3,6-trimethylbenzensulfonyl) is a chemical blocking agent used in the synthesis of the peptide library. A single Mtr substituent on the peptide backbone was required for chemosensitization and inhibition of ScPdr5p ATPase. Although KN20 had attributes expected of a chemosensitizer of its target efflux pump and showed useful apparent inhibition and chemosensitization of CaCdr1p and CaCdr2p, the peptide concentrations required for chemosensitization also permeabilized yeast cells to R6G. For example TRITC-labelled KN20 preferentially bound the plasma membrane of yeast cells overexpressing Pdr5p, but chemosensitization appeared indirect and at least partially mediated through non-lethal permeabilization of the plasma membrane (Niimi *et al.*, 2004).

The non-specific chemosensitization obtained with KN20 caused a re-evaluation of our approach to chemosensitizer discovery and the introduction of a counter-screen that monitored more subtle effects in cell growth caused by the presence of azole drug. A primary chemosensitization screen of the combinatorial peptide library was undertaken using *S. cerevisiae* AD expressing CaCdr1p (AD/CaCDR1) with an agarose diffusion growth assay in the presence and absence of FLC at 0.25 MIC (75 μg/ml). An *in vitro* secondary screen of plasma membrane oligomycin-sensitive ATPase activity in a 96-well microtitre plate format was used. *S. cerevisiae* cells expressing the MFS transporter CaMdr1p provided a counter-screen that eliminated non-selective chemosensitization to FLC. These screens identified the CaCdr1p-specific chemosensitizer RC21 (K. Niimi, D.R.K. Harding, A.R. Holmes, E. Lamping, M. Niimi, J.D.A. Tyndall, R.D. Cannon and B.C. Monk, unpublished data). This Mtr derivative of the D-octapeptide D-NH_2-FFKWQRRR-$CONH_2$ (at 1.5 μM) chemosensitized strain AD/CaCDR1 and inhibited CaCdr1p ATPase activity with a 50% inhibitory concentration of ~1.5 μM. RC21 was found to be a stereospecific inhibitor of CaCdr1p: D-RC21 but not L-RC21-chemosensitized CaCdr1p. D-RC21 failed to chemosensitize strains expressing other PDR drug efflux pumps or the human ABCB1 drug efflux pump to FLC. The stereospecificity of RC21 indicated that its target was likely to be a protein, and its specificity for CaCdr1p helped demonstrate that the CaCdr1p drug efflux pump was the dominant contributor to drug efflux in FLC-resistant clinical isolates of *C. albicans* overexpressing both Cdr1p and Cdr2p (Holmes *et al.*, 2008). RC21 was also found to be a highly specific inhibitor of R6G efflux from *S. cerevisiae* and *C. albicans* cells overexpressing CaCdr1p. Importantly, RC21 made an azole-resistant *C. albicans* isolate susceptible to FLC or itraconazole in a mouse model of oral candidiasis (Hayama *et al.*, 2012).

An advantage of heterologous expression of drug targets in *S. cerevisiae* is the tractability of its genetics. For example, when *S. cerevisiae* cells expressing an efflux pump are exposed to an antifungal pump substrate and an efflux pump inhibitor, they can acquire suppressor mutations that increase their resistance to pump inhibitors. Often these mutations are within the efflux pump gene, and mapping these mutations can give valuable information about the mechanism of pump inhibition. Agarose diffusion assays were used to identify suppressor mutants that gave stable resistance to RC21. For each of the 12 mutants analysed, SDS-PAGE analysis and measurements of CaCdr1p-specific ATPase activity showed that these strains had normal amounts of functional CaCdr1p in the yeast plasma membrane. DNA sequence analysis demonstrated that each suppressor mutant involved a single nucleotide mutation in the CaCdr1p open reading frame. Of the six mutations identified, five introduced a positive charge into CaCdr1p that was mapped to surface-exposed extracellular sites on the target enzyme using a homology model of CaCdr1p based on the Pdr5p model of Rutledge *et al.* (2011). The other mutation introduced a large aromatic group near the extracellular end of transmembrane segment 5 at a buried site that could modify the closed conformation of the enzyme. These studies identified CaCdr1p as the molecular target of RC21. Some of the chemosensitization suppressor mutants showed another interesting characteristic. Specific groups of the suppressor mutants demonstrated resistance to known drug-like chemosensitizers of CaCdr1p including the immunosuppressant FK506, the depsipeptide enniatin and the macrolides milbemycin β9 and α11. The suppressor mutations on CaCdr1p provided a provisional map of amino acids that affected the binding, either directly or indirectly, of these chemosensitizers. We therefore consider that peptide derivatives such as RC21 provide a model for the discovery of fungal-specific chemosensitizers.

5.5 High-throughput Screening

HTS is a valuable tool for drug discovery, as it allows rapid testing of large numbers of compounds. HTS assays are usually micro-volume and can be carried out in microtitre plates with robotic control. Given the paucity of antifungal drug classes (Ostrosky-Zeichner *et al.*, 2010), most applications of HTS to antifungal drug development have been focused on the discovery of novel antifungal compounds using assays of fungal-specific target enzymes or fungal viability functions (DiDone *et al.*, 2010).We have demonstrated, however, that HTS can be applied to the discovery of pump inhibitors that chemosensitize resistant cells to existing antifungals.

Cell-suspension HTS assays can utilize flow cytometry (Sklar *et al.*, 2007), with identification of hits based on differential fluorescence detection using signals generated from whole cells or from membrane vesicles. Indeed, flow cytometry-based assays of fluorescently tagged whole cells can be adapted readily for automated HTS. Quantification of ABC transporter activity is particularly amenable to the use of fluorescence-based assays using substrates including R6G, R123 (Nakamura *et al.*, 2001), fluorescein diacetate (FDA) and tetramethylrosamine (A.R. Holmes and R.D. Cannon, unpublished observations). FDA has been used in a fluorescence-based HTS for inhibitors of fungal ABC transporters in recombinant yeast cells (Kolaczkowski *et al.*, 2009).

We have used a similar approach to search for fungal PDR pump inhibitors, and developed a multiplex HTS assay to screen simultaneously for inhibitors to multiple pumps. The choice of fluorescent substrate in these HTS screens is important. Ideally the fluorescent substrate will show the same transport properties as the clinically important substrates, for example FLC. For multiplex screens, the fluorescent compound must clearly be a substrate of each pump. Our initial HTS for inhibitors of CaCdr1p used R6G as the fluorescent substrate. Enniatin B is a Cdr1p inhibitor; it reverses the FLC resistance of AD/CaCDR1 and the FLC resistance of *C. albicans* clinical isolates (Holmes *et al.*, 2008). Enniatin B also inhibits R6G efflux from AD/CaCDR1. Thus, R6G can be considered a good FLC surrogate, and enniatin B can be used as a positive (inhibitor) control in the HTS assay. In our triplex HTS, we screened for inhibitors of CaCdr1p, CaCdr2p and CaMdr1p. R6G is not, however, a substrate of Mdr1p. Instead, Nile red was used as the fluorescent multiplex substrate because it is pumped by all three pumps and its efflux by AD/CaCDR1 is also inhibited by enniatin B (Ivnitski-Steele *et al.*, 2009).

During HTS development, we showed that accumulation of both R6G and Nile red in the yeast cells could be measured in the HyperCyt® flow cytometry system and that *S. cerevisiae* AD strains expressing individual *C. albicans* efflux pumps were easily distinguished from the negative-control AD/pABC3 strain in single-strain assays. In a trial HTS, the Prestwick Chemical Library (PCL; Illkirch, France; a collection of 1200 off-patent small-molecule drugs) was screened for inhibitors of CaCdr1p or CaCdr2p by using flow cytometric analysis of R6G accumulation in strains AD/CaCDR1 and AD/CaCDR2 (Holmes *et al.*, 2012). Nine compounds were identified in the primary screen as inhibitors of CaCdr1p or CaCdr2p; seven were active against one or the other transporter and two inhibited both pumps. One of the hits, ebselen, is a known antifungal with activity against the *C. albicans* plasma membrane ATPase (Billack *et al.*, 2009), and therefore was considered to act indirectly on the efflux pumps. Disulfiram, a hit that was specific to CaCdr2p, had been reported previously to chemosensitize a Cdr2p-expressing strain to FLC (Holmes *et al.*, 2008). Another hit against the Cdr2p-expressing strain was the azole econazole. This demonstrates that compounds identified in screens for efflux inhibition may also be pump substrates that compete with the fluorescent substrate. The clinical use of an efflux inhibitor that is a pump substrate may be unwise because many pump substrates actually induce pump expression (e.g. fluphenazine). Induction of Cdr1p and Cdr2p expression would be an undesirable attribute of a pump inhibitor selected to reverse efflux-induced resistance. Hence, we use secondary assays to measure the sensitivity of strains to hits on their own, and the chemosensitization of strains to antifungal substrates. One of the hits from the R6G-based HTS using AD/CaCDR1 and AD/CaCDR2 was not an efflux substrate, and counter-screens showed that it did not inhibit human ABCB1. It is currently being investigated as a possible azole resistance reversal drug.

Nile red was used in the CaCdr1p-, CaCdr2p- and CaMdr1p multiplex HTS where inhibition of one or more pumps would give an increase in fluorescence of cells within the microtitre plate well. Nile red has the added advantage for the whole-cell, flow cytometry-based HTS assay that only intracellular, accumulated Nile red exhibits fluorescence. A trial multiplex assay using a portion of the PCL identified three hits: the antifungal tolnaftate, the fungal efflux pump substrate antimycin A and the human ABC transporter substrate ivermectin (J.J. Strouse, D. Perez, A. Waller, I. Ivnitski-Steele, M.J. Garcia, M.B. Carter, A.R. Holmes, B.C. Monk, K. Niimi, R.D. Cannon and L.A. Sklar, unpublished data). When individual pump-expressing strains were screened separately, the same three hits identified in the multiplex were also found. This validates the multiplex screening for fungal PDR pump inhibitors. The Nile red triplex HTS assay is currently being used to screen the Molecular Libraries Small Molecule Repository (MLSMR) (Strouse *et al.*, 2010). We are also genetically labelling *S. cerevisiae* strains that express different pumps by fusing different fluorescent proteins to housekeeping genes. This will enable the inclusion of more strains in a multiplex HTS that will generate cytometric read-out capable of identifying the individual pumps inhibited within the multiplex.

5.6 Future Prospects

The discovery of chemosensitizers targeting fungal drug efflux pumps by using compound libraries such as the MLSMR, the PCL and our in-house D-octapeptide combinatorial library, together with either low-, medium- or high-throughput screens, was an academic response to the problem of fungal resistance to the azole drugs. The identification of fungal PDR inhibitors is important for the study of ABC transporter function because they can also be used as probes of the biological roles of these proteins. We have demonstrated that PDR pump inhibitors can chemosensitize resistant clinical isolates to azole antifungal drugs and thus have potential value in protecting immunosuppressed transplant and cancer patients. Despite major successes achieved using drug cocktails in the treatment of diseases such as AIDS, malaria and bacterial infections, obtaining regulatory approval for drug cocktails can be a barrier to therapeutic development. The barrier is lower if at least one of the drugs has already been approved for the particular clinical application. There is also the question of pump specificity. Commercial viability requires a significant market, and thus inhibition of a range of efflux pumps is desirable. It is difficult to inhibit a range of fungal efflux pumps, however, without inhibiting human ABC pumps such as ABCB1, which play important physiological roles in protecting tissues from toxic compounds. We argue that targeting regions of low pump homology, such as the transmembrane segments or extracellular loops, of fungal ABC transporters is less likely to produce chemosensitizers that affect mammalian ABC transporters. This issue may be addressed for drug candidates in toxicity testing and by detecting drug interactions in animal trials. In addition, the over-expression of functional and phenotypically detectable human efflux pumps in yeast can provide counter-screens to eliminate inhibitors of transporters such as ABCB1 (Lamping *et al.*, 2007).

Single-molecule drugs rather than drug cocktails may provide another strategy to prevent and overcome efflux pump-mediated drug resistance. We have proposed a strategy for the discovery of triazole drug analogues that not only bind and inactivate their target Erg11p but also bind to Pdr1p or Pdr3p and block overexpression of the PDR genes responsible for azole efflux (Monk and

Goffeau, 2008). Triazole scaffolds are already available for chemical modification by substituents that are found to be Pdr1p inhibitors.

The discovery of drug targets that are not susceptible to drug resistance, including drug efflux, is a difficult task. Often resistance is due to mutations in the target gene. The chance of such a mutation being selected should be diminished if the target protein is produced in limiting quantities and is turned over rapidly. Inactivation of a growth-limiting essential gene product should give rapid cell death. If more than one spontaneous mutation is required for drug resistance, the opportunity for drug resistance should be reduced even more. These considerations provide opportunities to choose superior drug targets that will significantly delay or reduce the opportunity for antifungal resistance. An example of a target that may meet these criteria is glucan synthase, the target of the echinocandin antifungals. This enzyme is produced in limiting quantities in the growing tips of vegetatively dividing yeast cells. In the diploid pathogen *C. albicans*, the two *GSC1* alleles encoding glucan synthase behave independently, giving rise to a semi-dominant genotype when a mutation in one allele confers micafungin resistance (Niimi *et al.*, 2010). Full resistance to micafungin requires that both alleles contain resistance-conferring mutations. An analogous situation occurs in the haploid pathogen *C. glabrata*, where mutations in the two genes encoding glucan synthase (*FKS1* and *FKS2*) may be required for high-level echinocandin resistance (Niimi *et al.*, 2012). We therefore argue that families of functionally redundant genes that are modestly expressed, show synthetic lethality and can confer recessive or semi-dominant resistance may rarely give rise to clinically significant drug resistance.

The choice of targets for drug discovery is critical, especially with the industry preference for broad-spectrum fungicides. There is a relatively limited number of fungal genes that are essential in *S. cerevisiae*, conserved across a broad range of fungal species (> 40% amino acid similarity), and have low (< 40%) amino acid similarity with any human homologues (Liu *et al.*, 2006). We estimate for the dominant fungal pathogens that about 50 genes fall into this category. For this set of these genes, about 30 protein structures can be found in the protein database at resolutions suitable for structure-directed drug discovery (B.C. Monk, unpublished observations). We anticipate that some of these structures may enable the design of inhibitors that are less prone to the evolution of target-based drug resistance. Such inhibitors should also be fast acting, preferably completely blocking growth, and kill yeast cells on contact to avoid opportunity for the development of drug tolerance (Roemer *et al.*, 2003). Another option may be to select inhibitors that bind to consecutive essential enzymes in a metabolic pathway (i.e. where an inhibitory product analogue of the first target is also an inhibitory substrate analogue of the second target). This approach may dramatically reduce the incidence of target-based drug resistance and provides a rationale for the discovery of inhibitors of the riboflavin pathway in fungal pathogens.

Finally, our yeast expression system can contribute to antifungal drug discovery in several ways. It could be used to screen for inhibitors of new drug targets, as long as appropriate HTS assays are available. We have demonstrated how it can be used to identify inhibitors of pumps responsible for drug resistance. It can also be used as a counter-screen to eliminate drug candidates that are susceptible to drug efflux. Improved understanding of the substrate specificity of individual fungal PDR efflux pumps at the level of the structural fragments that contribute to pump/drug binding, such as from our recent study of CaCdr1p/CaCdr2p chimeras (Tanabe *et al.*, 2011), would also be of considerable value to antifungal discovery projects.

Acknowledgements

The authors gratefully acknowledge funding from the National Institutes of Health, USA (R01DE016885-01; R03MH087406-01, U54 MH084690), the Health Research Council of New Zealand, the Japan Health Science Foundation and the University of Otago Research Committee.

References

Balzi, E. and Goffeau, A. (1995) Yeast multidrug resistance: the PDR network. *Journal of Bioenergetics and Biomembranes* 27, 71–76.

Billack, B., Santoro, M. and Lau-Cam, C. (2009) Growth inhibitory action of ebselen on fluconazole-resistant *Candida albicans*: role of the plasma membrane H^+-ATPase. *Microbial Drug Resistance* 15, 77–83.

Cannon, R.D., Lamping, E., Holmes, A.R., Niimi, K., Tanabe, K., Niimi, M. and Monk, B.C. (2007) *Candida albicans* drug resistance another way to cope with stress. *Microbiology* 153, 3211–3217.

Cannon, R.D., Lamping, E., Holmes, A.R., Niimi, K., Baret, P.V., Keniya, M.V., Tanabe, K., Niimi, M., Goffeau, A. and Monk, B.C. (2009) Efflux-mediated antifungal drug resistance. *Clinical Microbiology Reviews* 22, 291–321.

Carvajal, E., Van Den Hazel, H.B., Cybularz-Kolaczkowska, A., Balzi, E. and Goffeau, A. (1997) Molecular and phenotypic characterization of yeast *PDR1* mutants that show hyperactive transcription of various ABC multidrug transporter genes. *Molecular and General Genetics* 256, 406–415.

Dean, M. (2005) The genetics of ATP-binding cassette transporters. *Methods in Enzymology* 400, 409–429.

Decottignies, A., Grant, A.M., Nichols, J.W., De Wet, H., Mcintosh, D.B. and Goffeau, A. (1998) ATPase and multidrug transport activities of the overexpressed yeast ABC protein Yor1p. *Journal of Biological Chemistry* 273, 12612–12622.

DiDone, L., Scrimale, T., Baxter, B.K. and Krysan, D.J. (2010) A high-throughput assay of yeast cell lysis for drug discovery and genetic analysis. *Nature Protocols* 5, 1107–1114.

Ferreira-Pereira, A., Marco, S., Decottignies, A., Nader, J., Goffeau, A. and Rigaud, J.L. (2003) Three-dimensional reconstruction of the *Saccharomyces cerevisiae* multidrug resistance protein Pdr5p. *Journal of Biological Chemistry* 278, 11995–11999.

Golin, J., Ambudkar, S.V., Gottesman, M.M., Habib, A.D., Sczepanski, J., Ziccardi, W. and May, L. (2003) Studies with novel Pdr5p substrates demonstrate a strong size dependence for xenobiotic efflux. *Journal of Biological Chemistry* 278, 5963–5969.

Golin, J., Ambudkar, S.V. and May, L. (2007) The yeast Pdr5p multidrug transporter: how does it recognize so many substrates? *Biochemical and Biophysical Research Communications* 356, 1–5.

Hayama, K., Ishibashi, H., Ishijima, S.A., Niimi, K., Tansho, S., Ono, Y., Monk, B.C., Holmes, A.R., Harding, D.R.K., Cannon, R.D. and Abe, S. (2012) A D-octapeptide drug efflux pump inhibitor acts synergistically with azoles in a murine oral candidiasis infection model. *FEMS Microbiology Letters* doi:10.1111/j.1574-6968.2011.02490.x (e-pub ahead of print).

Holmes, A.R., Tsao, S., Ong, S.W., Lamping, E., Niimi, K., Monk, B.C., Niimi, M., Kaneko, A., Holland, B.R., Schmid, J. and Cannon, R.D. (2006) Heterozygosity and functional allelic variation in the *Candida albicans* efflux pump genes *CDR1* and *CDR2*. *Molecular Microbiology* 62, 170–186.

Holmes, A.R., Lin, Y.H., Niimi, K., Lamping, E., Keniya, M., Niimi, M., Tanabe, K., Monk, B.C. and Cannon, R.D. (2008) ABC transporter Cdr1p contributes more than Cdr2p does to fluconazole efflux in fluconazole-resistant *Candida albicans* clinical isolates. *Antimicrobial Agents and Chemotherapy* 52, 3851–3862.

Holmes, A.R., Keniya, M.V., Ivnitski-Steele, I., Monk, B.C., Lamping, L.A. and Cannon, R.D. (2012) The monoamine oxidase A inhibitor clorgyline is a broad-spectrum inhibitor of fungal ABC and MFS transporter efflux pump activities which reverses the azole resistance of *Candida albicans* and *Candida glabrata* clinical isolates. *Antimicrobial Agents and Chemotherapy* doi:10.1128/AAC.05706-11 (e-pub ahead of print).

Ivnitski-Steele, I., Holmes, A.R., Lamping, E., Monk, B.C., Cannon, R.D. and Sklar, L.A. (2009) Identification of Nile red as a fluorescent substrate of the *Candida albicans* ATP-binding cassette transporters Cdr1p and Cdr2p and the major facilitator superfamily transporter Mdr1p. *Analytical Biochemistry* 394, 87–91.

Kolaczkowski, M., Kolaczowska, A., Luczynski, J., Witek, S. and Goffeau, A. (1998) *In vivo* characterization of the drug resistance profile of the major ABC transporters and other components of the yeast pleiotropic drug resistance network. *Microbial Drug Resistance* 4, 143–158.

Kolaczkowski, M., Kolaczkowska, A., Motohashi, N. and Michalak, K. (2009) New high-throughput screening assay to reveal similarities and differences in inhibitory sensitivities of multidrug ATP-binding cassette transporters. *Antimicrobial Agents and Chemotherapy* 53, 1516–1527.

Lamping, E., Monk, B.C., Niimi, K., Holmes, A.R., Tsao, S., Tanabe, K., Niimi, M., Uehara, Y. and Cannon, R.D. (2007) Characterization of three classes of membrane proteins involved in fungal azole resistance by functional hyperexpression in *Saccharomyces cerevisiae*. *Eukaryotic Cell* 6, 1150–1165.

Lamping, E., Ranchod, A., Nakamura, K., Tyndall, J.D., Niimi, K., Holmes, A.R., Niimi, M. and

Cannon, R.D. (2009) Abc1p is a multidrug efflux transporter that tips the balance in favor of innate azole resistance in *Candida krusei*. *Antimicrobial Agents and Chemotherapy* 53, 354–369.

Lamping, E., Baret, P.V., Holmes, A.R., Monk, B.C., Goffeau, A. and Cannon, R.D. (2010) Fungal PDR transporters: phylogeny, topology, motifs and function. *Fungal Genetics and Biology* 47, 127–142.

Liu, M., Healy, M.D., Dougherty, B.A., Esposito, K.M., Maurice, T.C., Mazzucco, C.E., Bruccoleri, R.E., Davison, D.B., Frosco, M., Barrett, J.F. and Wang, Y.K. (2006) Conserved fungal genes as potential targets for broad-spectrum antifungal drug discovery. *Eukaryotic Cell* 5, 638–649.

Monk, B.C. and Goffeau, A. (2008) Outwitting multidrug resistance to antifungals. *Science* 321, 367–369.

Monk, B.C., Cannon, R.D., Nakamura, K., Niimi, M., Niimi, K., Harding, D.R.K, Holmes, A.R., Lamping, E., Goffeau, A. and Decottignies, A. (2002) Membrane protein expression system and its application. International patent PCT/NZ02/00163.

Monk, B.C., Niimi, K., Lin, S., Knight, A., Kardos, T.B., Cannon, R.D., Parshot, R., King, A., Lun, D. and Harding, D.R. (2005) Surface-active fungicidal D-peptide inhibitors of the plasma membrane proton pump that block azole resistance. *Antimicrobial Agents and Chemotherapy* 49, 57–70.

Nakamura, K., Niimi, M., Niimi, K., Holmes, A.R., Yates, J.E., Decottignies, A., Monk, B.C., Goffeau, A. and Cannon, R.D. (2001) Functional expression of *Candida albicans* drug efflux pump Cdr1p in a *Saccharomyces cerevisiae* strain deficient in membrane transporters. *Antimicrobial Agents and Chemotherapy* 45, 3366–3374.

Niimi, K., Harding, D.R., Parshot, R., King, A., Lun, D.J., Decottignies, A., Niimi, M., Lin, S., Cannon, R.D., Goffeau, A. and Monk, B.C. (2004) Chemosensitization of fluconazole resistance in *Saccharomyces cerevisiae* and pathogenic fungi by a D-octapeptide derivative. *Antimicrobial Agents and Chemotherapy* 48, 1256–1271.

Niimi, K., Monk, B.C., Hirai, A., Hatakenaka, K., Umeyama, T., Lamping, E., Maki, K., Tanabe, K., Kamimura, T., Ikeda, F., Uehara, Y., Kano, R., Hasegawa, A., Cannon, R.D. and Niimi, M. (2010) Clinically significant micafungin resistance in *Candida albicans* involves modification of a glucan synthase catalytic subunit *GSC1* (*FKS1*) allele followed by loss of heterozygosity. *Journal of Antimicrobial Chemotherapy* 65, 842–852.

Niimi, K., Woods, M.A., Maki, K., Nakayama, H., Hatakenaka, K., Chibana, H., Ikeda, F., Ueno, K., Niimi, M., Cannon, R.D. and Monk, B.C. (2012) Reconstitution of high-level micafungin resistance detected in a clinical isolate of *Candida glabrata* identifies functional homozygosity in glucan synthase gene expression. *Journal of Antimicrobial Chemotherapy* 67, 1666–1676.

Odds, F.C., Brown, A.J. and Gow, N.A. (2003) Antifungal agents: mechanisms of action. *Trends in Microbiology* 11, 272–279.

Ostrosky-Zeichner, L., Casadevall, A., Galgiani, J.N., Odds, F.C. and Rex, J.H. (2010) An insight into the antifungal pipeline: selected new molecules and beyond. *Nature Reviews Drug Discovery* 9, 719–727.

Roemer, T., Jiang, B., Davison, J., Ketela, T., Veillette, K., Breton, A., Tandia, F., Linteau, A., Sillaots, S., Marta, C., Martel, N., Veronneau, S., Lemieux, S., Kauffman, S., Becker, J., Storms, R., Boone, C. and Bussey, H. (2003) Large-scale essential gene identification in *Candida albicans* and applications to antifungal drug discovery. *Molecular Microbiology* 50, 167–181.

Rutledge, R.M., Esser, L., Ma, J. and Xia, D. (2011) Toward understanding the mechanism of action of the yeast multidrug resistance transporter Pdr5p: a molecular modeling study. *Journal of Structural Biology* 173, 333–344.

Sanglard, D. and Bille, J. 2002. Current understanding of the modes of action of and resistance mechanisms to conventional and emerging antifungal agents for treatment of *Candida* infections. In: Calderone, R.A. (ed.) Candida *and Candidiasis*. ASM Press, Washington, DC.

Sklar, L.A., Carter, M.B. and Edwards, B.S. (2007) Flow cytometry for drug discovery, receptor pharmacology and high-throughput screening. *Current Opinion in Pharmacology* 7, 527–534.

Strouse, J.J., Young, S.M., Sedillo, S.E., Perez, D., Garcia, M.J., Houston, T., Ahghar, K., Foutz, T.D., Waller, A., Evangelisti, A.M., Carter, M.B., Salas, V.M., Lindsley, C.W., Cannon, R.D. and Sklar, L.A. (2010) *Summary Report for Phenotypic HTS Multiplex for Antifungal Efflux Pump Inhibitors*. National Center for Biotechnology Information, PubChem BioAssay Database, AID 485335. Available at: http://pubchem.ncbi.nlm.nih.gov/assay/assay.cgi?aid=485335 (accessed 6 March 2012).

Tanabe, K., Lamping, E., Nagi, M., Okawada, A., Holmes, A.R., Miyazaki, Y., Cannon, R.D., Monk, B.C. and Niimi, M. (2011) Chimeras of *Candida albicans* Cdr1p and Cdr2p reveal features of pleiotropic drug resistance transporter structure and function. *Molecular Microbiology* 82, 416–433.

Tsao, S., Rahkhoodaee, F. and Raymond, M. (2009) Relative contributions of the *Candida albicans* ABC transporters Cdr1p and Cdr2p to clinical azole resistance. *Antimicrobial Agents and Chemotherapy* 53, 1344–1352.

6 Vacuolar ATPase: a Model Proton Pump for Antifungal Drug Discovery

Karlett J. Parra
Department of Biochemistry and Molecular Biology, University of New Mexico, Albuquerque, New Mexico, USA

6.1 Introduction

Systemic fungal infections are emerging as major causes of human disease, especially among the immunocompromised (Pfaller and Diekema, 2010). Populations of immunologically suppressed individuals predisposed to the development of life-threatening fungal infections include cancer patients undergoing chemotherapy, organ transplantation patients and AIDS patients. The majority of the life-threatening infections are associated with *Candida*, *Aspergillus* and *Cryptococcus* spp., with *Candida* being the single most important cause of opportunistic mycoses-related deaths worldwide (Miceli *et al.*, 2011). The most commonly used antifungal agents for the treatment of systemic mycoses are the azoles. However, acquired resistance of many pathogens to azole therapy is a frequent cause of refractory infections, and novel drug therapies inhibiting fungal virulence factors and other targets are required (Ostrosky-Zeichner *et al.*, 2010).

Vacuolar ATPase (V-ATPase) proton pumps are emerging as new drug targets. V-ATPases participate in many aspects of fungus biology (Kane, 2006) and, as described in this chapter, their inactivation leads to a network of catastrophic events that prevent virulence with high efficiency. We are beginning to understand the mechanisms of action of V-ATPases and their implication for fungus survival. V-ATPase activity is involved in adaptation to stress conditions such as those encountered by fungal pathogens in host environments, including neutral-to-alkaline pH, low iron and elevated copper concentrations. V-ATPases confer protection against drugs and oxidative stress, and are essential for maintaining pH, calcium and metal homeostasis.

6.2 V-ATPase Pumps: Structure and Catalytic Mechanism of a Molecular Motor

The V-ATPase proton pump is a multisubunit protein complex that consists of peripheral subunits (subunits A–H) and membrane-bound subunits (subunits a, c, c′, c″, d and e) with a defined stoichiometry ($A_3B_3CDE_3FG_3Ha(c\text{–}c')_{4\text{–}5}c''de$) (Zhang *et al.*, 2008). Subunits are organized into two domains: V_1 and V_0 (Fig. 6.1a). V_1, the peripheral domain, forms a hexameric structure (A_3B_3) at the cytosolic side of the membrane. It houses three catalytic sites where ATP binds and is hydrolysed. V_0 is the membrane-bound domain. It forms the passageway transited by protons moving from the cytosol to the other side of the membrane against a concentration

 Antimicrobial Drug Discovery: Emerging Strategies (eds G. Tegos and E. Mylonakis)

gradient. Structural and functional coupling of V_1 and V_0 is maintained by one central and three peripheral stalk structures composed of V_1 and V_0 subunits.

Coupling of ATP hydrolysis and proton translocation entails relative rotation of subunits during catalysis (Forgac, 2007). Hydrolysis of ATP in A_3B_3 drives rotation of a 'rotor' formed by the central stalk (subunits D, F and d), which extends from the centre of A_3B_3 to a proteolipid ring structure in V_0 (c-ring) (Fig. 6.1a). Cytosolic protons are recruited by the V_0 subunit a and transferred to an essential glutamate residue located in each of the proteolipid subunits of the rotating c-ring (V_0 subunits c, c′ and c″). Exit of each proton at the other side of the membrane is facilitated by subunit a and requires 360° rotation of the rotor propelled by hydrolysis of three molecules of ATP. The peripheral stalks (V_1 subunits C, E, G, H and V_0 subunit a) function as 'stators' allowing rotation of rotor subunits relative to the steady catalytic sites in A_3B_3.

Each V-ATPase subunit is critical for assembly and function of the complex. In fungi, each subunit is encoded by a single gene, with the exception of V_0 subunit a, which is encoded by two genes (*VPH1* and

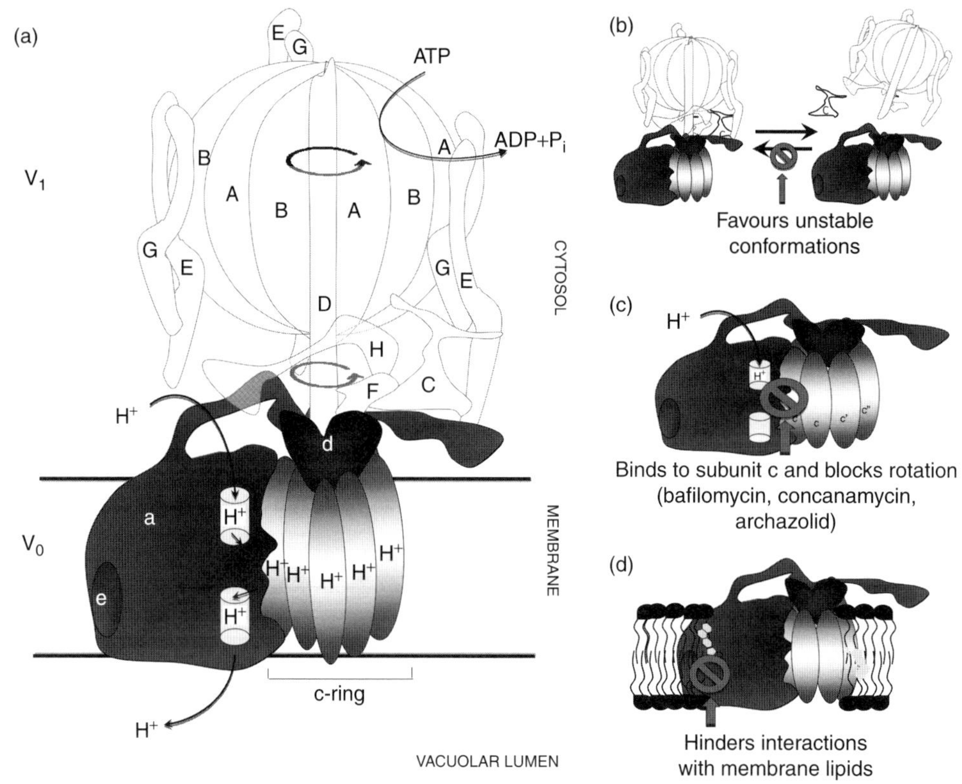

Fig. 6.1. V-ATPase pumps as antifungal drug targets. (a) A molecular motor. The V-ATPase proton pump is a large multisubunit protein complex with a molecular mass of approximately 850 kDa. Its two domains (V_1 and V_0) couple ATP hydrolysis and proton transport via rotation of a central rotor (subunits D, F, d, c, c′ and c″), which transports protons from the cytosol to the vacuolar lumen. (b) Inhibition by disassembly. V-ATPase inhibitors can provoke disassembly of V_1 from V_0, mimicking the mechanism that naturally inactivates the pumps *in vivo* when glucose is limiting. (c) Inhibition by stopping rotation. V-ATPase inhibitors such as bafilomycin, concanamycin and archazolid bind to the rotor c-ring blocking rotation. (d) Inhibition by disturbing interactions with membrane lipids. Antifungal drugs can affect interactions between V_0 and membrane lipids such as ergosterol and sphingolipids.

STV1). Two populations of V-ATPase pumps exist in fungi. Vph1p-containing V-ATPases are primarily localized in the vacuolar membrane and Stv1p-containing V-ATPases are present in Golgi and pre-vacuolar membranes. Complexes containing Vph1p and Stv1p differ in their kinetic properties and regulatory mechanisms (Kawasaki-Nishi *et al.*, 2001), suggesting isoform-specific roles in maintaining the differential pH of these intracellular compartments.

In contrast, multiple isoforms are expressed for most V-ATPase subunits in mammalian cells (two isoforms for subunits B, E, H and d, three isoforms for subunits C and G, and four isoforms for subunit a) (Toei *et al.*, 2010). These isoforms combine to yield different populations of V-ATPase pumps. The fact that heterologous expression of several mammalian subunit isoforms can rescue assembly and functional defects in yeast V-ATPase null mutant strains (Nishi *et al.*, 2003) shows a high level of conservation among V-ATPase pumps. Other subunits such as yeast subunit c′ (*VMA11*) do not have mammalian orthologues. Subunit c′ is a component of the c-ring found exclusively in V-ATPases of fungi.

6.3 V-ATPase Regulation: Proton Transport on a Leash

Essential cellular processes rely on V-ATPase function. Thus multiple mechanisms exist to efficiently regulate these pumps. These mechanisms include product inhibition, inhibition by disulfide bond formation between cysteines at the catalytic centres, and glucose-mediated reversible disassembly of V_1 and V_0, which is an important mechanism used by yeast to reset the V-ATPase assembly set point in response to nutritional changes (Kane, 2006).

Inactivation of V-ATPases by disassembly is a rapid response to glucose starvation (Kane and Parra, 2000). It helps maintain cellular pH homeostasis when glycolytic protons are not produced and prevents energy depletion when glucose, the preferred carbon source, is limiting. In the absence of glucose, the complex dissociates into three parts: V_1 subunit C, V_1 (without subunit C) and V_0 (Fig. 6.1b). Disassembly is reversible and the three components reassociate immediately after glucose addition, restoring proton transport and ATP hydrolysis. Because a fraction of the V-ATPase complexes never disassemble (about 30%; Parra and Kane, 1998), basal levels of V-ATPase activity are maintained, which support critical cellular functions in the absence of a carbon source.

Reversible disassembly is an elegant mechanism to fine tune V-ATPase proton transport in yeast. However, the cellular mechanisms that modulate assembly in response to glucose are incompletely understood. The level of extracellular glucose dictates the level of assembled V_1V_0 (Parra and Kane, 1998). When glucose is limiting, the need for functional V_1V_0 pumps decreases. As V_1V_0 disassembles, a new equilibrium between assembled and disassembled pumps ($V_1V_0 \leftrightarrow V_1 + V_0$) is reached. Therefore V-ATPases alternate between stable conformations that support mechanical rotation during catalysis and unstable conformations that support disassembly of V_1 and V_0. The dynamic nature of the V-ATPase complex opens a window of opportunity to develop a new kind of V-ATPase inhibitor. V-ATPase-targeted drugs that induce or favour the unstable conformations will generate disassembled and inactive pumps (Fig. 6.1b).

6.4 V-ATPase in Vacuolar Biogenesis: the Main Player

Proton-translocating V-ATPase pumps are present throughout the endomembrane system, where they are responsible for organelle acidification (Kane, 2006; Forgac, 2007). V-ATPases are found in endosomes, lysosomes, Golgi-derived vesicles, clathrin-coated vesicles, secretory vesicles and central vacuoles of fungi and plants. The lysosome-like vacuole of fungi is a highly dynamic compartment. Its acidic lumen is adapted to suit vital cellular functions. Vacuolar functions include absorption and degradative processes; storage of amino acids, calcium and polyphosphates; pH, ion and metal homeostasis; resistance to stress conditions; and cell differentiation (Palmer *et al.*, 2005; Kane, 2006). As more detailed analyses are conducted, it is becoming clear that V-ATPases control acidification and proper functioning of vacuoles in yeast and other fungi.

Organelle acidification and membrane energization are the primary functions of V-ATPases (Fig. 6.2). In addition to lowering the luminal pH of the vacuole and endosomal compartments, proton translocation by V-ATPases produces a membrane potential that drives secondary transporters. Among the secondary transporters energized by V-ATPases are the vacuolar Ca^{2+}/H^{+} (Vcx1p) and K^{+}/H^{+} (Vnx1p) antiporters, and the endosomal Na^{+}/H^{+} (Nhx1p) exchanger (Klionsky *et al.*, 1990). Vph1p- and Stv1p-containing V-ATPases energize different compartments and help sustain the differential luminal pH found at vacuolar and endosomal membranes that is critical for trafficking processes (Kawasaki-Nishi *et al.*, 2001). Therefore, active V-ATPase pumps are necessary for membrane and cargo trafficking across the endomembrane system. These trafficking pathways include pathways that sort degradative proteins from the Golgi apparatus to the vacuole, endocytic and autophagocytic pathways that deliver material for degradation in the vacuole, and secretory pathways that traffic proteins for extracellular export (Klionsky *et al.*, 1990; Bowers and Stevens, 2005).

Vacuolar biogenesis and pathogenesis are intimately related, and fungi need vacuolar functions to infect their hosts. Vacuoles are central for switching between morphogenic forms that are involved in the transition from commensal to pathogenic lifestyles (yeast-to-hyphal), for infection of macrophages and wild-type virulence in a mouse model of disseminated candidiasis (Palmer *et al.*, 2005; Palmer, 2010). Likewise, protein trafficking pathways and the cellular processes that they support are essential for virulence. Mutations in vacuolar protein sorting (*vps*) pathways disrupt vesicle-mediated trafficking leading to defective virulence traits, including aberrant filamentous growth, defective biofilm formation and reduced secretion of virulence-associated enzymes such as aspartyl proteases (Bernardo *et al.*, 2008; Lee *et al.*, 2009).

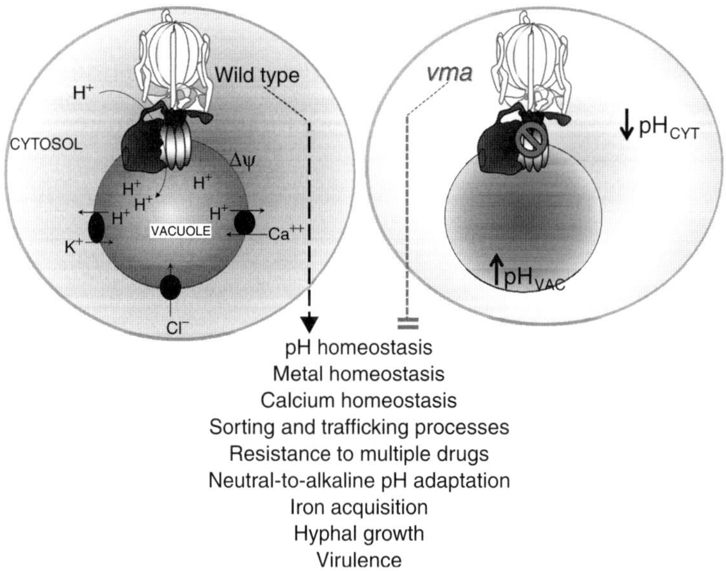

Fig. 6.2. Disruption of V-ATPase proton transport prevents virulence. V-ATPase proton transport is fundamental for vacuolar and endosomal acidification and membrane energization. V-ATPase is required for proper functioning and its inactivation alters vacuolar- and endosomal-dependent processes essential for fungi survival and virulence. *vma*, vacuolar membrane ATPase mutants.

Given the central role of vacuoles and vesicle-mediated transport during infections, it seems very likely that V-ATPase proton transport should be a necessary pathogenic determinant. A number of studies strongly support this notion. Fungi vacuolar membrane ATPase deletion (*vma*Δ) mutant strains, which lack all V-ATPase function because one structural gene of the V-ATPase complex has been deleted, exhibit profound defects in virulence. Defects include aberrant hyphal growth in *Neurospora crassa*, *Candida albicans*, *Histoplasma capsulatum* and *Aspergillus nidulans* (Bowman *et al.*, 2000; Melin *et al.*, 2004; Poltermann *et al.*, 2005; Hilty *et al.*, 2008); abnormally shrunken vacuoles at neutral-to-alkaline pH in *Aspergillus oryzae* (Kuroki *et al.*, 2002); and aberrant iron and copper homeostasis in *H. capsulatum* and *C. albicans* (Poltermann *et al.*, 2005; Hilty *et al.*, 2008). Importantly, V-ATPase deletion mutant strains are avirulent. *H. capsulatum* V-ATPase deletion mutants that lack the gene encoding the catalytic subunit A (*VMA1*) are avirulent in human and mouse macrophages, and in mouse models of pulmonary histoplasmosis (Hilty *et al.*, 2008). *C. albicans* strains that lack the gene *VMA7* encoding the V_1 subunit F are innocuous in animal models of systemic candidiasis (Poltermann *et al.*, 2005). The extent of these defects underscores the central role of V-ATPase proton transport in fungal survival and pathogenesis, and shows that V-ATPase inhibition will compromise the ability of pathogens to cause disease.

6.5 V-ATPase Functions: Long-reaching Connections

While the primary function of V-ATPases is to acidify vacuoles and other intracellular organelles, the scope and number of cellular processes that require functional V-ATPase pumps goes beyond their compartmentalized role (Fig. 6.2). Genetic and pharmacological inhibition of V-ATPases alters global pH and ion homeostasis (Martínez-Muñoz and Kane, 2008). Yeast V-ATPase null mutants (*vma*Δ) show a conditionally lethal growth phenotype. Cells grow in acidic pH but cannot grow in medium buffered to neutral pH or above. By contrast, most organisms die at an early stage of development if they do not have functional V-ATPases. This sensitivity to pH has made yeast an ideal system to study V-ATPase pumps. By growing *vma*Δ mutant strains at low pH, the downstream consequences of inhibiting V-ATPase function can be studied in fungi (Kane, 2006).

*Saccharomyces cerevisiae vma*Δ mutants cannot redistribute protons from the cytosol to the vacuole, and as a result cells have greater vacuolar and lower cytosolic pH than wild-type cells (Martínez-Muñoz and Kane, 2008). Yeast *vma*Δ mutants are hypersensitive to calcium (Kane, 2007). They exhibit defective calcium homeostasis and elevated cytosolic calcium concentrations. Yeast *vma*Δ mutants do not grow in the presence of heavy metals and are intolerant of non-fermentable carbon sources (Kane, 2007). This collection of traits, known as the *vma* growth phenotype, illustrates the central role that V-ATPase proton transport plays in maintaining pH, calcium and metal homeostasis. Like *S. cerevisiae* null mutants, V-ATPase null mutants of *N. crassa*, *C. albicans*, *H. capsulatum*, *A. nidulans* and *A. oryzae* are hypersensitive to alkaline pH, ions and metals (Bowman *et al.*, 2000; Kuroki *et al.*, 2002; Melin *et al.*, 2004; Poltermann *et al.*, 2005; Hilty *et al.*, 2008), showing that the physiological functions of V-ATPases are broadly conserved in fungi.

Genome-wide analyses of *S. cerevisiae* deletion libraries have revealed far more phenotypes associated with V-ATPase function (Kane, 2007). Yeast *vma*Δ mutants are over represented in genetic screenings that challenge cells with multiple drugs, DNA-damaging reagents, oxidative stress, alcohols or low iron. The molecular mechanisms that underlie the dependence on V-ATPases for survival under these conditions have yet to be established. Some of the phenotypes observed may be direct outcomes of deficient vacuolar functions, and others could result from cargo-specific missorting intrinsic to *vma* mutants. Regardless of the mechanism, it is evident that V-ATPases play important protective roles against oxidative stress, metals and multiple drugs. Far-reaching physiological roles of similar scope can be expected for other fungi, given the high degree of conservation among V-ATPases.

6.6 Fungal Adaptation to Host Environments: Participation of V-ATPases in Low Iron Conditions

Iron transport and homeostasis genes are heavily upregulated in *vma*Δ mutants of *S. cerevisiae* (Milgrom *et al.*, 2007), and *vma*Δ mutants of *S. cerevisiae*, *C. albicans* and *H. capsulatum* are not capable of growing in an iron-restricted medium (Davis-Kaplan *et al.*, 2004; Hilty *et al.*, 2008; Weissman *et al.*, 2008). These phenotypes indicate that fungi are iron starved in the absence of functional V-ATPase pumps. V-ATPase proton transport may give fungi a competitive edge to obtain iron, a scarce but essential element.

Iron uptake and homeostasis are attributes of virulence during fungal infection (Almeida *et al.*, 2009). Iron levels are extremely low in the mammalian host, and its acquisition is a challenge for fungi, which compete for iron. Iron assimilation depends primarily on two factors: iron availability within the host and effective iron-acquisition mechanisms within the pathogen. Fungi have developed specialized mechanisms to obtain iron from the host. These mechanisms include iron acquisition via high-affinity chelators (siderophores) and iron obtained from haemoglobin and other iron-containing proteins from the host (Almeida *et al.*, 2009). Both mechanisms involve cellular events that require active V-ATPase proton transport, i.e. endocytosis and vacuolar function.

To recover iron from siderophores, fungi express siderophore transporters at the plasma membrane, to internalize iron-loaded siderophores by endocytosis. To obtain iron from haemoglobin, fungi use specific haemoglobin receptors that are internalized by endocytic trafficking to the vacuole for degradation and haem release. Inactivation of V-ATPase pumps prevents siderophore- and haemoglobin-iron utilization, consistent with the V-ATPase playing a critical role in iron uptake. A V-ATPase null mutant strain of *C. albicans* lacking the gene *VMA11*, which encodes the V_0 subunit c′, cannot grow in medium supplemented with either iron-loaded siderophore or haemoglobin as the sole iron source (Weissman *et al.*, 2008). Turnover of the haemoglobin receptor (Rbt5p) is significantly reduced in this mutant because endosomal trafficking and vacuolar functions are greatly suppressed. Thus, the major pathways used by *C. albicans* to assimilate iron require V-ATPase proton transport.

Another mechanism of iron uptake in fungi that requires V-ATPase function is its acquisition via high-affinity transporters (Almeida *et al.*, 2009). One such transporter is the multicopper oxidase Fet3p, a functionally conserved iron transporter that is defective in *vma*Δ mutants. Interestingly, *C. albicans* strains lacking the gene that encodes Fet3p (Eck *et al.*, 1999) or the haemoglobin transporter Rbt5p (Braun *et al.*, 2000) display wild-type virulence, indicating that blockage of single iron-uptake pathways does not lead to iron assimilation defects. Therefore, the severe phenotype of *vma*Δ mutants is probably the outcome of multiple faulty iron-uptake systems and extensive endocytic and vacuolar defects caused by lack of V-ATPase proton transport.

6.7 Fungal Adaptation to Host Environments: Participation of V-ATPases in Neutral-to-Alkaline Environments

Host environments show major differences in pH, and fungal adaptation to environmental pH changes is crucial for life (Davis, 2009). It influences fungal growth and differentiation and, within the host tissue, adaptation to neutral-to-alkaline pH is essential for pathogenesis. Neutral-to-alkaline pH triggers the yeast-to-hyphal transition that is required for tissue damage (Biswas *et al.*, 2007). It also imposes nutritional stress because it affects membrane proton gradients preventing uptake of many nutrients. In fact, fungi grow more rapidly in acidic than in neutral-to-alkaline medium. When V-ATPase pumps are inactive (*vma* mutants), yeast growth is significantly slower at acidic pH, and growth at neutral pH or above is inhibited (Kane, 2006).

Lack of growth at neutral-to-alkaline pH is the hallmark trait of the *vma* phenotype. Although the physiological basis for pH conditional lethality is not fully understood, the involvement of V-ATPases in neutral-to-alkaline pH adaptation is critical at multiple levels.

V-ATPase proton transport give fungi a survival advantage in neutral-to-alkaline environments. Vacuolar membranes isolated from yeast cells grown in neutral-to-alkaline medium show enhanced V-ATPase activity (Diakov and Kane, 2010). In addition, down-regulation of V-ATPase pumps in response to glucose deprivation is suppressed. It appears that V-ATPase proton transport protects acidification of intracellular compartments such as the vacuole and endosomes in neutral-to-alkaline pH environments. The fact that *vps* mutants present defective alkaline tolerance in *S. cerevisiae* and *C. albicans* (Serrano *et al.*, 2004; Cornet *et al.*, 2005) shows that altered membrane trafficking can lead to pH growth defects similar to those found in *vma* mutants. However, *vma* mutations lead to a much more dramatic effect on alkaline tolerance than *vps* mutations, perhaps because *vma* cells exhibit widespread trafficking and pH defects.

The central role of V-ATPases in sustaining cellular pH homeostasis cannot be overlooked. Cytosolic and vacuolar pH are maintained through a concerted movement of protons out of the cytosol, which is achieved by the V-ATPase and Pma1p pumps, the major electrogenic pumps at the vacuolar and plasma membranes, respectively (Martínez-Muñoz and Kane, 2008). While the V-ATPase transfers protons into the vacuolar lumen, Pma1p moves cytosolic protons out of the cell, helping to sustain a favourable acidic growth environment. Not only are both transporters stimulated by glucose, but V-ATPase and Pma1p are functionally interdependent (Bowman *et al.*, 1997). Pma1p-mediated extracellular acidification is altered in *vma* mutants because sorting of Pma1p to the cell surface from the Golgi is defective (Huang and Chang, 2011). Thus, V-ATPase participation in both protein sorting and pH homeostasis helps fungi to adapt to neutral-to-alkaline environments.

In addition to supporting vesicular trafficking, V-ATPase pumps may influence vesicular membrane-associated signal transduction events not related to trafficking (Mitchell, 2008). The RIM101 pathway is the major signalling pathway known to be involved in fungal adaptation to neutral-to-alkaline pH (Peñalva *et al.*, 2008). In the RIM101 pathway, neutral-to-alkaline pH sensing promotes endocytosis. Endocytosis provides a membrane surface for transient association of regulatory proteins and activation of the transcription factor Rim101p. Activated Rim101p promotes transcriptional responses required for growth at neutral-to-alkaline pH and for pathogenesis. These responses include activation of iron-acquisition genes, because the solubility of iron decreases and becomes less accessible in neutral-to-alkaline environments (Davis, 2009). In neutral-to alkaline pH, V-ATPase genes and RIM101 genes become necessary for growth in low iron conditions.

Although there has not yet been a thorough dissection of the role of V-ATPases in the pH signals transmitted through this pathway, RIM101 signalling and V-ATPase proton transport are interconnected. Maps on a genome-wide level have revealed genetic interactions between a number of *vma* and *rim* mutants in yeast (Costanzo *et al.*, 2010), indicating that V-ATPase pumps and the RIM101 pathway belong to the same biological process. Additional analyses will be necessary to unravel the network of events that connect V-ATPases with the signalling pathways involved in pH adaptation and pH homeostasis. Nevertheless, V-ATPase function is required for these vital processes.

6.8 Inhibitors of V-ATPase Pumps: to the Core and Beyond

V-ATPase inhibition disrupts vital cell functions. It is probably for this reason that natural products have evolved to inhibit V-ATPases. These inhibitors, however, lack therapeutic human applications because they show poor selectivity and/or potency *in vivo* (Bowman and Bowman, 2005; Huss and Wieczorek, 2009). Bafilomycin and concanamycin, which are inhibitors broadly used to study V-ATPases, cannot discriminate between fungal and mammalian V-ATPases. Other compounds preferentially inhibit the mammalian V-ATPases (salicylihalamides, lobatamides and archazolid) but cannot discriminate between V-ATPase tissue-specific isoforms. Finally, the compounds that preferentially inhibit fungal V-ATPases (chondropsins) have low potency *in vivo*.

Bafilomycin and concanamycin are macrolide antibiotics that inhibit fungal V-ATPases with remarkable potency in vacuolar membrane fractions (50% inhibitory concentration (IC_{50}) = 1–5 nM; Bowman and Bowman, 2005), but require micromolar concentrations *in vivo* (Johnson *et al.*, 2010). Binding studies have mapped the binding site of bafilomycin and concanamycin to the V_0 subunit c (Vma3p) of the c-ring (Fig. 6.1c). They presumably bind at the interface of two adjacent c subunits in the cytosolic half of the membrane bilayer (Bowman *et al.*, 2006) in close proximity to subunit a (Wang *et al.*, 2005), blocking rotation. The macrolactone archazolid also binds to subunit c (Bockelmann *et al.*, 2010). The fact that these antibiotics bind to subunit c, a component in all V-ATPases, may explain their high potency *in vitro* against yeast and mammalian V-ATPases. It also may explain their poor discrimination against tissue-specific mammalian V-ATPases, which express only one form of subunit c.

Like subunit c, the other two proteolipid subunits forming the c-ring of the V-ATPase (subunits c′ and c″) are essential for activity. The three proteolipid subunits are homologous to each other and each proteolipid contains a buried glutamic acid residue critical for proton transport during rotation. The proteolipid subunits are arranged in a unique order in the ring, and the actual helical contacts between proteolipid subunits may be important in defining selectivity (Bowman *et al.*, 2006). As a number of subunit c mutants resistant to bafilomycin and concanamycin are available (Bowman and Bowman, 2002; Bockelmann *et al.*, 2010), antifungal drugs that recognize a binding site different from bafilomycin and concanamycin may be achievable. Equivalent mutations in subunit c′ cannot confer resistance to the drugs regardless of the fact that the sequence of subunits c′ and c from the host and fungi are 60% identical. Highly selective antifungal V-ATPase inhibitors could perhaps bind to subunit c′ (found only in fungi or at the interface between c′ and other proteolipid subunits), enabling target specificity.

The recent discovery that V-ATPase activity and vacuolar acidification are disturbed by azoles (Zhang *et al.*, 2010), the largest class of antifungal drugs, further highlights the therapeutic value of V-ATPase-targeted drugs. Because azole drugs inhibit ergosterol biosynthesis, these studies have revealed a new link between V-ATPase proton transport and ergosterol metabolism. Likewise, sphingolipid biosynthesis has been found to affect V-ATPase function (Chung *et al.*, 2003). Mutations in either ergosterol or sphingolipid biosynthetic pathways lead to *vma* growth phenotypes, suggesting that V-ATPases are exquisitely sensitive to the integrity of cellular membranes. In light of these observations, V-ATPase inhibitors can be designed to hinder interactions of V_0 subunits with membrane lipids (Fig. 6.1d). The absence of ergosterol in mammals might be exploited to enhance antifungal selectivity.

6.9 The Search for V-ATPase-targeted Antifungal Drugs: a High-throughput Screening Approach

Yeast vacuolar pH changes can be measured *in vivo* using pH-sensitive fluorescent probes such as 2,7 bis(2 carboxyethyl)-5(6)-carboxyfluorescein (BCECF). The membrane-permeable acetoxymethyl ester derivative (BCECF-AM) selectively labels the vacuoles, which trap florescent BCECF in the lumen. BCECF-loaded yeast yield stable fluorescence signals under steady-state conditions, making it desirable for high-throughput screening. A variety of high-throughput platforms can be used to screen for V-ATPase inhibitors using BCECF stained cells. We have used the HyperCyt platform technology that interfaces a flow cytometer and an autosampler (Edwards *et al.*, 2004). As BCECF fluorescence intensity increases when the pH increases from 5.0 to 8.0, V-ATPase inhibitors are expected to increase the fluorescence signals.

Using the HyperCyt high-throughput flow cytometry platform, we screened the Prestwick Chemical Library, which is a collection of bioactive structurally diverse compounds. These studies found that disulfiram (tetraethylthiuram disulfide) inhibits vacuolar acidification *in vivo* and ATP hydrolysis in vacuolar membrane fractions *in vitro* (Johnson *et al.*, 2010). Disulfiram is a cysteine-modifying compound (Sauna *et al.*, 2005). V-ATPases are sensitive to cysteine-modifying reagents because disulfide bond formation between residues in the catalytic subunit A of V_1 inhibits ATP hydrolysis (Feng and Forgac, 1994). Moreover, disulfiram has antifungal activity. *C. albicans* forms an abnormal biofilm in the presence of disulfiram (Mukherjee *et al.*, 2006). Disulfiram also inhibits Cdr1p, the ATP-binding cassette (ABC) transporter drug efflux pump involved in azole resistance (Shukla *et al.*, 2004). However, disulfiram lacks antifungal selectivity because it inhibits the mammalian ABC transporter and multidrug resistance pump P-glycoprotein (Sauna *et al.*, 2005).

BCECF-based high-throughput screening demonstrates that monitoring of vacuolar pH can be used to search for V-ATPase inhibitors. Screening efforts aimed at developing V-ATPase-specific antifungal drugs will require more advanced tactics. V-ATPase inhibitors alkalinize the vacuolar lumen and acidify the cytosol simultaneously. Thus, ideal screening tools should detect alterations in both vacuolar and cytosolic pH. Measuring cytosolic pH in yeast has long been a challenge, as commercially available pH-sensitive probes that work in mammalian cell systems cannot be used to measure cytosolic pH in yeast. They accumulate in the vacuole, underscoring the protective role of vacuoles in fungi.

Access to pHluorin, a pH-sensitive variant of green fluorescent protein, has facilitated yeast cytosolic pH measurements in recent years. These studies have considerably advanced our understanding of the central role played by V-ATPases in cytosolic pH homeostasis (Brett *et al.*, 2005; Martínez-Muñoz and Kane, 2008; Zhang *et al.*, 2010). pHluorin is retained solely in the cytosol of wild-type and a variety of mutant yeast strains including *vma*Δ. Like BCECF, pHluorin is a ratiometric probe and yields stable fluorescence signals. We have recently found that yeast cells carrying pHluorin are suitable for high-throughput screening. High-throughput screening of the Prestwick Chemical Library using cytosolic pHluorin also identified disulfiram as capable of lowering the cytosolic pH (Chan *et al.*, 2012). To help increase selectivity against V-ATPase pumps *in vivo*, vacuolar and cytosolic pH assays could be used separately in two consecutive high-throughput screenings. Hits that increase vacuolar pH can be interrogated further for their ability to lower the cytosolic pH, or vice versa. Alternatively, vacuolar and cytosolic probes with different emission filters could be used simultaneously, in the same cell, and vacuolar and cytosolic pH-dependent fluorescence concurrently monitored using multiplex formats.

The fact that *S. cerevisiae* V-ATPases have been thoroughly characterized is a valuable resource. Existing V-ATPase mutants can be used to enhance target selectivity. The *vma*Δ strains can help reduce the number of false positives. Yeast *vma* mutants that are resistant to bafilomycin and concanamycin could be used to identify inhibitors that mimic these drugs and block mammalian and fungal enzymes. This allows the discovery of novel inhibitors that operate by different mechanisms. Novel V-ATPase-targeted antifungal drugs may directly affect catalysis by stopping V-ATPase rotation, blocking proton transport and ATP hydrolysis (Fig. 6.1c). They may be catalytic uncouplers that prevent proton transport but not ATP hydrolysis, thus depleting cells of energy (Chan *et al.*, 2012). Other drugs may provoke disassembly of V_1V_0 by interfering with critical subunit interactions, thereby mimicking glucose-regulated V-ATPase inactivation (Fig. 6.1b).

Human V-ATPases have already been tested as potential targets to prevent and control infectious diseases, cancer metastasis and osteoporosis. Despite major efforts, drug discovery and development targeted at human V-ATPases have failed thus far due to the ubiquitous cellular and tissue distribution of V-ATPases and the lack of sufficiently selective pharmacological inhibitors. Therefore, the fungal V-ATPases remain our most promising drug targets. Tissue and isoform specificity are not a concern in fungi. Furthermore, the availability of high-resolution structures of yeast subunits (Zhang *et al.*, 2008), and ongoing structure–function studies are facilitating out understanding of structure–activity relationships and the mechanism-of-action studies that will be needed to develop highly selective V-ATPase-targeted antifungal drugs.

Acknowledgements

The author gratefully acknowledges funding from the National Institutes of Health, Bethesda, Maryland, USA (1R01GM086495-01).

References

Almeida, R.S., Wilson, D. and Hube, B. (2009) *Candida albicans* iron acquisition within the host. *FEMS Yeast Research* 9, 1000–1012.

Bernardo, S.M., Khalique, Z., Kot, J., Jones, J.K. and Lee, S.A. (2008) *Candida albicans* VPS1 contributes to protease secretion, filamentation, and biofilm formation. *Fungal Genetics and Biology* 45, 861–877.

Biswas, S., Van Dijck, P. and Datta, A. (2007) Environmental sensing and signal transduction pathways regulating morphopathogenic determinants of *Candida albicans*. *Microbiology and Molecular Biology Reviews* 71, 348–376.

Bockelmann, S., Menche, D., Rudolph, S., Bender, T., Grond, S., von Zezschwitz, P., Muench, S.P., Wieczorek, H. and Huss, M. (2010) Archazolid A binds to the equatorial region of the c-ring of the vacuolar H^+-ATPase. *Journal of Biological Chemistry* 285, 38304–38314.

Bowman, B.J. and Bowman, E.J. (2002) Mutations in subunit c of the vacuolar ATPase confer resistance to bafilomycin and identify a conserved antibiotic binding site. *Journal of Biological Chemistry* 277, 3965–3972.

Bowman, B.J., McCall, M.E., Baertsch, R. and Bowman, E.J. (2006) A model for the proteolipid ring and bafilomycin/concanamycin-binding site in the vacuolar ATPase of *Neurospora crassa*. *Journal of Biological Chemistry* 281, 31885–31893.

Bowman, E.J. and Bowman, B.J. (2005) V-ATPases as drug targets. *Journal of Bioenergetics and Biomembranes* 37, 431–435.

Bowman, E.J., O'Neill, F.J. and Bowman, B.J. (1997) Mutations of *pma-1*, the gene encoding the plasma membrane H^+-ATPase of *Neurospora crassa*, suppress inhibition of growth by concanamycin A, a specific inhibitor of vacuolar ATPases. *Journal of Biological Chemistry* 272, 14776–14786.

Bowman, E.J., Kendle, R. and Bowman, B.J. (2000) Disruption of *vma-1*, the gene encoding the catalytic subunit of the vacuolar H^+-ATPase, causes severe morphological changes in *Neurospora crassa*. *Journal of Biological Chemistry* 275, 167–176.

Bowers, K. and Stevens, T.H. (2005) Protein transport from the late Golgi to the vacuole in the yeast *Saccharomyces cerevisiae*. *Biochimica et Biophysica Acta* 1744, 438–454.

Braun, B.R., Head, W.S., Wang, M.X. and Johnson, A.D. (2000) Identification and characterization of TUP1-regulated genes in *Candida albicans*. *Genetics* 156, 31–44.

Brett, C.L., Tukaye, D.N., Mukherjee, S. and Rao, R. (2005) The yeast endosomal Na^+K^+/H^+ exchanger Nhx1 regulates cellular pH to control vesicle trafficking. *Molecular Biology of the Cell* 16, 1396–1405.

Chan, C.Y., Prudom, C., Raines, S.M., Charkhzarrin, S., Melman, S.D., De Haro, L.P., Allen, C., Lee, S.A., Sklar, L.A. and Parra, K.J. (2012) Inhibitors of V-ATPase proton transport reveal uncoupling functions of the tether linking cytosolic and membrane domains of the Vo subunit a (Vph1p). *Journal of Biological Chemistry* 287, 10236–10250.

Chung, J.H., Lester, R.L. and Dickson, R.C. (2003) Sphingolipid requirement for generation of a functional V_1 component of the vacuolar ATPase. *Journal of Biological Chemistry* 278, 28872–28881.

Cornet, M., Bidard, F., Schwarz, P., Da Costa, G., Blanchin-Roland S., Dromer, F. and Gaillardin, C. (2005) Deletions of endocytic components VPS28 and VPS32 affect growth at alkaline pH and virulence through both RIM101-dependent and RIM101-independent pathways in *Candida albicans*. *Infection and Immunity* 73, 7977–7987.

Costanzo, M., Baryshnikova, A., Bellay, J., Kim, Y., Spear, E.D., Sevier, C.S., Ding, H., Koh, J.L., Toufighi, K., Mostafavi, S., Prinz, J., St Onge, R.P., VanderSluis B., Makhnevych, T., Vizeacoumar, F.J., Alizadeh, S., Bahr, S., Brost, R.L., Chen, Y., Cokol, M., Deshpande, R., Li Z., Lin, Z.Y., Liang, W., Marback, M., Paw, J., San

Luis, B.J., Shuteriqi, E., Tong, A.H., van Dyk, N., Wallace, I.M., Whitney, J.A., Weirauch, M.T., Zhong, G., Zhu, H., Houry, W.A., Brudno, M., Ragibizadeh, S., Papp, B., Pál, C., Roth, F.P., Giaever, G., Nislow, C., Troyanskaya, O.G., Bussey, H., Bader, G.D., Gingras, A.C., Morris, Q.D., Kim, P.M., Kaiser, C.A., Myers, C.L., Andrews, B.J. and Boone, C. (2010) The genetic landscape of a cell. *Science* 327, 425–431.

Davis, D. (2009) How human pathogenic fungi sense and adapt to pH: the link to virulence. *Current Opinion in Microbiology* 12, 365–370.

Davis-Kaplan, S.R., Ward, D.M., Shiflett, S.L. and Kaplan, J. (2004) Genome-wide analysis of iron-dependent growth reveals a novel yeast gene required for vacuolar acidification. *Journal of Biological Chemistry* 279, 4322–4329.

Diakov, T.T. and Kane, P.M. (2010) Regulation of vacuolar proton-translocating ATPase activity and assembly by extracellular pH. *Journal of Biological Chemistry* 285, 23771–23778.

Eck, R., Hundt, S., Härtl, A., Roemer, E. and Künkel, W. (1999) A multicopper oxidase gene from *Candida albicans*: cloning, characterization and disruption. *Microbiology* 145, 2415–2422.

Edwards, B.S., Oprea, T., Prossnitz, E.R. and Sklar, L.A. (2004) Flow cytometry for high-throughput, high-content screening. *Current Opinion in Chemical Biology* 8, 392–398.

Feng, Y. and Forgac, M. (1994) Inhibition of vacuolar H^+-ATPase by disulfide bond formation between cysteine 254 and cysteine 532 in subunit A. *Journal of Biological Chemistry* 269, 13224–13230.

Forgac, M. (2007) Vacuolar ATPases: rotary proton pumps in physiology and pathophysiology. *Nature Reviews Molecular Cell Biology* 8, 917–929.

Hilty, J., Smulian, A.G. and Newman, S.L. (2008) The *Histoplasma capsulatum* vacuolar ATPase is required for iron homeostasis, intracellular replication in macrophages and virulence in a murine model of histoplasmosis. *Molecular Microbiology* 70, 127–139.

Huang, C. and Chang, A. (2011) pH dependent cargo sorting from the Golgi. *Journal of Biological Chemistry* 286, 10058–10065.

Huss, M. and Wieczorek, H. (2009) Inhibitors of V-ATPases: old and new players. *Journal of Experimental Biology* 212, 341–346.

Johnson, R.M., Allen, C., Melman, S.D., Waller, A., Young, S.M., Sklar, L.A. and Parra, K.J. (2010) Identification of inhibitors of vacuolar proton-translocating ATPase pumps in yeast by high-throughput screening flow cytometry. *Analytical Biochemistry* 398, 203–211.

Kane, P.M. (2006) The where, when, and how of organelle acidification by the yeast vacuolar H^+-ATPase. *Microbiology and Molecular Biology Reviews* 70, 177–191.

Kane, P.M. (2007) The long physiological reach of the yeast vacuolar H^+-ATPase. *Journal of Bioenergetics and Biomembranes* 39, 415–421.

Kane, P.M. and Parra, K.J. (2000) Assembly and regulation of the yeast vacuolar H^+-ATPase. *Journal of Experimental Biology* 203, 81–87.

Kawasaki-Nishi, S., Nishi, T. and Forgac, M. (2001) Yeast V-ATPase complexes containing different isoforms of the 100-kDa a-subunit differ in coupling efficiency and *in vivo* dissociation. *Journal of Biological Chemistry* 276, 17941–17948.

Klionsky, D.J., Herman, P.K. and Emr, S.D. (1990) The fungal vacuole: composition, function, and biogenesis. *Microbiological Reviews* 54, 266–292.

Kuroki, Y., Juvvadi, P.R., Arioka, M., Nakajima, H. and Kitamoto, K. (2002) Cloning and characterization of *vmaA*, the gene encoding a 69-kDa catalytic subunit of the vacuolar H^+-ATPase during alkaline pH mediated growth of *Aspergillus oryzae*. *FEMS Microbiology Letters* 209, 277–282.

Lee, S.A., Jones, J., Hardison, S., Kot, J., Khalique, Z., Bernardo, S.M., Lazzell, A., Monteagudo, C. and Lopez-Ribot J. (2009) *Candida albicans* VPS4 is required for secretion of aspartyl proteases and *in vivo* virulence. *Mycopathologia* 167, 55–63.

Martínez-Muñoz, G.A. and Kane, P. (2008) Vacuolar and plasma membrane proton pumps collaborate to achieve cytosolic pH homeostasis in yeast. *Journal of Biological Chemistry* 283, 20309–20319.

Melin, P., Schnürer, J. and Wagner, E.G. (2004) Disruption of the gene encoding the V-ATPase subunit A results in inhibition of normal growth and abolished sporulation in *Aspergillus nidulans*. *Microbiology* 150, 743–748.

Miceli, M.H., Díaz, J.A. and Lee, S.A. (2011) Emerging opportunistic yeast infections. *Lancet Infectious Diseases* 11, 142–151.

Milgrom, E., Diab, H., Middleton, F. and Kane, P.M. (2007) Loss of vacuolar proton-translocating ATPase activity in yeast results in chronic oxidative stress. *Journal of Biological Chemistry* 282, 7125–7136.

Mitchell, A.P. (2008) A VAST staging area for regulatory proteins. *Proceedings of the National Academy of Sciences USA* 105, 7111–7112.

Mukherjee, P.K., Mohamed, S., Chandra, J., Kuhn, D., Liu, S., Antar, O.S., Munyon, R., Mitchell, A.P., Andes, D., Chance, M.R., Rouabhia, M. and Ghannoum, M.A. (2006) Alcohol dehydrogenase restricts the ability of the pathogen *Candida albicans* to form a biofilm on catheter surfaces through an ethanol-based mechanism. *Infection and Immunity* 74, 3804–3816.

Nishi, T., Kawasaki-Nishi, S. and Forgac, M. (2003) Expression and function of the mouse V-ATPase d subunit isoforms. *Journal of Biological Chemistry* 278, 46396–46402.

Ostrosky-Zeichner, L., Casadevall, A., Galgiani, J.N., Odds, F.C. and Rex, J.H. (2010) An insight into the antifungal pipeline: selected new molecules and beyond. *Nature Reviews Drug Discovery* 9, 719–727.

Palmer, G.E. (2010) Endosomal and AP-3-dependent vacuolar trafficking routes make additive contributions to *Candida albicans* hyphal growth and pathogenesis. *Eukaryotic Cell* 9, 1755–1765.

Palmer, G.E., Kelly, M.N. and Sturtevant, J.E. (2005) The *Candida albicans* vacuole is required for differentiation and efficient macrophage killing. *Eukaryotic Cell* 4, 1677–1686.

Parra, K.J. and Kane, P.M. (1998) Reversible association between the V_1 and V_0 domains of yeast vacuolar H^+-ATPase is an unconventional glucose-induced effect. *Molecular and Cellular Biology* 18, 7064–7074.

Peñalva, M.A., Tilburn, J., Bignell, E. and Arst, H.N. Jr (2008) Ambient pH gene regulation in fungi: making connections. *Trends in Microbiology* 16, 291–300.

Pfaller, M.A. and Diekema, D.J. (2010) Epidemiology of invasive mycoses in North America. *Critical Reviews in Microbiology* 36, 1–53.

Poltermann, S., Nguyen, M., Günther, J., Wendland, J., Härtl, A., Künkel, W., Zipfel, P.F. and Eck, R. (2005) The putative vacuolar ATPase subunit Vma7p of *Candida albicans* is involved in vacuole acidification, hyphal development and virulence. *Microbiology* 151, 1645–1655.

Sauna, Z.E., Shukla, S. and Ambudkar, S.V. (2005) Disulfiram, an old drug with new potential therapeutic uses for human cancers and fungal infections. *Molecular Biosystems* 1, 127–134.

Serrano, R., Bernal, D., Simón, E. and Ariño, J. (2004) Copper and iron are the limiting factors for growth of the yeast *Saccharomyces cerevisiae* in an alkaline environment. *Journal of Biological Chemistry* 279, 19698–19704.

Shukla, S., Sauna, Z.E., Prasad, R. and Ambudkar, S.V. (2004) Disulfiram is a potent modulator of multidrug transporter Cdr1p of *Candida albicans. Biochemical and Biophysical Research Communications* 322, 520–525.

Toei, M., Saum, R. and Forgac, M. (2010) Regulation and isoform function of the V-ATPases. *Biochemistry* 49, 4715–4723.

Wang, Y., Inoue, T. and Forgac, M. (2005) Subunit a of the yeast V-ATPase participates in binding of bafilomycin. *Journal of Biological Chemistry* 280, 40481–40488.

Weissman, Z., Shemer, R., Conibear, E. and Kornitzer, D. (2008) An endocytic mechanism for haemoglobin-iron acquisition in *Candida albicans. Molecular Microbiology* 69, 201–217.

Zhang, Y.Q., Gamarra, S., Garcia-Effron G., Park, S., Perlin, D.S. and Rao, R. (2010) Requirement for ergosterol in V-ATPase function underlies antifungal activity of azole drugs. *PLoS Pathogens* 6, e1000939.

Zhang, Z., Zheng, Y., Mazon, H., Milgrom, E., Kitagawa, N., Kish-Trier, E., Heck, A.J., Kane, P.M. and Wilkens, S. (2008) Structure of the yeast vacuolar ATPase. *Journal of Biological Chemistry* 283, 35983–35995.

7 Drug Tolerance, Persister Cells and Drug Discovery

Kim Lewis
Antimicrobial Discovery Center and the Department of Biology, Northeastern University, Boston, Massachusetts, USA

7.1 The Nature of Threat: Persisters

It is a given fact that new antibiotics are needed to combat drug-resistant pathogens. However, this is only part of the need – we actually never had antibiotics capable of eradicating an infection. Currently used antibiotics have been developed against rapidly growing bacteria, and most of them have no activity against stationary-state organisms, and none is effective against dormant persister cells. The relative effectiveness of antibiotics in treating disease is largely a result of cooperation with the immune system, which mops up after antibiotics have eliminated the bulk of a growing population. However, the deficiency of existing antibiotics against supposedly drug-susceptible pathogens is becoming increasingly apparent with the rise of immunocompromised patients (e.g. those infected with human immunodeficiency virus or those undergoing chemotherapy) and the wide use of indwelling devices (e.g. catheters, prostheses and heart valves), where the pathogen forms biofilms protecting its cells from the components of the immune system. The ineffectiveness of the immune system leads to chronic diseases, which make up approximately half of all infectious disease cases in the developed world. The main culprits responsible for tolerance of pathogens to antibiotics are specialized survivors, known as persister cells (Lewis, 2007, 2010).

Persisters represent a small subpopulation of cells that spontaneously enter a dormant, non-dividing state. When a population is treated with a bactericidal antibiotic, regular cells die, while persisters survive. In order to kill, antibiotics require active targets, which explains the tolerance of persisters. Taking samples and plating them for colony counts over time from a culture treated with antibiotic produces a biphasic pattern, with a distinct plateau of surviving persisters. By contrast, resistance mechanisms prevent antibiotics from binding to their targets.

Infectious disease is often untreatable, even when caused by a pathogen that is not resistant to antibiotics. This is the essential paradox of chronic infections. In most cases, chronic infections are accompanied by the formation of biofilms, which seems to point to the source of the problem (Costerton *et al.*, 1999; Del Pozo and Patel, 2007). Biofilms have been linked to dental disease, endocarditis, cystitis, urinary tract infections, deep-seated infections, indwelling device and catheter infections, and the incurable disease of cystic fibrosis. In the case of indwelling devices such as prostheses and heart valves, re-operation is the method of choice for treating the infection. Biofilms do not generally restrict penetration of antibiotics (Walters *et al.*, 2003) but do form a barrier for the larger components of the immune system (Leid *et al.*, 2002; Jesaitis *et al.*,

 Antimicrobial Drug Discovery: Emerging Strategies (eds G. Tegos and E. Mylonakis)

2003; Vuong *et al.*, 2004). The bulk of cells in the biofilm are actually highly susceptible to killing by antibiotics; only a small fraction of persisters remains alive (Spoering and Lewis, 2001). Based on these findings, we have proposed a simple model of a relapsing chronic infection – antibiotics kill the majority of cells, and the immune system eliminates both regular cells and persisters from the bloodstream (Lewis, 2001). The only remaining live cells are then persisters in the biofilm. Once the level of antibiotic drops, persisters repopulate the biofilm and the infection relapses. While this is a plausible model, it is not the only one. A simpler possibility is that antibiotics fail to effectively reach at least some cells *in vivo*, resulting in a relapsing infection.

Establishing potential causality between persisters and therapy failure is not trivial, as these cells form a small subpopulation with a temporary phenotype, which precludes introducing them into an animal model of infection. We have reasoned that causality can be tested based on what we know about selection for high persister (*hip*) mutants *in vitro*. Periodic application of high doses of bactericidal antibiotics leads to the selection of strains that produce increased levels of persisters (Moyed and Bertrand, 1983; Wolfson *et al.*, 1990). This is precisely what happens in the course of treating chronic infections – the patient is periodically exposed to high doses of antibiotics, which may select for *hip* mutants. However, *hip* mutants will only gain advantage if the drugs effectively reach and kill the regular cells of the pathogen.

Patients with cystic fibrosis (CF) may be treated for decades for an incurable *Pseudomonas aeruginosa* infection to which they eventually succumb (Gibson *et al.*, 2003). The periodic application of high doses of antibiotics provides some relief by decreasing the pathogen burden but does not clear the infection. If *hip* strains of pathogens were selected *in vivo*, they would most likely be present in a CF patient. We took advantage of a set of longitudinal *P. aeruginosa* isolates from a single patient, collected over the course of many years (Smith *et al.*, 2006). Testing persister levels by monitoring survival after challenge with a high dose of ofloxacin showed a dramatic 100-fold increase in surviving cells in the last four isolates (Mulcahy *et al.*, 2010). Testing paired strains from additional patients showed that, in most cases, there was a considerable increase in persister levels in the late isolate from a patient. Interestingly, most of the *hip* isolates had no increase in minimum inhibitory concentration (MIC) compared with their clonal parental strain to ofloxacin, carbenicillin and tobramycin, suggesting that classical acquired resistance plays little to no role in the recalcitrance of CF infection. These experiments directly link persisters to the clinical manifestation of the disease and suggest that persisters are responsible for the therapy failure of chronic CF infection. This begs the question, why have the *hip* mutants with their striking survival phenotype evaded detection for such a long time?

The main focus of research in antimicrobials has been on drug resistance, and the basic starting experiment is to test a clinical isolate for its ability to grow in the presence of elevated levels of different antibiotics, and to record any increases in the MIC. This is also the standard test employed by clinical microbiology laboratories. *hip* mutants are, of course, missed by this test, which explains why they have remained undetected, despite a major effort aimed at understanding pathogen survival to antimicrobial chemotherapy. Given that *hip* mutants are the probable main culprit responsible for morbidity and mortality of CF infection, it makes sense to test for their presence. Testing for persister levels is not that much more difficult compared with an MIC test.

Is selection for *hip* mutants a general feature of chronic infections? We recently examined patients with chronic oral thrush caused by *Candida albicans* (Lafleur *et al.*, 2010). These were cancer patients undergoing chemotherapy, and suppression of the immune system caused the fungal infection. In patients where the disease did not resolve, the *C. albicans* isolates were almost invariably *hip* mutants, compared with patients where the disease cleared within 3 weeks of treatment with chlorhexidine. The eukaryotic *C. albicans* forms persisters (Lafleur *et al.*, 2006; Harrison *et al.*, 2007; Al-Dhaheri and Douglas, 2008) through mechanisms that are probably analogous, rather than homologous, to that of their bacterial counterparts. Given the similar lifestyles of the unrelated *P. aeruginosa* and *C. albicans*, we may expect that the survival advantage of a *hip* mutation is universal. Just as multidrug resistance has become the prevalent danger in acute infections, multidrug tolerance of persisters and *hip* mutants may be the main but largely overlooked culprit of chronic infectious disease.

Biofilms apparently serve as a protective habitat for persisters (Spoering and Lewis, 2001; Harrison *et al.*, 2005a,b, 2009; Lafleur *et al.*, 2006), allowing them to evade the immune response. However, a more general paradigm is that persisters will be critical for pathogens to survive antimicrobial chemotherapy whenever the immune response is limited. Such cases would include disseminating infections in immunocompromised patients undergoing cancer chemotherapy or infected with human immunodeficiency virus. Persisters are also likely to play an important role in immunocompetent individuals in cases where the pathogen is located at sites poorly accessible by components of the immune system. These include the central nervous system, where pathogens cause debilitating meningitis and brain abscesses (Honda and Warren, 2009), and the gastrointestinal tract, where the hard-to-eradicate *Helicobacter pylori* causes gastroduodenal ulcers and gastric carcinoma (Peterson *et al.*, 2000). Tuberculosis is perhaps the most prominent case of a chronic infection by a pathogen evading the immune system. The acute infection may resolve spontaneously or as a result of antimicrobial therapy, but the pathogen often remains in a 'latent' form (Barry *et al.*, 2009). It is estimated that one in every three people carry latent *Mycobacterium tuberculosis*, and 10% of carriers develop an acute infection at some stage in their lives. Virtually nothing is known about this latent form that serves as the main reservoir of tuberculosis. Similar to other pathogens, *M. tuberculosis* forms persisters (Keren *et al.*, 2011), and one simple possibility is that they are equivalent to the latent form of the pathogen.

The above analysis underscores the significance of drug tolerance as a barrier to effective antimicrobial chemotherapy. Given its significance – roughly half of all cases of infection – the number of studies dedicated to tolerance is tiny compared with publications on resistance. The difficulty in pinpointing the mechanism of biofilm recalcitrance and the formidable barriers to studying persister cells account for the lack of parity between these two comparably significant fields. Hopefully, a better balance will be achieved, and the following discussion summarizes recent advances in our understanding of the mechanism of tolerance.

Persisters were initially discovered in 1944, but the mechanism of their formation eluded us for a very long time. Only recently has the molecular mechanism of dormancy begun to emerge.

The most straightforward approach to finding an underlying mechanism of a complex function is by screening a library of transposon insertion mutants. This produces a set of candidate genes, and subsequent analysis leads to a pathway and a mechanism. This is indeed how the basic mechanisms of sporulation, flagellation, chemotaxis, virulence and many other functions have been established. However, screening a transposon insertion library of *Escherichia coli* for the ability to tolerate high doses of antibiotics produced no mutants completely lacking persisters (Hu and Coates, 2005; Spoering, 2006). With the development of a complete, ordered *E. coli* gene-knockout library by the Mori group (the Keio collection; Baba *et al.*, 2006), it seemed reasonable to revisit the screening approach. Indeed, there always remains a possibility that transposons missed a critical gene, or that the library was not large enough. The use of the Keio collection largely resolves this uncertainty.

This advanced screen (Hansen *et al.*, 2008), similar to previous efforts, did not produce a single mutant lacking persisters, suggesting a high degree of redundancy. The screen did identify a number of interesting genes, with knockouts showing about a tenfold decrease in persister formation. The majority of hits were in global regulators, such as DksA, DnaKJ, HupAB and IhfAB. This is an independent indication of redundancy – a global regulator can affect expression of several persister genes simultaneously, resulting in a phenotype. The screen also produced two interesting candidate genes that may be more directly involved in persister formation – YgfA, which can inhibit nucleotide synthesis, and YigB, which may block metabolism by depleting the pool of flavin mononucleotide.

A similar screen of a *P. aeruginosa* mutant library was reported recently (De Groote *et al.*, 2009). As in *E. coli*, no persisterless mutant was identified, pointing to a similar redundancy theme.

The main conclusion from the screens is that persister formation does not follow the main design theme of complex cellular functions – a single linear regulatory pathway controlling an execution mechanism. By contrast, persisters are apparently formed through a number of independent parallel mechanisms. There is a considerable adaptive advantage in this redundant design, as no single compound will disable persister formation.

Screens for persister genes were useful in finding some possible candidate genes and pointing to redundancy of function. It seemed that a method better suited to uncover redundant elements would be transcriptome analysis. For this, persisters had to be isolated.

Persisters form a small and temporary population, making isolation challenging. The simplest approach is to lyse a population of growing cells with a β-lactam antibiotic and collect surviving persisters (Keren *et al.*, 2004). This allows isolation of enough *E. coli* cells to perform a transcriptome analysis. A more advanced method aimed at isolating native persisters was developed, based on a guess that these are dormant cells with diminished protein synthesis (Shah *et al.*, 2006). If the strain expressed degradable green fluorescent protein (GFP), then cells that stochastically enter into dormancy will become less fluorescent. In a population of *E. coli* expressing degradable GFP under the control of a ribosomal promoter that is only active in dividing cells, a small number of cells indeed appeared to be less fluorescent. The difference in fluorescence allowed sorting of the two subpopulations. The cells with reduced fluorescence were tolerant to ofloxacin, confirming that they were persisters.

Transcriptomes obtained by both methods point to downregulation of biosynthesis genes, confirming the dormant nature of persisters. A very similar downregulation of biosynthetic operons is seen in *M. tuberculosis* persisters as well (Keren *et al.*, 2011). *E. coli* persisters have increased expression of several toxin/antitoxin modules (RelBE, MazEF, DinJ-YafQ and YgiU). Toxin–antitoxin (TA) modules are found on plasmids where they constitute a maintenance mechanism (Gerdes *et al.*, 1986b; Hayes, 2003). Typically, the toxin is a protein that inhibits an important cellular function such as translation or replication, and forms an inactive complex with the antitoxin. The toxin is stable, while the antitoxin is degradable. If a daughter cell does not receive a plasmid after segregation, the antitoxin level decreases due to proteolysis, leaving a toxin that either kills the cell or inhibits propagation. TA modules are also commonly found on bacterial chromosomes, but their role is largely unknown. In *E. coli*, MazF and an unrelated toxin, RelE, induce stasis by cleaving mRNA, which, of course, inhibits translation, a condition that can be reversed by expression of the corresponding antitoxins (Pedersen *et al.*, 2002; Christensen and Gerdes, 2003). This property of toxins makes them excellent candidates for persister genes.

Ectopic expression of RelE (Keren *et al.*, 2004) or MazF (Vazquez-Laslop *et al.*, 2006) strongly increased tolerance to antibiotics. The first gene linked to persisters, *hipA* (Moyed and Bertrand, 1983), is also a toxin, and its ectopic expression also causes multidrug tolerance (Falla and Chopra, 1998; Correia *et al.*, 2006; Korch and Hill, 2006). Interestingly, a bioinformatics analysis indicated that HipA is a member of the Tor family of kinases, which have been studied extensively in eukaryotes (Schmelzle and Hall, 2000) but have not previously been identified in bacteria. HipA is indeed a kinase: it autophosphorylates on Ser150, and site-directed mutagenesis replacing it, or other conserved amino acids, in the catalytic and Mg^{2+}-binding sites abolishes its ability to stop cell growth and confer drug tolerance (Correia *et al.*, 2006). The crystal structure of HipA in complex with its antitoxin HipB was recently resolved, and a pull-down experiment showed that the substrate of HipA is elongation factor EF-Tu (Schumacher *et al.*, 2009). Phosphorylated EF-Tu is inactive, which leads to a block in translation and dormancy.

Deletion of potential candidate persister genes noted above does not produce a discernible phenotype affecting persister production, possibly due to the high degree of redundancy of these elements. In *E. coli*, there are at least 15 TA modules (Pedersen and Gerdes, 1999; Pandey and Gerdes, 2005; Alix and Blanc-Potard, 2009), and more than 80 in *M. tuberculosis* (Ramage *et al.*, 2009).

The high redundancy of TA genes would explain the lack of a multidrug tolerance phenotype in knockout mutants, and therefore it seemed useful to search for conditions where a particular toxin would be highly expressed in a wild-type strain and then examine a possible link to persister formation.

Several TA modules contain the Lex box and are induced by the SOS response. These are *symER*, *hokE*, *yafN/yafO* and *tisAB/istr1* (Pedersen and Gerdes, 1999; Fernandez De Henestrosa *et al.*, 2000; Courcelle *et al.*, 2001; McKenzie *et al.*, 2003; Vogel *et al.*, 2004; Kawano *et al.*, 2007; Motiejunaite *et al.*, 2007; Singletary *et al.*, 2009). Fluoroquinolones induce the SOS response (Phillips *et al.*, 1987), and we tested the ability of ciprofloxacin to induce persister formation (Dorr *et al.*, 2009).

Examination of deletion strains showed that the level of persisters dropped dramatically, by ten- to 100-fold, in a Δ*tisAB* mutant. This suggested that TisB was responsible for the formation of the majority of persisters under conditions of SOS induction. The level of persisters was unaffected in strains deleted in the other Lex box containing TA modules. Persister levels observed in time-dependent killing experiments with ampicillin or streptomycin that do not cause DNA damage were unchanged in the Δ*tisAB* strain. TisB only had a phenotype in the presence of a functional RecA protein, confirming the dependence on the SOS pathway.

Ectopic overexpression of *tisB* sharply increased the level of persisters. A drop in the level of persisters in a deletion strain and an increase following overexpression gives reasonable confidence in the functionality of a persister gene. The dependence of TisB-induced persisters on a particular regulatory pathway, the SOS response, further strengthens the case for TisB as a specialized persister protein. Incidentally, a *tisB* mutant is not present in the otherwise fairly complete Keio knockout library, and the small open reading frame might easily have been missed by transposon mutagenesis as well, evading detection by the generalized screens for persister genes.

The role of TisB in persister formation is unexpected based on what we know about this type of protein. TisB is a small 29 amino acid hydrophobic peptide that binds to the membrane and disrupts the proton motive force, which leads to a drop in ATP levels (Unoson and Wagner, 2008). Bacteria, plants and animals all produce antimicrobial membrane-acting peptides (Garcia-Olmedo *et al.*, 1998; Sahl and Bierbaum, 1998; Zasloff, 2002). Toxins of many TA loci found on plasmids belong to this type as well. If a daughter cell does not inherit a plasmid, the concentration of a labile antitoxin decreases, and the toxin, such as the membrane-acting *hok*, kills the cell (Gerdes *et al.*, 1986a). High-level artificial overexpression of TisB also causes cell death (Unoson and Wagner, 2008). It is remarkable from this perspective that the membrane-acting TisB under conditions of natural (mild) expression has the exact opposite effect of protecting the cell from antibiotics.

Fluoroquinolones such as ciprofloxacin are widely used broad-spectrum antibiotics, and their ability to induce multidrug-tolerant cells is unexpected and a cause of considerable concern. Induction of persister formation by fluoroquinolones may contribute to the ineffectiveness of antibiotics in eradicating infections. Indeed, pre-exposure with a low dose of ciprofloxacin drastically increases tolerance to subsequent exposure with a high dose, and TisB persisters are multidrug tolerant.

The finding of the role of TisB in tolerance opens an intriguing possibility of a wider link between other stress responses and persister formation. Pathogens are exposed to many stress factors in the host environment in addition to DNA damaging agents, such as oxidants, high temperature, low pH and membrane-acting agents. It is possible that all stress responses induce the formation of surviving persisters.

While resistance and tolerance are mechanistically distinct, there is sufficient reason to believe that tolerance may be a major cause for developing resistance. Indeed, the probability of resistance development is proportional to the size of the pathogen population, and a lingering chronic infection that cannot be eradicated due to tolerance will go on to produce resistant mutants and strains acquiring resistant determinants by transmission from other bacteria (Levin and Rozen, 2006). Combating tolerance then becomes a major component in preventing resistance.

7.2 The Discovery Challenge: Source Compounds

The discovery of penicillin was an isolated event, but development of screening for antimicrobial activity from soil actinomycetes by Salman Waxman produced the first and also the only known effective platform technology for antibiotic discovery (Schatz *et al.*, 1944). Cultivable actinomycetes are, however, a limited resource: 99% of microbes do not grow readily in the laboratory and are known as 'uncultured' (Lewis *et al.*, 2010). Overmining of actinomycetes by the early 1960s replaced the discovery of novel compounds with rediscovery of known compounds.

In response to the dwindling returns in natural product antibiotic discovery, the industry responded by focusing on synthetic compounds. A number of antimicrobials are synthetic (e.g. metronidazole, trimethoprim, isoniazid, ethionamide, pyrazinamide, ethambutol), and there is one highly effective class of synthetic broad-spectrum antibiotics, the fluoroquinolones. Encouraged by these examples, and by dramatic advances in synthetic and combinatorial chemistry, high-throughput robotics, genomics and proteomics, a new discovery platform was proposed. Combinatorial chemistry provided a large number of test compounds, which were screened in high-throughput format against isolated essential target proteins determined by genomics. However, this platform failed to produce a new class of broad-spectrum antibiotics, leading to the closure of anti-infectives divisions in many of the Big Pharma companies. The main reasons for failure is well understood – high-throughput screening hits were literally running into the penetration barrier of Gram-negative bacteria, which is made of *trans*-envelope multidrug-resistant (MDR) pumps that extrude amphipathic compounds across the outer-membrane barrier (Lomovskaya *et al.*, 2008). Drugs have to be amphipathic in order to penetrate the hydrophobic inner membrane, but this is precisely the feature that the outer membrane restricts and that MDR pumps recognize. There are few compounds that pass this seemingly impenetrable barrier effectively – the broad-spectrum aminoglycosides, tetracyclines, fluoroquinolones, some β-lactams, chloramphenicol and azithromycin. Fluoroquinolones are the only synthetics on this list, and they were discovered 50 years ago.

But what about less challenging narrow-spectrum drugs, with good activity against at least Gram-positive species? Seventy high-throughput screens performed by Glaxo SmithKline, for example, against a large number of targets produced no viable leads (Payne *et al.*, 2007). Glaxo scientists realized that penetration is a serious problem, and therefore also performed *in vivo* screens against *E. coli*, but only obtained 'nuisance' hits, such as membrane-acting compounds. One obvious conclusion from this negative experience is that the libraries do not contain good starting compounds. In part, this is due to the fact that libraries are based on Lipinski rules (Lipinski, 2003), which are good for predicting drug-like properties for compounds acting against mammalian cell targets but do not work well for bacteria because of peculiarities of permeation (O'Shea and Moser, 2008; Silver, 2008). Another important consideration is the probability of resistance development. Pathogen populations produce 10^9 cells in an infected patient, which means that the probability of resistance development should be $< 10^9$. This is readily achieved with most of the antibiotic classes currently in use, as they hit more than one target (fluoroquinolones attack DNA gyrase and topoisomerase, β-lactams inhibit several penicillin-binding proteins and ribosomal inhibitors bind to rRNA, which is encoded by multiple genes)

(Silver, 2007). This requirement severely limits the number of realistic targets for antimicrobial drug discovery.

The above analysis presents an extremely bleak picture – if we cannot even discover compounds acting against rapidly growing Gram-positive bacteria, what are the prospects of finding broad-spectrum antimicrobials acting against non-growing stationary cells and persisters?

7.3 Opportunities

There are many steps in the drug-discovery pipeline, but if there are no viable leads, there is no pipeline. Indeed, at the last Interscience Conference on Antimicrobial Agents and Chemotherapy (ICAAC) meeting in 2010, there was not a single broad-spectrum lead presented. This means that the number of realistic broad-spectrum leads in the global antimicrobial drug-discovery pipeline is zero. This is where the process needs to be restarted, and this is where allocation of resources will make a tangible impact.

7.3.1 A fresh look at potential sources of compounds

Natural products

There are two largely untapped and potentially enormous new sources of natural products – uncultured microorganisms and silent operons encoding secondary metabolites.

A recent resurgence in cultivation efforts aimed at gaining access to uncultured microorganisms has been sparked by the vast diversity of uncultured bacterial groups revealed by environmental surveys of 16S rRNA (Bruns *et al.*, 2002; Connon and Giovannoni, 2002; Kaeberlein *et al.*, 2002; Rappe *et al.*, 2002; Zengler *et al.*, 2002; Stevenson *et al.*, 2004; Davis *et al.*, 2005; Ferrari *et al.*, 2005; Bollmann *et al.*, 2007; Gavrish *et al.*, 2008; Nichols *et al.*, 2008; Aoi *et al.*, 2009). While some novel bacterial species were successfully cultured by varying media and growth conditions (Joseph *et al.*, 2003), significant departures from conventional techniques were clearly in order, and indeed the new technologies substantially diverged from traditional cultivation methods by adopting single-cell and high-throughput strategies (Connon and Giovannoni, 2002; Rappe *et al.*, 2002; Zengler *et al.*, 2002; Nichols *et al.*, 2008), better mimicking the natural milieu (Bruns *et al.*, 2002; Stevenson *et al.*, 2004; Ferrari *et al.*, 2005; Aoi *et al.*, 2009), increasing the length of incubation and lowering the concentration of nutrients (Davis *et al.*, 2005). High-throughput extinction culturing is based on the dilution of natural communities of bacteria to one to ten cells per well in low-nutrient, filtered marine water. This strategy resulted in cultivation of the first member of the ubiquitous, previously uncultured clade, SAR11 (Rappe *et al.*, 2002). Our research group contributed to the effort by developing three cultivation methodologies (Kaeberlein *et al.*, 2002; Gavrish *et al.*, 2008; Nichols *et al.*, 2008). All three strategies aim to provide microorganisms with their natural growth conditions by incubating them in simulated natural environments.

The diffusion chamber is designed to essentially 'trick' cells by creating an incubation strategy that closely mimics their natural habitat (Kaeberlein *et al.*, 2002). The diffusion chamber consists of a stainless steel washer and 0.03 μm pore-size membranes. After gluing a membrane to one side of the washer, the inoculum (a mix of environmental cells and warm agar) is introduced, and the second membrane seals the chamber. Nutrients from the environment can diffuse into the chamber, and therefore it is not necessary to add them to the medium. Once inoculated and assembled, the chamber can be returned to the original location of sampling or in a simulated natural environment such as a block of sediment kept in an aquarium. Microcolonies grow in the chamber during such incubation. A mean recovery rate of 22% was observed in the diffusion chambers. In this study and in follow-up research (Bollmann *et al.*, 2007; Nichols *et al.*, 2008), we isolated numerous species that did not grow in Petri dishes inoculated with environmental samples but were grown successfully in the diffusion chambers.

Reinoculation of material from both marine and soil environments from chamber to chamber produces 'domesticated' variants that grow on regular media on a Petri dish and can be exploited for secondary metabolite production (Bollmann *et al.*, 2007; Nichols *et al.*, 2008, 2010).

Microorganisms that are particularly important for drug discovery – microscopic fungi and actinomycetes – grow by forming filaments capable of penetrating soft substrates. As actinomycetes can pass through 0.2 μm pores, we reasoned this could be used to design a trap for the specific capture of these organisms (Gavrish *et al.*, 2008). The trap is similar in design to the diffusion chamber, except that the membranes have larger pores and the agar inside the trap is initially sterile when placed in the environment. Any growth observed afterwards inside the trap is due to the movement of cells into the trap during incubation. The majority of organisms grown in the traps proved to be actinomycetes, some of which represented rare and unusual species from the genera *Dactylosporangium*, *Catellatospora*, *Catenulispora*, *Lentzea* and *Streptacidiphilus*.

We noticed that some organisms forming colonies in the diffusion chamber can grow on a Petri dish, but only in the presence of other species from the same environment (Kaeberlein *et al.*, 2002; Nichols *et al.*, 2008) and suggested that uncultured bacteria only commit to division in a familiar environment, which they recognize by the presence of growth factors released by their neighbours. In order to assess the commonality of the growth dependence of uncultured organisms on neighbouring species and pick good models for study, we chose an environment where bacteria live in a tightly packed community (D'Onofrio *et al.*, 2010). This is a biofilm that envelopes sand particles of a tidal ocean beach. There were disproportionately more colonies appearing on densely inoculated plates compared with more dilute plates. This indicated that some of the cells that grew on the densely seeded plates were receiving growth factors from neighbouring colonies. To test the possible growth dependence of microorganisms on neighbouring species, pairs of colonies growing within a short distance of each other were restreaked in close proximity to each other. Potential uncultured isolates were identified by their diminishing growth with increasing distance from the cultivable 'helper' strain on the cross-streak plates. Colonies of the culturable organism *M. luteus* KLE1011 (a marine sand sediment isolate 99.5% identical to *M. luteus* DSM 200030^T according to the 16S rRNA gene sequence) grew larger as their distance from other colonies increased. Approximately 100 randomly picked pairs of colonies were restreaked from the high-density plates, and 10% of these pairs showed this pattern of growth induction on cross-streaked plates.

In order to isolate growth factors, spent medium from the helper *M. luteus* KLE1011 was tested and shown to induce growth of the uncultured *Micrococcus polysiphoniae* KLE1104. An assay-guided fractionation led to isolation and structure determination of five different siderophores, each of which was able to induce growth of *M. polysiphoniae* KLE1104. This demonstrated that siderophores represent the growth factors responsible for the helping activity. The siderophores consisted of a central core with alternating *N*-hydroxycadaverine and succinic acid units and were of the desferrioxamine class (Challis, 2005). Both close relatives of known microorganisms and novel species were isolated by this approach. This study identified the first class of growth factors for uncultured bacteria and suggests that additional ones will come from analysing organisms growing in co-culture.

Silent operons

Whole-genome sequencing of several actinomycetes has shown that there are many more potential biosynthetic pathways for the production of secondary metabolites than there are known antibiotics made by these organisms (Ikeda *et al.*, 2003). Ecopia Biosciences has used fermentation in 40 different media to entice the production of additional compounds, and discovered a novel type of enediyne with anticancer activity (Zazopoulos *et al.*, 2003). No novel antimicrobials emerged from this effort. However, in order to be effective, one needs to develop a high-throughput approach to induce production of such compounds. This is entirely doable.

Synthetics

Are existing libraries, both commercially available and proprietary collections in the Big Pharma, useless for antibiotic discovery? It does seem so, as they have obviously already been screened for actives, including non-biased screens for growth inhibition of whole cells, and produced no viable leads. But does it not seem strange that a screen of a collection of 600 dyes by Gerhard Domagk produced the first viable antibiotic, while a screen of the total global library of 10^7 compounds produced nothing at all? As the libraries grew, a number of innovations were introduced aimed at improving the screening outcome – *in vitro* screening, targeted screens, Lipinski rules and specificity validation. Each time we tried to improve things, the result was to discard valuable compounds. I believe that the existing libraries do harbour useful molecules; the question is how to identify them.

7.3.2 Good compounds from bad libraries

Back to Domagk

The first screen was also perfect – Domagk tested compounds against mice infected with streptococci. The result was the discovery of prontosil, a sulfa drug that has no activity *in vitro*. The compound is cleaved in the intestine by gut bacteria, releasing the active sulfonamide moiety, which inhibits dehydropteroate synthase in the folate pathway. An *in vitro* test would have missed prontosil. There are obvious advantages to testing compounds *in situ* – this automatically eliminates the significant burden of toxic molecules, and demonstrates efficacy, again automatically eliminating substances with problems of action in an animal, such as serum binding, instability or poor tissue distribution. In addition, different types of compound may be uniquely uncovered, such as those requiring activation *in situ* and those hitting targets that are only important in an infection but not *in vitro*. While this would theoretically be the perfect way to go, testing in 10^7 mice is not an option for a variety of reasons, including ethical considerations and the large amounts of required test compound. We therefore considered a useful intermediate between *in vitro* and a mammal – an animal that, unlike mice, can be dispersed in microtitre wells. *Caenorhabditis elegans* can be infected with human pathogens by simply ingesting them, and we found that the worm can be cured by common antibiotics such as tetracycline and vancomycin, and at concentrations typically achieved in human plasma (Moy *et al.*, 2006). Worms infected with a pathogen such as *Enterococcus faecalis* die and stop moving, their shape changes from curved to straight and they can be detected by typical eukaryotic vital dyes. Using these parameters, an automated approach was developed, and a large pilot screen of compound libraries uncovered hits, some of which had no activity *in vitro* (Moy *et al.*, 2006, 2009). This approach shows that *C. elegans* points us in the right direction – back to Domagk, but with larger libraries.

Better libraries and rules of penetration

Of course it would be great to have a better library, constructed based not on Lipinski rules but on 'rules of penetration'. We have a small number of broad-spectrum compounds that are largely able to bypass the MDR pumps and get across the impermeable barrier of Gram-negative membranes – tetracycline, chloramphenicol, aminoglycosides, trimethoprim, fluoroquinolones, metronidazole and β-lactams (the latter only need to traverse the outer membrane). This set is too small to enable us to discern rules of penetration. However, testing a large number of unbiased compounds from a library for their ability to enter into the cytoplasm of Gram-negative bacteria should allow us to deduce general rules that favour penetration. Once these are available, this would drive the synthesis/ combinatorial chemistry of new compound libraries specifically geared towards antimicrobial discovery.

Prodrugs

It is useful to consider the theoretically perfect antibiotic from first principles and then decide whether it is realistic. Approaches we have discussed so far do not address the daunting challenge of killing persister cells while at the same time showing broad-spectrum activity. It is useful to start with the end result, a highly reactive compound that will kill all cells, including persisters. In order to spare the host, the compound must be delivered as a pro-drug, and then a bacteria-specific enzyme will activate it into a generally reactive molecule that will bind covalently to unrelated targets. Importantly, this mechanism creates an irreversible sink, largely resolving the issue of MDR pump efflux, so the antimicrobial is automatically a broad-spectrum drug. Is this realistic? Several existing antimicrobials closely match the properties of this idealized pro-drug antibiotic. These are isoniazid, pyrazinamide, ethionamide and metronidazole. The first three are anti-*M. tuberculosis* drugs, while metronidazole is a broad-spectrum compound acting against anaerobic bacteria. All four compounds convert into active antiseptic-type molecules inside the cell that covalently bind to their targets. It seems to be no accident that pro-drug antibiotics make up the core of the anti-*M. tuberculosis* drug arsenal, as the ability to kill the pathogen is critical for treating the disease. Preferred targets have been identified for isoniazid and ethionamide (Vilcheze *et al.*, 2005), suggesting a relatively limited reactivity of these compounds. The existence of preferred targets indicates that the pro-drug products are not that reactive, and there is considerable room for developing better sterilizing antibiotics based on the same principle.

References

Al-Dhaheri, R.S. and Douglas, L.J. (2008) Absence of amphotericin B-tolerant persister cells in biofilms of some *Candida* species. *Antimicrobial Agents and Chemotherapy* 52, 1884–1887.

Alix, E. and Blanc-Potard, A. (2009) Hydrophobic peptides: novel regulators within bacterial membranes. *Molecular Microbiology* 72, 5–11.

Aoi, Y., Kinoshita, T., Hata, T., Ohta, H., Obokata, H. and Tsuneda, S. (2009) Hollow-fiber membrane chamber as a device for in situ environmental cultivation. *Applied and Environmental Microbiology* 75, 3826–3833.

Baba, T., Ara, T., Hasegawa, M., Takai, Y., Okumura, Y., Baba, M., Datsenko, K.A., Tomita, M., Wanner, B.L. and Mori, H. (2006) Construction of *Escherichia coli* K-12 in-frame, single-gene knockout mutants: the Keio collection. *Molecular Systematic Biology* 2, 2006.0008.

Barry, C.E. III, Boshoff, H.I., Dartois, V., Dick, T., Ehrt, S., Flynn, J., Schnappinger, D., Wilkinson, R.J. and Young, D. (2009) The spectrum of latent tuberculosis: rethinking the biology and intervention strategies. *Nature Reviews Microbiology* 7, 845–855.

Bollmann, A., Lewis, K. and Epstein, S.S. (2007) Incubation of environmental samples in a diffusion chamber increases the diversity of recovered isolates. *Applied and Environmental Microbiology* 73, 6386–6390.

Bruns, A., Cypionka, H. and Overmann, J. (2002) Cyclic AMP and acyl homoserine lactones increase the cultivation efficiency of heterotrophic bacteria from the central Baltic Sea. *Applied and Environmental Microbiology* 68, 3978–3987.

Challis, G.L. (2005) A widely distributed bacterial pathway for siderophore biosynthesis independent of nonribosomal peptide synthetases. *ChemBioChem* 6, 601–611.

Christensen, S.K. and Gerdes, K. (2003) RelE toxins from bacteria and Archaea cleave mRNAs on translating ribosomes, which are rescued by tmRNA. *Molecular Microbiology* 48, 1389–1400.

Connon, S.A. and Giovannoni, S.J. (2002) High-throughput methods for culturing microorganisms in very-low-nutrient media yield diverse new marine isolates. *Applied and Environmental Microbiology* 68, 3878–3885.

Correia, F.F., D'Onofrio, A., Rejtar, T., Li, L., Karger, B.L., Makarova, K., Koonin, E.V. and Lewis, K. (2006) Kinase activity of overexpressed *HipA* is required for growth arrest and multidrug tolerance in *Escherichia coli*. *Journal of Bacteriology*188, 8360–8367.

Costerton, J.W., Stewart, P.S. and Greenberg, E.P. (1999) Bacterial biofilms: a common cause of persistent infections. *Science* 284, 1318–1322.

Courcelle, J., Khodursky, A., Peter, B., Brown, P. and Hanawalt, P. (2001) Comparative gene expression profiles following UV exposure in wild type and SOS-deficient *Escherichia coli*. *Genetics* 158, 41–64.

Davis, K.E., Joseph, S.J. and Janssen, P.H. (2005) Effects of growth medium, inoculum size, and incubation time on culturability and isolation of soil bacteria. *Applied and Environmental Microbiology* 71, 826–834.

De Groote, V.N., Verstraeten, N., Fauvart, M., Kint, C.I., Verbeeck, A.M., Beullens, S., Cornelis, P.

and Michiels, J. (2009) Novel persistence genes in *Pseudomonas aeruginosa* identified by high-throughput screening. *FEMS Microbiology Letters* 297, 73–79.

Del Pozo, J. and Patel, R. (2007) The challenge of treating biofilm-associated bacterial infections. *Clinical Pharmacology and Therapeutics* 82, 204–209.

D'Onofrio, A., Crawford, J.M., Stewart, E.J., Witt, K., Gavrish, E., Epstein, S., Clardy, J. and Lewis, K. (2010) Siderophores from neighboring organisms promote the growth of uncultured bacteria. *Chemistry and Biology* 17, 254–264.

Dorr, T., Lewis, K. and Vulic, M. (2009) SOS response induces persistence to fluoroquinolones in *Escherichia coli. PLoS Genetics* 5, e1000760.

Falla, T.J. and Chopra, I. (1998) Joint tolerance to β-lactam and fluoroquinolone antibiotics in *Escherichia coli* results from overexpression of *hipA. Antimicrobial Agents and Chemotherapy* 42, 3282–3284.

Fernandez De Henestrosa, A.R., Ogi, T., Aoyagi, S., Chafin, D., Hayes, J.J., Ohmori, H. and Woodgate, R. (2000) Identification of additional genes belonging to the LexA regulon in *Escherichia coli. Molecular Microbiology* 35, 1560–1572.

Ferrari, B.C., Binnerup, S.J. and Gillings, M. (2005) Microcolony cultivation on a soil substrate membrane system selects for previously uncultured soil bacteria. *Applied and Environmental Microbiology* 71, 8714–8720.

Garcia-Olmedo, F., Molina, A., Alamillo, J.M. and Rodriguez-Palenzuela, P. (1998) Plant defense peptides. *Biopolymers* 47, 479–491.

Gavrish, E., Bollmann, A., Epstein, S. and Lewis, K. (2008) A trap for *in situ* cultivation of filamentous actinobacteria. *Journal of Microbiological Methods* 72, 257–262.

Gerdes, K., Bech, F.W., Jorgensen, S.T., Lobner-Olesen, A., Rasmussen, P.B., Atlung, T., Boe, L., Karlstrom, O., Molin, S. and Von Meyenburg, K. (1986a) Mechanism of postsegregational killing by the *hok* gene product of the parB system of plasmid R1 and its homology with the *relF* gene product of the *E. coli relB* operon. *EMJO Journal* 5, 2023–2029.

Gerdes, K., Rasmussen, P.B. and Molin, S. (1986b) Unique type of plasmid maintenance function: postsegregational killing of plasmid-free cells. *Proceedings of the National Academy of Sciences USA,* 83, 3116–3120.

Gibson, R.L., Burns, J.L. and Ramsey, B.W. (2003) Pathophysiology and management of pulmonary infections in cystic fibrosis. *American Journal of Respiratory and Critical Care Medicine* 168, 918–951.

Hansen, S., Lewis, K. and Vuli , M. (2008) The role of global regulators and nucleotide metabolism in antibiotic tolerance in *Escherichia coli. Antimicrobial Agents and Chemotherapy* 52, 2718–2726.

Harrison, J.J., Ceri, H., Roper, N.J., Badry, E.A., Sproule, K.M. and Turner, R.J. (2005a) Persister cells mediate tolerance to metal oxyanions in *Escherichia coli. Microbiology* 151, 3181–3195.

Harrison, J.J., Turner, R.J. and Ceri, H. (2005b) Persister cells, the biofilm matrix and tolerance to metal cations in biofilm and planktonic *Pseudomonas aeruginosa. Environmental Microbiology* 7, 981–994.

Harrison, J.J., Turner, R.J. and Ceri, H. (2007) A subpopulation of *Candida albicans* and *Candida tropicalis* biofilm cells are highly tolerant to chelating agents. *FEMS Microbiology Letters* 272, 172–181.

Harrison, J.J., Wade, W.D., Akierman, S., Vacchi-Suzzi, C., Stremick, C.A., Turner, R.J. and Ceri, H. (2009) The chromosomal toxin gene *yafQ* is a determinant of multidrug tolerance for *Escherichia coli* growing in a biofilm. *Antimicrobial Agents and Chemotherapy* 53, 2253–2258.

Hayes, F. (2003) Toxins–antitoxins: plasmid maintenance, programmed cell death, and cell cycle arrest. *Science* 301, 1496–1499.

Honda, H. and Warren, D.K. (2009) Central nervous system infections: meningitis and brain abscess. *Infectious Disease Clinics of North America* 23, 609–623.

Hu, Y. and Coates, A.R. (2005) Transposon mutagenesis identifies genes which control antimicrobial drug tolerance in stationary-phase *Escherichia coli. FEMS Microbiology Letters* 243, 117–124.

Ikeda, H., Ishikawa, J., Hanamoto, A., Shinose, M., Kikuchi, H., Shiba, T., Sakaki, Y., Hattori, M. and Omura, S. (2003) Complete genome sequence and comparative analysis of the industrial microorganism *Streptomyces avermitilis. Nature Biotechnology* 21, 526–531.

Jesaitis, A.J., Franklin, M.J., Berglund, D., Sasaki, M., Lord, C.I., Bleazard, J.B., Duffy, J.E., Beyenal, H. and Lewandowski, Z. (2003) Compromised host defense on *Pseudomonas aeruginosa* biofilms: characterization of neutrophil and biofilm interactions. *Journal of Immunology* 171, 4329–4339.

Joseph, S.J., Hugenholtz, P., Sangwan, P., Osborne, C.A. and Janssen, P.H. (2003) Laboratory cultivation of widespread and previously uncultured soil bacteria. *Applied and Environmental Microbiology* 69, 7210–7215.

Kaeberlein, T., Lewis, K. and Epstein, S.S. (2002) Isolating "uncultivable" microorganisms in pure culture in a simulated natural environment. *Science* 296, 1127–1129.

Kawano, M., Aravind, L. and Storz, G. (2007) An antisense RNA controls synthesis of an SOS-induced toxin evolved from an antitoxin. *Molecular Microbiology* 64, 738–754.

Keren, I., Shah, D., Spoering, A., Kaldalu, N. and Lewis, K. (2004) Specialized persister cells and the mechanism of multidrug tolerance in *Escherichia coli. Journal of Bacteriology* 186, 8172–8180.

Keren, I., Minami, S., Rubin, E. and Lewis, K. (2011) Characterization and transcriptome analysis of *Mycobacterium tuberculosis* persisters. *MBio* 2, e00100-11.

Korch, S.B. and Hill, T.M. (2006) Ectopic overexpression of wild-type and mutant *hipA* genes in *Escherichia coli*: effects on macromolecular synthesis and persister formation. *Journal of Bacteriology* 188, 3826–3836.

Lafleur, M.D., Kumamoto, C.A. and Lewis, K. (2006) *Candida albicans* biofilms produce antifungal-tolerant persister cells. *Antimicrobial Agents and Chemotherapy* 50, 3839–3846.

Lafleur, M.D., Qi, Q. and Lewis, K. (2010) Patients with long-term oral carriage harbor high-persister mutants of *Candida albicans. Antimicrobial Agents and Chemotherapy* 54, 39–44.

Leid, J.G., Shirtliff, M.E., Costerton, J.W. and Stoodley, A.P. (2002) Human leukocytes adhere to, penetrate, and respond to *Staphylococcus aureus* biofilms. *Infection and Immunity* 70, 6339–6345.

Levin, B.R. and Rozen, D.E. (2006) Non-inherited antibiotic resistance. *Nature Reviews Microbiology* 4, 556–562.

Lewis, K. (2001) Riddle of biofilm resistance. *Antimicrobial Agents and Chemotherapy* 45, 999–1007.

Lewis, K. (2007) Persister cells, dormancy and infectious disease. *Nature Reviews Microbiology* 5, 48–56.

Lewis, K. (2010) Persister cells. *Annual Reviews in Microbiology* 64, 357–372.

Lewis, K., Epstein, S., D'Onofrio, A. and Ling, L.L. (2010) Uncultured microorganisms as a source of secondary metabolites. *Journal of Antibiotics* 63, 468–476.

Lipinski, C.A. (2003) *The Practice of Medicinal Chemistry.* Academic Press, Amsterdam.

Lomovskaya, O., Zgurskaya, H.I., Bostian, K.A. and Lewis, K. (2008) Multidrug efflux pumps: structure, mechanism, and inhibition. In: Wax, R.G., Lewis, K., Salyers, A.A. and Taber, H. (eds) *Bacterial Resistance to Antimicrobials*, 2nd edn. CRC Press, Boca Raton, Florida, pp. 45–69.

McKenzie, G.J., Magner, D.B., Lee, P.L. and Rosenberg, S.M. (2003) The *dinB* operon and spontaneous mutation in *Escherichia coli. Journal of Bacteriology* 185, 3972–3977.

Motiejunaite, R., Armalyte, J., Markuckas, A. and Suziedeliene, E. (2007) *Escherichia coli dinJ-yafQ* genes act as a toxin–antitoxin module. *FEMS Microbiology Letters* 268, 112–119.

Moy, T.I., Ball, A.R., Anklesaria, Z., Casadei, G., Lewis, K. and Ausubel, F.M. (2006) Identification of novel antimicrobials using a live-animal infection model. *Proceedings of the National Academy of Sciences USA* 103, 10414–10419.

Moy, T.I., Conery, A.L., Larkins-Ford, J., Wu, G., Mazitschek, R., Casadei, G., Lewis, K., Carpenter, A.E. and Ausubel, F.M. (2009) High-throughput screen for novel antimicrobials using a whole animal infection model. *ACS Chemical Biology* 4, 527–533.

Moyed, H.S. and Bertrand, K.P. (1983) *hipA*, a newly recognized gene of *Escherichia coli* K-12 that affects frequency of persistence after inhibition of murein synthesis. *Journal of Bacteriology* 155, 768–775.

Mulcahy, L.R., Burns, J.L., Lory, S. and Lewis, K. (2010) Emergence of *Pseudomonas aeruginosa* strains producing high levels of persister cells in patients with cystic fibrosis. *Journal of Bacteriology* 192, 6191–6199.

Nichols, D., Lewis, K., Orjala, J., Mo, S., Ortenberg, R., O'Connor, P., Zhao, C., Vouros, P., Kaeberlein, T. and Epstein, S.S. (2008) Short peptide induces an 'uncultivable' microorganism to grow *in vitro. Applied and Environmental Microbiology* 74, 4889–4897.

Nichols, D., Cahoon, N., Trakhtenberg, E.M., Pham, L., Mehta, A., Belanger, A., Kanigan, T., Lewis, K. and Epstein, S.S. (2010) Use of ichip for high-throughput *in situ* cultivation of "uncultivable" microbial species. *Applied and Environmental Microbiology* 76, 2445–2450.

O'Shea, R. and Moser, H.E. (2008) Physicochemical properties of antibacterial compounds: implications for drug discovery. *Journal of Medicinal Chemistry* 51, 2871–2878.

Pandey, D.P. and Gerdes, K. (2005) Toxin–antitoxin loci are highly abundant in free-living but lost from host-associated prokaryotes. *Nucleic Acids Research* 33, 966–976.

Payne, D.J., Gwynn, M.N., Holmes, D.J. and Pompliano, D.L. (2007) Drugs for bad bugs: confronting the challenges of antibacterial discovery. *Nature Reviews Drug Discovery* 6, 29–40.

Pedersen, K. and Gerdes, K. (1999) Multiple *hok* genes on the chromosome of *Escherichia coli. Molecular Microbiology* 32, 1090–1102.

Pedersen, K., Christensen, S.K. and Gerdes, K. (2002) Rapid induction and reversal of a bacteriostatic condition by controlled expression of toxins and antitoxins. *Molecular Microbiology* 45, 501–510.

Peterson, W.L., Fendrick, A.M., Cave, D.R., Peura, D.A., Garabedian-Ruffalo, S.M. and Laine, L. (2000) *Helicobacter pylori*-related disease: guidelines for testing and treatment. *Archives of Internal Medicine* 160, 1285–1291.

Phillips, I., Culebras, E., Moreno, F. and Baquero, F. (1987) Induction of the SOS response by new 4-quinolones. *Journal of Antimicrobial Chemotherapy* 20, 631–638.

Ramage, H.R., Connolly, L.E. and Cox, J.S. (2009) Comprehensive functional analysis of *Mycobacterium tuberculosis* toxin–antitoxin systems: implications for pathogenesis, stress responses, and evolution. *PLoS Genetics* 5, e1000767.

Rappe, M.S., Connon, S.A., Vergin, K.L. and Giovannoni, S.J. (2002) Cultivation of the ubiquitous SAR11 marine bacterioplankton clade. *Nature* 418, 630–633.

Sahl, H.G. and Bierbaum, G. (1998) Lantibiotics: biosynthesis and biological activities of uniquely modified peptides from Gram-positive bacteria. *Annual Reviews in Microbiology* 52, 41–79.

Schatz, A., Bugie, E. and Waxman, S.A. (1944) Streptomycin, a substance exhibiting antibiotic activity against Gram positive and Gram negative bacteria. *Proceedings of the Society for Experimental Biology and Medicine* 55, 66.

Schmelzle, T. and Hall, M.N. (2000) TOR, a central controller of cell growth. *Cell* 103, 253–262.

Schumacher, M.A., Piro, K.M., Xu, W., Hansen, S., Lewis, K. and Brennan, R.G. (2009) Molecular mechanisms of HipA-mediated multidrug tolerance and its neutralization by HipB. *Science* 323, 396–401.

Shah, D., Zhang, Z., Khodursky, A., Kaldalu, N., Kurg, K. and Lewis, K. (2006) Persisters: a distinct physiological state of *E. coli*. *BMC Microbiology* 6, 53–61.

Silver, L.L. (2007) Multi-targeting by monotherapeutic antibacterials. *Nature Reviews Drug Discovery* 6, 41–55.

Silver, L.L. (2008) Are natural products still the best source for antibacterial discovery? The bacterial entry factor. *Expert Opinion in Drug Discovery* 3, 487–500.

Singletary, L.A., Gibson, J.L., Tanner, E.J., McKenzie, G.J., Lee, P.L., Gonzalez, C. and Rosenberg, S.M. (2009) An SOS-regulated type 2 toxin-antitoxin system. *Journal of Bacteriology* 191, 7456–7465.

Smith, E.E., Buckley, D.G., Wu, Z., Saenphimmachak, C., Hoffman, L.R., D'argenio, D.A., Miller, S.I., Ramsey, B.W., Speert, D.P., Moskowitz, S.M., Burns, J.L., Kaul, R. and Olson, M.V. (2006) Genetic adaptation by *Pseudomonas aeruginosa* to the airways of cystic fibrosis patients. *Proceedings of the National Academy of Sciences USA* 103, 8487–8492.

Spoering, A. (2006) GlpD and PlsB participate in persister cell formation in *Escherichia coli*. *Journal of Bacteriology* 188, 5136–5144.

Spoering, A.L. and Lewis, K. (2001) Biofilms and planktonic cells of *Pseudomonas aeruginosa* have similar resistance to killing by antimicrobials *Journal of Bacteriology* 183, 6746–6751.

Stevenson, B.S., Eichorst, S.A., Wertz, J.T., Schmidt, T.M. and Breznak, J.A. (2004) New strategies for cultivation and detection of previously uncultured microbes. *Applied and Environmental Microbiology* 70, 4748–4755.

Unoson, C. and Wagner, E. (2008) A small SOS-induced toxin is targeted against the inner membrane in *Escherichia coli*. *Molecular Microbiology* 70, 258–270.

Vazquez-Laslop, N., Lee, H. and Neyfakh, A.A. (2006) Increased persistence in *Escherichia coli* caused by controlled expression of toxins or other unrelated proteins. *Journal of Bacteriology* 188, 3494–3497.

Vilcheze, C., Weisbrod, T.R., Chen, B., Kremer, L., Hazbon, M.H., Wang, F., Alland, D., Sacchettini, J.C. and Jacobs, W.R. Jr (2005) Altered NADH/NAD^+ ratio mediates coresistance to isoniazid and ethionamide in mycobacteria. *Antimicrobial Agents and Chemotherapy* 49, 708–720.

Vogel, J., Argaman, L., Wagner, E.G. and Altuvia, S. (2004) The small RNA IstR inhibits synthesis of an SOS-induced toxic peptide. *Current Biology* 14, 2271–2276.

Vuong, C., Voyich, J.M., Fischer, E.R., Braughton, K.R., Whitney, A.R., Deleo, F.R. and Otto, M. (2004) Polysaccharide intercellular adhesin (PIA) protects *Staphylococcus epidermidis* against major components of the human innate immune system. *Cell Microbiology* 6, 269–275.

Walters, M.C. III, Roe, F., Bugnicourt, A., Franklin, M.J. and Stewart, P.S. (2003) Contributions of antibiotic penetration, oxygen limitation, and low metabolic activity to tolerance of *Pseudomonas aeruginosa* biofilms to ciprofloxacin and tobramycin. *Antimicrobial Agents and Chemotherapy* 47, 317–323.

Wolfson, J.S., Hooper, D.C., McHugh, G.L., Bozza, M.A. and Swartz, M.N. (1990) Mutants of *Escherichia coli* K-12 exhibiting reduced killing by both quinolone and β-lactam antimicrobial agents. *Antimicrobial Agents and Chemotherapy* 34, 1938–1943.

Zasloff, M. (2002) Antimicrobial peptides of multicellular organisms. *Nature* 415, 389–395.

Zazopoulos, E., Huang, K., Staffa, A., Liu, W., Bachmann, B.O., Nonaka, K., Ahlert, J., Thorson, J.S., Shen, B. and Farnet, C.M. (2003) A genomics-guided approach for discovering and expressing cryptic metabolic pathways. *Nature Biotechnology* 21, 187–190.

Zengler, K., Toledo, G., Rappe, M., Elkins, J., Mathur, E.J., Short, J.M. and Keller, M. (2002) Cultivating the uncultured. *Proceedings of the National Academy of Sciences USA* 99, 15681–15686.

8 Inhibition of Quorum Sensing as a Novel Antimicrobial Strategy

Gilles Brackman, Hans J. Nelis and Tom Coenye
Laboratory of Pharmaceutical Microbiology, Ghent University, Ghent, Belgium

8.1 Introduction

Although antibiotic resistance in bacteria is a growing problem, relatively few novel antibacterials have been developed in recent years (Projan, 2003; Tenover, 2006). In addition, killing of bacteria or the inhibition of their growth results in selective pressure, making antimicrobial resistance an inevitable consequence of antimicrobial use (Tenover, 2006). For this reason, innovative antimicrobials with novel targets and modes of action are needed. One alternative approach is targeting the bacterial communication system, known as quorum sensing (QS). QS is a process by which bacteria produce and detect signal molecules and thereby coordinate their behaviour in a cell-density-dependent manner (Waters and Bassler, 2005). Three main QS systems can be distinguished: the acylhomoserine lactone (AHL) QS system in Gram-negative bacteria, the autoinducing peptide (AIP) QS system in Gram-positive bacteria and the Autoinducer-2 (AI-2) QS system in both Gram-negative and Gram-positive bacteria (Fig. 8.1). Gram-negative bacteria use AHL signalling molecules (Fig. 8.1), which are produced by a LuxI-type synthase and are perceived by a DNA-binding LuxR-type transcriptional activator (Waters and Bassler, 2005). The QS system of Gram-positive bacteria typically consists of signal peptides (Fig. 8.1), such as Agr and RNA-III activating/inhibiting peptides (RAP/RIP) in *Staphylococcus aureus*, and a two-component regulatory system made up of a membrane-bound sensor and an intracellular response regulator (Thoendel and Horswill, 2009). A third QS system is shared by many Gram-positive and Gram-negative bacteria and is based on a mixture of interconvertible molecules collectively referred to as AI-2 (Fig. 8.1) (Vendeville *et al.*, 2005; Waters and Bassler, 2005). A key enzyme in the production of AI-2 is LuxS. LuxS catalyses the cleavage of *S*-ribosylhomocysteine to homocysteine and 4,5 dihydroxy-2,3-pentanedione (DPD). DPD will subsequently undergo spontaneous rearrangements and modifications, forming a mixture of molecules, collectively called AI-2. Although LuxS is encoded in more than half of all sequenced bacterial genomes, AI-2 receptors and signal transduction systems have only been described in *Vibrio* spp., *Salmonella enterica* serovar Typhimurium and *Escherichia coli* (Sun *et al.*, 2004; Vendeville *et al.*, 2005). In *Vibrio* spp., binding of AI-2 to LuxP, a periplasmic AI-2 receptor associated with the LuxQ sensor kinase, results in the production of LuxR, and ultimately in changes in gene expression. In *S. enterica* serovar Typhimurium and *E. coli*, AI-2 is first transported into the cell prior to initiating a signalling cascade (Vendeville *et al.*, 2005).

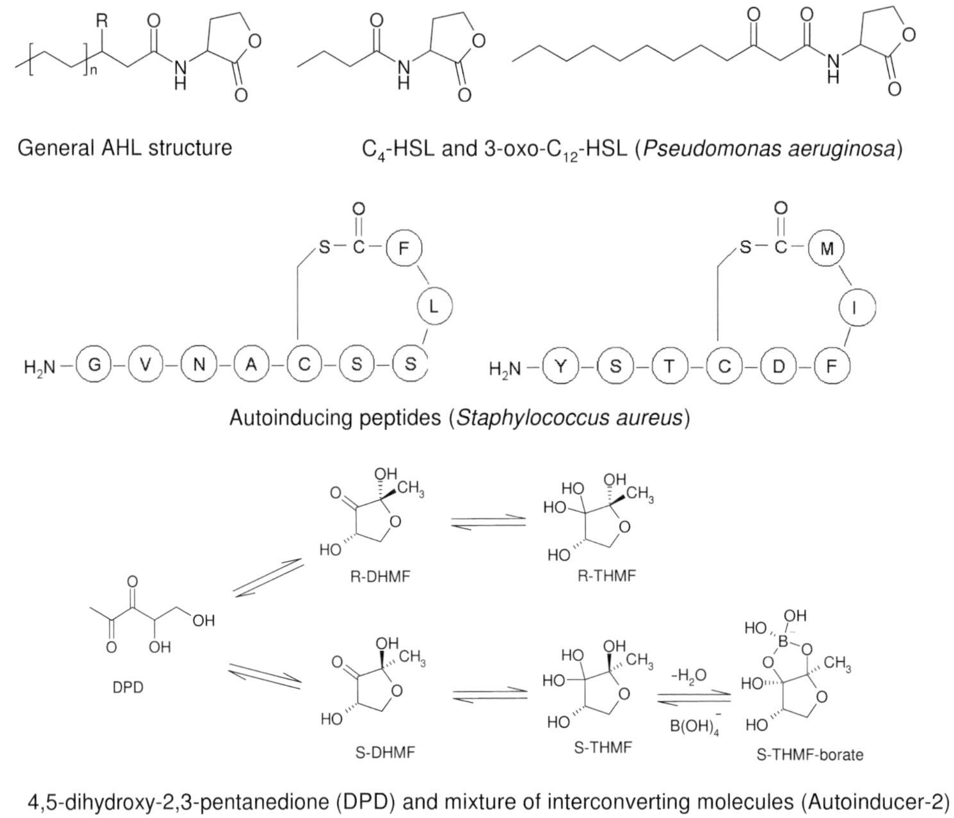

Fig. 8.1. QS signal molecules. HSL, homoserine lactone.

Various bacteria use their QS systems for the regulation of the production of virulence factors. For this reason, QS inhibition has been proposed as an attractive antipathogenic strategy. QS inhibition can be achieved by inhibiting the synthesis of signal molecules, interference with signal transport/secretion, degradation of the signal, inhibition of binding of the signal molecule to the receptor and/or inhibition of the signal transduction cascade. In this chapter, we will discuss the different QS inhibitors (QSIs).

8.2 Inhibition of Signal Molecule Synthesis

8.2.1 Inhibition of AHL synthesis

AHL signal molecules are formed when an acyl carrier protein (ACP)-bound fatty acyl derivative is transferred to the amino group of *S*-adenosylmethionine (SAM) by LuxI. Given the nature of this reaction and the precursors involved, inhibitors of SAM or fatty acid biosynthesis may be used as AHL QSIs. *S*-adenosylhomocysteine (SAH), sinefungin, 5′-methylthioadenosine (MTA), various SAM analogues and the SAM biosynthesis inhibitor cycloleucine inhibit AHL production (Fig. 8.2) (Hanzelka and Greenberg, 1996; Parsek *et al.*, 1999). Azithromycin, ceftazidime and tobramycin (Fig. 8.2) inhibit the synthesis of C_4-homoserine lactone (C_4-HSL) and 3-oxo-C_{12}-HSL in *Pseudomonas aeruginosa* when used at subinhibitory concentrations (Garske *et al.*, 2004; Tateda *et al.*, 2007).

AHL synthesis can also be inhibited at the level of fatty acid biosynthesis by the use of cerulenin (Fig. 8.2) and diazoborine. Cerulenin is a specific and irreversible inhibitor of the β-keto-acyl-ACP synthases I and II, while diazoborine inhibits fatty acid synthesis

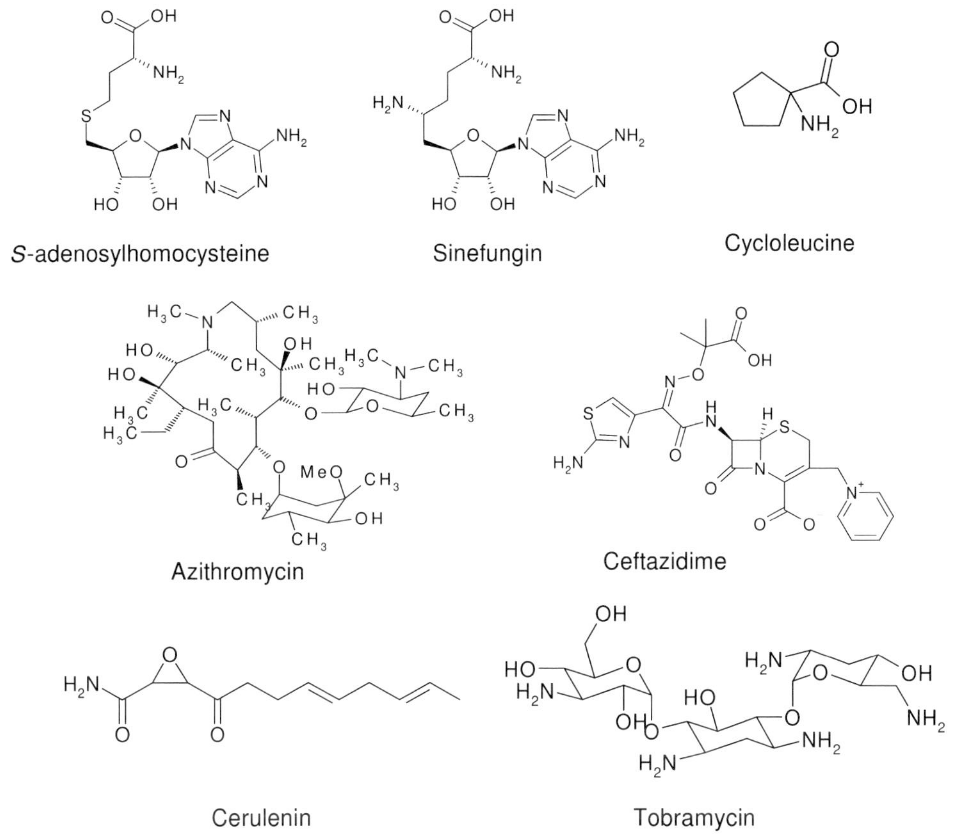

Fig. 8.2. Examples of QSIs targeting AHL signal synthesis.

by blocking the active sites of the NADH-dependent enoyl-ACP reductase. Cerulenin decreases AHL production in *Vibrio harveyi*, and cerulenin and diazoborine abolish AHL production in an *E. coli* strain carrying the AHL synthase gene (Cao and Meighen, 1993; Val and Cronan, 1998). However, SAM and fatty acids are ubiquitous in humans and animals, which makes it unlikely that these can be applied *in vivo*.

8.2.2 Inhibition of AI-2 synthesis

AI-2 synthesis involves two major enzymatic steps. First, adenine is removed from SAH by MTA nucleosidase (MTAN) (encoded by *pfs*), resulting in the production of *S*-ribosylhomocysteine (SRH). Next, SRH is cleaved by LuxS to form DPD and homocysteine. In addition, MTAN is also involved in the AHL QS system, and LuxS and MTAN are only found in bacteria, making them attractive targets. Several inhibitors of LuxS and MTAN have been described. *S*-Anhydroribosyl-L-homocysteine (Fig. 8.3) and *S*-homoribosyl-L-cysteine block the initial and final steps of the LuxS reaction mechanism, respectively (Zhao *et al.*, 2003; Alfaro *et al.*, 2004). Based on these molecules, Shen *et al.* (2006) synthesized several more potent LuxS inhibitors. Different peptides capable of inhibiting LuxS have also been developed (Han and Lu, 2009; Zhang *et al.*, 2009). The naturally occurring (5Z)-4-bromo-5-(bromomethylene)-3-butyryl-2(5H)-furanone, produced by the red algae *Delisea pulchra*, was recently shown to bind covalently to and inactivate LuxS, as well as decrease LuxS expression (Kuehl *et al.*, 2009). Starting from immucillin and DADMe-immucillin (Fig. 8.3), several other MTAN

S-anhydroribosyl-L-homocysteine DADME-immucillin

Fig. 8.3. Examples of QSIs targeting AI-2 signal synthesis.

inhibitors (e.g. BuT-DADMe-immucillin-A and *p*-Cl-PhT-DADMe-immucillin-A), active in pico- and femtomolar concentrations, were developed (Lee *et al.*, 2005; Gutierrez *et al.*, 2009; Longshaw *et al.*, 2010).

8.2.3 Inhibition of QS signal synthesis in Gram-positive bacteria

Proteins involved in peptide signal synthesis and post-translational modifications of the peptide in Gram-positive bacteria are interesting targets. Molecular characterization of AgrD and AgrB demonstrated that Glu34 and Leu41 of the AgrD C-terminal tail are essential for AgrB endopeptidase activity and AIP biosynthesis. In addition, a cysteine in AgrB proved essential for the formation of the AgrD–AgrB complex (Thoendel and Horswill, 2009). However, to date no inhibitors specifically targeting these proteins have been reported. In contrast, different linear peptide inhibitors targeting the type I signal peptidase SpsB reportedly reduce AIP-I production (Kavanaugh *et al.*, 2007; Buzder-Lantos *et al.*, 2009).

8.3 Quorum Quenching of Signalling Molecules

Once synthesized, QS signal molecules can be degraded to prevent their accumulation and subsequent activation of the QS system. This so-called 'quorum quenching' (QQ) can be non-enzymatic or enzymatic.

8.3.1 Non-enzymatic QQ of signalling molecules

Although QS inhibition has been studied extensively, little attention has been paid to the stability of AHL signal molecules with respect to the pH and temperature of the surrounding environment, although both factors influence the activity of AHL signal molecules. The lactone ring of AHL can be hydrolysed to the corresponding acylhomoserine under alkaline conditions, resulting in inactivation of the signal molecule (Yates *et al.*, 2002). This hydrolysis is highly chain length and pH dependent. Yates *et al.* (2002) showed that the HSL ring was hydrolysed above pH 2, while for a C_4-HSL ring opening only occurred between pH 5 and 8. For other AHLs, the rate of hydrolysis decreased as the length of the acyl side chain of the AHL signal molecule increased (Yates *et al.*, 2002).

Temperature also plays an important role. The rate of hydrolysis was much higher at 37 than at 22°C, again with the tendency for AHLs with the longest side chain to be more stable at higher temperatures (Yates *et al.*, 2002). In addition, C_6-HSL is more stable at –20 than at 37°C and is inactivated by boiling (Byers *et al.*, 2002; Delalande *et al.*, 2005).

Besides temperature and pH, other environmental conditions can also affect AHL stability. AHLs were found to be more stable in anaerobic conditions than in aerobic conditions (Byers *et al.*, 2002). In addition, HOBr and HOCl are able to inactivate 3-oxo-C_6-HSL signal molecules unlike 3-unsubstituted AHLs such as C_6-HSL (Michels *et al.*, 2000; Borchardt *et al.*, 2001).

8.3.2 Enzymatic QQ of signalling molecules

QS signal molecules can also be degraded enzymatically. Several bacterial species, including *Bacillus* spp., *Acinetobacter* spp., *Bosea* spp., *Delftia acidovorans*, *Sphingomonas* spp. and *Sphingopyxis* spp. produce enzymes capable of degrading AHLs (Uroz *et al.*, 2009). This degradation can occur in four different ways. AHL lactonases and AHL acylases hydrolyse the HSL ring and the amide bonds of the AHL molecule, respectively. The first hydrolysis is identical to pH-mediated lactonolysis and can be reversed by acidification, while the second hydrolysis is irreversible. AHL oxidases and AHL reductases do not degrade the AHL molecule but modify it and change its activity.

AHL lactonases

Different bacterial lactonases have been identified. Dong *et al.* (2000) first reported the presence of a gene coding for autoinducer inactivation (*aiiA*) in *Bacillus* spp. Expression of this gene in *E. coli* resulted in lactonolysis of different AHLs (Dong *et al.*, 2000). Different homologues of the *aiiA* gene are found in several *Bacillus* spp., including *B. thuringiensis, B. cereus, B. mycoides* and *B. anthracis*, suggesting that these species may also be able to enzymatically degrade AHLs (Dong *et al.*, 2002; Lee *et al.*, 2002; Lu *et al.*, 2006). However, the presence of AHL lactonase is not restricted to *Bacillus* spp. AHL lactonases have been found to be widely distributed and include AttM and AiiB in *Agrobacterium tumefaciens*, AhlD in *Arthrobacter* spp. and AhlK in *Klebsiella pneumoniae* (Zhang *et al.*, 2002; Carlier *et al.*, 2003). In addition, *ahlD* homologues are also present in *Burkholderia fungorum Bradyrhizobium japonicum*, *Thermoplasma volcanium* and *Sulfolobus solfataricus* (Park *et al.*, 2003). The AHL lactonases QsdA and QlcA are both members of the metallohydrolase-related enzyme family but are only distantly related to the other AHL lactonases. QsdA and QlcA have been found in *Rhodococcus* spp. and *Acidobacterium* spp., respectively (Park *et al.*, 2006; Riaz *et al.*, 2008). These enzymes have a broad AHL-degrading spectrum. Another AHL lactonase was recently discovered in *Ochrobactrum* spp. (Mei *et al.*, 2010). AHL-degrading activity of *Ochrobactrum* spp. was previously reported, but the genes responsible for this AHL-degrading activity were unknown (Jafra *et al.*, 2006). Mei *et al.* (2010) demonstrated the presence of an AidH protein with AHL lactonase degrading activity. AidH has no detectable homology with any of the known AHL-degrading enzymes, but is allegedly a member of the α/b hydrolase fold family (Mei *et al.*, 2010). Members of this enzyme family share little sequence similarity and do not act on similar substrates, making it difficult to predict whether AidH homologues, present in *Mesorhizobium* spp. are also capable of inactivating AHLs. However, at least one predicted member of this protein family, AiiM in *Microbacterium testaceum* was shown to have lactonase activity (Morohoshi *et al.*, 2009; Wang *et al.*, 2010). These data indicate that AHL lactonase activity is common in many bacterial genera. In addition, AHL lactonase activity can also be detected in eukaryotes. Uroz and Heinonsalo (2008) showed that several root-associated fungi are able to degrade AHL signal molecules. Lactonase activity was also observed in mycorrhizal basidiomycetes and in a *Meliniomyces variabilis* isolate (Uroz *et al.*, 2009). Several plants, including *Hordeum vulgare, Lotus corniculatus* and *Pachyrhizus erosus* can degrade AHL signal molecules, although the exact mechanism remains unknown (Delalande *et al.*, 2005; Götz *et al.*, 2007). AHL inactivation by several human cell lines and mammalian serum was also observed (Chun *et al.*, 2004; Yang *et al.*, 2005). Paraoxonases (PONs) were observed to be involved in AHL degradation (Yang *et al.*, 2005; Teiber *et al.*, 2008). PONs, including PON1, PON2 and PON3, are enzymes that play a key role in organophosphate detoxification and in the prevention of atherosclerosis. PON1 and PON3 are synthesized in the liver and secreted into the blood, whereas PON2 is not detected in plasma but expressed widely in certain tissues, including lungs and kidney (Yang *et al.*, 2005; Teiber *et al.*, 2008).

AHL acylases

AHL acylases hydrolyse the AHL amide bond, which results in the formation of the corresponding fatty acid and HSL. Leadbetter and Greenberg (2000) were the first to report AHL acylase activity (in *V. paradoxus*). AHL acylases share many of the known characteristics of N-terminal nucleophile (Ntn) hydrolases. Four domains can be distinguished: the signal peptide followed by an α subunit, spacer sequence and b subunit (Hewitt *et al.*, 2000). The AHL acylase pro-enzyme has to be processed into an active enzyme by autoproteolysis. Despite these overall similarities, substrate specificity may differ between the different AHL acylases. It was demonstrated previously that *P. aeruginosa* and closely related pseudomonads isolated from soil were able to degrade and utilize long-chain but not short-chain AHLs as sole sources of carbon and energy (Huang *et al.*, 2003). This degradation is mediated by the AHL acylase PvdQ. However, studies of *pvdQ* revealed that, although this gene was sufficient to degrade long-chain acyl AHLs, it was not necessary. A diversity of *pvdQ* mutants remains capable of degrading and utilizing AHLs (Huang *et al.*, 2003; Sio *et al.*, 2006). This indicates that *P. aeruginosa* encodes at least one additional acylase. Huang *et al.* (2006) identified the QuiP acylase as a second AHL acylase of *P. aeruginosa* PAO1. Multiple AHL-degrading enzymes were also observed to be present in *Rhodococcus erythropolis* and *Pseudomonas syringae* (Uroz *et al.*, 2005; Shepherd and Lindow, 2009). QuiP has specificity for the degradation of long-chain AHLs, similar to that of PvdQ and AhlM from *Streptomyces* spp. (Park *et al.*, 2005). In contrast, other PvdQ homologues, including AiiD in *Ralstonia euthropa*, AiiC in *Anabaena* spp. and AaC in *Shewanella* spp., degrade long-chain as well as short-chain AHLs (Lin *et al.*, 2003; Morohoshi *et al.*, 2008; Romero *et al.*, 2008). Interestingly, besides AhlM, only one other AHL acylase was reportedly secreted. The *P. syringae* genome contains two genes encoding AHL acylases, *hacA* and *hacB* (Shepherd and Lindow, 2009). While HacB is cell bound, HacA is secreted. In addition, HacA is capable of degrading long-chain AHLs only, while HacB degrades a broader range of AHLs (Shepherd and Lindow, 2009). AHL acylase activity was also observed in *Comamonas* spp., *Tenacibaculum maritimum* and *Bacillus pumilus* (Uroz *et al.*, 2007; Nithya *et al.*, 2010; Romero *et al.*, 2010). However, the genes encoding this activity have not yet been identified.

Degradation of AHLs by other enzymes

AHL signalling molecules can also be modified by AHL oxidases and reductases (Uroz *et al.*, 2009). Unlike acylases or lactonases, these enzymes do not degrade the AHL molecules but modify them, and change their activity. To date, only two bacterial enzymes with an AHL oxido-reductase activity have been reported. *R. erythropolis* produces an AHL oxido-reductase capable of reducing the keto group of 3-oxo-AHLs (Uroz *et al.*, 2005). It is active against a broad range of 3-oxo-substituted AHLs but has no effect on 3-hydroxylated or unsubstituted AHLs (Uroz *et al.*, 2005). In addition, Chowdhary *et al.* (2007) reported the presence of a P450 monooxygenase enzyme in *Bacillus megaterium*, capable of oxidizing long-chain AHLs.

Antibodies with QQ activity

The QS signal molecule can also be affected by the immune system. Immunization of mice with an AHL protein conjugate prevented lethality in a *P. aeruginosa* infection model (Miyairi *et al.*, 2006). However, as mentioned above, AHLs may be prone to degradation due to their instability. To overcome this problem, Kaufmann *et al.* (2006) replaced the lactone ring of the hapten with a more stable lactam moiety. Three different haptens, closely resembling 3-oxo-C_{12}-HSL and C_4-HSL yielded several monoclonal antibodies (Kaufmann *et al.*, 2006). All antibodies effectively inhibited QS signalling in *P. aeruginosa*. Recently, the concept of QQ using antibody catalysis has been introduced (De Lamo Marin *et al.*, 2007). This approach uses small molecules as haptens to induce the production of antibodies capable of catalysing AHL hydrolysis and thus inhibit QS. In a first study, haptens not specifically designed as structural mimics of the transition state for AHL hydrolysis were used (De Lamo Marin *et al.*, 2007). Consequently, only moderate levels of activity were observed. Kapadnis *et al.* (2009) synthesized sulfones resembling the transition state structure for

AHL-ring hydrolysis and demonstrated that these could be used to detect human transition state binders capable of degrading AHLs. In addition, an anti-autoinducer monoclonal antibody affected AIPs produced by *S. aureus* and AI-2 produced by *S. enterica* serovar Typhimurium (Chan *et al.*, 2004; Park *et al.*, 2007). These strategies may have some important advantages over other QS inhibition approaches. Monoclonal antibodies have predictable pharmacodynamic and pharmacokinetic properties, and these properties can be improved through design. In addition, although the manufacturing cost may represent a major disadvantage, only small amounts of these monoclonal antibodies will be needed. Furthermore, only AHLs coupled to an immunogenic carrier protein would be needed for active vaccination. This makes active and passive immunotherapeutic strategies to combat QS possible in the future. However, further optimization of antibody–ligand activity and improved hapten design are necessary.

8.4 QSIs Targeting Signal Transport and Signal Secretion

In some bacteria, QS and resistance–nodulation–cell division (RND) efflux pump expression are linked. For example, the extracellular autoinducer concentration was significantly reduced when BpeAB-OprM in *Burkholderia pseudomallei* and MexAB-OprM in *P. aeruginosa* were knocked out (Pearson *et al.*, 1999; Chan *et al.*, 2007), suggesting that inhibition of these efflux pumps could be useful therapeutically. Carbonyl cyanide *m*-chlorophenyl hydrazone (CCCP), an uncoupler that dissipates the transmembrane proton gradient necessary as a driving force for efflux pumps, and phenyl-arginine-β-naphthylamide (PAbN) have both been described as efficient efflux pump inhibitors (Pumbwe *et al.*, 2008; Liu *et al.*, 2010). In addition, andrographolide was reported to repress the transcription of MexAB-OprM in *P. aeruginosa* (Wu *et al.*, 2008). Andrographolide was clearly shown to decrease the production of QS-regulated virulence factors in *P. aeruginosa* (Li *et al.*, 2006). Azithromycin also suppresses the production of MexAB-OprM, in a concentration-dependent manner (Sugimura *et al.*, 2008). Although low levels of this macrolide may directly affect protein synthesis and consequently result in a lowered production of MexAB-OprM, other mechanisms of action are more likely, as streptomycin and chloramphenicol (also acting on protein synthesis) only exerted a limited effect on MexAB-OprM synthesis (Sugimura *et al.*, 2008). Finally, spermidine synthase inhibitors, such as dicyclohexylamine, can affect the expression of RND efflux pumps and consequently QS (Chan and Chua, 2010). Dicyclohexylamine significantly downregulates the transcription of several RND efflux pump genes, including BpeAB-OprM in *B. pseudomallei* (Chan and Chua, 2010).

8.5 QSIs Targeting Signal Receptors or Affecting Signal Transduction

The search for new antagonists has focused largely on the development of structurally modified AHL, AIP or AI-2 QS signals. In addition, different natural and synthetic structurally unrelated antagonists also block the different QS systems.

8.5.1 QSIs targeting AHL signal receptors and AHL signal transduction

Several AHL QS systems can be found in a single bacterial species, and several species can use similar AHL signalling molecules. For instance, *P. aeruginosa* uses two AHL-type QS systems, LasI/R and RhlI/R, both activated by their own signalling molecules, 3-oxo-C_{12}-HSl and C_4-HSL, respectively. Despite promoting *rhlR* expression, 3-oxo-C_{12}-HSL is an antagonist of the C_4-HSL signalling molecule, both competing for binding to RhlR (Pesci *et al.*, 1997). AHLs produced by a particular species can also inhibit the AHL QS system of other bacteria (Schaefer *et al.*, 1996; Geske *et al.*, 2007a,b).

Most of the research on receptor antagonists has focused on modifying either the acyl side chain or the lactone ring of AHLs, or both. However, interpretation of the results of these studies is not straightforward, and results obtained in one species should not be extrapolated to other species. First, despite binding similar AHL molecules and similarities in their binding region, various LuxR homologues exhibit differences in DNA-binding activity and in the accessibility of their AHL binding site. For example, LuxR–AHL binding in *Vibrio fischeri* is weaker than AHL binding to TraR in *A. tumefaciens*, as the former can be inactivated by dilution, while the latter is known to completely embed the AHL into a narrow cavity without solvent contact (Vannini *et al.*, 2002; Zhang *et al.*, 2002; Urbanowski *et al.*, 2004).

Secondly, differences in the expression of the LuxR homologue can alter the AHL response. For example, overexpression of TraR allows the detection of a broad range of AHLs but abolishes the ability of several AHLs to act as potent antagonists, while TraR, when expressed normally, clearly discriminates between its cognate AHL signal and other AHLs (Zhu *et al.*, 1998). In addition, 3-hydroxy-C_4-HSL fails to activate LuxR in *V. fischeri* but does so when LuxR is overexpressed in a mutant *E. coli* strain (Sitnikov *et al.*, 1995).

QSIs targeting V. fischeri *LuxR*

Eberhard *et al.* (1986) were the first to explore the effect of AHLs with varying 3-oxo substituents and varying length and saturation of the acyl chains on QS in *V. fischeri*. Later, Schaefer *et al.* (1996) evaluated similar AHL analogues in an *E. coli* reporter strain overexpressing LuxR. Both studies indicated that the 3-oxo substituent was essential for strong agonist activity, but was non-essential for binding in ligand displacement assays. The optimal length of the acyl side chain for agonistic activity was six carbons. Shorter or longer chains lead to inhibition (Eberhard *et al.*, 1986; Schaefer *et al.*, 1996; Castang *et al.*, 2004). In addition, changing the flexibility of the acyl side chain through the introduction of ramified substituents also affects the activity of the AHLs (Reverchon *et al.*, 2002). Introduction of alkene subunits, a phenyl group or a phenyl group bearing a heteroatom in para position results in antagonistic activity. However, the antagonistic activity disappears when the phenyl group is replaced by a thiophenyl group, indicating that specific interactions play an important role (Reverchon *et al.*, 2002). In addition, naphthyl, biphenyl or adamantylalkyl groups show no activity. In accordance with the previous data, 3-oxo-C_6-HSL analogues are only slightly more effective than their corresponding C_6-HSL analogues (Reverchon *et al.*, 2002). In their pursuit of finding new AHL QSIs, Castang *et al.* (2004) observed that replacing the carboxyamide functional group by a sulfonamide function resulted in a new group of AHL antagonists. The inhibitory activity of these compounds was explained by the presence of a tetrahedral geometry around the sulfone, allowing the formation of additional hydrogen bonds with a tyrosine residue of the LuxR ligand pocket (Frezza *et al.*, 2008). In addition, phenyl-substituted ureas and alkyl-substituted ureas bearing an alkyl chain of at least four carbon atoms displayed strong inhibitory activity (Frezza *et al.*, 2006). The presence of the free amine group of the substituted ureas enforced hydrogen bonding with an aspartic acid residue in the LuxR ligand-binding pocket (Frezza *et al.*, 2008). The effect of both modifications together was also investigated (Frezza *et al.*, 2008). Several AHL derivatives containing the two amine groups of the urea function and maintaining the tetrahedral geometry of the sulfonamide function had antagonistic effects (Frezza *et al.*, 2008). In addition, compounds bearing a phenyl group at the end also displayed good inhibitory activity (Frezza *et al.*, 2008). In recent studies, Geske *et al.* (2007a,b, 2008) developed more than 90 additional AHL analogues by changing acyl chain length, lactone stereochemistry and functional groups on the AHL molecule. It was observed that several phenylacetyl homoserine lactone (PHL) compounds with an electron-withdrawing group and a lipophilic group in the 4-position displayed antagonistic activity towards LuxR. In addition, replacement of the carbonyl group by a sulfonyl group did not alter the antagonistic effects of these compounds. Finally, several *N*-acyl-cyclopentylamide (*N*-C_n-CPA) compounds had antagonistic activity (Morohoshi *et al.*, 2007; Wang *et al.*, 2008). *N*-C_n-CPA with an acyl side chain ranging from five to ten carbons showed strong inhibitory effects on LuxR QS.

QSIs targeting *P. aeruginosa* LasR

Passador *et al.* (1996) showed that several AHL analogues were able to antagonize and agonize *lasR*-dependent QS (Eberhard *et al.*, 1986; Schaefer *et al.*, 1996). The acyl chain length proved crucial for effective binding to LasR. AHLs with a shorter chain length (six carbons or less) were unable to bind competitively to LasR, while AHL analogues with 12 carbons were agonists. In addition, removal of the 3-oxo group decreases activity, indicating the importance of this group for effective binding to LasR (Passador *et al.*, 1996). The role of the ring structure in binding is not yet clear. No difference in activity was observed upon switching to a thiolactone ring, while lactam derivatives had no activity (Passador *et al.*, 1996). This attempt to develop *P. aeruginosa* LasR autoinducer antagonists focused mainly on modifying the length of the acyl chain while retaining its flexibility. Kline *et al.* (1999) investigated the effects of locking the flexibility of the β-ketoamide system, while retaining the full atom content of the LasR-dependent signalling molecule. The Z-enol tautomer was investigated using β-nitrones and salicylamides, and the E-enol tautomer using furan and oxazoles and gem-difluoronated analogues (Kline *et al.*, 1999). Only the non-enolizable analogues were weak agonists, indicating that, in order to activate LasR, a certain degree of flexibility must be retained (Kline *et al.*, 1999). In addition, D-isomers of 3-oxo-C_{12}-HSL and C_4-HSL could not activate LasR and RhlR, respectively. In order to investigate the role of the lactone ring, different AHL analogues in which the HSL moiety was replaced by amines or alcohols were synthesized (Smith *et al.*, 2003). Several aniline derivatives had antagonistic activity. This set of molecules contained a hydroxyl, carboxyamide or pyridyl group in the ortho or meta position, which can act as a H-bond acceptor. The position of these substituents was proven to be important and depended on the type of substitution, ortho for hydroxyl or pyridyl and ortho/meta for carboxyamide. Structurally similar compounds differing only in the position of these substituents were inactive. In addition, C_n-CPA lacking the lactone ring has strong antagonistic activity against LasR (Ishida *et al.*, 2007). A C_{10}-CPA (Fig. 8.4) was the most potent inhibitor. Substitution of the ring of this compound by related cyclopropane, cyclobutane, cyclohexane or cyclooctane structures decreased activity (Ishida *et al.*, 2007). In addition, PHL and indole-AHL showed good inhibitory activity towards LasR (Geske *et al.*, 2005, 2007a; Oliver *et al.*, 2009). Similar trends were observed for these compounds and for the ones blocking LuxR. Several unrelated compounds, such as lumichrome, riboflavin, andrographolide derivatives, salicylic acid, nifuroxazide and chlorzoxazone (Fig. 8.4) also inhibit QS at the level of the LasR QS receptor (Rajamani *et al.*, 2008; Jiang *et al.*, 2009).

QSIs targeting other AHL receptors

Only a few studies have focused on the use of AHL analogues to block LuxR homologues other than those from *V. fischeri* or *P. aeruginosa*.

Zhu *et al.* (1998) evaluated a set of AHL analogues of the ones previously evaluated by Schaefer *et al.* (1996) and Eberhard *et al.* (1986) for their binding to TraR of *A. tumefaciens*. TraR tolerated acyl groups of one carbon shorter and up to four carbons longer than the cognate autoinducer, as well as a triple bond at the C_7–C_8 position. Antagonistic activity was observed for a compound similar to the native signal molecule but lacking the 3-oxo group (Zhu *et al.*, 1998). Hydroxyl substitution at the 3-position or C_2–C_3 unsaturated bonds also resulted in antagonism. The best antagonistic effect was observed for 3-oxo-C_6-HSL (Zhu *et al.*, 1998). This indicates that, although the 3-oxo group is not required for binding to TraR, it may play an important role in converting TraR to its active conformation (Zhu *et al.*, 1998). Geske *et al.* (2007a) also investigated the effect of their compounds on TraR. While none of the non-natural AHL compounds activated TraR, several PHL analogues inhibited TraR QS.

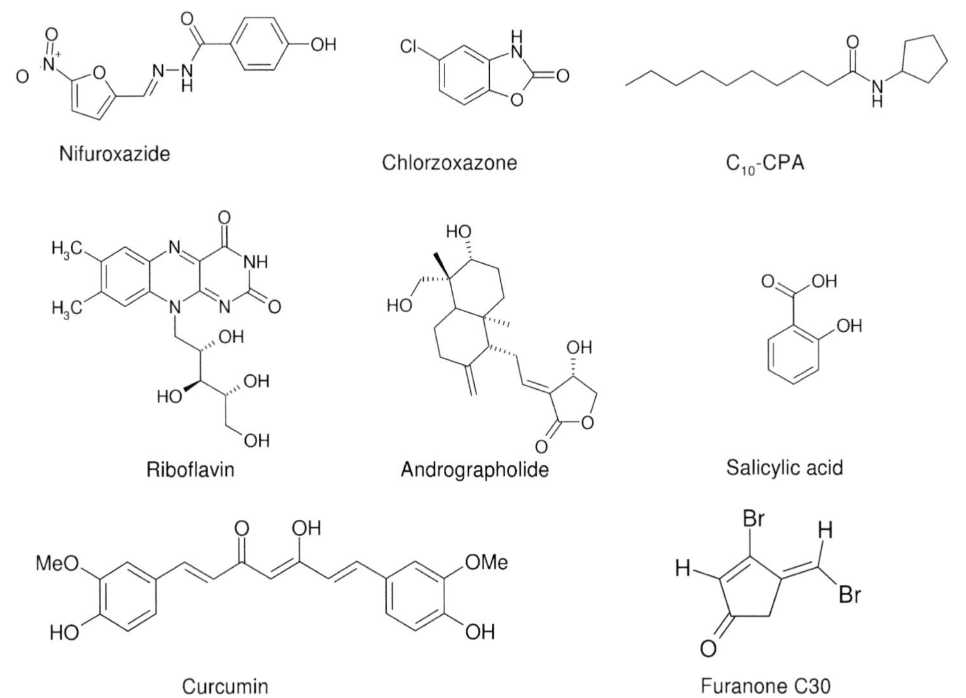

Fig. 8.4. Examples of QSIs targeting AHL receptor/signal transduction.

In line with previous results, PHLs carrying an electron-withdrawing group in the para position were the most active antagonists (Geske *et al.*, 2007a). It is, however, important to mention that several antagonists were also partially agonistic.

Morohoshi *et al.* (2007) found that C_9-CPA was capable of blocking QS in *Serratia marcescens* and Janssens *et al.* (2007) found that *N*-3-oxo-acyl-homocysteine thiolactone and 3-oxo-acyl-(*E*)-2-aminocyclohexanols were strong activators of SdiA of *S. enterica* serovar Typhimurium. Several unrelated compounds, such as cinnamaldehyde, curcumin (Fig. 8.4) and components from garlic were found to have an effect on different AHL QS systems (Persson *et al.*, 2005; Rasmussen *et al.*, 2005; Niu *et al.*, 2006; Brackman *et al.*, 2009a). In addition, several extracts from honey, fruits and plants, as well as secondary metabolites from fungi, nematodes, marine sponges and bryozoans, also block different AHL-type QS systems (Peters *et al.*, 2003; Vattem *et al.*, 2007; Adonizio *et al.*, 2008; Zhu and Sun, 2008; Singh *et al.*, 2009; Teasdale *et al.*, 2009; Truchado *et al.*, 2009; Szabó *et al.*, 2010).

Furanones targeting AHL QS receptors

De Nys *et al.* (1993) isolated several natural furanone compounds from the red alga *D. pulchra*. One of these compounds, (5Z)-4-bromo-5-(bromomethylene)-3-butyryl-2(5H)-furanone, inhibited AHL-based QS in several Gram-negative bacteria. Due to its structural similarity with AHL molecules, it was initially hypothesized that the furanone would compete with AHLs at the level of the binding site. However, this is highly uncertain (Koch *et al.*, 2005; Taha *et al.*, 2006; Bottomley *et al.*, 2007). Manefield *et al.* (2002) demonstrated that this furanone and several analogues promoted a rapid turnover of the LuxR protein. To date, many furanone analogues, such as furanone C30 (Fig. 8.4), capable of blocking AHL QS, have been described (Manefield *et al.*, 2002; Hjelmgaard *et al.*, 2003; Martinelli *et al.*, 2004; Estephane *et al.*, 2008; Janssens *et al.*, 2008; Kim *et al.*, 2008).

8.5.2 QSIs targeting QS receptors and signal transduction in Gram-positive bacteria

AIPs are typically recognized by an AgrC receptor histidine kinase. Four different AIP groups can be distinguished in *S. aureus* (Novick and Geisinger, 2008). The AIP of one group can block the AgrC receptor of another group (Dunman *et al.*, 2001). Besides the inhibition by natural AIPs, several other AIP receptor inhibitors have been described (Chan *et al.*, 2004). A truncated version of AIP-II (TrAIP-II) and different AIP-II analogues inhibit QS in different *Staphylococcus* spp. (Lyon *et al.*, 2000; Scott *et al.*, 2003; George *et al.*, 2008). In addition, several analogues of the AIP precursor AgrD blocked QS in Gram-positive bacteria (Mayville *et al.*, 1999).

Although targeting AIP receptors looks appealing due to their location and the lack of outer-membrane barriers in Gram-positive bacteria, the diversity in AIP receptors among the different *Staphylococcus* spp. would limit the therapeutic potential of compounds targeting these receptors (Thoendel and Horswill, 2010).

Finally, RIP, RIP-peptide analogues and its non-peptide analogue hamamelitannin inhibit QS-regulated virulence in staphylococci (Balaban *et al.*, 2005; Kiran *et al.*, 2008). These compounds compete with RAP and inhibit the phosphorylation of a TRAP (target of RAP) protein, leading to the inactivation of QS in these Gram-positive bacteria.

8.5.3 QSIs targeting the AI-2 receptor and signal transduction

To date, two distinct AI-2 receptors, LuxPQ and LsrB, have been shown to bind a mixture of AI-2 molecules. This AI-2 mixture is synthesized through several enzymatic steps. In the final step, LuxS converts SRH into DPD. This DPD will then react to form a mixture of molecules. Frezza *et al.* (2007) developed an Ac_2-DPD precursor that is stable and easy to purify. This precursor was shown to be an active agonist (but a less active agonist than DPD) of the AI-2 QS system. Several other DPD derivatives including alkyl-DPD, carbonate-DPD, trifluoro-*S*-THMF-borate and structures resembling DPD such as laurencione and 4-hydroxy-5-methyl-3-(2H)-furanone (MHF) (Fig. 8.5) also activate the AI-2 QS system (McKenzie *et al.*, 2005; Lowery *et al.*, 2005, 2008, 2009; Frezza *et al.*, 2006). In addition, oxazaborilidines (Fig. 8.5) (heterocyclic hydrated complexes containing a negatively charged boron atom) are agonists of the AI-2 QS system (Aharoni *et al.*, 2008).

AI-2 QS antagonists have also been reported. Several diol-containing compounds (including pyrogallol), boronic acids (Fig. 8.5) and sulfones have been shown to be potent antagonists of AI-2–LuxP binding (Ni *et al.*, 2008a,b, 2009; Peng *et al.*, 2009). In addition, several other non-related compounds block the AI-2 QS pathway. From a random screening for compounds targeting LuxPQ, it was discovered that phenothiazine (Fig. 8.5) had an AI-2 QS inhibitory effect (Ni *et al.*, 2009). Furthermore, an adenosine derivative with a *p*-methoxyphenylpropionamide moiety at C-3′, ursolic acid, 7-hydroxyindole, isatin and several fatty acids blocked the production of AI-2-regulated virulence factors (Ren *et al.*, 2005; Lee *et al.*, 2007; Widmer *et al.*, 2007; Brackman *et al.*, 2009b).

The AI-2 QS system can also be blocked at the level of the signal transduction cascade. Although in theory AI-2 QS could be blocked at the level of the kinase activity of LuxQ, no such QSIs have yet been reported. Cinnamaldehyde (Fig. 8.5) and several of its derivatives inhibit AI-2 QS in *V. harveyi* (Niu *et al.*, 2006; Brackman *et al.*, 2008, 2011) and a natural furanone compound, (5Z)-4-bromo-5-(bromomethylene)3-butyryl-2(5H)-furanone (Fig. 8.5), inhibits AI-2 QS in *Vibrio* spp., *B. subtilis* and *E. coli* (Ren *et al.*, 2001, 2002, 2004). Both cinnamaldehyde and furanone block the AI-2 signal transduction by decreasing the DNA-binding ability of the transcriptional regulator LuxR (Defoirdt *et al.*, 2007; Brackman *et al.*, 2008).

To date, several studies have demonstrated the QS inhibitory effects of furanones on AI-2 QS (Manefield *et al.*, 2000; Ren *et al.*, 2001; Defoirdt *et al.*, 2006; Lönn-Stensrud *et al.*, 2009). However, the toxicity of these compounds will probably limit their use (Han *et al.*, 2008; Janssens *et al.*, 2008).

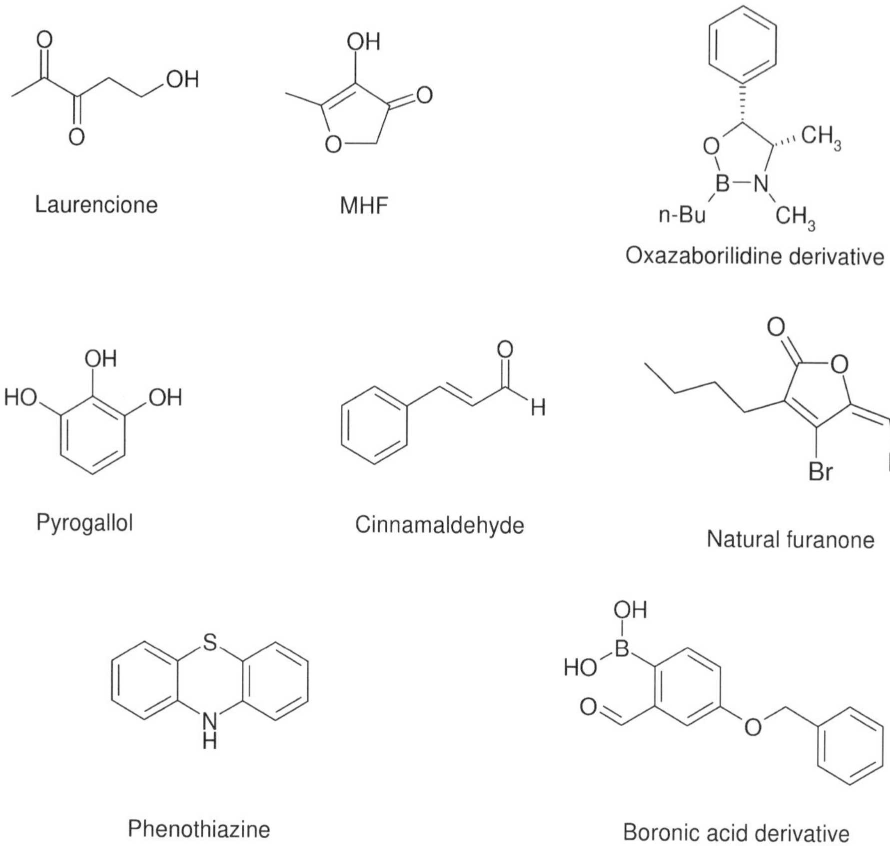

Fig. 8.5. Examples of compounds targeting AI-2 receptor/signal transduction.

8.6 Conclusion

Since the discovery that QS is used by bacteria to coordinate the expression of several genes involved in virulence, biofilm formation and pathogenicity, QS inhibition has gained increasing attention as a potential alternative antipathogenic strategy. A major advantage compared with antibiotic therapy is that QSIs are used in concentrations not affecting bacterial growth. For this reason, it is expected that these compounds would exert less pressure towards the development of resistance. However, some important answers still need to be addressed. Although several inhibitors have proven to be active antipathogenic agents *in vitro* and in various *in vivo* models, it is still unknown whether these compounds will also be useful in humans. Furthermore, many known QSIs are cytotoxic, and several fundamental mechanisms by which the different QS systems exert their regulatory functions and are inhibited by QSIs are still poorly understood. In order to achieve real-life applications with QSIs, these challenges should be addressed and more research will be needed. Despite this, QS inhibition remains an exciting and promising strategy to combat bacterial infections in the future.

Acknowledgements

The authors gratefully acknowledge funding by the Institute for the Promotion of Innovation through Science and Technology in Flanders (IWT-Vlaanderen), by the Fund for Scientific Research – Flanders (FWO-Vlaanderen) and by the Special Research Fund (BOF) of Ghent University, Belgium.

References

Adonizio, A., Kong, K.F. and Mathee, K. (2008) Inhibition of quorum sensing-controlled virulence factor production in *Pseudomonas aeruginosa* by South Florida plant extracts. *Antimicrobial Agents and Chemotherapy* 52, 198–203.

Aharoni, R., Bronstheyn, M., Jabbour, A., Zaks, B., Srebnik, M. and Steinberg, D. (2008) Oxazaborolidine derivatives inducing autoinducer-2 signal transduction in *Vibrio harveyi*. *Bioorganic and Medicinal Chemistry* 16, 1596–1604.

Alfaro, J.F., Zhang, T., Wynn, D.P., Karschner, E.L. and Zhou, Z.S. (2004) Synthesis of LuxS inhibitors targeting bacterial cell–cell communication. *Organic Letters* 6, 3043–3046.

Balaban, N., Stoodley, P., Fux, C.A., Wilson, S., Costerton, J.W. and Dell'Acqua, G. (2005) Prevention of staphylococcal biofilm-associated infections by the quorum sensing inhibitor RIP. *Clinical Orthopaedics and Related Research* 437, 48–54.

Borchardt, S.A., Allain, E.J., Michels, J.J., Stearns, G.W., Kelly, R.F. and McCoy, W.F. (2001) Reaction of acylated homoserine lactone bacterial signalling molecules with oxidized halogen antimicrobials. *Applied and Environmental Microbiology* 67, 3174–3179.

Bottomley, M.J., Muraglia, E., Bazzo, R. and Carfì, A. (2007) Molecular insights into quorum sensing in the human pathogen *Pseudomonas aeruginosa* from the structure of the virulence regulator LasR bound to its autoinducer. *Journal of Biological Chemistry* 282, 13592–13600.

Brackman, G., Defoirdt, T., Miyamoto, C., Van Calenbergh, S., Bossier, P., Nelis, H..J. and Coenye, T. (2008) Cinnamaldehyde and cinnamaldehyde derivatives reduce virulence in *Vibrio* spp. by decreasing the DNA-binding activity of the quorum sensing response regulator LuxR. *BMC Microbiology* 8, 149.

Brackman, G., Hillaert, U., Van Calenbergh, S., Nelis, H.J. and Coenye, T. (2009a) Use of quorum sensing inhibitors to interfere with biofilm formation and development in *Burkholderia multivorans* and *Burkholderia cenocepacia*. *Research in Microbiology* 160, 144–151.

Brackman, G., Celen, S., Baruah, K., Bossier, P., Van Calenbergh, S., Nelis, H.J. and Coenye, T. (2009b) AI-2 quorum-sensing inhibitors affect the starvation response and reduce virulence in several *Vibrio* species, most likely by interfering with LuxPQ. *Microbiology* 155, 4114–4122.

Brackman, G., Celen, S., Hillaert, U., Van Calenbergh, S., Cos, P., Maes, L., Nelis, H.J. and Coenye, T. (2011) Structure–activity relationship of cinnamaldehyde analogs as inhibitors of AI-2 based quorum sensing and their effect on virulence of *Vibrio* spp. *PloS One* 6, e16084.

Buzder-Lantos, P., Bockstael, K., Anné, J. and Herdewijn, P. (2009) Substrate based peptide aldehyde inhibits bacterial type I signal peptidase. *Bioorganic and Medicinal Chemistry Letters* 19, 2880–2883.

Byers, J.T., Lucas, C., Salmond, G.P. and Welch, M. (2002) Nonenzymatic turnover of an *Erwinia carotovora* quorum-sensing signalling molecule. *Journal of Bacteriology* 184, 1163–1171.

Cao, J.G. and Meighen, E.A. (1993) Biosynthesis and stereochemistry of the autoinducer controlling luminescence in *Vibrio harveyi*. *Journal of Bacteriology* 175, 3856–3862.

Carlier, A., Uroz, S., Smadja, B., Fray, R., Latour, X., Dessaux, Y. and Faure, D. (2003) The Ti plasmid of *Agrobacterium tumefaciens* harbors an *attM*-paralogous gene, *aiiB*, also encoding *N*-acyl homoserine lactonase activity. *Applied and Environmental Microbiology* 69, 4989–4993.

Castang, S., Chantegrel, B., Deshayes, C., Dolmazon, R., Gouet, P., Haser, R., Reverchon, S., Nasser, W., Hugouvieux-Cotte-Pattat, N. and Doutheau, A. (2004) *N*-Sulfonyl homoserine lactones as antagonists of bacterial quorum sensing. *Bioorganic and Medicinal Chemistry Letters* 14, 5145–5149.

Chan, W.C., Coyle, B.J. and Williams, P. (2004) Virulence regulation and quorum sensing in staphylococcal infections: competitive AgrC antagonists as quorum sensing inhibitors. *Journal of Medicinal Chemistry* 47, 4633–4641.

Chan, Y.Y. and Chua, K.L. (2010) Growth-related changes in intracellular spermidine and its effect on efflux pump expression and quorum sensing in *Burkholderia pseudomallei*. *Microbiology* 156, 1144–1154.

Chan, Y.Y., Bian, H.S., Tan, T.M., Mattmann, M.E., Geske, G.D., Igarashi, J., Hatano, T., Suga, H., Blackwell, H.E. and Chua, K.L. (2007) Control of quorum sensing by a *Burkholderia pseudomallei* multidrug efflux pump. *Journal of Bacteriology* 189, 4320–4324.

Chowdhary, P.K., Keshavan, N., Nguyen, H.Q., Peterson, J.A., González, J.E. and Haines, D.C. (2007) *Bacillus megaterium* CYP102A1 oxidation of acyl homoserine lactones and acyl homoserines. *Biochemistry* 46, 14429–14437.

Chun, C.K., Ozer, E.A., Welsh, M.J., Zabner, J. and Greenberg, E.P. (2004) Inactivation of a *Pseudomonas aeruginosa* quorum-sensing signal by human airway epithelia. *Proceedings of the National Academy of Sciences USA* 101, 3587–3590.

Defoirdt, T., Crab, R., Wood, T.K., Sorgeloos, P., Verstraete, W. and Bossier, P. (2006) Quorum sensing-disrupting brominate furanones protect the gnotobiotic brine shrimp *Artemia franciscana* from pathogenic *Vibrio harveyi*, *Vibrio campbellii* and *Vibrio parahaemolyticus* isolates. *Applied and Environmental Microbiology* 72, 6419–6423.

Defoirdt, T., Miyamoto, C.M., Wood, T.K., Meighen, E.A., Sorgeloos, P., Verstraete, W. and Bossier, P. (2007) The natural furanone (5Z)-4-bromo-5-(bromomethylene)-3-butyl-2(5H)-furanone disrupts quorum sensing-regulated gene expression in *Vibrio harveyi* by decreasing the DNA-binding activity of the transcriptional regulator protein luxR. *Environmental Microbiology* 9, 2486–2495.

Delalande, L., Faure, D., Raffoux, A., Uroz, S., D'Angelo-Picard, C., Elasri, M., Carlier, A., Berruyer, R., Petit, A., Williams, P. and Dessaux, Y. (2005) N-hexanoyl-L-homoserine lactone, a mediator of bacterial quorum-sensing regulation, exhibits plant-dependent stability and may be inactivated by germinating *Lotus corniculatus* seedlings. *FEMS Microbiology Ecology* 52, 13–20.

De Lamo Marin, S., Xu, Y., Meijler, M.M. and Janda, K.D. (2007) Antibody catalyzed hydrolysis of a quorum sensing signal found in Gram-negative bacteria. *Bioorganic and Medicinal Chemistry Letters* 17, 1549–1552.

De Nys, R., Wright, A.D., Konig, G.M. and Sticher, O. (1993) New halogenated furanones from the marine alga *Delisea pulchra* (cf. *fimbriata*). *Tetrahedron* 49, 11213–11220

Dong, Y.H., Xu, J.L., Li, X.Z. and Zhang, L.H. (2000) AiiA, an enzyme that inactivates the acylhomoserine lactone quorum-sensing signal and attenuates the virulence of *Erwinia carotovora*. *Proceedings of the National Academy of Sciences USA* 97, 3526–3531.

Dong, Y.H., Gusti, A.R., Zhang, Q., Xu, J.L. and Zhang, L.H. (2002) Identification of quorum-quenching *N*-acyl homoserine lactonases from *Bacillus* species. *Applied and Environmental Microbiology* 68, 1754–1759.

Dunman, P.M., Murphy, E., Haney, S., Palacios, D., Tucker-Kellogg, G., Wu, S., Brown, E.L., Zagursky, R.J., Shlaes, D. and Projan, S.J. (2001) Transcription profiling-based identification of *Staphylococcus aureus* genes regulated by the *agr* and/or *sarA* loci. *Journal of Bacteriology* 183, 7341–7353.

Eberhard, A., Widrig, C.A., McBath, P. and Schineller, J.B. (1986) Analogs of the autoinducer of bioluminescence in *Vibrio fischeri*. *Archives of Microbiology* 146, 35–40.

Estephane, J., Dauvergne, J., Soulère, L., Reverchon, S., Queneau, Y. and Doutheau, A. (2008) *N*-Acyl-3-amino-5H-furanone derivatives as new inhibitors of LuxR-dependent quorum sensing: synthesis, biological evaluation and binding mode study. *Bioorganic and Medicinal Chemistry Letters* 18, 4321–4324.

Frezza, M., Castang, S., Estephane, J., Soulère, L., Deshayes, C., Chantegrel, B., Nasser, W., Queneau, Y., Reverchon, S. and Doutheau, A. (2006) Synthesis and biological evaluation of homoserine lactone derived ureas as antagonists of bacterial quorum sensing. *Bioorganic and Medicinal Chemistry* 14, 4781–4791.

Frezza, M., Soulère, L., Balestrino, D., Gohar, M., Deshayes, C., Queneau, Y., Forestier, C. and Doutheau, A. (2007) Ac2-DPD, the bis-(*O*)-acetylated derivative of 4,5-dihydroxy-2,3-pentanedione (DPD) is a convenient stable precursor of bacterial quorum sensing autoinducer AI-2. *Bioorganic and Medicinal Chemistry Letters* 17, 1428–1431.

Frezza, M., Soulère, L., Reverchon, S., Guiliani, N., Jerez, C., Queneau, Y. and Doutheau, A. (2008) Synthetic homoserine lactone-derived sulfonylureas as inhibitors of *Vibrio fischeri* quorum sensing regulator. *Bioorganic and Medicinal Chemistry* 16, 3550–3556.

Garske, L.A., Beatson, S.A., Leech, A.J., Walsh, S.L. and Bell, S.C. (2004) Sub-inhibitory concentrations of ceftazidime and tobramycin reduce the quorum sensing signals of *Pseudomonas aeruginosa*. *Pathology* 36, 571–575.

George, E.A., Novick, R.P. and Muir, T.W. (2008) Cyclic peptide inhibitors of staphylococcal virulence prepared by Fmoc-based thiolactone peptide synthesis. *Journal of the American Chemical Society* 130, 4914–4924.

Geske, G.D., Wezeman, R.J., Siegel, A.P. and Blackwell, H.E. (2005) Small molecule inhibitors of bacterial quorum sensing and biofilm formation. *Journal of the American Chemical Society* 127, 12762–12763.

Geske, G.D., O'Neill, J.C. and Blackwell, H.E. (2007a) *N*-phenylacetanoyl-L-homoserine lactones can strongly antagonize or superagonize quorum sensing in *Vibrio fischeri*. *ACS Chemical Biology* 2, 315–319.

Geske, G.D., O'Neill, J.C., Miller, D.M., Mattmann, M.E. and Blackwell, H.E. (2007b) Modulation of bacterial quorum sensing with synthetic ligands: systematic evaluation of *N*-acylated homoserine lactones in multiple species and new insights into their mechanisms of action. *Journal of the American Chemical Society* 129, 13613–13625.

Geske, G.D., Mattmann, M.E. and Blackwell, H.E. (2008) Evaluation of a focused library of *N*-aryl L-homoserine lactones reveals a new set of potent quorum sensing modulators. *Bioorganic and Medicinal Chemistry Letters* 18, 5978–5981.

Götz, C., Fekete, A., Gebefuegi, I., Forczek, S.T., Fuksová, K., Li, X., Englmann, M., Gryndler, M., Hartmann, A., Matucha, M., Schmitt-Kopplin, P. and Schröder, P. (2007) Uptake, degradation and chiral discrimination of *N*-acyl-D/L-homoserine lactones by barley (*Hordeum vulgare*) and yam bean (*Pachyrhizus erosus*) plants. *Analytical and Bioanalytical Chemistry* 389, 1447–1457.

Gutierrez, J.A., Crowder, T., Rinaldo-Matthis, A., Ho, M.C., Almo, S.C. and Schramm, V.L. (2009) Transition state analogs of 5′-methylthioadenosine nucleosidase disrupt quorum sensing. *Nature Chemical Biology* 5, 251–257.

Han, X. and Lu, C. (2009) Biological activity and identification of a peptide inhibitor of LuxS from *Streptococcus suis* serotype 2. *FEMS Microbiology Letters* 294, 16–23.

Han, Y., Hou, S., Simon, K.A., Ren, D. and Luk, Y.Y. (2008) Identifying the important structural elements of brominated furanones for inhibiting biofilm formation by *Escherichia coli*. *Bioorganic and Medicinal Chemistry Letters* 18, 1006–1010.

Hanzelka, B.L. and Greenberg, E.P. (1996) Quorum sensing in *Vibrio fischeri*: evidence that *S*-adenosylmethionine is the amino acid substrate for autoinducer synthesis. *Journal of Bacteriology* 178, 5291–5294.

Hewitt, L., Kasche, V., Lummer, K., Lewis, R.J., Murshudov, G.N., Verma, C.S., Dodson, G.G. and Wilson, K.S. (2000) Structure of a slow processing precursor penicillin acylase from *Escherichia coli* reveals the linker peptide blocking the active-site cleft. *Journal of Molecular Biology* 302, 887–898.

Hjelmgaard, T., Persson, T., Rasmussen, T.B., Givskov, M. and Nielsen, J. (2003) Synthesis of furanone-based natural product analogues with quorum sensing antagonist activity. *Bioorganic and Medicinal Chemistry* 11, 3261–3271.

Huang, J.J., Han, J.I., Zhang, L.H. and Leadbetter, J.R. (2003) Utilization of acyl-homoserine lactone quorum signals for growth by a soil pseudomonad and *Pseudomonas aeruginosa* PAO1. *Applied and Environmental Microbiology* 69, 5941–5949.

Huang, J.J., Petersen, A., Whiteley, M. and Leadbetter, J.R. (2006) Identification of QuiP, the product of gene PA1032, as the second acyl-homoserine lactone acylase of *Pseudomonas aeruginosa* PAO1. *Applied and Environmental Microbiology* 72, 1190–1197.

Ishida, T., Ikeda, T., Takiguchi, N., Kuroda, A., Ohtake, H. and Kato, J. (2007) Inhibition of quorum sensing in *Pseudomonas aeruginosa* by *N*-acyl cyclopentylamides. *Applied and Environmental Microbiology* 73, 3183–3188.

Jafra, S., Przysowa, J., Czajkowski, R., Michta, A., Garbeva, P. and van der Wolf, J.M. (2006) Detection and characterization of bacteria from the potato rhizosphere degrading *N*-acyl-homoserine lactone. *Canadian Journal of Microbiology* 52, 1006–1015.

Janssens, J.C., Metzger, K., Daniels, R., Ptacek, D., Verhoeven, T., Habel, L.W., Vanderleyden, J., De Vos, D.E. and De Keersmaecker, S.C. (2007) Synthesis of *N*-acyl homoserine lactone analogues reveals strong activators of SdiA, the *Salmonella enterica* serovar Typhimurium LuxR homologue. *Applied and Environmental Microbiology* 73, 535–544.

Janssens, J.C., Steenackers, H., Robijns, S., Gellens, E., Levin, J., Zhao, H., Hermans, K., De Coster, D., Verhoeven, T.L., Marchal, K., Vanderleyden, J., De Vos, D.E. and De Keersmaecker, S.C. (2008) Brominated furanones inhibit biofilm formation by *Salmonella enterica* serovar Typhimurium. *Applied and Environmental Microbiology* 74, 6639–6648.

Jiang, X., Yu, P., Jiang, J., Zhang, Z., Wang, Z., Yang, Z., Tian, Z., Wright, S.C., Larrick, J.W. and Wang, Y. (2009) Synthesis and evaluation of antibacterial activities of andrographolide analogues. *European Journal of Medicinal Chemistry* 44, 2936–2943.

Kapadnis, P.B., Hall, E., Ramstedt, M., Galloway, W.R., Welch, M. and Spring, D.R. (2009) Towards quorum-quenching catalytic antibodies. *Chemical Communications (Cambridge)* 5, 538–540.

Kaufmann, G.F., Sartorio, R., Lee, S.H., Mee, J.M., Altobell, L.J. III., Kujawa, D.P., Jeffries, E., Clapham, B., Meijler, M.M. and Janda, K.D. (2006) Antibody interference with *N*-acyl homoserine lactone-mediated bacterial quorum sensing. *Journal of the American Chemical Society* 128, 2802–2803.

Kavanaugh, J.S., Thoendel, M. and Horswill, A.R. (2007) A role for type I signal peptidase in *Staphylococcus aureus* quorum sensing. *Molecular Microbiology* 65, 780–798.

Kim, C., Kim, J., Park, H.Y., Park, H.J., Lee, J.H., Kim, C.K. and Yoon, J. (2008) Furanone

derivatives as quorum-sensing antagonists of *Pseudomonas aeruginosa*. *Applied Microbiology and Biotechnology* 80, 37–47
Kiran, M.D., Adikesavan, N.V., Cirioni, O., Giacometti, A., Silvestri, C., Scalise, G., Ghiselli, R., Saba, V., Orlando, F., Shoham, M. and Balaban, N. (2008) Discovery of a quorum sensing inhibitor of drug-resistant staphylococcal infections by structure-based virtual screening. *Molecular Pharmacology* 73, 1578–1586.
Kline, T., Bowman, J., Iglewski, B.H., de Kievit, T., Kakai, Y. and Passador, L. (1999) Novel synthetic analogs of the *Pseudomonas* autoinducer. *Bioorganic and Medicinal Chemistry Letters* 9, 3447–3452.
Koch, B., Liljefors, T., Persson, T., Nielsen, J., Kjelleberg, S. and Givskov, M. (2005) The LuxR receptor: the sites of interaction with quorum-sensing signals and inhibitors. *Microbiology* 151, 3589–3602.
Kuehl, R., Al-Bataineh, S., Gordon, O., Luginbuehl, R., Otto, M., Textor, M. and Landmann, R. (2009) Furanone at subinhibitory concentrations enhances staphylococcal biofilm formation by *luxS* repression. *Antimicrobial Agents and Chemotherapy* 53, 4159–4166
Leadbetter, J.R. and Greenberg, E.P. (2000) Metabolism of acyl-homoserine lactone quorum-sensing signals by *Variovorax paradoxus*. *Journal of Bacteriology* 182, 6921–6926.
Lee, J., Bansal, T., Jayaraman, A., Bentley, WE. and Wood, T.K. (2007) Enterohemorrhagic *Escherichia coli* biofilms are inhibited by 7-hydroxyindole and stimulated by isatin. *Applied and Environmental Microbiology* 73, 4100–4109.
Lee, J.E., Singh, V., Evans, G.B., Tyler, P.C., Furneaux, R.H., Cornell, K.A., Riscoe, M.K., Schramm, V.L. and Howell, P.L. (2005) Structural rationale for the affinity of pico- and femtomolar transition state analogues of *Escherichia coli* 5′-methylthioadenosine/*S*-adenosylhomocysteine nucleosidase. *Journal of Biological Chemistry* 280, 18274–18282.
Lee, S.J., Park, S.Y., Lee, J.J., Yum, D.Y., Koo, B.T. and Lee, J.K. (2002) Genes encoding the *N*-acyl homoserine lactone-degrading enzyme are widespread in many subspecies of *Bacillus thuringiensis*. *Applied and Environmental Microbiology* 68, 3919–3924.
Li, H.T., Qin, H.M., Wang, W.H., Li, G.J., Wu, C.M. and Song, J.X. (2006) Effect of andrographolide on QS regulating virulence factors production in *Pseudomonas aeruginosa*. *Zhongguo Zhong Yao Za Zhi* 31, 1015–1017.
Lin, Y.H., Xu, J.L., Hu, J., Wang, L.H., Ong, S.L., Leadbetter, J.R. and Zhang, L.H. (2003) Acyl-homoserine lactone acylase from *Ralstonia* strain XJ12B represents a novel and potent class of quorum-quenching enzymes. *Molecular Microbiology* 47, 849–860.
Liu, Y., Yang, L. and Molin, S. (2010) Synergistic activities of an efflux pump inhibitor and iron chelators against *Pseudomonas aeruginosa* growth and biofilm formation. *Antimicrobial Agents and Chemotherapy* 54, 3960–3963.
Longshaw, A.I., Adanitsch, F., Gutierrez, J.A., Evans, G.B., Tyler, P.C. and Schramm, V.L. (2010) Design and synthesis of potent “sulfur-free” transition state analogue inhibitors of 5′-methylthioadenosine nucleosidase and 5′-methylthioadenosine phosphorylase. *Journal of Medicinal Chemistry* 53, 6730–6746.
Lönn-Stensrud, J., Landin, M.A., Benneche, T., Petersen, F.C. and Scheie, A.A. (2009) Furanones, potential agents for preventing *Staphylococcus epidermidis* biofilm infections? *Journal of Antimicrobial Chemotherapy* 63, 309–316.
Lowery, C.A., McKenzie, K.M., Qi, L., Meijler, M.M. and Janda, K.D. (2005) Quorum sensing in *Vibrio harveyi*: probing the specificity of the LuxP binding site. *Bioorganic and Medicinal Chemistry Letters* 15, 2395–2398.
Lowery, C.A., Park, J., Kaufmann, G.F. and Janda, K.D. (2008) An unexpected switch in the modulation of AI-2-based quorum sensing discovered through synthetic 4,5-dihydroxy-2,3-pentanedione analogues. *Journal of the American Chemistry Society* 130, 9200–9201.
Lowery, C.A., Abe, T., Park, J., Eubanks, L.M., Sawada, D., Kaufmann, G.F. and Janda, K.D. (2009) Revisiting AI-2 quorum sensing inhibitors: direct comparison of alkyl-DPD analogues and a natural product fimbrolide. *Journal of the American Chemistry Society* 131, 15584–15585.
Lu, X., Yuan, Y., Xue, X.L., Zhang, G.P. and Zhou, S.N. (2006) Identification of the critical role of Tyr-194 in the catalytic activity of a novel *N*-acyl-homoserine lactonase from marine *Bacillus cereus* strain Y2. *Current Microbiology* 53, 346–350.
Lyon, G.J., Mayville, P., Muir, T.W. and Novick, R.P. (2000) Rational design of a global inhibitor of the virulence response in *Staphylococcus aureus*, based in part on localization of the site of inhibition to the receptor-histidine kinase, AgrC. *Proceedings of the National Academy of Sciences USA* 97, 13330–13335.
Manefield, M., Harris, L., Rice, S.A., de Nys, R. and Kjelleberg, S. (2000) Inhibition of luminescence and virulence in the black tiger prawn (*Penaeus monodon*) pathogen *Vibrio harveyi*

by intercellular signal antagonists. *Applied Environmental Microbiology* 66, 2079–2084.

Manefield, M., Rasmussen, T.B., Henzter, M., Andersen, J.B., Steinberg, P., Kjelleberg, S. and Givskov, M. (2002) Halogenated furanones inhibit quorum sensing through accelerated LuxR turnover. *Microbiology* 148, 1119–1127.

Martinelli, D., Grossmann, G., Séquin, U., Brandl, H. and Bachofen, R. (2004) Effects of natural and chemically synthesized furanones on quorum sensing in *Chromobacterium violaceum*. *BMC Microbiology* 4, 25.

Mayville, P., Ji, G., Beavis, R., Yang, H., Goger, M., Novick, R.P. and Muir, T.W. (1999) Structure–activity analysis of synthetic autoinducing thiolactone peptides from *Staphylococcus aureus* responsible for virulence. *Proceedings of the National Academy of Sciences USA* 96, 1218–1223.

McKenzie, K.M., Meijler, M.M., Lowery, C.A., Boldt, G.E. and Janda, K.D. (2005) A furanosyl-carbonate autoinducer in cell-to-cell communication of *V. harveyi*. *Chemical Communications (Cambridge)* 38, 4863–4865.

Mei, G.Y., Yan, X.X., Turak, A., Luo, Z.Q. and Zhang, L.Q. (2010) AidH, an α/β-hydrolase fold family member from an *Ochrobactrum* sp. strain, is a novel *N*-acylhomoserine lactonase. *Applied Environmental Microbiology* 76, 4933–4942.

Michels, J.J., Allain, E.J., Borchardt, S.A., Hu, P. and McCoy, W.F. (2000) Degradation pathway of homoserine lactone bacterial signal molecules by halogen antimicrobials identified by liquid chromatography with photodiode array and mass spectrometric detection. *Journal of Chromatography A* 898, 153–165.

Miyairi, S., Tateda, K., Fuse, E.T., Ueda, C., Saito, H., Takabatake, T., Ishii, Y., Horikawa, M., Ishiguro, M., Standiford, T.J. and Yamaguchi, K. (2006) Immunization with 3-oxododecanoyl-L-homoserine lactone-protein conjugate protects mice from lethal *Pseudomonas aeruginosa* lung infection. *Journal of Medical Microbiology* 55, 1381–1387.

Morohoshi, T., Shiono, T., Takidouchi, K., Kato, M., Kato, N., Kato, J. and Ikeda, T. (2007) Inhibition of quorum sensing in *Serratia marcescens* AS-1 by synthetic analogs of *N*-acylhomoserine lactone. *Applied and Environmental Microbiology* 73, 6339–6344.

Morohoshi, T., Nakazawa, S., Ebata, A., Kato, N. and Ikeda, T. (2008) Identification and characterization of *N*-acylhomoserine lactone-acylase from the fish intestinal *Shewanella* sp. strain MIB015. *Bioscience, Biotechnology and Biochemistry* 72, 1887–1893.

Morohoshi, T., Someya, N. and Ikeda, T. (2009) Novel *N*-acylhomoserine lactone-degrading bacteria isolated from the leaf surface of *Solanum tuberosum* and their quorum-quenching properties. *Bioscience, Biotechnology and Biochemistry* 73, 2124–2127.

Ni, N., Chou, H.T., Wang, J., Li, M., Lu, C.D., Tai, P.C. and Wang, B. (2008a) Identification of boronic acids as antagonists of bacterial quorum sensing in *Vibrio harveyi*. *Biochemical and Biophysical Research Communications* 369, 590–594.

Ni, N., Choudhary, G., Li, M. and Wang, B. (2008b) Pyrogallol and its analogs can antagonize bacterial quorum sensing in *Vibrio harveyi*. *Bioorganic and Medicinal Chemistry Letters* 18, 1567–1572.

Ni, N., Li, M., Wang, J. and Wang, B. (2009) Inhibitors and antagonists of bacterial quorum sensing. *Medical Research Reviews* 29, 65–124.

Nithya, C., Aravindraja, C. and Pandian, S.K. (2010) *Bacillus pumilus* of Palk Bay origin inhibits quorum-sensing-mediated virulence factors in Gram-negative bacteria. *Research in Microbiology* 161:293–304.

Niu, C., Afre, S. and Gilbert, E.S. (2006) Subinhibitory concentrations of cinnamaldehyde interfere with quorum sensing. *Letters in Applied Microbiology* 43, 489–494.

Novick, R.P. and Geisinger, E. (2008) Quorum sensing in staphylococci. *Annual Review of Genetics* 42, 541–564.

Oliver, C.M., Schaefer, A.L., Greenberg, E.P. and Sufrin, J.R. (2009) Microwave synthesis and evaluation of phenacylhomoserine lactones as anticancer compounds that minimally activate quorum sensing pathways in *Pseudomonas aeruginosa*. *Journal of Medicinal Chemistry* 52, 1569–1575.

Park, J., Jagasia, R., Kaufmann, G.F., Mathison, J.C., Ruiz, D.I., Moss, J.A., Meijler, M.M., Ulevitch, R.J. and Janda, K.D. (2007) Infection control by antibody disruption of bacterial quorum sensing signalling. *Chemistry and Biology* 14, 1119–1127.

Park, S.Y., Lee, S.J., Oh, T.K., Oh, J.W., Koo, B.T., Yum, D.Y. and Lee, J.K. (2003) AhlD, an *N*-acylhomoserine lactonase in *Arthrobacter* sp., and predicted homologues in other bacteria. *Microbiology* 149, 1541–1550.

Park, S.Y., Kang, H.O., Jang, H.S., Lee, J.K., Koo, B.T. and Yum, D.Y. (2005) Identification of extracellular *N*-acylhomoserine lactone acylase from a *Streptomyces* sp. and its application to quorum quenching. *Applied and Environmental Microbiology* 71, 2632–2641.

Park, S.Y., Hwang, B.J., Shin, M.H., Kim, J.A., Kim, H.K. and Lee, J.K. (2006) *N*-Acylhomoserine lactonase producing *Rhodococcus* spp. with

different AHL-degrading activities. *FEMS Microbiology Letters* 261, 102–108.
Parsek, M.R., Val, D.L., Hanzelka, B.L., Cronan, J.E. Jr and Greenberg, E.P. (1999) Acyl homoserine-lactone quorum-sensing signal generation. *Proceedings of the National Academy of Sciences USA* 96, 4360–4365.
Passador, L., Tucker, K.D., Guertin, K.R., Journet, M.P., Kende, A.S. and Iglewski, B.H. (1996) Functional analysis of the *Pseudomonas aeruginosa* autoinducer PAI. *Journal of Bacteriology* 178, 5995–6000.
Pearson, J.P., Van Delden, C. and Iglewski, B.H. (1999) Active efflux and diffusion are involved in transport of *Pseudomonas aeruginosa* cell-to-cell signals. *Journal of Bacteriology* 181, 1203–1210.
Peng, H., Cheng, Y., Ni, N., Li, M., Choudhary, G., Chou, H.T., Lu, C.D., Tai, P.C. and Wang, B. (2009) Synthesis and evaluation of new antagonists of bacterial quorum sensing in *Vibrio harveyi. ChemMedChem* 4, 1457–1468.
Persson, T., Hansen, T.H., Rasmussen, T.B., Skindersø, M.E., Givskov, M. and Nielsen, J. (2005) Rational design and synthesis of new quorum-sensing inhibitors derived from acylated homoserine lactones and natural products from garlic. *Organic and Biomolecular Chemistry* 3, 253–262.
Pesci, E.C., Pearson, J.P., Seed, P.C. and Iglewski, B.H. (1997) Regulation of *las* and *rhl* quorum sensing in *Pseudomonas aeruginosa. Journal of Bacteriology* 179, 3127–3132.
Peters, L., König, G.M., Wright, A.D., Pukall, R., Stackebrandt, E., Eberl, L. and Riedel, K. (2003) Secondary metabolites of *Flustra foliacea* and their influence on bacteria. *Applied and Environmental Microbiology* 69, 3469–3475.
Projan, S.J. (2003) Why is big Pharma getting out of antibacterial drug discovery? *Current Opinion in Microbiology* 6, 1–4.
Pumbwe, L., Skilbeck, C.A. and Wexler, H.M. (2008) Presence of quorum-sensing systems associated with multidrug resistance and biofilm formation in *Bacteroides fragilis. Microbial Ecology* 56, 412–419.
Rajamani, S., Bauer, W.D., Robinson, J.B., Farrow, J.M. III, Pesci, E.C., Teplitski, M., Gao, M., Sayre, R.T. and Phillips, D.A. (2008) The vitamin riboflavin and its derivative lumichrome activate the LasR bacterial quorum-sensing receptor. *Molecular Plant–Microbe Interactions* 21, 1184–1192.
Rasmussen, T.B., Bjarnsholt, T., Skindersoe, M.E., Hentzer, M., Kristoffersen, P., Köte, M., Nielsen, J., Eberl, L. and Givskov, M. (2005) Screening for quorum-sensing inhibitors (QSI) by use of a novel genetic system, the QSI selector. *Journal of Bacteriology* 187, 1799–1814.
Ren, D., Sims, J.J. and Wood, T.K. (2001) Inhibition of biofilm formation and swarming of *Escherichia coli* by (5Z)-4-bromo-5-(bromomethylene)-3-butyl-2(5H)-furanone. *Environmental Microbiology* 3, 731–736.
Ren, D., Sims, J.J. and Wood, T.K. (2002) Inhibition of biofilm formation and swarming of *Bacillus subtilis* by (5Z)-4-bromo-5-(bromomethylene)-3-butyl-2(5H)-furanone. *Letters in Applied Microbiology* 34, 293–299.
Ren, D., Bedzyk, L.A., Ye, R.W., Thomas, S.M. and Wood, T.K. (2004) Differential gene expression shows natural brominated furanones interfere with the autoinducer-2 bacterial signalling system of *Escherichia coli. Biotechnology and Bioengineering* 88, 630–642.
Ren, D., Zuo, R., González Barrios, A.F., Bedzyk, L.A., Eldridge, G.R., Pasmore, M.E. and Wood, T.K. (2005) Differential gene expression for investigation of *Escherichia coli* biofilm inhibition by plant extract ursolic acid. *Applied and Environmental Microbiology* 71, 4022–4034.
Reverchon, S., Chantegrel, B., Deshayes, C., Doutheau, A. and Cotte-Pattat, N. (2002) New synthetic analogues of *N*-acyl homoserine lactones as agonists or antagonists of transcriptional regulators involved in bacterial quorum sensing. *Bioorganic and Medicinal Chemistry Letters* 12, 1153–1157.
Riaz, K., Elmerich, C., Raffoux, A., Moreira, D., Dessaux, Y. and Faure, D. (2008) Metagenomics revealed a quorum quenching lactonase QlcA from yet unculturable soil bacteria. *Communications in Agricultural and Applied Biological Sciences* 73, 3–6.
Romero, M., Diggle, S.P., Heeb, S., Cámara, M. and Otero, A. (2008) Quorum quenching activity in *Anabaena* sp. PCC 7120: identification of AiiC, a novel AHL-acylase. *FEMS Microbiology Letters* 280, 73–80.
Romero, M., Avendaño-Herrera, R., Magariños, B., Cámara, M. and Otero, A. (2010) Acylhomoserine lactone production and degradation by the fish pathogen *Tenacibaculum maritimum*, a member of the Cytophaga-Flavobacterium-Bacteroides (CFB) group. *FEMS Microbiology Letters* 304, 131–139.
Schaefer, A.L., Hanzelka, B.L., Eberhard, A. and Greenberg, E.P. (1996) Quorum sensing in *Vibrio fischeri*: probing autoinducer-LuxR interactions with autoinducer analogs. *Journal of Bacteriology* 178, 2897–2901.
Scott, R.J., Lian, L.Y., Muharram, S.H., Cockayne, A., Wood, S.J., Bycroft, B.W., Williams, P. and Chan, W.C. (2003) Side-chain-to-tail thiolactone

peptide inhibitors of the staphylococcal quorum-sensing system. *Bioorganic and Medicinal Chemistry Letters* 13, 2449–2453.

Shen, G., Rajan, R., Zhu, J., Bell, C.E. and Pei, D. (2006) Design and synthesis of substrate and intermediate analogue inhibitors of *S*-ribosylhomocysteinase. *Journal of Medicinal Chemistry* 49, 3003–3011

Shepherd, R.W. and Lindow, S.E. (2009) Two dissimilar *N*-acyl-homoserine lactone acylases of *Pseudomonas syringae* influence colony and biofilm morphology. *Applied and Environmental Microbiology* 75, 45–53.

Singh, B.N., Singh, B.R., Singh, R.L., Prakash, D., Sarma, B.K. and Singh, H.B. (2009) Antioxidant and anti-quorum sensing activities of green pod of *Acacia nilotica* L. *Food and Chemical Toxicology* 47, 778–786.

Sio, C.F., Otten, L.G., Cool, R.H., Diggle, S.P., Braun, P.G., Bos, R., Daykin, M., Cámara, M., Williams, P. and Quax, W.J. (2006) Quorum quenching by an *N*-acyl-homoserine lactone acylase from *Pseudomonas aeruginosa* PAO1. *Infection and Immunity* 74, 1673–1682.

Sitnikov, D.M., Schineller, J.B. and Baldwin, T.O. (1995) Transcriptional regulation of bioluminesence genes from *Vibrio fischeri. Molecular Microbiology* 17, 801–812.

Smith, K.M., Bu, Y. and Suga, H. (2003) Induction and inhibition of *Pseudomonas aeruginosa* quorum sensing by synthetic autoinducer analogs. *Chemistry and Biology* 10, 81–89.

Sugimura, M., Maseda, H., Hanaki, H. and Nakae, T. (2008) Macrolide antibiotic-mediated downregulation of MexAB-OprM efflux pump expression in *Pseudomonas aeruginosa. Antimicrobial Agents and Chemotherapy* 52, 4141–4144.

Sun, J., Daniel, R., Wagner-Döbler, I. and Zeng, A.P. (2004) Is autoinducer-2 a universal signal for interspecies communication: a comparative genomic and phylogenetic analysis of the synthesis and signal transduction pathways. *BMC Evolutionary Biology* 4, 36.

Szabó, M.A., Varga, G.Z., Hohmann, J., Schelz, Z., Szegedi, E., Amaral, L. and Molnár, J. (2010) Inhibition of quorum-sensing signals by essential oils. *Phytotherapy Research* 24, 782–786.

Taha, M.O., Al-Bakri, A.G. and Zalloum, W.A. (2006) Discovery of potent inhibitors of pseudomonal quorum sensing via pharmacophore modeling and in silico screening. *Bioorganic and Medicinal Chemistry Letters* 16, 5902–5906.

Tateda, K., Ishii, Y., Kimura, S., Horikawa, M., Miyairi, S. and Yamaguchi, K. (2007) Suppression of *Pseudomonas aeruginosa* quorum-sensing systems by macrolides: a promising strategy or an oriental mystery? *Journal of Infection and Chemotherapy* 13, 357–367.

Teasdale, M.E., Liu, J., Wallace, J., Akhlaghi, F. and Rowley, D.C. (2009) Secondary metabolites produced by the marine bacterium *Halobacillus salinus* that inhibit quorum sensing-controlled phenotypes in Gram-negative bacteria. *Applied and Environmental Microbiology* 75, 567–572.

Teiber, J.F., Horke, S., Haines, D.C., Chowdhary, P.K., Xiao, J., Kramer, G.L., Haley, R.W. and Draganov, D.I. (2008) Dominant role of paraoxonases in inactivation of the *Pseudomonas aeruginosa* quorum-sensing signal *N*-(3-oxododecanoyl)-L-homoserine lactone. *Infection and Immunity* 76, 2512–2519.

Tenover, F.C. (2006) Mechanisms of antimicrobial resistance in bacteria. *American Journal of Medicine* 119, S3–S10.

Thoendel, M. and Horswill, A.R. (2009) Identification of *Staphylococcus aureus* AgrD residues required for autoinducing peptide biosynthesis. *Journal of Biological Chemistry* 284, 21828–21838.

Thoendel, M. and Horswill, A.R. (2010) Biosynthesis of peptide signals in Gram-positive bacteria. *Advances in Applied Microbiology* 71, 91–112.

Truchado, P., Gil-Izquierdo, A., Tomás-Barberán, F. and Allende, A. (2009) Inhibition by chestnut honey of *N*-Acyl-L-homoserine lactones and biofilm formation in *Erwinia carotovora, Yersinia enterocolitica,* and *Aeromonas hydrophila. Journal of Agricultural and Food Chemistry* 57, 11186–11193.

Urbanowski, M.L., Lostroh, C.P. and Greenberg, E.P. (2004) Reversible acyl-homoserine lactone binding to purified *Vibrio fischeri* LuxR protein. *Journal of Bacteriology* 186, 631–637.

Uroz, S. and Heinonsalo, J. (2008) Degradation of *N*-acyl homoserine lactone quorum sensing signal molecules by forest root-associated fungi. *FEMS Microbiological Ecology* 65, 271–278.

Uroz, S., Chhabra, S.R., Cámara, M., Williams, P., Oger, P. and Dessaux, Y. (2005) *N*-Acylhomoserine lactone quorum-sensing molecules are modified and degraded by *Rhodococcus erythropolis* W2 by both amidolytic and novel oxidoreductase activities. *Microbiology* 151, 3313–3322.

Uroz, S., Oger, P., Chhabra, S.R., Cámara, M., Williams, P. and Dessaux, Y. (2007) *N*-Acyl homoserine lactones are degraded via an amidolytic activity in *Comamonas* sp. strain D1. *Archives of Microbiology* 187, 249–256.

Uroz, S., Dessaux, Y. and Oger, P. (2009) Quorum sensing and quorum quenching: the yin and yang of bacterial communication. *ChemBioChem* 10, 205–216.

Val, D.L. and Cronan, J.E. Jr (1998) *In vivo* evidence that *S*-adenosylmethionine and fatty acid synthesis intermediates are the substrates for the

LuxI family of autoinducer synthases. *Journal of Bacteriology* 180, 2644–2651.

Vannini, A., Volpari, C., Gargioli, C., Muraglia, E., Cortese, R., De Francesco, R., Neddermann, P. and Marco, D. (2002) The crystal structure of the quorum sensing protein TraR bound to its autoinducer and target DNA. *EMBO Journal* 21, 4393–4401.

Vattem, D.A., Mihalik, K., Crixell, S.H. and McLean, R.J. (2007) Dietary phytochemicals as quorum sensing inhibitors. *Fitoterapia* 78, 302–310.

Vendeville, A., Winzer, K., Heurlier, K., Tang, C.M. and Hardie, K.R. (2005) Making 'sense' of metabolism: autoinducer-2, LuxS and pathogenic bacteria. *Nature Reviews Microbiology* 3, 383–396.

Wang, W., Morohoshi, T., Ikeda, T. and Chen, L. (2008) Inhibition of Lux quorum-sensing system by synthetic *N*-acyl-L-homoserine lactone analogous. *Acta Biochimica et Biophysica Sinica (Shanghai)* 40, 1023–1028.

Wang, W.Z., Morohoshi, T., Ikenoya, M., Someya, N. and Ikeda, T. (2010) AiiM, a novel class of *N*-acylhomoserine lactonase from the leaf-associated bacterium *Microbacterium testaceum*. *Applied and Environmental Microbiology* 76, 2524–2530.

Waters, C.M. and Bassler, B.L. (2005) Quorum sensing: cell-to-cell communication in bacteria. *Annual Review of Cell and Developmental Biology* 21, 319–346.

Widmer, K.W., Soni, K.A., Hume, M.E., Beier, R.C., Jesudhasan, P. and Pillai, S.D. (2007) Identification of poultry meat-derived fatty acids functioning as quorum sensing signal inhibitors to autoinducer-2 (AI-2). *Journal of Food Science* 72, M363–M368.

Wu, C.M., Cao, J.L., Zheng, M.H., Ou, Y., Zhang, L., Zhu, X.Q. and Song, J.X. (2008) Effect and mechanism of andrographolide on the recovery of *Pseudomonas aeruginosa* susceptibility to several antibiotics. *Journal of International Medical Research* 36, 178–186.

Yang, F., Wang, L.H., Wang, J., Dong, Y.H., Hu, J.Y. and Zhang, L.H. (2005) Quorum quenching enzyme activity is widely conserved in the sera of mammalian species. *FEBS Letters* 579, 3713–3717.

Yates, E.A., Philipp, B., Buckley, C., Atkinson, S., Chhabra, S.R., Sockett, R.E., Goldner, M., Dessaux, Y., Cámara, M., Smith, H. and Williams, P. (2002) *N*-Acylhomoserine lactones undergo lactonolysis in a pH-, temperature-, and acyl chain length-dependent manner during growth of *Yersinia pseudotuberculosis* and *Pseudomonas aeruginosa*. *Infection and Immunity* 70, 5635–5646.

Zhang, M., Jiao, X.D., Hu, Y.H. and Sun, L. (2009) Attenuation of *Edwardsiella tarda* virulence by small peptides that interfere with LuxS/autoinducer type 2 quorum sensing. *Applied and Environmental Microbiology* 75, 3882–3890.

Zhang, R.G., Pappas, T., Brace, J.L., Miller, P.C., Oulmassov, T., Molyneaux, J.M., Anderson, J.C., Bashkin, J.K., Winans, S.C. and Joachimiak, A. (2002) Structure of a bacterial quorum-sensing transcription factor complexed with pheromone and DNA. *Nature* 417, 971–974.

Zhao, G., Wan, W., Mansouri, S., Alfaro, J.F., Bassler, B.L., Cornell, K.A. and Zhou, Z.S. (2003) Chemical synthesis of *S*-ribosyl-L-homocysteine and activity assay as a LuxS substrate. *Bioorganic and Medicinal Chemistry Letters* 13, 3897–3900.

Zhu, H. and Sun, S.J. (2008) Inhibition of bacterial quorum sensing-regulated behaviors by *Tremella fuciformis* extract. *Current Microbiology* 57, 418–422.

Zhu, J., Beaber, J.W., Moré, M.I., Fuqua, C., Eberhard, A. and Winans, S.C. (1998) Analogs of the autoinducer 3-oxooctanoyl-homoserine lactone strongly inhibit activity of the TraR protein of *Agrobacterium tumefaciens*. *Journal of Bacteriology* 180, 5398–5405.

9 Filamentous Temperature-sensitive Mutant Z (FtsZ) Protein as an Antibacterial Target

Jaroslaw M. Boberek,[1] Shan Goh,[1] Jem Stach[2] and Liam Good[1]
[1]*Department of Pathology and Infectious Diseases, The Royal Veterinary College, University of London, London, UK;*[2] *School of Biology, University of Newcastle, Newcastle upon Tyne, UK*

9.1 FtsZ and its Function in the Bacterial Cell

Prokaryotic cell division is a vital and tightly regulated process that has been most thoroughly studied in the rod-shaped bacteria *Escherichia coli* and *Bacillus subtilis*. In *E. coli*, cell division is driven by at least 12 proteins that co-localize at the division site. Among these 12 proteins, filamentous temperature-sensitive mutant Z protein (FtsZ) plays perhaps the most central role and has been the most rigorously studied. FtsZ undergoes dynamic assembly into a contractile ring (the Z-ring) at the mid-cell, which marks the site of the future septum (Bi and Lutkenhaus, 1991). The Z-ring consists of protofilaments of polymerized FtsZ subunits. Formation of the Z-ring is the earliest known step in bacterial cytokinesis, yet the exact signal and mechanism of Z-ring contraction remains unclear. Assembly of FtsZ into the ring is required for the recruitment and interactions of other essential division proteins such as FtsA, ZipA, FtsQ, FtsK, FtsL, FtsB, FtsI and FtsW (Errington *et al.*, 2003; Goehring and Beckwith, 2005; Margolin, 2005; Harry *et al.*, 2006).

ftsZ is as an essential gene (Beall and Lutkenhaus, 1991; Dai and Lutkenhaus, 1991; Dziadek *et al.*, 2003) and is highly conserved among both the bacteria and Archaea. It is present in almost all species of bacteria. The exceptions include *Chlamydia* spp., Planctomycetes and *Ureaplasma urealyticum* (Erickson, 2000; Vaughan *et al.*, 2004; Lindås *et al.*, 2008; Samson *et al.*, 2008). In *Mycoplasma genitalium ftsZ* was recently found to be non-essential through the creation of an *ftsZ* null mutant (Lluch-Senar *et al.*, 2010). FtsZ is the ancestor of eukaryotic tubulin; the three-dimensional structures of both proteins are remarkably similar despite low-level (10–18%) similarity at the amino acid level (Mukherjee and Lutkenhaus, 1994; de Pereda *et al.*, 1996; Romberg and Levin, 2003). In *E. coli*, FtsZ is a protein of approximately 40 kDa consisting of 383 amino acids. Like eukaryotic tubulin, it is a GTPase and polymerizes in a GTP-dependent manner (de Boer *et al.*, 1992; RayChaudhuri and Park, 1992; Mukherjee *et al.*, 1993; Mukherjee and Lutkenhaus, 1994).

In addition to transcriptional regulation, FtsZ activity is regulated at the mRNA and protein levels by at least seven endogenous *trans*-acting cell division inhibitory factors in *E. coli* (Table 9.1; Joseleau-Petit *et al.*, 1999). Most notably, inhibition of FtsZ by SulA is an element of the bacterial SOS response to DNA damage (Bi and Lutkenhaus, 1993). Division arrest in this case gives cells time to repair

Table 9.1. Endogenous inhibitors of FtsZ in *E. coli*.

FtsZ inhibitor	Level of regulation	Comment	Reference
SulA	Protein	SOS-mediated cell division inhibition	Lutkenhaus (1983)
SfiC	Protein	SOS-mediated cell division inhibition	D'Ari and Huisman (1983)
MinC-MinD	Protein	Site-specific septation regulation	Bi and Lutkenhaus (1993)
MinC-DicB	Protein	Site-specific septation regulation	de Boer *et al.* (1990)
Kil^{Rac}	Protein	Rac prophage-mediated cell killing	Conter *et al.* (1996)
DicF	mRNA	Antisense RNA	Bouché and Bouché (1989)
StfZ	mRNA	Antisense RNA	Dewar and Donachie (1993)

DNA lesions and if necessary induce an alternative mutagenic DNA repair polymerase V, although at the risk of introducing errors to the genome (Foster, 2007; Janion, 2008). The central role of FtsZ in assembly of the cell-division machinery and its tight regulation strongly suggest that FtsZ polymerization is essential to bacterial cytokinesis.

9.2 FtsZ as a Promising Target for Antibacterial Discovery

The rise and rapid spread of antibiotic resistance necessitates not only the modification of known antimicrobial classes but also the discovery of novel targets and new drug classes. FtsZ is a novel, previously underexploited target for drug discovery, and many of its properties suggest it could provide a successful strategy. Although no compound that targets cell division is currently used in clinical antibacterial chemotherapy, tubulin inhibitors are widely applied in anticancer therapy (Jordan *et al.*, 1998; Dumontet and Jordan, 2010). The structural similarity of tubulin and FtsZ suggest that these anticancer compounds could be used as a basis for the development of FtsZ inhibitors (Kinnings *et al.*, 2010). Moreover, a number of agents that target FtsZ have been identified (Table 9.2).

FtsZ amino acid sequence conservation among diverse prokaryotes is consistent with broad-spectrum antibacterial development. Importantly, FtsZ is absent in the mitochondria of higher eukaryotes, where its function is fulfilled by dynamin (Erickson, 2000). Despite the similarities between FtsZ and tubulin, sufficient structural differences exist to enable selective inhibition. Indeed, none of the classic tubulin inhibitors (3methoxybenzamide, albendazole, colchicine, nocodazole, paclitaxel and thiabendazole) significantly perturbs FtsZ *in vitro*, and inhibitors specific for FtsZ are also known (Wang *et al.*, 2003). However, the *in vivo* efficacy of compounds targeting FtsZ or tubulin may differ significantly from predictions based on *in vitro* data. For instance, 3-methoxybenzamide (3-MBA; Table 9.2) is a weak FtsZ inhibitor *in vivo*, despite poor inhibition of FtsZ polymerization and GTPase activity *in vitro*, and has been used to development several compounds that target FtsZ with much improved efficacy, such as PC190723 (Jaiswal *et al.*, 2007; Haydon *et al.*, 2008, 2010; Plaza *et al.*, 2010). Overall, FtsZ appears to be sufficiently conserved in bacteria and divergent from mammalian homologues to enable broad-spectrum antibacterial development.

Extensive structural and biochemical data on FtsZ are available to aid the design and modification of new inhibitors (Löwe and Amos, 1998). The structure of the protein reveals at least two 'druggable' domains. The N-terminal domain is essential for GTP binding (de Boer *et al.*, 1992; RayChaudhuri and Park, 1992; Mukherjee *et al.*, 1993; Hopkins and Groom, 2002). The C-terminal domain is responsible for crucial interactions with other essential division proteins, ZipA and FtsA (Ma *et al.*, 1997; Wang *et al.*, 1997; Din

Table 9.2. Examples of described inhibitors of FtsZ.

Inhibitor	Origin	MIC data	MBC data	Activity against Gram +/– or mycobacteria	Morphology effect reported	Polymerization inhibition	GTPase activity effect	Z-ring effect	Genetic evidence	*In silico* docking prediction	Reference(s)
16.a.4	Synthetic			+, –	Y						Inhibitor of ZipA–FtsZ binding; Jennings *et al.*(2004)
A189	Synthetic	Y		+, –	Y	Y	Y	Y	Y		Ito *et al.* (2006)
2-Alkoxycarbonylamino-pyridines	Synthetic	Y	Y	*Mycobacterium tuberculosis*		Y	Y				White *et al.* (2002)
8-Bromoguanosine 5′-triphosphate (BrGTP)	Synthetic					Y	Y				GTP analogue; Läppchen *et al.* (2005)
3-Methoxybenzamide (3-MBA)	Synthetic	Y		+	Y				Y		Ohashi *et al.* (1999)
Benzimidazoles	Synthetic	Y		*M. tuberculosis*	Y	Y	Y				Slayden *et al.* (2006); Kumar *et al.* (2010)
N-Benzyl-3-sulfonamidopyrrolidines	Synthetic	Y		–	Y		Y		Y		Mukherjee *et al.* (2007)
Berberine	Plant	Y		+, –	Y	Y	Y	Y	Y	Y	Domadia *et al.* (2008); Boberek *et al.* (2010)
Chrysophaentins	Algal	Y		+		Y	Y			Y	Plaza *et al.* (2010)
Cinnamaldehyde	Plant	Y	Y	+, –	Y	Y	Y	Y		Y	Domadia *et al.* (2007)
Compounds 12 and 14 (carboxybiphenyl-indoles)	Synthetic	Y		+							Inhibitor of ZipA–FtsZ binding; Sutherland *et al.* (2003)

Continued

Table 9.2. Continued.

Inhibitor	Origin	MIC data	MBC data	Activity against Gram +/– or mycobacteria	Morphology effect reported	Polymerization inhibition	GTPase activity effect	Z-ring effect	Genetic evidence	*In silico* docking prediction	Reference(s)
Curcumin	Plant	Y		+, –	Y	Y	Y	Y	Y		Rai *et al.* (2008)
Dichamenetin and 2‴-hydroxy-5″-benzylisouvarinol	Plant	Y		+, –, *Mycobacterium smegmatis*			Y				Urgaonkar *et al.* (2005)
GAL core compound 14	Synthetic			+			Y				GTP analogue; Paradis-Bleau *et al.* (2007)
PC58538, PC170942, PC190723[a], 8j[a]	Synthetic	Y		+, –	Y	Y	Y	Y	Y	Y	Stokes *et al.* (2005); Haydon *et al.* (2008, 2010); Adams *et al.* (2011)
Sanguinarine	Plant	Y		+, –	Y	Y		Y	Y		Godowski (1989); Beuria *et al.* (2005)
Totarol	Plant	Y		+, *M. tuberculosis*	Y	Y	Y	Y			Jaiswal *et al.* (2007)
TRA 10 series	Synthetic	Y		*M. tuberculosis*	Y						Huang *et al.* (2006)
Viriditoxin	Fungal	Y		+	Y	Y	Y		Y		Wang *et al.* (2003)
Zantrins (Z1–Z3)	Synthetic	Y		+, –	Y	Y	Y	Y	Y		Margalit *et al.* (2004)

MIC, minimal inhibitory concentration; MBC, minimal bactericidal concentration.
[a]Successfully tested *in vivo* in a murine septicaemia model of staphylococcal infection.

et al., 1998; Mosyak *et al.*, 2000; Yan *et al.*, 2000; Haney *et al.*, 2001), and with the essential *E. coli* chaperonin system GroEL/S (Ogino *et al.*, 2004; Fujiwara and Taguchi, 2007). However, a known FtsZ inhibitor, PC190723 (Haydon *et al.*, 2008), has been predicted to bind to a different part of the protein, namely a cleft between the N- and C-terminal domains. Furthermore, as the residues involved in interactions between ZipA and FtsA proteins and FtsZ have been identified, this knowledge can be used to design inhibitors (Liu *et al.*, 1999; Mosyak *et al.*, 2000; Moy *et al.*, 2000; Haney *et al.*, 2001; Pichoff and Lutkenhaus, 2005, 2007).

Bacterial cells are very sensitive to both under- and overexpression of *ftsZ* (Haney *et al.*, 2001; Dziadek *et al.*, 2002, 2003; Honrubia-Marcos *et al.*, 2005; Goh *et al.*, 2009), suggesting a tight regulatory control of the gene/protein, perhaps due to the central role it plays in cell viability. Indeed, recent evidence shows that *ftsZ* is more stringently required than two other essential genes in *E. coli*, *murA* and *fabI*, whose products are established targets for clinically used antimicrobials (Goh *et al.*, 2009). It appears that only a modest reduction in the activity of FtsZ through specific inhibitor interaction is needed to inhibit growth.

There is a substantial amount of data on the effect of inhibition of FtsZ on bacterial growth. In the case of rod-shaped bacteria such as *E. coli* and *B. subtilis*, successful FtsZ inhibitors are likely to be bacteriostatic. These bacteria have two spatially distinct modes of peptidoglycan synthesis, one involved in cell elongation and shape maintenance and one responsible for septal-wall synthesis, which is dependent on FtsZ. Inhibition of cell division causes formation of long filamentous cells with decreased viability (Fig. 9.1) (Scheffers and Pinho, 2005). However, in *Staphylococcus aureus* and possibly in other cocci, depletion of functional FtsZ results in significant cell enlargement, inhibition of growth and rapid cell lysis. This is due to peptidoglycan synthesis being restricted mainly to the division septum in these bacteria and thereby growth of the cells being limited to septal-wall synthesis. Following inhibition of FtsZ, the cell-wall synthesis machinery becomes dispersed and new peptidoglycan is incorporated in patches

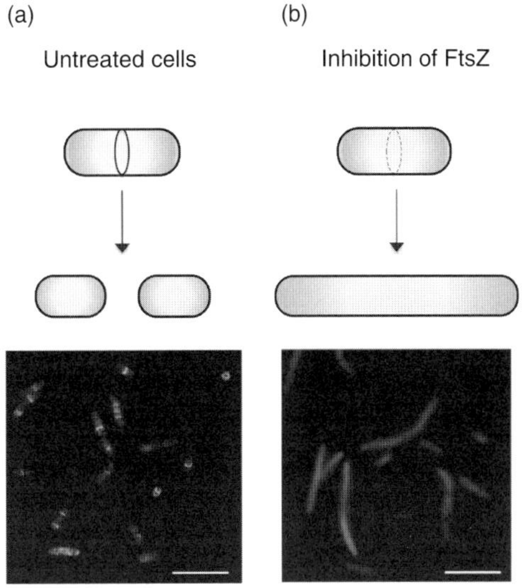

Fig. 9.1. Effect of FtsZ inhibition on the morphology of rod-shaped bacteria. (a) Normal course of cell division with formation of the Z-ring at the mid-cell. By the expression of *ftsZ* fused to a yellow fluorescent protein (*yfp*) gene, the Z-rings in *E. coli* were visualized by fluorescence microscopy. (b) Cell morphology under inhibition of FtsZ resulted in visible cell elongation and perturbation of Z-ring formation. Bars, 10 μm. (Based on Boberek *et al.*, 2010.)

over the entire surface of the cells, resulting in increased cell volume before lysis. Therefore, in the case of cocci such as *S. aureus* and *Enterococcus faecalis*, FtsZ inhibitors are likely to be bactericidal (Pinho and Errington, 2003; Stokes *et al.*, 2005).

9.3 Arguments Against FtsZ as a Target for Antibacterials

The arguments for FtsZ as a viable target for the development of new antibacterials are substantial, but at an early stage it is also necessary to consider counterarguments that raise doubts about the validity of FtsZ as a target.

First, as with any other single-target inhibitor, resistance to the new drug targeting bacterial FtsZ may appear rapidly. However, this could potentially be prevented or postponed by wise and responsible usage of the drug or its application in combination therapy. Moreover, FtsZ inhibitors are likely to be broad-spectrum antibacterials due to the high level of conservation of the target protein. For many reasons, broad-spectrum antibiotics are favoured by clinicians. However, broad-spectrum anti-infective treatments should be discouraged where possible, as they exert widespread selective pressure and cause widespread damage to the natural flora of the host. On the other hand, broad-spectrum antibiotics are more likely to give an investment return for pharmaceutical companies looking into possibilities of developing novel antibacterials.

Secondly, growth arrest in bacteria often involves regulated inhibition of FtsZ. Indeed, cell-division inhibition is often associated with stress and survival responses. The best-known example is the bacterial SOS response. Such a response is known to be involved in resistance to certain antibiotics such as ciprofloxacin and some β-lactams (Hastings *et al.*, 2004; Miller *et al.*, 2004; Cirz *et al.*, 2005; Michel, 2005). Therefore, it is possible that FtsZ inhibitors could augment bacterial stress responses. For example, it is has been suggested that cell elongation is one of the mechanisms that may aid bacterial evasion of the host innate immune responses (Justice *et al.*, 2004, 2006). Highly elongated cells could potentially resist engulfment by neutrophils and other phagocytes. Furthermore, it may be necessary to learn whether bacteria are able to resume normal cell division upon removal of the inhibitor through simple fragmentation of the filaments into individual, viable cells (Maier *et al.*, 1999).

Thirdly, targeting FtsZ implies the necessity of thoroughly testing whether the drug candidate perturbs tubulin function of the host cells, as both proteins are structurally similar. Moreover, the number of FtsZ molecules in the cytoplasm of a typical *E. coli* cell is relatively high, around 15,000 (Lu *et al.*, 1998), and although a fraction is incorporated into the Z-ring, it may be important to know what percentage of these molecules needs to be inhibited for a drug to be effective. However, ribosomes are highly abundant in cells and are proven successful targets in antibacterial therapy.

Furthermore, recent evidence suggested that functional cell division might be required for the activity of other antibiotics. For instance, some β-lactams require successful assembly of the cell-division machinery in order for rapid cell lysis to occur (Chung *et al.*, 2009), which could be compromised if used in combination with FtsZ inhibitors.

Overall, while an antibacterial approach based on FtsZ as a target has many advantages, there are also reasons to be cautious when developing FtsZ inhibitors for antibacterial therapy. A better understanding of the cell-division process in bacteria and the role that FtsZ inhibition plays in stress responses seem critical if successful FtsZ inhibitors are to be developed for the clinic.

9.4 FtsZ Inhibitors

Many examples of FtsZ inhibitors can be found in the literature. They vary greatly in origin, development stage and strength of evidence supporting their inhibition of FtsZ. Table 9.2 summarizes the data available on some of the established FtsZ-targeting agents.

9.5 Strategies for the Identification of FtsZ Inhibitors

Various methods have been developed to describe novel inhibitors of FtsZ, ranging from *in silico* predictions, to *in vitro* studies and even to live-cell-based, target-selective screening. These techniques (Table 9.3) can help to better understand established FtsZ inhibitors and possibly to identify new compounds.

One approach derives from the fact that eukaryotic tubulin and FtsZ share many characteristics. Knowledge about their structure, biochemistry and interactions with other proteins makes it possible to exploit their differences for development of inhibitors specific for FtsZ. In such an approach, new molecules can be designed *in silico* based on the structural data of already known inhibitors of either FtsZ or tubulin, and applied in docking studies or in screening specific

Table 9.3. Summary of screens and techniques useful for discovery and validation of putative FtsZ inhibitors.

Method	Nature of the screen	Throughput	Examples of compounds identified/tested	Reference
Molecule design and docking studies based on previously known inhibitors	*In silico/in vitro*	High	PC190723	Haydon *et al.* (2008)
Design of GTP analogues	*In silico/in vitro*	High	BrGTP	Läppchen *et al.* (2005)
GTP hydrolysis assays (malachite – ammonium molybdate)	*In vitro*	Low–medium	Curcumin	Rai *et al.* (2008)
GTP hydrolysis (real-time coupled enzyme assay)	*In vitro*	High	Zantrins	Margalit *et al.* (2004)
Fluorescently labelled FtsZ polymerization assay	*In vitro*	High	Viriditoxin	Wang *et al.* (2003)
FtsZ light-scattering assay	*In vitro*	Low–medium	Cinnamaldehyde	Domadia *et al.* (2007)
FtsZ polymer sedimentation assay	*In vitro*	Low–medium	OTBA	Beuria *et al.* (2009)
Electron microscopy FtsZ polymer analysis	*In vitro*	Low	Totarol	Jaiswal *et al.* (2007)
Cell-morphology studies	*In vivo*	Low	16.a.4	Jennings *et al.* (2004)
Reporter-based *Bacillus subtilis* sporulation assay	*In vivo*	High	PC58538	Stokes *et al.* (2005)
Anucleate cell blue assay	*In vivo*	Medium–high	A189	Ito *et al.* (2006)
Antisense sensitization assay	*In vivo*	Medium	Berberine	Boberek *et al.* (2010)

compound libraries using other assays (White *et al.*, 2002; Huang *et al.*, 2006). As exemplified by 3-MBA, a modest inhibitor of FtsZ *in vivo* can be used successfully as a lead for the development of a series of compounds with highly improved potency (Stokes *et al.*, 2005; Haydon *et al.*, 2008).

Another example is *in silico* and *in vitro* screening for GTP analogues that have the potential to inhibit the enzymatic activity of FtsZ and prevent formation of the Z-ring. This approach led to the design of GAL core compound 14 (GAL is a guanine moiety linked to alanine) and 8-bromoguanosine 5′-triphosphate (BrGTP; Läppchen *et al.*, 2005; Paradis-Bleau *et al.*, 2007). Both inhibit FtsZ GTPase activity, and BrGTP also perturbs FtsZ polymerization without affecting tubulin assembly *in vitro*. However, additional studies are required to assess the antimicrobial potential of these compounds. Furthermore, various methods (e.g. the established malachite green/ammonium molybdate colorimetric assay, or the novel real-time assay based on enzyme-coupled reactions involving pyruvate kinase and lactate dehydrogenase) allow quantitative measurement of FtsZ GTPase activity. They have been used for high-throughput screening of compound libraries to identify synthetic compounds, such as the polyphenols called zantrins as novel inhibitors of FtsZ, and to test the antibacterial mode of action of some natural products, such as the plant alkaloid berberine (Margalit *et al.*, 2004; Domadia *et al.*, 2007, 2008; Rai *et al.*, 2008).

A high-throughput method measuring inhibition of fluorescently labelled FtsZ polymerization was used to screen a library of over 100,000 extracts from microbial fermentation broths and plants. This revealed viriditoxin as an FtsZ inhibitor (Trusca and Bramhill, 2002; Wang *et al.*, 2003). First reported in 1971 from the fungus *Aspergillus viridinutans*, viriditoxin is a novel inhibitor of FtsZ polymerization and GTPase activity. Moreover, the standard FtsZ light-scattering assay and electron microscopy have also proven very useful to validate whether an inhibitor is able to affect the GTP-initiated polymerization of FtsZ (Mukherjee and Lutkenhaus, 1999; Domadia *et al.*, 2007; Andreu *et al.*, 2010).

Quantitative increases in polymerization of FtsZ may also be used in screening assays to identify inhibitors. Promotion of FtsZ assembly and stability of monomers, determined by comparing sedimentation mass of FtsZ polymers in the absence and presence of inhibitors, enabled the identification of 3-(5-[4-oxo-2-thioxo-3-(3-trifluoromethylphenyl)-thiazolidin-5-ylidenemethyl]-furan-2-yl)-benzoic acid (OTBA). OTBA promoted FtsZ assembly *in vitro* and inhibited bacterial cell division through increased monomer bundling and a decreased rate of GTP hydrolysis (Beuria *et al.*, 2009). While a strictly *in vitro*-based approach can be very effective, it can also provide positive hits for compounds that do not enter the cells. It is therefore important to validate these with the help of *in vivo* and cell-morphology studies.

Several types of cell-based assays have been used for compound screening and often involve the use of reporter genes. For example, an elegant assay that used β-glucuronidase/β-galactosidase-based reporters of *B. subtilis* asymmetric septation during sporulation (Stokes *et al.*, 2005) allowed identification of PC58538. This compound was also later used as a lead for development of analogues with improved potency. Another example is the anucleate cell blue assay, where the production of anucleate cells is visible as a blue zone around the growth inhibition zone on a plate. This method, originally developed for identification of inhibitors of chromosome partitioning in *E. coli*, led to the discovery of four 4-aminofurazan derivatives that showed good inhibitory activity against FtsZ (Ito *et al.*, 2006). As *ftsZ* is typically essential in bacteria, knock-out mutants are not viable and thus *ftsZ* mutants cannot be used in cell assays. However, antisense RNA silencing of *ftsZ* can provide titratable reduction of *ftsZ* expression and has enabled novel cell-based assays to be carried out (Kaur *et al.*, 2009). RNA silencers (either expressed antisense RNA or antisense peptide nucleic acid) specific for *ftsZ* have been utilized in an assay where a knockdown of *ftsZ* expression sensitized bacteria to compounds targeting FtsZ (Boberek *et al.*, 2010). This approach provided genetic evidence for inhibition of FtsZ by berberine. Such live-cell-based methods, combined with cell-morphology studies using, for example, phase-contrast microscopy, allow putative FtsZ inhibitors to be tested *in vivo*.

A wealth of knowledge is available on the structure, biochemistry and function of FtsZ in bacteria. The protein is a promising target in antibacterial discovery. Potent inhibitors of FtsZ have been identified and claimed in patent applications, and some have been tested in animal model studies and have shown promising potential in ADMET (absorption, distribution, metabolism, excretion and toxicity) evaluations (Haydon *et al.*, 2010; Awasthi *et al.*, 2011). Nevertheless, further work is required to establish the efficacy and feasibility of FtsZ as a target in the clinical setting.

References

Adams, D.W., Wu, L.J., Czaplewski, L.G. and Errington, J. (2011) Multiple effects of benzamide antibiotics on FtsZ function. *Molecular Microbiology* 80, 68–84.

Andreu, J.M., Schaffner-Barbero, C., Huecas, S., Alonso, D., Lopez-Rodriguez, M.L., Ruiz-Avila, L.B., Núñez-Ramírez, R., Llorca, O. and Martín-Galiano, A.J. (2010) The antibacterial cell division inhibitor PC190723 is an FtsZ polymer-stabilizing agent that induces filament assembly and condensation. *Journal of Biological Chemistry* 285, 14239–14246.

Awasthi, D., Kumar, K. and Ojima, I. (2011) Therapeutic potential of FtsZ inhibition: a patent perspective. *Expert Opinion on Therapeutic Patents* 21, 657–679.

Beall, B. and Lutkenhaus, J. (1991) FtsZ in *Bacillus subtilis* is required for vegetative septation and for asymmetric septation during sporulation. *Genes & Development* 5, 447–455.

Beuria, T.K., Santra, M.K. and Panda, D. (2005) Sanguinarine blocks cytokinesis in bacteria by inhibiting FtsZ assembly and bundling. *Biochemistry* 44, 16584–16593.

Beuria, T.K., Singh, P., Surolia, A. and Panda, D. (2009) Promoting assembly and bundling of FtsZ as a strategy to inhibit bacterial cell division: a new approach for developing novel antibacterial drugs. *Biochemical Journal* 423, 61–69.

Bi, E.F. and Lutkenhaus, J. (1991) FtsZ ring structure associated with division in *Escherichia coli*. *Nature* 354, 161–164.

Bi, E. and Lutkenhaus, J. (1993) Cell division inhibitors SulA and MinCD prevent formation of the FtsZ ring. *Journal of Bacteriology* 175, 1118–1125.

Boberek, J.M., Stach, J. and Good, L. (2010) Genetic evidence for inhibition of bacterial division protein FtsZ by berberine. *PLoS ONE* 5, e13745.

Bouché, F. and Bouché, J.P. (1989) Genetic evidence that DicF, a second division inhibitor encoded by *the Escherichia coli dicB* operon, is probably RNA. *Molecular Microbiology* 3, 991–994.

Chung, H.S., Yao, Z., Goehring, N.W., Kishony, R., Beckwith, J. and Kahne, D. (2009) Rapid β-lactam-induced lysis requires successful assembly of the cell division machinery. *Proceedings of the National Academy of Sciences USA* 106, 21872–21877.

Cirz, R.T., Chin, J.K., Andes, D.R., de Crécy-Lagard, V., Craig, W.A. and Romesberg, F.E. (2005) Inhibition of mutation and combating the evolution of antibiotic resistance. *PLoS Biology* 3, e176.

Conter, A., Bouché, J.P. and Dassain, M. (1996) Identification of a new inhibitor of essential division gene *ftsZ* as the *kil* gene of defective prophage Rac. *Journal of Bacteriology* 178, 5100–5104.

Dai, K. and Lutkenhaus, J. (1991) *ftsZ* is an essential cell division gene in *Escherichia coli*. *Journal of Bacteriology* 173, 3500–3506.

D'Ari, R. and Huisman, O. (1983) Novel mechanism of cell division inhibition associated with the SOS response in *Escherichia coli*. *Journal of Bacteriology* 156, 243–250.

de Boer, P.A., Crossley, R.E. and Rothfield, L.I. (1990) Central role for the *Escherichia coli minC* gene product in two different cell division-inhibition systems. *Proceedings of the National Academy of Sciences USA* 87, 1129–1133.

de Boer, P., Crossley, R. and Rothfield, L. (1992) The essential bacterial cell-division protein FtsZ is a GTPase. *Nature* 359, 254–256.

de Pereda, J.M., Leynadier, D., Evangelio, J.A., Chacón, P. and Andreu, J.M. (1996) Tubulin secondary structure analysis, limited proteolysis sites, and homology to FtsZ. *Biochemistry* 35, 14203–14215.

Dewar, S.J. and Donachie, W.D. (1993) Antisense transcription of the *ftsZ–ftsA* gene junction inhibits cell division in *Escherichia coli*. *Journal of Bacteriology* 175, 7097–7101.

Din, N., Quardokus, E.M., Sackett, M.J. and Brun, Y.V. (1998) Dominant C-terminal deletions of FtsZ that affect its ability to localize in *Caulobacter* and its interaction with FtsA. *Molecular Microbiology* 27, 1051–1063.

Domadia, P., Swarup, S., Bhunia, A., Sivaraman, J. and Dasgupta, D. (2007) Inhibition of bacterial cell division protein FtsZ by cinnamaldehyde. *Biochemical Pharmacology* 74, 831–840.

Domadia, P.N., Bhunia, A., Sivaraman, J., Swarup, S. and Dasgupta, D. (2008) Berberine targets assembly of *Escherichia coli* cell division protein FtsZ. *Biochemistry* 47, 3225–3234.

Dumontet, C. and Jordan, M.A. (2010) Microtubule-binding agents: a dynamic field of cancer therapeutics. *Nature Reviews Drug Discovery* 9, 790–803.

Dziadek, J., Madiraju, M.V.V.S., Rutherford, S.A., Atkinson, M.A.L. and Rajagopalan, M. (2002) Physiological consequences associated with overproduction of *Mycobacterium tuberculosis* FtsZ in mycobacterial hosts. *Microbiology* 148, 961–971.

Dziadek, J., Rutherford, S.A., Madiraju, M.V., Atkinson, M.A.L. and Rajagopalan, M. (2003) Conditional expression of *Mycobacterium smegmatis ftsZ*, an essential cell division gene. *Microbiology* 149, 1593–1603.

Erickson, H.P. (2000) Dynamin and FtsZ. *Journal of Cell Biology* 148, 1103–1106.

Errington, J., Daniel, R.A. and Scheffers, D.J. (2003) Cytokinesis in bacteria. *Microbiology and Molecular Biology Reviews* 67, 52–65.

Foster, P.L. (2007) Stress-induced mutagenesis in bacteria. *Critical Reviews in Biochemistry and Molecular Biology* 42, 373–397.

Fujiwara, K. and Taguchi, H. (2007) Filamentous morphology in GroE-depleted *Escherichia coli* induced by impaired folding of FtsE. *Journal of Bacteriology* 189, 5860–5866.

Godowski, K.C. (1989) Antimicrobial action of sanguinarine. *Journal of Clinical Dentistry* 1, 96–101.

Goehring, N.W. and Beckwith, J. (2005) Diverse paths to midcell: assembly of the bacterial cell division machinery. *Current Biology* 15, R514–526.

Goh, S., Boberek, J.M., Nakashima, N., Stach, J. and Good, L. (2009) Concurrent growth rate and transcript analyses reveal essential gene stringency in *Escherichia coli*. *PLoS ONE* 4, e6061.

Haney, S.A., Glasfeld, E., Hale, C., Keeney, D., He, Z., de Boer, P. (2001) Genetic analysis of the *Escherichia coli* FtsZ.ZipA interaction in the yeast two-hybrid system. Characterization of FtsZ residues essential for the interactions with ZipA and with FtsA. *The Journal of Biological Chemistry* 276, 11980–11987.

Harry, E., Monahan, L. and Thompson, L. (2006) Bacterial cell division: the mechanism and its precision. *International Review of Cytology* 253, 27–94.

Hastings, P.J., Rosenberg, S.M. and Slack, A. (2004) Antibiotic-induced lateral transfer of antibiotic resistance. *Trends in Microbiology* 12, 401–404.

Haydon, D.J., Stokes, N.R., Ure, R., Galbraith, G., Bennett, J.M., Brown, D.R., Baker, P.J., Barynin, V.V., Rice, D.W., Sedelnikova, S.E., Heal, J.R., Sheridan, J.M., Aiwale, S.T., Chauhan, P.K., Srivastava, A., Taneja, A., Collins, I., Errington, J. and Czaplewski, L.G. (2008) An inhibitor of FtsZ with potent and selective anti-staphylococcal activity. *Science* 321, 1673–1675.

Haydon, D.J., Bennett, J.M., Brown, D., Collins, I., Galbraith, G., Lancett, P., Macdonald, R., Stokes, N.R., Chauhan, P.K., Sutariya, J.K., Nayal, N., Srivastava, A., Beanland, J., Hall, R., Henstock, V., Noula, C., Rockley, C. and Czaplewski, L. (2010) Creating an antibacterial with in vivo efficacy: synthesis and characterization of potent inhibitors of the bacterial cell division protein FtsZ with improved pharmaceutical properties. *Journal of Medicinal Chemistry* 53, 3927–3936.

Honrubia-Marcos, M.P., Ramos, A. and Gil, J.A. (2005) Overexpression of the *ftsZ* gene from *Corynebacterium glutamicum* (*Brevibacterium lactofermentum*) in *Escherichia coli*. *Canadian Journal of Microbiology* 51, 85–89.

Hopkins, A.L. and Groom, C.R. (2002) The druggable genome. *Nature Reviews Drug Discovery* 1, 727–730.

Huang, Q., Kirikae, F., Kirikae, T., Pepe, A., Amin, A., Respicio, L., Slayden, R.A., Tonge, P.J. and Ojima, I. (2006) Targeting FtsZ for antituberculosis drug discovery: noncytotoxic taxanes as novel antituberculosis agents. *Journal of Medicinal Chemistry* 49, 463–466.

Ito, H., Ura, A., Oyamada, Y., Tanitame, A., Yoshida, H., Yamada, S., Wachi, M., Yamagishi, J. (2006) A 4-aminofurazan derivative-A189-inhibits assembly of bacterial cell division protein FtsZ *in vitro* and *in vivo*. *Microbiology and Immunology* 50, 759–764.

Jaiswal, R., Beuria, T.K., Mohan, R., Mahajan, S.K. and Panda, D. (2007) Totarol inhibits bacterial cytokinesis by perturbing the assembly dynamics of FtsZ. *Biochemistry* 46, 4211–4220.

Janion, C. (2008) Inducible SOS response system of DNA repair and mutagenesis in *Escherichia coli*. *International Journal of Biological Sciences* 4, 338–344.

Jennings, L.D., Foreman, K.W., Rush, T.S., III, Tsao, D.H.H., Mosyak, L., Kincaid, S.L., Sukhdeo, M.N., Sutherland, A.G., Ding, W., Kenny, C.H., Sabus, C.L., Liu, H., Dushin, E.G., Moghazeh, S.L., Labthavikul, P., Petersen, P.J., Tuckman, M., Haney, S.A. and Ruzin, A.V. (2004) Combinatorial synthesis of substituted 3-(2-indolyl)piperidines and 2-phenyl indoles as inhibitors of ZipA–FtsZ interaction. *Bioorganic & Medicinal Chemistry* 12, 5115–5131.

Jordan, A., Hadfield, J.A., Lawrence, N.J. and McGown, A.T. (1998) Tubulin as a target for anticancer drugs: agents which interact with the mitotic spindle. *Medicinal Research Reviews* 18, 259–296.

Joseleau-Petit, D., Vinella, D. and D'Ari, R. (1999) Metabolic alarms and cell division in *Escherichia coli*. *Journal of Bacteriology* 181, 9–14.

Justice, S.S., Hung, C., Theriot, J.A., Fletcher, D.A., Anderson, G.G., Footer, M.J. and Hultgren, S.J. (2004) Differentiation and developmental pathways of uropathogenic *Escherichia coli* in urinary tract pathogenesis. *Proceedings of the National Academy of Sciences USA* 101, 1333–1338.

Justice, S.S., Hunstad, D.A., Seed, P.C. and Hultgren, S.J. (2006) Filamentation by *Escherichia coli* subverts innate defenses during urinary tract infection. *Proceedings of the National Academy of Sciences USA* 103, 19884–19889.

Kaur, P., Agarwal, S. and Datta, S. (2009) Delineating bacteriostatic and bactericidal targets in mycobacteria using IPTG inducible antisense expression. *PLoS ONE* 4, e5923.

Kinnings, S.L., Xie, L., Fung, K.H., Jackson, R.M., Xie, L. and Bourne, P.E. (2010) The *Mycobacterium tuberculosis* drugome and its polypharmacological implications. *PLoS Computational Biology* 6, e1000976.

Kumar, K., Awasthi, D., Lee, S.Y., Zanardi, I., Ruzsicska, B., Knudson, S., Tonge, P.J., Slayden, R.A. and Ojima, I. (2010) Novel trisubstituted benzimidazoles, targeting Mtb FtsZ, as a new class of antitubercular agents. *Journal of Medicinal Chemistry* 54, 374–381.

Läppchen, T., Hartog, A.F., Pinas, V.A., Koomen, G.-J. and den Blaauwen, T. (2005) GTP analogue inhibits polymerization and GTPase activity of the bacterial protein FtsZ without affecting its eukaryotic homologue tubulin. *Biochemistry* 44, 7879–7884.

Lindås, A.-C., Karlsson, E.A., Lindgren, M.T., Ettema, T.J.G. and Bernander, R. (2008) A unique cell division machinery in the Archaea.

Proceedings of the National Academy of Sciences USA 105, 18942 -18946.
Liu, Z., Mukherjee, A. and Lutkenhaus, J. (1999) Recruitment of ZipA to the division site by interaction with FtsZ. *Molecular Microbiology* 31, 1853–1861.
Lluch-Senar, M., Querol, E. and Piñol, J. (2010) Cell division in a minimal bacterium in the absence of ftsZ. *Molecular Microbiology* 78, 278–289.
Löwe, J. and Amos, L.A. (1998) Crystal structure of the bacterial cell-division protein FtsZ. *Nature* 391, 203–206.
Lu, C., Stricker, J. and Erickson, H.P. (1998) FtsZ from *Escherichia coli*, *Azotobacter vinelandii*, and *Thermotoga maritima* – quantitation, GTP hydrolysis, and assembly. *Cell Motility and the Cytoskeleton* 40, 71–86.
Lutkenhaus, J.F. (1983) Coupling of DNA replication and cell division: sulB is an allele of *ftsZ*. *Journal of Bacteriology* 154, 1339–1346.
Ma, X., Sun, Q., Wang, R., Singh, G., Jonietz, E.L. and Margolin, W. (1997) Interactions between heterologous FtsA and FtsZ proteins at the FtsZ ring. *Journal of Bacteriology* 179, 6788–6797.
Maier, S.K., Scherer, S. and Loessner, M.J. (1999) Long-chain polyphosphate causes cell lysis and inhibits *Bacillus cereus* septum formation, which is dependent on divalent cations. *Applied and Environmental Microbiology* 65, 3942–3949.
Margalit, D.N., Romberg, L., Mets, R.B., Hebert, A.M., Mitchison, T.J., Kirschner, M.W., RayChaudhuri, D. (2004) Targeting cell division: small-molecule inhibitors of FtsZ GTPase perturb cytokinetic ring assembly and induce bacterial lethality. *Proceedings of the National Academy of Sciences USA* 101, 11821–11826.
Margolin, W. (2005) FtsZ and the division of prokaryotic cells and organelles. *Nature Reviews Molecular Cell Biology* 6, 862–871.
Michel, B. (2005) After 30 years of study, the bacterial SOS response still surprises us. *PLoS Biology* 3, e255.
Miller, C., Thomsen, L.E., Gaggero, C., Mosseri, R., Ingmer, H. and Cohen, S.N. (2004) SOS response induction by β-lactams and bacterial defense against antibiotic lethality. *Science* 305, 1629–1631.
Mosyak, L., Zhang, Y., Glasfeld, E., Haney, S., Stahl, M., Seehra, J. and Somers, W.S. (2000) The bacterial cell-division protein ZipA and its interaction with an FtsZ fragment revealed by X-ray crystallography. *EMBO Journal* 19, 3179–3191.
Moy, F.J., Glasfeld, E., Mosyak, L. and Powers, R. (2000) Solution structure of ZipA, a crucial component of *Escherichia coli* cell division. *Biochemistry* 39, 9146–9156.
Mukherjee, A. and Lutkenhaus, J. (1994) Guanine nucleotide-dependent assembly of FtsZ into filaments. *Journal of Bacteriology* 176, 2754–2758.
Mukherjee, A. and Lutkenhaus, J. (1999) Analysis of FtsZ assembly by light scattering and determination of the role of divalent metal cations. *Journal of Bacteriology* 181, 823–832.
Mukherjee, A., Dai, K. and Lutkenhaus, J. (1993) *Escherichia coli* cell division protein FtsZ is a guanine nucleotide binding protein. *Proceedings of the National Academy of Sciences USA* 90, 1053–1057.
Mukherjee, S., Robinson, C.A., Howe, A.G., Mazor, T., Wood, P.A., Urgaonkar, S., Hebert, A.M., RayChaudhuri, D. and Shaw, J.T. (2007) *N*-Benzyl-3-sulfonamidopyrrolidines as novel inhibitors of cell division in *E. coli*. *Bioorganic and Medicinal Chemistry Letters* 17, 6651–6655.
Ogino, H., Wachi, M., Ishii, A., Iwai, N., Nishida, T., Yamada, S., Nagai, K. and Sugai, M. (2004) FtsZ-dependent localization of GroEL protein at possible division sites. *Genes to Cells* 9, 765–771.
Ohashi, Y., Chijiiwa, Y., Suzuki, K., Takahashi, K., Nanamiya, H., Sato, T., Hosoya, Y., Ochi, K. and Kawamura, F. (1999) The lethal effect of a benzamide derivative, 3-methoxybenzamide, can be suppressed by mutations within a cell division gene, *ftsZ*, in *Bacillus subtilis*. *Journal of Bacteriology* 181, 1348–1351.
Paradis-Bleau, C., Beaumont, M., Sanschagrin, F., Voyer, N. and Levesque, R.C. (2007) Parallel solid synthesis of inhibitors of the essential cell division FtsZ enzyme as a new potential class of antibacterials. *Bioorganic and Medicinal Chemistry* 15, 1330–1340.
Pichoff, S. and Lutkenhaus, J. (2005) Tethering the Z ring to the membrane through a conserved membrane targeting sequence in FtsA. *Molecular Microbiology* 55, 1722–1734.
Pichoff, S. and Lutkenhaus, J. (2007) Identification of a region of FtsA required for interaction with FtsZ. *Molecular Microbiology* 64, 1129–1138.
Pinho, M.G. and Errington, J. (2003) Dispersed mode of *Staphylococcus aureus* cell wall synthesis in the absence of the division machinery. *Molecular Microbiology* 50, 871–881.
Plaza, A., Keffer, J.L., Bifulco, G., Lloyd, J.R. and Bewley, C.A. (2010) Chrysophaentins A–H, antibacterial bisdiarylbutene macrocycles that inhibit the bacterial cell division protein FtsZ. *Journal of the American Chemical Society* 132, 9069–9077.
Rai, D., Singh, J.K., Roy, N. and Panda, D. (2008) Curcumin inhibits FtsZ assembly: an attractive mechanism for its antibacterial activity. *Biochemical Journal* 410, 147–155.

RayChaudhuri, D. and Park, J.T. (1992) *Escherichia coli* cell-division gene *ftsZ* encodes a novel GTP-binding protein. *Nature* 359, 251–254.

Romberg, L. and Levin, P.A. (2003) Assembly dynamics of the bacterial cell division protein FtsZ: poised at the edge of stability. *Annual Review of Microbiology* 57, 125–154.

Samson, R.Y., Obita, T., Freund, S.M., Williams, R.L. and Bell, S.D. (2008) A role for the ESCRT system in cell division in Archaea. *Science* 322, 1710–1713.

Scheffers, D.-J. and Pinho, M.G. (2005) Bacterial cell wall synthesis: new insights from localization studies. *Microbiology and Molecular Biology Reviews* 69, 585–607.

Slayden, R.A., Knudson, D.L. and Belisle, J.T. (2006) Identification of cell cycle regulators in *Mycobacterium tuberculosis* by inhibition of septum formation and global transcriptional analysis. *Microbiology* 152, 1789–1797.

Stokes, N.R., Sievers, J., Barker, S., Bennett, J.M., Brown, D.R., Collins, I., Errington, V.M., Foulger, D., Hall, M., Halsey, R., Johnson, H., Rose, V., Thomaides, H.B., Haydon, D.J., Czaplewski, L.G. and Errington, J. (2005) Novel inhibitors of bacterial cytokinesis identified by a cell-based antibiotic screening assay. *Journal of Biological Chemistry* 280, 39709–39715.

Sutherland, A.G., Alvarez, J., Ding, W., Foreman, K.W., Kenny, C.H., Labthavikul, P., Mosyak, L., Petersen, P.J., Rush, T.S. III, Ruzin, A., Tsao, D.H.H. and Wheless, K.L. (2003) Structure-based design of carboxybiphenylindole inhibitors of the ZipA–FtsZ interaction. *Organic & Biomolecular Chemistry* 1, 4138–4140.

Trusca, D. and Bramhill, D. (2002) Fluorescent assay for polymerization of purified bacterial FtsZ cell-division protein. *Analytical Biochemistry*, 307, 322–329.

Urgaonkar, S., La Pierre, H.S., Meir, I., Lund, H., RayChaudhuri, D. and Shaw, J.T. (2005) Synthesis of antimicrobial natural products targeting FtsZ: (+/-)-dichamanetin and (+/-)-2′-hydroxy-5″-benzylisouvarinol-B. *Organic Letters* 7, 5609–5612.

Vaughan, S., Wickstead, B., Gull, K. and Addinall, S.G. (2004) Molecular evolution of FtsZ protein sequences encoded within the genomes of Archaea, Bacteria, and Eukaryota. *Journal of Molecular Evolution* 58, 19–29.

Wang, J., Galgoci, A., Kodali, S., Herath, K.B., Jayasuriya, H., Dorso, K., Vicente, F., González, A. and Cully, D. (2003) Discovery of a small molecule that inhibits cell division by blocking FtsZ, a novel therapeutic target of antibiotics. *Journal of Biological Chemistry* 278, 44424–44428.

Wang, X., Huang, J., Mukherjee, A., Cao, C. and Lutkenhaus, J. (1997) Analysis of the interaction of FtsZ with itself, GTP, and FtsA. *Journal of Bacteriology* 179, 5551–5559.

White, E.L., Suling, W.J., Ross, L.J., Seitz, L.E. and Reynolds, R.C. (2002) 2-Alkoxycarbonylaminopyridines: inhibitors of *Mycobacterium tuberculosis* FtsZ. *Journal of Antimicrobial Chemotherapy* 111–114.

Yan, K., Pearce, K.H. and Payne, D.J. (2000) A conserved residue at the extreme C-terminus of FtsZ is critical for the FtsA–FtsZ interaction in *Staphylococcus aureus*. *Biochemical and Biophysical Research Communications* 270, 387–392.

10 Lysostaphin: a Silver Bullet for Staph

John F. Kokai-Kun
Biosynexus Incorporated, Gaithersburg, Maryland, USA

10.1 Discovery and the Early Years

The discovery of lysostaphin in the early 1960s was one of those serendipitous scientific discoveries similar to the discovery of penicillin. During a series of attempted transduction experiments with staphylococci, Charles Schindler, working in the laboratory of Vernon Schuhardt at the University of Texas, noticed a small white colony surrounded by an area of growth inhibition on a *Staphylococcus aureus* lawn (Schindler and Schuhardt, 1964). Upon further incubation, it was observed that the area of growth inhibition actually continued to spread. The colony, designated K-6-WI, was isolated and determined to be of the genus *Staphylococcus*. The bacteriolytic factor produced by this colony was called 'lysostaphin', and was found to lyse all staphylococcal strains tested, including numerous strains of *S. aureus* as well as *Staphylococcus epidermidis*, albeit at a slower rate. Lysostaphin was found not to have activity against any other genus of bacteria but was effective against heat-killed *S. aureus*, suggesting that lysostaphin itself was sufficient for the lytic activity and that the activities of endogenous bacterial factors were not required.

The earliest published *in vivo* work with lysostaphin examined it as a treatment for mice that had been challenged with *S. aureus* and found that it significantly improved mouse survival (Schuhardt and Schindler, 1964). The purification of lysostaphin from its natural host strain of staphylococci by ammonium sulfate precipitation and a series of column chromatography steps was published in 1965 (Schindler and Schuhardt, 1965), and lysostaphin was shown to be a heat-sensitive protein of 20–30 kDa.

Shortly after its discovery, lysostaphin was licensed to Mead Johnson & Co. of Evansville, Indiana (see Fig. 10.1 for a timeline of lysostaphin development). Scientists at Mead Johnson begin a development program using lysostaphin purified from its natural staphylococcal host, which was designated *Staphylococcus staphylolyticus* (Zygmunt and Tavormina, 1972). It was shown that lysostaphin was lytic for 252 strains of *S. aureus* from various clinical sources (Cropp and Harrison, 1964), and a lysostaphin index was established based on the capacity of lysostaphin to clear the turbidity of *S. aureus* suspensions within 10 min. The mechanism of the lytic activity of lysostaphin was determined in 1965 to be associated primarily with the loss of the peptide structure of the staphylococcal cell wall, apparently through the cleavage of alanine and glycine peptide bonds (Browder *et al.*, 1965). The early preparations of lysostaphin appeared to have been a mixture of two enzymatic activities, a peptidase

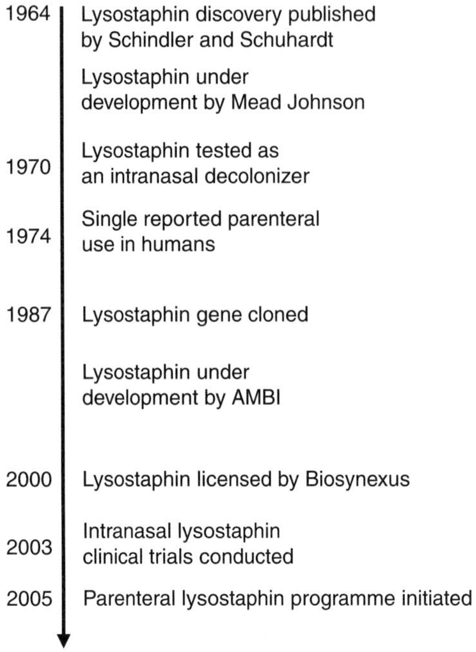

Fig. 10.1. A timeline of lysostaphin development.

and hexosaminidase. Further studies determined that it was the glycine-liberating activity of lysostaphin that was responsible for bacterial lysis through cleavage of the genus-specific polyglycine bridges of the staphylococcal cell wall (Schaffner *et al.*, 1967a). As more sophisticated analytical methods were used, lysostaphin was found to be a zinc metalloprotease of between 24.5 and 25 kDa (Trayer and Buckley, 1970). Lysostaphin was also determined to be a single polypeptide with an unusual single cystine residue.

Pre-clinical development of lysostaphin continued at Mead Johnson into the early 1970s, where it was found that human serum did not substantially inhibit lysostaphin activity (Zygmunt *et al.*, 1966b) and that lysostaphin was lytic against metabolically inactive staphylococci. Lysostaphin also could not enter polymorphonuclear leukocytes to kill engulfed *S. aureus* (Schaffner *et al.*, 1967a).

The earliest discussions of the development of resistance to lysostaphin considered the absence of polyglycine structures within the staphylococcal cell wall as a likely scenario for generation of resistance (Schaffner *et al.*, 1967a). Following repeat passage in the presence of lysostaphin, *S. aureus* variants were isolated that were less susceptible to lysostaphin and, as predicted, these variants appeared to have less glycine in their cell walls (Zygmunt *et al.*, 1966a). At the time, however, the mechanism that led to the changes in glycine content and thus resistance was unclear. These lysostaphin-resistant *S. aureus* variants appeared to be less virulent in mice and had an increased lag phase of growth. These early resistant variants appeared not to be totally lysostaphin resistant and were instead lysed at a slower rate than their parental strains (Zygmunt *et al.*, 1966a). It was also determined that there was no cross-resistance between lysostaphin and other antibiotics. Additional testing of 400 clinical isolates of *S. aureus* failed to isolate naturally occurring lysostaphin-resistant variants (Zygmunt *et al.*, 1966a).

Pre-clinical animal studies continued with studies in *S. aureus*-infected mice (Schaffner *et al.*, 1967b). A single treatment of 12.5 mg/kg of lysostaphin 4 h after *S. aureus* challenge significantly improved the survival of the lysostaphin-treated mice compared with penicillin-treated mice and untreated control animals (100 versus 53 and 6%, respectively) (Schaffner *et al.*, 1967b). Lysostaphin was also significantly better than oxacillin for protecting intravenously challenged mice against *S. aureus* and for clearing kidney infection in these mice.

Goldberg *et al.* (1967) tested lysostaphin in an experimental endocarditis model in dogs and found that courses of between 1 and 23 doses of lysostaphin, from 5 to 50 mg/kg, at intervals of 1–24 h, administered for up to 6.5 days after initiation of infection, significantly improved the clinical condition of the infected dogs. These treatments also decreased the numbers of staphylococci in lung, liver, spleen, kidney, and aortic and mitral valves. Some lysostaphin-resistant *S. aureus* colonies were isolated following treatment, and these appeared to be more common in dogs that relapsed during treatment with repeated smaller doses of lysostaphin. There were no apparent adverse reactions to any of the lysostaphin treatment courses in the dogs.

Lysostaphin was found to be immunogenic in mice and rabbits (Schaffner *et al.*, 1967b). Rabbits were administered single or multiple intravenous injections of lysostaphin at approximately 13 mg/kg with four injections at intervals of 3–4 days. There was no discernible adverse reaction to these infusions, but serum obtained from animals with multiple infusions was shown to significantly interfere with lysostaphin activity. The rabbits with the anti-lysostaphin titres were administered two additional intravenous injections of lysostaphin without any observed negative effects. While it was shown that lysostaphin could induce anti-lysostaphin antibodies in animal models, these antibodies did not appear to be associated with any toxicity or neutralization of the drug and thus were not considered an impediment to further development of the drug for use.

The earliest reported clinical use for lysostaphin was as a topical application for nasal carriage of staphylococci (Harris *et al.*, 1967; Martin and White, 1967; Quickel *et al.*, 1971). In these studies, lysostaphin was administered to infants and children (Harris *et al.*, 1967; Quickel *et al.*, 1971) and adults (Martin and White, 1967; Quickel *et al.*, 1971) in the form of a spray administered for 5–14 days. When the 0.5% lysostaphin spray was administered to children four times a day, the *S. aureus* carrier state was promptly eradicated in all subjects and there were no apparent clinical side effects (Harris *et al.*, 1967). In adults, a 0.5% lysostaphin solution administered for 7–12 days reduced *S. aureus* carriage by 80% and there was a good correlation between *in vitro* susceptibility to lysostaphin and *in vivo* efficacy for clearance of nasal colonization (Martin and White, 1967). Reacquisition of *S. aureus* carriage was considerably slower after lysostaphin treatment than was seen with previous topical antibiotics used to treat *S. aureus* nasal carriage. The authors attributed this to the selective effect of lysostaphin for *S. aureus*, which allowed the remaining nasal flora to interfere with repopulation of the nares by *S. aureus*. In the largest of the three studies (Quickel *et al.*, 1971), 152 subjects were treated intranasally with lysostaphin, Neosporin® or no treatment. Five days of three treatments a day with lysostaphin appeared to be more effective than Neosporin for eradication and prevention of recolonization by *S. aureus*. No lysostaphin-resistant *S. aureus* variants were isolated following treatments and there were no local or systemic reactions to lysostaphin. However, antibody formation to lysostaphin was reported in most of the treated subjects.

The early development of lysostaphin (reviewed by Zygmunt and Tavormina, 1972) culminated in the publication in 1974 of the single reported parenteral use of lysostaphin in a human (Stark *et al.*, 1974). A young soldier suffering from myelocytic leukaemia and several associated complications developed staphylococcal pneumonia and multiple metastatic staphylococcal abscesses. These infections were unresponsive to 3 weeks of treatments with methicillin, cephalothin and vancomycin serially and in combination. A single 500 mg dose of lysostaphin was administered intravenously and levels in excess of 10 μg/ml lysostaphin were detected in the patient's serum for up to 4 h post-administration. No lysostaphin was detected at 24 h after administration. There was a brief episode of flushing and mild hypotension following lysostaphin administration; these were controlled with diphenhydramine and epinephrine. The patient had decreased pain and swelling in the abscesses and no staphylococci were cultured from blood, sputum or abscess fluid. Three days after lysostaphin administration, the patient died from congestive heart failure not associated with the lysostaphin administration, and at post-mortem no staphylococci were recovered from the blood, lungs or abscess sites.

The first 10 years of lysostaphin research were supportive of this unique enzyme as a potential therapy for staphylococcal infections, but despite this early flurry of research, several factors conspired to relegate lysostaphin to a laboratory reagent for lysis of *S. aureus*. These factors included the lack of reproducible purified lots of lysostaphin coupled with the availability of many relatively inexpensive and easy-to-manufacture effective antibiotics at the time. Methicillin-resistant *S. aureus* (MRSA) were only beginning to emerge (Hiramatsu *et al.*, 2001), and it would be several years before the gene for lysostaphin was cloned and recombinant lysostaphin became available for further study.

10.2 Recombinant Lysostaphin and Manufacturing

In 1986, the structural gene for lysostaphin was cloned and sequenced from its natural host strain of *Staphylococcus simulans* (renamed from *S. staphylolyticus*) in the laboratory of Dr Richard Novick (Recsei *et al.*, 1987). The gene, which was present on a large penicillinase plasmid called pACK1 (Gargis *et al.*, 2010b) in *S. simulans* biovar *staphylolyticus*, encodes a preproenzyme of 42 kDa. The N-terminal sequence of prolysostaphin consists of a signal peptide followed by seven tandem repeats of a 13 amino acid sequence. Conversion of the proenzyme to mature, fully active lysostaphin involves proteolytic cleavage of this tandem repeat region. This proform of lysostaphin was determined to be one of the ways in which the host strain of *S. simulans* that produces lysostaphin protects itself from the enzymatic effects. During this cloning and sequencing work, lysostaphin was also found to be structurally related to the autolytic enzymes of staphylococci.

Early work with lysostaphin was conducted with lysostaphin purified from its natural host *S. simulans* biovar *staphylolyticus*, which yielded fairly low amounts of lysostaphin of inconsistent purity (Federov *et al.*, 2003). The cloning and sequencing of the lysostaphin gene allowed lysostaphin to be produced recombinantly in higher amounts that could be purified to lots of consistent purity from various expression systems. This sparked a renewed interest in the development of lysostaphin as a therapeutic agent for *S. aureus*. Applied Microbiology Inc. (AMBI) of New York licensed the rights to the lysostaphin gene in the late 1980s and produced recombinant mature lysostaphin in *Bacillus sphaericus* (Recsei, 1990) under the trade name Ambicin® L. AMBI also developed a colorimetric assay for determination of lysostaphin activity using a hexaglycine substrate (Kline *et al.*, 1994), which allowed a more consistent determination of lysostaphin activity in recombinant lots. Much of the next 20 years of lysostaphin development was conducted using Ambicin L produced in *B. sphaericus*.

In 2000, Biosynexus Inc. of Gaithersburg, Maryland, licensed the rights to the lysostaphin patents from AMBI and began producing lysostaphin in a *Lactococcus lactis* system, which used a nisin-controlled gene expression system called NICE (Mierau *et al.*, 2005a). In this system, the nisin peptide was used to induce expression of recombinant protein under the control of the nisin production system and the *nisA* promoter. The gene for mature lysostaphin with the first two alanines of its sequence truncated (Fig. 10.2) was cloned into the NICE vector. Lysostaphin was expressed intracellularly in the lactococcal cells and released by homogenization. The recombinant lysostaphin was purified by a series of column chromatography steps and found to be highly active, seemingly more so than Ambicin L (Stinson *et al.*, 2003). While the NICE expression system produced highly active lysostaphin that could be purified to homogeneity, this expression system was only capable of producing approximately 300 mg/l of lysostaphin (Mierau *et al.*, 2005b), which was considered to be insufficient for a commercially viable process.

Recombinant production of lysostaphin was moved into a commercial-grade pPOP expression system in *Escherichia coli* at Avecia in Stansted, UK (McCoy, 2004) for production of lysostaphin for clinical use. Expression of lysostaphin in *E. coli* allowed the production of more than 5 g/l of lysostaphin in culture. In this system, lysostaphin was produced intracellularly and then released by homogenization of the cells. The recombinant lysostaphin was purified to homogeneity by a series of chromatography steps. *E. coli* was capable of producing highly active lysostaphin with an activity similar to that produced by *L. lactis*, but it also appeared that *E. coli* produced some minor lysostaphin variants with somewhat reduced activity compared with *L. lactis* lysostaphin (J.F. Kokai-Kun, unpublished data). Production of these minor variants could be controlled by altering the fermentation conditions of the *E. coli*. These minor variants could also be removed during purification but at a loss to the overall yield of the

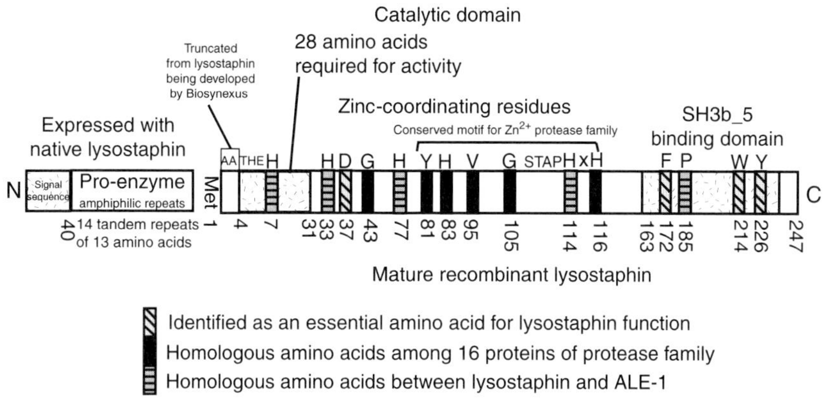

10 20 30 40 50 60
MAATHEHSAQ-WLNNYKKGYG-YGPYPLGING-GMHYGVDFFM-NIGTPVKAIS-SGKIVEAGWS-NYGGGNQIGL 70
IENDGVHRQW-YMHLSKYNVK-VGDYVKAGQI-IGWSGSTGYS-TAPHLHFQRM-VNSFSNSTAQ-DPMPFLKSAG 140
YGKAGGTVTP-TPNTGWKTNK-YGTLYKSESA-SFTPNTDIIT-RTTGPFRSMP-QSGVLKAGQT-IHYDEVMKQD 210
GHVWVGYTGN-SGQRIYLPVR-TWNKSTNTLG-VLWGTIK 247

Fig. 10.2. Structure–function relationships of lysostaphin. Lysostaphin is depicted as a linear structure showing the functional regions of the molecule. The catalytic domain is in the N-terminal portion of the molecule, while the SH3b_5 binding domain (Becker *et al.*, 2009) is in the C-terminal portion of the molecule (hashed). The prepro portion of native lysostaphin is also shown for reference. When mature lysostaphin is expressed from recombinant systems, an N-terminal methionine is sometimes added. Conserved and essential amino acids from various metalloproteases from the lysostaphin family are also displayed. The single-letter amino acid sequence of lysostaphin is displayed at the bottom. The 28 N-terminal amino acids that we have identified as essential to lysostaphin function (J.F. Kokai-Kun, unpublished data) as well as the conserved SHb3_5 domains are underlined. Essential zinc-coordinating amino acids are shaded in grey. We find it ironic that the single-letter amino acid sequence of lysostaphin spells 'STAPH' from amino acid 110 to 114.

process. Other groups have also reported success with expressing recombinant lysostaphin with an N terminal poly-histidine tag in *E. coli* followed by purification with metal-affinity chromatography (Szweda *et al.*, 2005; Sharma *et al.*, 2006).

A revised method of measuring lysostaphin activity was developed in conjunction with the transition to its production in *E. coli*. Freshly grown, non-pathogenic *Staphylococcus carnosus* cells were used as the substrate for the assay, and a reduction in turbidity of a cell suspension over time was used as a measure of lysostaphin activity. This method was qualified for use in manufacturing and found to be highly sensitive for differentiating lysostaphin activity from lot to lot, more so than using heat-killed *S. aureus* or the colorimetric assay (Stinson *et al.*, 2003).

In early work, lysostaphin was formulated at 0.5% in saline (Harris *et al.*, 1967), but it was later determined that lysostaphin was most stable and soluble at pH 6.5 in phosphate-buffered saline, (J.F. Kokai-Kun, unpublished data). Lysostaphin has also been linked to a polyethylene glycol (PEG) to reduce its antibody reactivity and improve its pharmacokinetics (Walsh *et al.*, 2003). While PEGylation of lysostaphin did reduce its immunoreactivity, the covalent attachment of a PEG moiety eliminated lysostaphin activity (S. Walsh, unpublished data). Lysostaphin is only active when reversibly bound to PEG (S. Walsh, unpublished data). The highly charged nature of lysostaphin also allows it to stick to medical materials, such as plastic catheters, and maintain its antibacterial activity (Shah *et al.*, 2004). This finding suggests another possible use for lysostaphin for prevention of infections of indwelling medical devices by pre-treatment of the device with lysostaphin (Kokai-Kun *et al.*, 2007).

10.3 Lysostaphin and *In Vitro* Anti-staphylococcal Activity

Lysostaphin is highly active against almost all strains of *S. aureus in vitro*. A turbid suspension of MRSA can be cleared within 10 min by the addition of lysostaphin (Fig. 10.3). Direct observation of *S. aureus* cell digestion by lysostaphin revealed major structural changes to the *S. aureus* cells in the form of cell swelling, splitting of the septum and creation of nanoscale perforations (Francius *et al.*, 2008). These modifications are consistent with the digestion of peptidoglycan by lysostaphin leading to osmotically fragile cells that rapidly lyse.

Several more recent studies have examined lysostaphin activity against various strains of *S. aureus* and report minimum inhibitory concentrations (MICs) of 0.001–2.0 µg/ml (Climo *et al.*, 1998; von Eiff *et al.*, 2003; Kusuma and Kokai-Kun, 2005; Yang *et al.*, 2007). Antibiotic-resistant strains of *S. aureus* including MRSA and vancomycin intermediately susceptible (VISA) strains of *S. aureus* were found to be as sensitive to lysostaphin as methicillin-sensitive strains (von Eiff *et al.*, 2003; Kusuma and Kokai-Kun, 2005; Yang *et al.*, 2007). A number of defined genetic mutations of *S. aureus* as well as stable small-colony variants were also highly susceptible to the lytic activity of lysostaphin (Kusuma and Kokai-Kun, 2005). It is questionable, however, whether an MIC is really the most relevant measure of lysostaphin activity. Lysostaphin is so extremely staphylolytic that when an MIC assay is performed with lysostaphin, the initial inoculum of staphylococci is lysed almost immediately after inoculation. Within 30 min of incubation with lysostaphin, there is a 3 $\log_{10}$ drop in all lysostaphin-susceptible *S. aureus* strains. In support of this, the MIC and minimum bactericidal concentration for *S. aureus* strains are generally the same or within a couple of dilutions of each other (Kusuma and Kokai-Kun, 2005; Yang *et al.*, 2007).

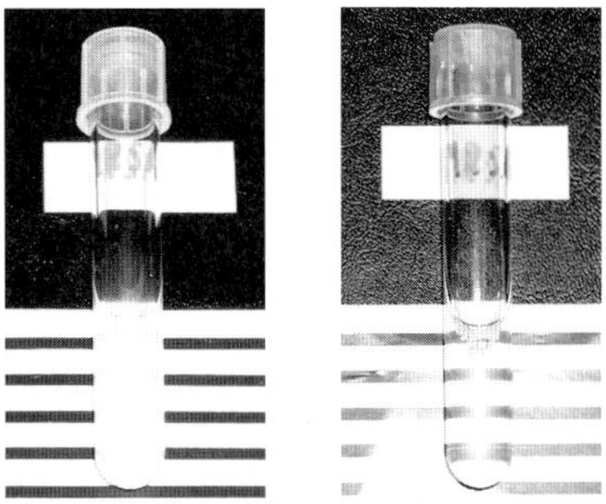

10^8 MRSA/ml +10 µg/ml lysostaphin 10 min

Fig. 10.3. *In vitro* lysostaphin activity. A turbid suspension of methicillin-resistant *Staphylococcus aureus* (MRSA; ~10^8 colony-forming units/ml) was treated with 10 µg/ml of lysostaphin and within 10 min the suspension was cleared and the *S. aureus* had been killed.

We examined four methods for determining lysostaphin susceptibility *in vitro* (Kusuma and Kokai-Kun, 2005) and found that a disk diffusion method was the simplest method for determination of susceptibility. All lysostaphin-susceptible strains of *S. aureus* had zones of inhibition of ≥ 11 mm at 20 h using a 50 µg lysostaphin disk, and, as previously reported (Schindler and Schuhardt, 1964), these zones of inhibition continued to expand with longer incubation times as the lysostaphin continued to diffuse through the agar and lyse the staphylococci. In a study of 429 well-characterized clinical *S. aureus* isolates, most strains demonstrated a zone of inhibition around a lysostaphin disk of ≥ 15 mm (von Eiff *et al.*, 2003). Lysostaphin-resistant reference strains of *S. aureus* had no zones of inhibition (Kusuma and Kokai-Kun, 2005). While lysostaphin-susceptible strains of *S. aureus* were found to be susceptible by all four methods used in the study, there was not a good correlation of the degree of susceptibility between the methods, suggesting that the local microenvironment may play a role in the degree of lysostaphin activity. Lysostaphin-resistant reference strains, however, were resistant to lysostaphin in all four methods.

Other species of staphylococci are less susceptible to lysostaphin than *S. aureus* (Zygmunt and Tavormina, 1972; Robinson *et al.*, 1979; Kiri *et al.*, 2002). The MIC for various strains of *S. epidermidis* range from 0.125 to > 64 µg/ml with an MIC_{50} of 4 µg/ml (Kiri *et al.*, 2002). This is probably due to *S. epidermidis* having fewer pure pentaglycine bridges and instead having more cell-wall bridges, which include other amino acids such as alanine (Climo *et al.*, 2001) or serine, as is the case for lysostaphin-producing *S. simulans* biovar *staphylolyticus* (Robinson *et al.*, 1979).

Bacteria growing in biofilms are less susceptible to most antibiotics (Donlan and Costerton, 2002), and this is true of staphylococci as well. The capacity of staphylococci to form biofilms is a major virulence factor, especially for the coagulase-negative staphylococci (Otto, 2008). When a staphylococcal infection occurs in the presence of an indwelling medical device like a catheter, the device is generally removed if possible on the assumption that a biofilm is present and would be resistant to antibiotic treatment. It is very difficult to treat a biofilm infection *in situ* with conventional antibiotics, but lysostaphin has the capacity to degrade staphylococcal biofilms *in vitro*, not only killing the staphylococci but also stripping the extracellular biofilm matrix from the artificial surface (Wu *et al.*, 2003). Even an enzyme as potent as lysostaphin requires higher concentrations to degrade biofilms, however. Lysostaphin at 50 μg/ml degrades static *S. aureus* biofilms *in vitro* within 3 h (Wu *et al.*, 2003). Higher concentrations of lysostaphin (200 μg/ml) are also able to degrade *S. epidermidis* biofilms (Wu *et al.*, 2003). This lysostaphin activity presents a new treatment option for patients with difficult-to-treat staphylococcal infections of indwelling devices such as artificial heart valves and other prosthetic devices. Rather than risking surgery to remove an infected heart valve, the option becomes available to treat *in situ* with lysostaphin.

10.4 Lysostaphin Resistance and Synergy with Antibiotics

As with most antibiotics, staphylococci also have the capacity to become resistant to lysostaphin. This resistance, when selected by lysostaphin pressure *in vitro* or *in vivo*, is usually a result of mutations to the *fem* genes (Stranden *et al.*, 1997; Climo *et al.*, 2001). The *femAB* operon is involved in the formation of the pentaglycine side chains of the peptidoglycan of staphylococci, while the *fmhB* gene encodes a protein that adds the first glycine to the ε-amino group of the lysine of the stem peptide and is essential to staphylococcal survival (Rohrer *et al.*, 1999). When the *femAB* operon is disrupted, the pentaglycine bridges are replaced with monoglycines (Stranden *et al.*, 1997). FemA adds the second and third glycine to the bridge, while the FemB adds the fourth and fifth glycine (Stranden *et al.*, 1997). FemB is not capable of substituting for FemA and vice versa (Ehlert *et al.*, 1997). Lysostaphin-resistant variants that were selected *in vitro* by incubation with increasing doses of lysostaphin have been mapped to mutations in *femA* and have monoglycine cross-bridges (Climo *et al.*, 2001; Kusuma *et al.*, 2007). Laboratory-selected, lysostaphin-resistant variants of two MRSA strains were mapped to an insertion/frame shift and a 66 bp deletion mutation in the *femA* gene (Kusuma *et al.*, 2007), while other changes in *femA* and *femB* leading to lysostaphin resistance have also been detected (Climo *et al.*, 2001).

There is a second mechanism of resistance to lysostaphin that can be found naturally in strains of staphylococci that produce lysostaphin and similar lytic enzymes. The lysostaphin endopeptidase resistance gene (*epr*, also called *lif*; Thumm and Gotz, 1997) modifies the peptidoglycan of staphylococci by substituting serines for glycines in the pentaglycine cross-bridges (DeHart *et al.*, 1995). The *epr* gene is found naturally in *S. simulans* biovar *staphylolyticus* that produces lysostaphin, and can be transferred to *S. aureus* in the laboratory to induce lysostaphin resistance leading to a greater than tenfold loss of susceptibility to lysostaphin (DeHart *et al.*, 1995). The increase in serine content of the peptidoglycan ranges from 2 to 35% (Thumm and Gotz, 1997). Interestingly, *epr* is homologous to the *femA* and *femB* genes (Sugai *et al.*, 1997b; Ehlert *et al.*, 2000). Serine is incorporated at positions 3 and 5 of the pentaglycine bridge (Ehlert *et al.*, 2000), but this does not affect the sorting of cell-wall-anchored proteins in strains expressing these resistance genes (Strauss *et al.*, 1998). This substitution does, however, also affect the binding of lysostaphin to the cell walls through its targeting domain (Gargis *et al.*, 2010a). Similar mechanisms of resistance can also be found in other species of staphylococci that express lytic enzymes with activities similar to lysostaphin. These include *Staphylococcus capitis* EPK1 expressing ALE-1 and an *epr*-like gene (Sugai *et al.*, 1997b) and *Staphylococcus sciuri* DD4747 expressing an *N*-acetylmuramyl-L-alanine amidase-like gene and its own *femABX*-like immunity factor (Heath *et al.*, 2005). The presence of the *epr* gene along with lysostaphin being expressed as a proenzyme requiring activation is how the host strain of *S. simulans* protects itself from the lysostaphin that it produces (Thumm and Gotz, 1997). Lysostaphin resistance genes have not been detected outside of lytic factor-expressing strains of staphylococci, however.

The combination of lysostaphin plus a β-lactam antibiotic has been shown to be synergistic against *S. aureus* and coagulase-negative staphylococci both *in vitro* and *in vivo* (Polack *et al.*, 1993; Climo *et al.*, 1998; Climo *et al.*, 2001; Kiri *et al.*, 2002; Kokai-Kun *et al.*, 2007, 2009). Interestingly, for both mechanisms of lysostaphin resistance described above, the lysostaphin-resistant staphylococcal variants actually become more susceptible to β-lactam antibiotics than their parental strains (DeHart *et al.*, 1995, Stranden *et al.*, 1997). Lysostaphin combined with β-lactams is more than 100-fold more active against *S. aureus*, including MRSA, than lysostaphin alone (Polack *et al.*, 1993), and this combination has a fractional inhibitory concentration index ranging from 0.0234 to 0.2656 against *S. epidermidis*, also indicating synergy (Kiri *et al.*, 2002). The synergy between lysostaphin and β-lactams, as well as the capacity of β-lactam antibiotics to suppress lysostaphin resistance (Climo *et al.*, 2001), can be better understood by examining the mechanism of β-lactam resistance in staphylococci. MRSA produce an alternative penicillin-binding protein called PBP2a or PBP2′ encoded by the *mecA* gene (Chambers, 1997). This alternative PBP has a low affinity for β-lactams and can substitute for the essential function of the β-lactam-susceptible PBPs. Methicillin-resistant strains of staphylococci continue to produce PBP2 along with PBP2a and the other penicillin-binding proteins. PBP2a performs cell-wall transpeptidation activity when the other PBPs are inactivated by the presence of β-lactams (Chambers, 1997). PBP2a, however, appears to have a requirement for pure pentaglycine muropeptide monomers for efficient cross-linking activity (Climo *et al.*, 2001), but in lysostaphin-resistant variants, these muropeptides are either mono- or triglycine or of mixed amino acids and thus cannot be used as a substrate for transpeptidation by PBP2a. Because of this, resistance to both lysostaphin and β-lactams is unlikely to coexist. Lysostaphin rapidly degrades the cell walls of all of the staphylococci with pentaglycine bridges, while any lysostaphin-resistant variants that are selected become susceptible to β-lactams because their PBP2a cannot use the altered muropeptide monomers caused by mutation of the *fem* genes as substrates for transpeptidation. Since lysostaphin and β-lactams are synergistic and resistance between these two antibiotics appears to be mutually exclusive, this supports the conclusion that their combination would be the best choice clinically for treatment of staphylococcal infections.

Lysostaphin has synergistic or additive effects with other antibiotics as well. Lysostaphin demonstrates synergy with bacitracin, polymixin B (Polack *et al.*, 1993) and ranalexin, a cationic peptide, both *in vitro* (Graham and Coote, 2007) and *in vivo* (Desbois *et al.*, 2010). Lysostaphin is also synergistic with antimicrobial peptides such as nisin and lactoferrin, and lipopeptides such as daptomycin (Desbois and Coote, 2011). Lysostaphin has additive effects with vancomycin, gentamycin, tetracycline and erythromycin (Polack *et al.*, 1993). The additive effect of lysostaphin and vancomycin has also been shown *in vivo* in two animal models (Climo *et al.*, 1998; Kokai-Kun *et al.*, 2007). In unpublished results, we also found that bacitracin appears to prevent the emergence of lysostaphin resistance *in vitro*. Beyond becoming susceptible to β-lactams, lysostaphin-resistant *S. aureus* variants also have increased susceptibility to several other cell-wall-active antibiotics including fosfomycin, bacitracin, teicoplanin and vancomycin, as well as other non-cell-wall-active antibiotics (Labschinski *et al.*, 1998; Ling and Berger-Bachi, 1998).

Not only do lysostaphin-resistant variants become more sensitive to other antibiotics, but there is also a significant fitness toll that accompanies the development of lysostaphin resistance (Kusuma *et al.*, 2007). Lysostaphin-resistant *S. aureus* grow as smaller colonies and display altered cellular morphology, growing as short chains rather than clusters and having larger cells with incomplete septation (Stranden *et al.*, 1997; Kusuma *et al.*, 2007). Lysostaphin-resistant variants also demonstrate increased temperature sensitivity and a fivefold reduction in virulence in mouse models compared with wild-type *S.aureus* (Kusuma *et al.*, 2007). During a 14-day serial passage, fitness-reduced lysostaphin-resistant variants failed to develop compensatory mutations to restore their fitness (Kusuma *et al.*, 2007). These findings suggest that if lysostaphin resistance should develop during clinical use of lysostaphin, the resistant variants may not contribute to pathogenesis in the treated patient.

There have been other reports regarding lysostaphin resistance, such as a report of development of vancomycin and lysostaphin resistance in a methicillin-resistant clinical *S. aureus* isolate that remained methicillin resistant (Boyle-Vavra *et al.*, 2001), but when this isolate was examined for lysostaphin sensitivity in a separate study, it was found to be susceptible to lysostaphin in all assays (Kusuma and Kokai-Kun, 2005). There was also a passage-selected VISA strain that appeared to have reduced susceptibility to lysostaphin for whole cells but increased susceptibility of purified cell walls (Koehl *et al.*, 2004). This was attributed to reduced autolysin activity in this strain and suggested that autolysin may contribute to lysostaphin activity, at least at low concentrations. Most recently, Grundling *et al.* (2006) reported a *S. aureus* strain Newman transposon mutant with a high degree of lysostaphin resistance. The transposon was inserted in a gene encoding a polytopic membrane protein with a predicted protease domain, which was called *lyrA*. This mutation did not lead to the increased β-lactam susceptibility as seen with *fem* mutations. Resistance in this transposon mutant appeared to be due to an increased abundance of altered cross-bridges in the cell envelope, but this resistance mutation has not been reported to have been isolated through selection by lysostaphin pressure *in vitro* or *in vivo*.

10.5 Structure–Function Relationships of Mature Lysostaphin

As mentioned above, native lysostaphin expressed by *S. simulans* is expressed as a preproenzyme with secretion and proenzyme sequences and is activated by proteolytic cleavage of the N-terminal tandem repeats of the proenzyme (Recsei *et al.*, 1987). Mature lysostaphin is a bacterial zinc metalloproteinase of 27 kDa in the family of peptidoglycan hydrolases, and is further subcategorized into the family of lysostaphin-type endopeptidases that also includes bacteriophage lytic enzymes (Bochtler *et al.*, 2004). Other bacterial hydrolases in this subfamily include LytM from *S. aureus* (Ramadurai *et al.*, 1999; Odintsov *et al.*, 2003) and ALE-1 from *S. capitis* (Sugai *et al.*, 1997a). Like lysostaphin, ALE-1 has one zinc atom per molecule (Sugai *et al.*, 1997a); unlike lysostaphin, however, ALE-1 is not processed from a proenzyme to the active form. While there is a report that lysostaphin can degrade elastin (Park *et al.*, 1995), ALE-1 does not appear have this activity (Sugai *et al.*, 1997a), and the relevance of this activity with regards to lysis of *S. aureus* in unclear. LytM is also a zinc-containing glycylglycine endopeptidase similar to lysostaphin, but LytM plays a role in staphylococcal growth (Ramadurai *et al.*, 1999). All three of these enzymes are part of the D-Ala-D-Ala metallopeptidases, having similar active sites and sharing a core folding motif (Bochtler *et al.*, 2004). The central Zn^{2+} is tetrahedrally coordinated by two histidines, an aspartate and a water molecule. This group of amino acids are said to have an LAS arrangement and have an HxH motif that is also found in other metalloproteases (Bochtler *et al.*, 2004).

The lysostaphin molecule consists of two discrete regions; binding activity is found in the C-terminal end of the molecule (Baba and Schneewind, 1996), while enzymatic activity can be found in the N-terminal portion (Fig. 10.3). The lysostaphin molecule has been difficult to crystallize, possibly because it is highly soluble, but some structural information can be gleaned from other similar proteases. The LytM structure has been solved to 1.3Å resolution and the Zn^{2+} is coordinated by the side chains of an asparagine, two histidines and an aspartate as predicted (Odintsov *et al.*, 2003). Of the two histidines of the HxH motif, however, only one is involved directly in the coordination of the zinc. The first histidine of the HxH motif does not actually coordinate the Zn^{2+} directly. It was also determined that a truncated form of LytM that corresponds roughly to the mature form of lysostaphin and has higher specific activity than full-length native LytM and may actually be processed *in vivo* in a similar fashion to lysostaphin (Odintsov *et al.*, 2003). The N-terminal sequence of mature lysostaphin is AATHE, but we found that truncating the N terminus to THE actually somewhat enhances lysostaphin activity *in vitro* (Stinson *et al.*, 2003); however, removal of any further amino acids from the N terminus eliminates its activity (J.F. Kokai-Kun, unpublished data). We also found that addition of an N-terminal methionine during expression of lysostaphin in some expression systems may have a small effect on reducing lysostaphin activity (J.F. Kokai-Kun, unpublished data).

The binding of ALE-1 to *S. aureus* cells occurs through its C-terminal 92 amino acids, known as the targeting domain (Lu *et al.*, 2006). This domain belongs to the SH3b domain family and its structure has been determined to a resolution of 1.74Å. The lysostaphin SH3b_5 domain confers specificity of lysostaphin for staphylococci, compared with other hydrolases (Becker *et al.*, 2009). The domain includes two strictly conserved residues, a tryptophan and a proline. This binding domain has an all β-fold structure and has patches of conserved residues with orthologous targeting domains that can potentially interact with the Gram-positive cell wall. Studies with this targeting domain have determined the length of the interpeptide bridge, as well as the amino acid composition of that bridge, determined the maximum binding of the targeting domain to *S. aureus* (Lu *et al.*, 2006). If the highly conserved first ten amino acids are removed from the C terminus of ALE-1, binding activity is lost. The C-terminal targeting domain of ALE-1 binds to *S. aureus*, but not *S. simulans*, suggesting that the targeting domain confers specificity (Lu *et al.*, 2006). Binding is reduced considerably when serines are substituted for glycines in the interpeptide bridges. More recently, it was shown that the C-terminal cell-wall-targeting domain of lysostaphin binds directly to cross-linked peptidoglycan, which also serves as the substrate for the glycylglycine endopeptidase activity (Grundling and Schneewind, 2006). Binding of the lysostaphin-targeting domain was reduced dramatically in lysostaphin-resistant organisms with shortened polyglycine bridges, as would be seen in *S. aureus* strains with mutated *fem* genes.

10.6 Pre-clinical Animal Studies

Since the early animal efficacy studies with natural lysostaphin described above, there have been many additional studies of the efficacy of recombinant lysostaphin in various animal models. Lysostaphin is extremely effective in eradicating staphylococcal infections in mouse models of systemic *S. aureus* infection for both methicillin-sensitive *S. aureus* (MSSA) and MRSA (Kokai-Kun *et al.*, 2007). In this model, mice develop bacteraemia and solid-organ infections. A 5 mg/kg dose of lysostaphin administered once a day over 3 days consistently cleared bacteraemia and solid-organ infections in the *S. aureus*-challenged mice. In this study, *in vivo* synergy between lysostaphin and oxacillin was also demonstrated, and this allowed the therapeutic dose to lysostaphin to be reduced to 1 mg/kg. Vancomycin also had additive activity with lysostaphin in this model. In this study, animals sacrificed 24 h after the final lysostaphin treatment had more *S. aureus* recovered from the solid organs than animals sacrificed 72 h after the final lysostaphin treatment. *S. aureus* can survive within phagocytic cells such as neutrophils (Lowy, 2000), but lysostaphin is unable to enter these cells (Craven and Anderson, 1980). Thus, bacteria recovered from the spleens and livers of lysostaphin-treated mice sacrificed 24 h after the final lysostaphin treatment may represent *S. aureus* recovered from within phagocytic cells that were protected from lysostaphin activity. When lysostaphin-treated mice were sacrificed 72h after the final treatment, the *S. aureus* sequestered within the neutrophils may already have been killed by these cells, thus resulting in a greater reduction in infection in all organs. Consistent with this possibility are data demonstrating that mice rendered neutropenic for the entire course of an experiment and then treated with lysostaphin were cleared of *S. aureus* infection significantly more than non-neutropenic animals sacrificed on day 4. In these neutropenic mice, there were no neutrophils to shield the *S. aureus* from lysostaphin. Lysostaphin was also more effective than vancomycin for the treatment of MRSA infection in a suckling mouse model (Placencia *et al.*, 2009), significantly improving the survival of the lysostaphin-treated pups versus vancomycin-treated pups.

As lysostaphin is so rapidly lytic, it could be a concern that treatment of systemic staphylococcal infections with lysostaphin might lead to the induction of shock, as the *S. aureus* are rapidly lysed, releasing immunomodulatory factors from the lysed bacteria that lead to induction of a cytokine storm. To the contrary, we found that treatment of systemic *S. aureus* with lysostaphin actually blunted the inflammatory cytokine-mediated response, leading to reduced expression of tumour necrosis factor-α and interleukin-6 in response to *S. aureus* challenge (Sei *et al.*, 2011). Lysostaphin treatment also was able to reverse the systemic shock caused by *S. aureus* as measured by changes in core body temperature. These findings may be explained by a recent publication (Ip *et al.*, 2010) that demonstrated that, prior to Toll-like receptor (TLR)-dependent cytokine production, whole staphylococci must be engulfed and delivered into acidic phagosomes where acid-activated host enzymes digest the internalized bacteria to liberate otherwise cryptic bacterial-derived ligands that initiate the response from vacuoles. Thus, whole bacteria need to be taken up by phagocytic cells, as the TLR signalling actually occurs within the phagosomes. Lysostaphin rapidly lyses all free bacteria, thus preventing their uptake in phagosomes.

In a more difficult-to-treat mouse model of *S. aureus* biofilm infection, lysostaphin proved highly efficacious for clearance of *S. aureus* infection (Kokai-Kun *et al.*, 2009). In this model, jugular vein-catheterized mice were challenged with *S. aureus* and a biofilm infection was allowed to form on the catheters over 5 days. These mice were then treated with lysostaphin with and without oxacillin. Consistent with the finding that higher concentrations of lysostaphin were required to degrade *S. aureus* in biofilms *in vitro* (Wu *et al.*, 2003), higher doses of lysostaphin were also required to clear biofilm infections in the mice. A dose of 20mg/kg of lysostaphin three times a day for 4 days cleared the biofilm infection from the implanted catheters (Fig. 10.4) and also cleared organ infections (Kokai-Kun *et al.*, 2009). This dose of lysostaphin could be reduced to 15mg/kg three times a day for 4 days when oxacillin was added to the treatment of MRSA biofilms. Pre-instillation of a single dose of 10mg/kg lysostaphin in the catheters 24h prior to *S. aureus* challenge also protected the catheterized mice from *S. aureus* infection consistent with lysostaphin's capacity to bind to artificial surfaces (Shah *et al.*, 2004).

Lysostaphin has also proven to be extremely effective as an agent against staphylococcal endocarditis in animal models. In a rabbit model of MRSA endocarditis, lysostaphin administered at 15mg/kg three times daily for 3 days sterilized the vegetations of 10 of 11 treated rabbits with a mean reduction in bacterial counts of 8.5 $\log_{10}$ (Climo *et al.*, 1998). In this model, vancomycin given twice daily did not sterilize the vegetations of any animals and only reduced the bacterial counts vegetations by 4.8 $\log_{10}$. The combination of lysostaphin plus vancomycin allowed the daily dosage of lysostaphin to be reduced to a single dose and reduced the bacterial vegetation count by 7.5 $\log_{10}$. The lysostaphin treatment regimen also appeared to be well tolerated by the rabbits. Lysostaphin is also effective in this endocarditis model against *S. aureus* strains with reduced susceptibility to vancomycin (Patron *et al.*, 1999). Lysostaphin can be administered either as a single dose of 100mg/kg or for 3 days at 30mg/kg twice a day. The single dose of lysostaphin sterilized

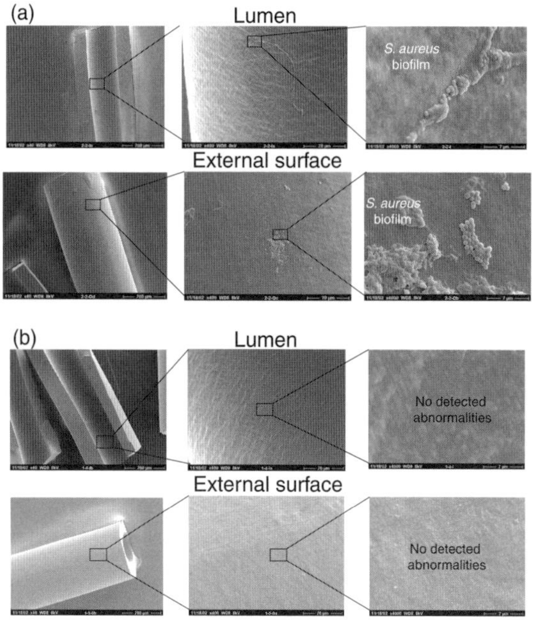

Fig. 10.4. Scanning electron microscopy of recovered catheters from mice challenged with methicillin-resistant *Staphylococcus aureus* (MRSA). Jugular vein-catheterized mice were challenged with MRSA and then treated with PBS alone (a) or with lysostaphin in PBS (b; 20 mg/kg, three times a day for 4 days). Three catheters from each group were cultured for *S. aureus* (mean number of colony-forming units of control = 67,780 and of lysostaphin treatment = 0), while three others were sent for scanning electron microscopy. Panels (a) and (b) are representative micrographs of the external surface and lumen of catheters from control and lysostaphin-treated samples, respectively. The magnifications are 40×, 400× and 4000× from left to right. (Reprinted from Kokai-Kun *et al.*, 2009.)

the valve vegetations of three of seven animals, while the twice a day dosing sterilized the valves of five of six rabbits. Vancomycin alone in this model had little effect. In another rabbit model of endocarditis, echocardiography showed that lysostaphin treatment of endocarditis actually causes a measurable reduction in the size of the staphylococcal cardiac vegetations (Kupferwasser *et al.*, 2003).

There has also been considerable research into the use of lysostaphin as a treatment for staphylococcal mastitis in dairy cows. In a mouse model of mastitis, infusion of lysostaphin into lactating murine mammary glands significantly reduced viable *S. aureus* within 30 min (Bramley and Foster, 1990). There has been considerable additional work in this area (reviewed by Bastos *et al.*, 2010). These studies have determined that lysostaphin may be an effective therapy for *S. aureus* mastitis in dairy cows.

In another novel application of lysostaphin, 0.28% lysostaphin was found to be highly effective for treating keratitis mediated by MSSA or MRSA in a rabbit model (Dajcs *et al.*, 2000). The lysostaphin was administered every 30 min up to 15 h post-infection and was found to be capable of penetrating the cornea to kill the staphylococci. Lysostaphin was also found to remain in the aqueous humour for days while maintaining its anti-staphylococcal activity (Balzli *et al.*, 2010).

As a bacterial protein, it is not surprising that lysostaphin induces an antibody response when administered by various routes. In the rabbit endocarditis model described above, rabbits treated with weekly doses of lysostaphin for 9 weeks developed antibodies to lysostaphin (Climo *et al.*, 1998). We also found anti-lysostaphin antibodies in mice administered repeat doses of lysostaphin (J.F. Kokai-Kun, unpublished data) and dairy cattle receiving intramammary infusions of lysostaphin developed significant serum titres against lysostaphin after 18–21 infusions (Daley and Oldham, 2000). Antibodies to lysostaphin could have several effects: they could neutralize lysostaphin activity, they could affect the clearance of lysostaphin from the system either by enhancing clearance or extending the half-life, or there could be toxicity associated with an immune response to lysostaphin. As has also been found with various phage lytic enzymes that are under development as possible therapeutic agents (Schuch *et al.*, 2002), antibodies against lysostaphin do not fully neutralize its activity. Rabbit serum with high-titre anti-lysostaphin raised the lysostaphin MIC about eightfold (Climo *et al.*, 1998), and in our hands, high-titre anti-lysostaphin serum reduces lysostaphin activity by about 50% in a turbidity reduction assay. Mice with anti-lysostaphin titres require approximately twice the dose of lysostaphin to clear systemic infection. In serum from dairy cattle administered intramammary lysostaphin, anti-lysostaphin antibodies did not affect the *in vitro* activity of lysostaphin (Daley and Oldham, 2000). There were also no deleterious symptoms (e.g. anaphylaxis) in the dairy cows with anti-lysostaphin titres upon subsequent infusions of lysostaphin. In the rabbits administered weekly doses of lysostaphin, there was no evidence of hypersensitivity or proteinuria, but upon autopsy and pathological examination, the kidneys one of two rabbits demonstrated non-specific plasma cellular interstitial nephritis (Climo *et al.*, 1998).

In our own pre-clinical studies with Ambicin L lysostaphin, rabbits in a repeat-dose toxicology study received 14 days of once-daily intravenous doses of 2, 10 or 20 mg/kg of lysostaphin. While no deleterious clinical observations were made while the animals were alive, upon autopsy, there was significant pathology observed including microscopic observations in the kidneys and heart and glomerulonephritis in all animals receiving the higher two doses of lysostaphin. Arteritis was also observed in these animals. In a follow-up study, however, when rabbits received 50 mg/kg of lysostaphin purified from *E. coli* twice a day for 5 or 7 days, there were no pathological findings in the tissues of rabbits receiving 5 days of lysostaphin treatment, but there were some mild pathological changes noted after 7 days of dosing with lysostaphin. This follow-up study demonstrated that it is possible to administered lysostaphin safely to rabbits for 5 days without inducing toxicity. In a similar 14-day repeat-dosing study in non-human primates where lysostaphin purified from *E. coli* was administered at 10 or 40 mg/kg twice a day, again there were no pathologies observed while the animals were alive, and no pathology was observed in animals sacrificed immediately after the dosing period (day 14). In a recovery group of animals sacrificed 14 days after dosing ended (day 28), however, minimal to mild vasculitis was observed in large arteries of the lysostaphin-treated animals in a dose-responsive manner. This potential toxicity of lysostaphin, which may be consistent with the formation of antigen–antibody complexes of lysostaphin, which can be deposited on the vascular walls leading to vasculitis, could complicate clinical development.

10.7 Lysostaphin as a Therapy for *S. aureus* Nasal Colonization

Nasal colonization with *S. aureus* has been shown to be a risk factor for subsequent *S. aureus* infection (Perl *et al.*, 2002). When Biosynexus first licensed the lysostaphin patents from AMBI, we pursued lysostaphin as a topical treatment for *S. aureus* nasal colonization. We developed a cotton rat model of *S. aureus* nasal colonization (Kokai-Kun, 2007) and demonstrated that a single dose of lysostaphin formulated at 0.5% in a semi-solid cream with enhanced nasal residence time (Walsh *et al.*, 2004) was effective in eradicating *S. aureus* nasal colonization in cotton rats (Kokai-Kun *et al.*, 2003). Lysostaphin dosed once was also more effective than a single dose of mupirocin for clearing *S. aureus* nasal colonization in the cotton rats. Lysostaphin formulated in cream could also be pre-administered in the nares and prevent nasal colonization. No lysostaphin-resistant variants of *S. aureus* were isolated following treatment with lysostaphin cream. Some cotton rats did, however, develop antibodies against lysostaphin following repeat administration, but 14-day repeat intranasal dosing in rabbits of lysostaphin purified from *L. lactis* formulated in cream demonstrated no pathological effects, although same animals did develop antibodies to lysostaphin. While most strains of *S. aureus* colonize cotton rat nares quite well, lysostaphin-resistant variants of *S. aureus* are not good colonizers of the nares.

Biosynexus has conducted two clinical trials with intranasal lysostaphin. The first trial was a phase I, double-blind, placebo-controlled, single-dose study for tolerability and pharmacokinetics in 18 healthy volunteers. Twelve subjects received 0.5% BSYX-L110 nasal lysostaphin cream, while six subjects received placebo cream. The 0.5% lysostaphin cream or placebo cream was administered twice daily for 3 days and then once on the fourth day (seven doses in total). The lysostaphin nasal cream was found to be safe and well tolerated with no adverse events directly attributed to the test article. There was no evidence of absorption of the lysostaphin, as serum concentrations of lysostaphin remained below detection in all volunteers. Of the 18 volunteers, seven were colonized nasally with MSSA prior to the trial. Four of these subjects randomly received active cream and three received placebo cream. Placebo cream had no consistent effect on *S. aureus* nasal colonization, but the 0.5% lysostaphin cream consistently reduced the *S. aureus* nasal colonization in all colonized subjects.

In the second phase I/II clinical trial, an open-label study was conducted to investigate the microbiological activity as well as safety and local tolerability of various dosing regimens for lysostaphin nasal cream. Sixteen volunteers who were pre-determined to be chronically nasally colonized with *S. aureus* by repeat nasal culture were dosed with 1% lysostaphin cream either by finger or swab twice a day for 1 or 2 days (two or four doses in total). Quantitative nasal cultures were taken from the dosed subjects at various time points to determine *S. aureus* nasal colonization, and safety and tolerability assessments were made. The BSYX-L210 1% lysostaphin nasal cream was safe and well tolerated, with no adverse events considered to be related to the cream. All subjects had a reduction in the number of colony-forming units of *S. aureus* from baseline following treatment with lysostaphin cream, and some subjects who received four doses of cream had the *S. aureus* in their nares eradicated. The method of application did not appear to affect the results. All subjects eventually returned to baseline *S. aureus* nasal colonization, usually within approximately 8 days of the end of treatment. Interestingly, when the *S. aureus* population in the nares was reduced by lysostaphin treatment, the coagulase-negative population of the nares increased and then, as the *S. aureus* colonization returned, the coagulase-negative population fell, suggesting that these bacteria may compete with each other in the nares (J.F. Kokai-Kun, unpublished data). Again, no absorption of lysostaphin was detected in the subjects, but two of the subjects who were administered lysostaphin cream had an increase in anti-lysostaphin titre over baseline within 2–3 weeks after administration. No lysostaphin-resistant variants were recovered from the nares of any of the treated subjects.

Lysostaphin formulated at 0.5 or 1% in cream was safe and well tolerated following repeat administration in the nares of healthy volunteers. There was some increase in anti-lysostaphin antibody titre in two of the volunteers but no associated pathology. Data from the animal model as well as the clinical studies suggested that administration of lysostaphin cream could reduce or eliminate *S. aureus* nasal colonization, but additional development as well as head-to-head studies against mupirocin would have been required to continue clinical development of lysostaphin nasal cream. Shortly after the conclusion of the second clinical trial, mupirocin (Bactroban Nasal®) went off patent, opening the door for generic mupirocin and greatly reducing the cost of the product. The strategic decision was made to halt the development of the lysostaphin nasal cream because it would not be cost effective to market a biological drug for this indication in the face of at least three generic alternatives.

10.8 Lysostaphin: What's Next?

Lysostaphin has been shown to be extremely effective for treating serious *S. aureus* infections in various animal models, and its efficacy appears to be superior to vancomycin and other antibiotics in most of the models. Lysostaphin has even been shown to be able to clear *S. aureus* in biofilm infections, something most antibiotics are not particularly effective against. The synergy between lysostaphin and β-lactam antibiotics, as well as the mutually exclusive nature of resistance to these two anti-bacterials, suggests that lysostaphin should be administered clinically with a β-lactam antibiotic for maximal efficacy. There are, however, concerns with lysostaphin toxicity. The pathology that was consistent with large vessel vasculitis associated with repeat lysostaphin dosing in rabbits and non-human primates may limit the usefulness of lysostaphin. One possible explanation for this toxicity could be the formation of antibody–antigen complexes in the presence of excess antigen, leading to deposition of the complexes on vessel walls and vasculitis. The finding that rabbits can be dosed twice a day for 5 days without evidence of toxicity suggests that it may be possible to dose lysostaphin safely on a limited basis, but redosing of lysostaphin in the same patient may not be possible. The one model for which lysostaphin has not been as effective as conventional antibiotics is skin and soft-tissue infections, probably due to its inability to permeate cells. This indication is often the most straightforward path for approval of drugs effective against staphylococci, thus adding to the challenge of development of lysostaphin. The clinical development plan needed to demonstrate the superiority of lysostaphin to current treatments coupled with the potential toxicity of lysostaphin make further development of this promising anti-staphylococcal challenging.

Acknowledgement

Thanks to Dr Jimmy Mond for his helpful review of this chapter.

References

Baba, T. and Schneewind, O. (1996) Target cell specificity of a bacteriocin molecule of C-terminal signal directs lysostaphin to the cell wall of *Staphylococcus aureus*. *EMBO Journal* 4789–4797.

Balzli, C.L., McCormick, C.C., Caballero, A.R. and O'Callaghan, R.J. (2010) Sustained anti-staphylococcal effect of lysostaphin in the rabbit aqueous humor. *Current Eye Research* 35, 480–486.

Bastos, M.C.F., Coutinho, B.G. and Coelho, M.L.V. (2010) Lysostaphin: a staphylococcal bacteriolysin with potential clinical applications. *Pharmaceuticals* 3, 1139–1161.

Becker, S.C., Foster-Frey, J., Stodola, A.J., Anacker, D. and Donovan, D.M. (2009) Differentially conserved staphylococcal SH3b_5 cell wall binding domains confer increased staphylolytic and streptolytic activity to a streptococcal prophage endolysin domain. *Gene* 443, 32–41.

Bochtler, M., Odintsov, S.G., Marcyjaniak, M. and Sabala, I. (2004) Similar active sites in lysostaphins and D-Ala-D-Ala metallopeptidases. *Protein Science* 13, 854–861.

Boyle-Vavra, S., Carey, R. and Daum, R. (2001) Development of vancomycin and lysostaphin resistance in a methicillin-resistant *Staphylococcus aureus* isolate. *Journal of Antimicrobial Chemotherapy* 48, 617–625.

Bramley, A.J. and Foster, R. (1990) Effects of lysostaphin on *Staphylococcus aureus* infections of the mouse mammary gland. *Research in Veterinary Science* 49, 120–121.

Browder, H.P., Zygmunt, W.A., Young, J.R. and Travormina, P.A. (1965) Lysostaphin: enzymatic mode of action. *Biochemical and Biophysical Research Communications* 19, 383–389.

Chambers, H.F. (1997) Methicillin resistance in staphylococci: molecular and biochemical basis and clinical implications. *Clinical Microbiological Review* 10, 781–791.

Climo, M., Ehlert, K. and Archer, G. (2001) Mechanism and suppression of lysostaphin-resistance in oxacillin-resistant *Staphylococcus aureus*. *Antimicrobial Agents and Chemotherapy* 45, 1431–1437.

Climo, M.W., Patron, R.L., Goldstein, B.P. and Archer, G.L. (1998) Lysostaphin treatment of experimental methicillin-resistant *Staphylococcus aureus* aortic valve endocarditis. *Antimicrobial Agents and Chemotherapy* 42, 1355–1360.

Craven, N. and Anderson, J.C. (1980) The selection *in vitro* of antibiotics with activity against intracellular *S. aureus*. *Journal of Veterinary Pharmacology and Therapy* 3, 221–226.

Cropp, C.B. and Harrison, E.F. (1964) The *in vitro* effect of lysostaphin on clinical isolates of *Staphylococcus aureus*. *Canadian Journal of Microbiology* 10, 823–828.

Dajcs, J.J., Hume, E.B., Moreau, J.M., Caballero, A.R., Cannon, B.M. and O'Callaghan, R.J. (2000) Lysostaphin treatment of methicillin-resistant *Staphylococcus aureus* keratitis in the rabbit. *Investigational Ophthalmology and Vision Science* 41, 1432–1437.

Daley, M.J. and Oldham, E.R. (2000) Lysostaphin: immunogenicity of locally administered recombinant protein used in mastitis therapy. *Veterinary Immunology and Immunopathology* 31, 301–312.

DeHart, H., Heath, H., Heath, L., LeBlanc, P. and Sloan, G. (1995) The lysostaphin endopeptidase resistance gene (*epr*) specifies modification of peptidoglycan cross bridges in *Staphylococcus simulans* and *Staphylococcus aureus*. *Applied and Environmental Microbiology* 61, 1475–1479.

Desbois, A.P. and Coote, P.J. (2011) Bactericidal synergy of lysostaphin in combination with antimicrobial peptides. *European Journal of Clinical Microbiology and Infectious Diseases* 30, 1015–1021.

Desbois, A.P., Gemmell, C.G. and Coote, P.J. (2010) *In vivo* efficacy of the antimicrobial peptide ranalexin in combination with the endopeptidase lysostaphin against wound and systemic methicillin-resistant *Staphylococcus aureus* (MRSA) infection. *International Journal of Antimicrobial Agents* 35, 559–565.

Donlan, R.M. and Costerton, W. (2002) Biofilms: survival mechanisms of clinically relevant microorganisms. *Clinical Microbiology Reviews* 15, 167–193.

Ehlert, K., Schroder, W. and Labischinski, H. (1997) Specificities of FemA and FemB for different glycine residues: FemB cannot substitute for FemA in staphylococcal peptidoglycan pentaglycine side chain formation. *Journal of Bacteriology* 179, 7573–7576.

Ehlert, K., Tschierske, M., Mori, C., Schroder, W. and Berger-Bachi, B. (2000) Site-specific serine incorporation by Lif and Epr into positions 3 and 5 of the staphylococcal peptidoglycan interpeptide bridge. *Journal of Bacteriology* 182, 2635–2638.

Federov, T.V., Surovtsev, V.I., Plentnev, V.Z., Borozdina, M.A. and Gusev, V.V. (2003) Purification and some properties of lysostaphin a glycylglycine endopeptidase from culture liquid of *Staphylococcus simulans* biovar *staphylolyticus*. *Biochemistry (Moscow)* 68, 61–65.

Francius, G., Domenech, O., Mingeot-Leclercq, M.P. and Dufrene, Y.F. (2008) Direct observation of *Staphylococcus aureus* cell wall digestion by lysostaphin. *Journal of Bacteriology* 190, 7904–7909.

Gargis, S.R., Heath, H.E., LeBlane, P.A., Dekker, L., Simmonds, R.S. and Sloan, G.L. (2010a) Inhibition of the activity of both domains of lysostaphin through peptide modification by the lysostaphin immunity protein. *Applied and Environmental Microbiology* 76, 6944–6946.

Gargis, S.R., Tate, A.H., Heath, L.S., Heath, H.E., LeBlanc, P.A. and Sloan, G.L. (2010b) Complete nucleotide sequences of plasmids pACK1 and pACK3 from *Staphylococcus simulans* biovar *staphylolyticus*. *Plasmid* 64, 104–109.

Goldberg, L.M., DeFranco, J.M., Watanakunakorn, C. and Hamburger, M. (1967) Studies in experimental staphylococcal endocarditis in dogs. VI. Treatment with lysostaphin. *Antimicrobial Agents and Chemotherapy* 7, 45–53.

Graham, S. and Coote, P.J. (2007) Potent, synergistic inhibition of *Staphylococcus aureus* upon exposure to a combination of the endopeptidase lysostaphin and the cationic peptide ranalexin. *Journal of Antimicrobial Chemotherapy* 59, 759–762.

Grundling, A. and Schneewind, O. (2006) Cross-linked peptidoglycan mediates lysostaphin binding to the cell wall envelop of *Staphylococcus aureus*. *Journal of Bacteriology* 188, 2463–2472.

Grundling, A., Missiakas, D.M. and Schneewind, O. (2006) *Staphylococcus aureus* mutants with increased lysostaphin resistance. *Journal of Bacteriology* 188, 6286–6297.

Harris, R.L., Nunnery, A.W. and Riley, H.D. (1967) Effect of lysostaphin on staphylococcal carriage in infants and children. *Antimicrobial Chemotherapy* 110–112.

Heath, L.S., Gargis, S.R., Smithberg, S.R., Johnson, H.P., Heath, H.E., LeBlanc, P.A. and Sloan, G.L. (2005) Plasmid-specific FemABX-like immunity factor in *Staphylococcus sciuri* DD 4747. *FEMS Microbiology Letters* 249, 227–231.

Hiramatsu, K., Cui, L., Kuroda, M. and Ito, T. (2001) The emergence and evolution of methicillin-resistant *Staphylococcus aureus*. *Trends in Microbiology* 9, 486–493.

Ip, W.K.E., Sokolovska, A., Charriere, G.M., Boyer, L., Dejardin, S., Cappillino, M.P., Yantosca, L.M., Takahashi, K., Moore, K.J., Lacy-Hubert, A. and Stuart, L.M. (2010) Phagocytosis and phagosome acidification are required for pathogen processing and MyD88-dependent responses to *Staphylococcus aureus*. *Journal of Immunology* 184, 7071–7081.

Kiri, N., Archer, G. and Climo, M. (2002) Combinations of lysostaphin with β-lactams are synergistic against oxacillin-resistant *Staphylococcus epidermidis*. *Antimicrobial Agents and Chemotherapy* 46, 2017–2020.

Kline, S.A., de la Harpe, J. and Blackburn, P. (1994) A colorimetric microtiter plate assay for lysostaphin using a hexaglycine substrate. *Analytical Biochemistry* 217, 329–331.

Koehl, J.L., Muthaiyan, A., Jayaswal, R.K., Ehlert, K., Labschinski, H. and Wilkinson, B.J. (2004) Call wall composition and decreased autolytic activity and lysostaphin susceptibility of glycopeptide-intermediate *Staphylococcus aureus*. *Antimicrobial Agents and Chemotherapy* 48, 3749–3757.

Kokai-Kun, J.F. (2007) The cotton rat as a model for *Staphylococcus aureus* nasal colonization in humans. In: DeLeo, F.R. and Otto, M. (eds) *Methods in Molecular Biology*, vol. 431. *Bacterial Pathogenesis*. Humana Press, Totowa, New Jersey, pp. 241–254.

Kokai-Kun, J.F., Walsh, S.M., Chanturiya, T. and Mond, J.J. (2003) Lysostaphin cream eradicates *Staphylococcus aureus* nasal colonization in a cotton rat model. *Antimicrobial Agents and Chemotherapy* 47, 1589–1597.

Kokai-Kun, J.F., Chanturiya, T. and Mond, J.J. (2007) Lysostaphin as a treatment for systemic *Staphylococcus aureus* infection in a mouse model. *Journal of Antimicrobial Chemotherapy* 60, 1051–1059.

Kokai-Kun, J.F., Chanturiya, T. and Mond, J.J. (2009) Lysostaphin eradicates established *Staphylococcus aureus* biofilms in jugular vein catheterized mice. *Journal of Antimicrobial Chemotherapy* 64, 94–100.

Kupferwasser, L.I., Shapiro, S.M., Nast, C.C. and Bayer, A.S. (2003) Microbiologic and cardiac functional impacts of lysostaphin in experimental *Staphylococcus aureus* endocarditis due to a methicillin-resistant strain. In: *103rd General Meeting of the American Society of Microbiology*, Washington, DC, abstract A027.

Kusuma, C.M. and Kokai-Kun, J.F. (2005) Comparison of four methods for determining lysostaphin susceptibility of various strains of *Staphylococcus aureus*. *Antimicrobial Agents and Chemotherapy* 49, 3256–3263.

Kusuma, C., Jadanova, A., Chanturiya, T. and Kokai-Kun, J.F. (2007) Lysostaphin-resistant variants of *Staphylococcus aureus* demonstrate reduced fitness *in vitro* and *in vivo*. *Antimicrobial Agents and Chemotherapy* 51, 475–482.

Labschinski, H., Ehlert, K. and Berger-Bachi, B. (1998) The targeting factors necessary for expression of methicillin resistance in staphylococci. *Journal of Antimicrobial Chemotherapy* 41, 581–584.

Ling, B. and Berger-Bachi, B. (1998) Increased overall antibiotic susceptibility in *Staphylococcus aureus femAB* null mutants. *Antimicrobial Agents and Chemotherapy* 42, 936–938.

Lowy, F.D. (2000) Is *Staphylococcus aureus* an intracellular pathogen? *Trends in Microbiology* 8, 341–344.

Lu, J.Z., Fujiwara, T., Komasuzawa, H., Sugai, M. and Sakon, J. (2006) Cell wall targeting domain of glycylglycine endopeptidase discriminates among peptidoglycan cross-bridges. *Journal of Biological Chemistry* 281, 549–558.

Martin, R.R. and White, A. (1967) The selective activity of lysostaphin *in vivo*. *Laboratory and Clinical Medicine* 70, 1–8.

McCoy, M. (2004) Killing staph together: start-up Biosynexus places fermentation project in newly started Avecia facility. *Chemical Engineering News* 82, 36–40.

Mierau, I., Leij, P., van Swam, I., Blommestein, B., Floris, E., Mond, J.J. and Smid, E.J. (2005a) Industrial-scale production and purification of a heterologous protein in *Lactococcus lactis* using the nisin-controlled gene expression system NICE: the case of lysostaphin. *Microbial Cell Factories* 4, 1–9.

Mierau, I., Olieman, K., Mond, J.J. and Smid, E.J. (2005b) Optimization of the *Lactococcus lactis* nisin-controlled gene expression system NICE for industrial applications. *Microbial Cell Factories* 4, 16–28.

Odintsov, S.G., Sabala, I., Marcyjaniak, M. and Bochtler, M. (2003) Latent LytM at 1.3Å resolution. *Journal of Molecular Biology* 335, 775–785.

Otto, M. (2008) Staphylococcal biofilms. *Current Topics in Microbiology and Immunology* 322, 207–228.

Park, P.W., Senior, R.M., Griffin, G.L., Broekelmann, T.J., Mudd, M.S. and Mecham, R.P. (1995) Binding and degradation of elastin by the staphylolytic enzyme lysostaphin. *International Journal of Biochemistry and Cellular Biology* 27, 139–146.

Patron, R.L., Climo, M.W., Goldstein, B.P. and Archer, G.L. (1999) Lysostaphin treatment of experimental aortic valve endocarditis caused by a *Staphylococcus aureus* isolates with reduced susceptibility to vancomycin. *Antimicrobial Agents and Chemotherapy* 43, 1754–1755.

Perl, T., Cullen, J., Wenzel, R., Zimmerman, B., Pfaller, M., Sheppard, D., Twombley, J., French, P. and Herwalt, L. (2002) Intranasal mupirocin to prevent postoperative *Staphylococcus aureus* infections. *New England Journal of Medicine* 24, 1871–1877.

Placencia, F.X., Kong, L. and Weisman, L.E. (2009) Treatment of methicillin-resistant *Staphylococcus aureus* in neonatal mice: lysostaphin versus vancomycin. *Pediatric Research* 65, 420–424.

Polack, J., Latta, P.D. and Blackburn, P. (1993) *In vitro* activity of recombinant lysostaphin–antibiotic combinations toward methicillin-resistant *Staphylococcus aureus*. *Diagnostic Microbiology and Infectious Diseases* 17, 265–270.

Quickel, K.E., Selden, R., Caldwell, J.R., Nora, N.F. and Schaffner, W. (1971) Efficacy and safety of topical lysostaphin treatment of persistent nasal carriage of *Staphylococcus aureus*. *Applied Microbiology* 22, 446–450.

Ramadurai, L., Lockwood, K.J., Nadakavukaren, M.J. and Jayaswal, R.K. (1999) Characterization of a chromosomally encoded glycylglycine endopeptidase of *Staphylococcus aureus*. *Microbiology* 145, 801–808.

Recsei, P.A. (1990) Expression of the cloned lysostaphin gene. US patent 49131390.

Recsei, P.A., Gruss, A.D. and Novick, R.P. (1987) Cloning, sequence and expression of the lysostaphin gene from *Staphylococcus simulans*. *Proceedings of the National Academy of Sciences USA* 84, 1127–1137.

Robinson, J.M., Hardman, J.K. and Sloan, G.L. (1979) Relationship between lysostaphin endopeptidase production and cell wall composition in *Staphylococcus staphylolyticus*. *Journal of Bacteriology* 137, 1158–1168.

Rohrer, S., Ehlert, K., Tscierske, M., Labschinski, H. and Berger-Bachi, B. (1999) The essential *Staphylococcus aureus* gene *fmhB* is involved in the first step of peptidoglycan pentaglycine interpeptide formation. *Proceedings of the National Academy of Sciences USA* 96, 9351–9356.

Schaffner, W., Melly, M.A., Hash, J.H. and Koenig, M.G. (1967a) Lysostaphin: an enzymatic approach to staphylococcal disease. I. *In vitro* studies. *Yale Journal of Biology and Medicine* 39, 215–229.

Schaffner, W., Melly, M.A. and Koenig, M.G. (1967b) Lysostaphin: an enzymatic approach to staphylococcal disease. II. *In vivo* studies. *Yale Journal of Biology and Medicine* 39, 230–244.

Schindler, C.A. and Schuhardt, V.T. (1964) Lysostaphin: a new bacteriolytic agent for the staphylococci. *Proceedings of the National Academy of Sciences USA* 51, 414–421.

Schindler, C.A. and Schuhardt, V.T. (1965) Purification and properties of lysostaphin – a lytic agent for *Staphylococcus aureus*. *Biochemical and Biophysical Acta* 97, 242–250.

Schuch, R., Nelson, D. and Fischetti, V.A. (2002) A bacteriolytic agent that detects and kills *Bacillus anthracis*. *Nature* 418, 884–889.

Schuhardt, V.T. and Schindler, C.A. (1964) Lysostaphin therapy in mice infected with *Staphylococcus aureus*. *Journal of Bacteriology* 88, 815–816.

Sei, C., Chanturiya, T., Mond, J.J. and Kokai-Kun, J.F. (2011) Lysostaphin reduces the production of inflammatory cytokines in *Staphylococcus aureus* challenged mice, and prevents systemic shock. *Open Antimicrobial Agents Journal* 3, 6–11.

Shah, A., Mond, J.J. and Walsh, S. (2004) Lysostaphin-coated catheters eradicate *Staphylococcus aureus* challenge and block surface colonization. *Antimicrobial Agents and Chemotherapy* 48, 2704–2707.

Sharma, R., Sharma, P.R., Choudhary, M.L., Pande, A. and Khatri, G.S. (2006) Cytoplasmic expression of mature glycylglycine endopeptidase lysostaphin with an amino terminal hexahistidine in a soluble and catalytically active form in *Escherichia coli*. *Protein Expression and Purification* 45, 206–215.

Stark, F.R., Thornsvard, C., Flannery, E.P. and Artenstein, M.S. (1974) Systemic lysostaphin in man – apparent antimicrobial activity in a neutropenic patient. *New England Journal of Medicine* 291, 239–240.

Stinson, J.R., Grinberg, L., Lees, A., Mond, J.J. and Kokai-Kun, J.F. (2003) Truncated lysostaphin molecule with enhanced staphylolytic activity. US PCT number PCT/US02/40924.

Stranden, A., Ehlert, K., Labischinski, H. and Berger-Bachi, B. (1997) Cell wall monoglycine cross-bridges and methicillin hypersusceptibility in a *femAB* null mutant of methicillin-resistant *Staphylococcus aureus*. *Journal of Bacteriology* 179, 9–16.

Strauss, A., Thumm, G. and Gotz, F. (1998) Influence of Lif, the lysostaphin immunity factor on acceptors of surface proteins and cell wall sorting efficiency in *Staphylococcus canosus*. *Journal of Bacteriology* 180, 4960–4962.

Sugai, M., Fujiwara, T., Akiyama, T., Ohara, M., Komatsuzawa, H., Inoue, S. and Suginaka, H. (1997a) Purification and molecular characterization of glycylglycine endopeptidase produced by *Staphylococcus capitis* EPK1. *Journal of Bacteriology* 179, 1193–1202.

Sugai, M., Fujiwara, T., Ohta, K., Komatsuzawa, H., Ohara, M. and Suginaka, H. (1997b) *epr*, which encodes glycylglycine endopeptidase resistance, is homologous to *femAB* and affects serine content of peptidoglycan cross bridges in *Staphylococcus capitis* and *Staphylococcus aureus*. *Journal of Bacteriology* 179, 4311–4318.

Szweda, P., Kotlowski, R. and Kur, J. (2005) New effective sources of the *Staphylococcus simulans* lysostaphin. *Journal of Biotechnology* 117, 203–213.

Thumm, G. and Gotz, F. (1997) Studies on pro-lysostaphin processing and characterization of the lysostaphin immunity factor (Lif) of *Staphylococcus simulans* biovar *staphylolyticus*. *Molecular Microbiology* 23, 1251–1265.

Trayer, H.R. and Buckley, C.E. (1970) Molecular properties of lysostaphin, a bacteriolytic agent specific for *Staphylococcus aureus*. *Journal of Biological Chemistry* 245, 4842–4846.

von Eiff, C., Kokai-Kun, J.F., Becker, K. and Peters, G. (2003) *In vitro* activity of recombinant lysostaphin against *Staphylococcus aureus* isolates from anterior nares and blood. *Antimicrobial Agents and Chemotherapy* 47, 3613–3615.

Walsh, S., Shah, A. and Mond, J.J. (2003) Improved pharmacokinetics and reduced antibody reactivity of lysostaphin conjugated to polyethylene glycol. *Antimicrobial Agents and Chemotherapy* 47, 554–558.

Walsh, S., Kokai-Kun, J.F., Shah, A. and Mond, J.J. (2004) Extended nasal residence time of lysostaphin and an anti-staphylococcal monoclonal antibody by delivery in semisolid or polymeric carriers. *Pharmacological Research* 21, 1770–1775.

Wu, J.A., Kusuma, C., Mond, J.J. and Kokai-Kun, J.F. (2003) Lysostaphin disrupts *Staphylococcus aureus* and *Staphylococcus epidermidis* biofilms on artificial surfaces. *Antimicrobial Agents and Chemotherapy* 47, 3407–3414.

Yang, X., Li, C., Lou, R., Wang, Y., Zhang, W., Chen, H., Huang, Q., Han, Y., Jiang, J. and You, X. (2007) *In vitro* activity of recombinant lysostaphin against *Staphylococcus aureus* isolates from hospitals in Beijing, China. *Journal of Medical Microbiology* 56, 71–76.

Zygmunt, W.A., Browder, H.P. and Tavormina, P.A. (1966a) Lytic action of lysostaphin on susceptible and resistant strains of *Staphylococcus aureus*. *Canadian Journal of Microbiology* 13, 845–853.

Zygmunt, W.A., Browder, H.P. and Tavormina, P.A. (1966b) Influence of blood and serum on the anti-staphylococcal activity of lysostaphin. *Journal of Bacteriology* 91, 725–728.

Zygmunt, W.A. and Tavormina, P.A. (1972) Lysostaphin: model for a specific enzymatic approach to infectious disease. *Progress in Drug Research* 16, 309–333.

11 Strategies to Identify Modified Ribosomally Synthesized Antimicrobials

Alan J. Marsh,[1] Colin Hill,[2] R. Paul Ross[1] and Paul D. Cotter[1]
[1]*Teagasc Food Research Centre, Moorepark, Fermoy, Cork, Ireland;*
[2]*Microbiology Department, University College Cork, Cork, Ireland*

11.1 Introduction

This chapter describes the different strategies that can be, and have been, employed to identify/create novel post-translationally modified, ribosomally synthesized antimicrobial peptides. These are peptides that are first synthesized as immature peptides and then undergo enzyme-mediated post-translational modification and cleavage of an N-terminal leader region to form fully functional, mature peptides. In recent years, the number of such antimicrobials has increased noticeably through the identification of novel forms of well-known families, such as the lantibiotics, and the inclusion of additional families of antimicrobials, such as the cyanobactins, thiopeptides, microviridins and amatoxins. Some of these are thought to be viable alternatives to the antibiotics that are currently used clinically, and indeed it is hoped that their use could stave off the issues arising as a consequence of resistance to existing antimicrobials. Here, we will review the strategies employed to identify a representative, and possibly the most extensively studied, family of modified antimicrobial peptides, the lantibiotics, and highlight how these have been and can be applied to screen for other modified peptides.

11.2 The Lantibiotics

Bacteriocins are small, heat-stable, antimicrobial peptides produced by bacteria and are typically active against species closely related to the producer but can also exhibit activity across genera. Bacteriocin producers are naturally immune to their own bacteriocins as a consequence of possessing specific self-protective mechanisms. There is a wide range of existing and potential commercial and medicinal applications for these peptides. Due to the continuous discovery of novel antimicrobial peptides, one of the original bacteriocin, and highly cited, classification systems, devised by Klaenhammer (1993) to classify bacteriocins produced by Gram-positive, lactic acid bacteria, has undergone several revisions. The most recent classification (Rea *et al.*, 2011) represents an updating of a system proposed by Cotter *et al.* (2005b) and recommends that Gram-positive bacteriocins, and indeed bacteriocins in general, could be divided into two classes, consisting of class I, the post-translationally modified bacteriocins, and class II, the unmodified bacteriocins. Class I Gram-positive bacteriocins can be subdivided into three groups: (i) the lantibiotics/lantipeptides; (ii) the labyrinthopeptides; and (iii) the sactibiotics, although further groups are likely to be added. These can be further subdivided according to amino acid composition and the number of peptides involved. Gram-positive bacteriocins from within class II can be divided into four groups, which can also be further subdivided (Rea *et al.*, 2011) (Fig. 11.1a).

The lantibiotics/lantipeptides, which are the primary focus of this chapter, contains four subgroups. Types 1 and 2 are the lantibiotics (so named because they are lanthionine-containing antibiotics), while types 3 and 4 are the lantipeptides, so named because they are lanthionine-containing peptides that exhibit no antimicrobial activity. The generic name given to lantibiotic structural prepropeptides is LanA encoded by the *lanA* gene, and they undergo subsequent modification via cleavage of an N-terminal leader region (required for export and directing post-translational modification) and modification of the C-terminal (propeptide) region. The modifications that are specifically associated with this family of peptides occur as follows. Specific serine and threonine residues contained within the propeptide are dehydrated to form dehydroalanine and dehydrobutyrine, respectively. When these modified residues interact with an intrapeptide cysteine, a thioether bond is formed resulting in the formation of the eponymous amino acids, lanthionine (Lan, from Dha) or β-methyl lanthionine (meLan, from Dhb), respectively (Fig. 11.1b). These structures play a critical role in the antimicrobial activity of the peptides, such as, in the case of the prototypical type 1 lantibiotic nisin, facilitating the binding to a

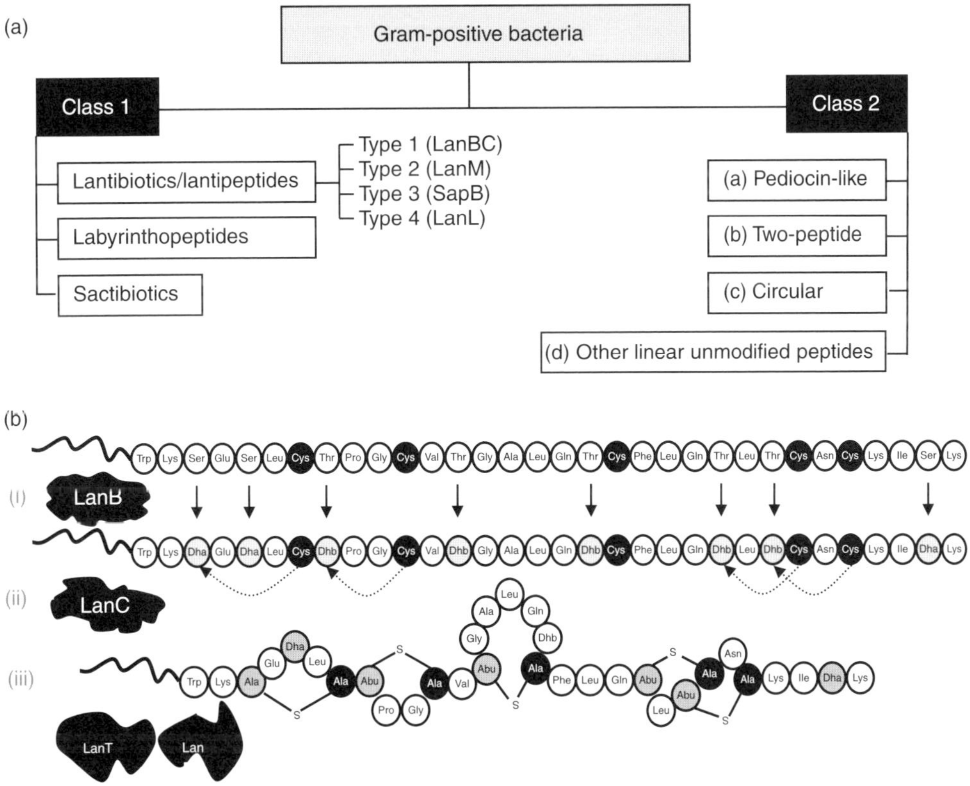

Fig. 11.1. (a) Classification of Gram-positive bacteriocins. (b) Enzyme-mediated synthesis of the lantibiotic subtilin. (i) Lanthionine dehydratase (LanB) catalyses the dehydration of serine and threonine residues to form Dha and Dhb, respectively. (ii) Lanthionine synthetase (LanC) catalyses a condensation reaction between the sulfhydryl group of cysteines and the dehydrated residues. (iii) Following the cleavage of the leader peptide by LanP, LanT transports the mature peptide across the cell membrane.

lipid II receptor (Hsu *et al.*, 2004). Similarly, the contribution of these structures to the resistance of lantibiotics to high temperature and proteolytic enzymes is also apparent (Suda *et al.*, 2010). The distinction between type 1 and type 2 lantibiotics is based on the modification enzymes involved. Type 1 peptides are modified by two catalytic enzymes, LanB, a lanthionine dehydratase, and LanC, a lanthionine synthetase. Type 2 lantibiotics are modified by LanM enzymes, which perform both the dehydratase and cyclase functions. The *lanM/lanBC* genes are the most highly conserved genes within lantibiotic gene clusters, a trait that has been utilized through the use of degenerate primers and *in silico* screens to identify novel lantibiotic-encoding clusters (see below). The type 1 and 2 lantibiotics can be further subdivided on the basis of homology with respect to the amino acid sequence of the prepropeptide. There also exist a number of two-peptide lantibiotics i.e. lantibiotics that are active through the combined activity of two lanthionine-containing peptides (Lawton *et al.*, 2007b).

The aforementioned nisin is currently the best studied of all bacteriocins and has been used as a food preservative in over 50 countries. However, as a consequence of the emergence of microbial resistance to therapeutic antibiotics, there have been a number of investigations into the use of nisin and novel lantibiotics against clinically relevant pathogens. This stems from the fact that the antimicrobial activity of lantibiotics can be greater than that of classical antibiotics and that they can target very sensitive components of the bacterial cell, such as lipid II, as mentioned above. To date, approximately 60 lantibiotics have been isolated from Gram-positive bacteria (Firmicutes and Actinobacteria) (Table 11.1). Although the majority of these have been identified using traditional bioactivity-based screens, we are at the dawn of a new age in technological advancements, in which *in silico*, molecular and bioengineering-based approaches can complement and potentially ultimately supersede the reliable but increasingly out-dated, culture-based methods employed for lantibiotic discovery. Here, we review the use of these various approaches (Fig. 11.2).

11.3 Traditional (Culture-based) Screening Methods

The first historical report of bacteriocin production dates back to 1877 when Pasteur and Joubert (1877) noticed that bacteria isolated from urine samples inhibited *Bacillus anthracis*. This was followed in 1925 by a report prompted by the observation that species of *Escherichia coli* inhibited the growth of one another. A 1928 study of the limiting factors in lactic acid fermentation concluded that cell inhibition was 'determined by the concentration of a definite, soluble and diffusible substance excreted by the cells'. Similarly, Whitehead (1933), by a process of elimination, deduced that the inability of a certain milk sample to accommodate the growth of starter lactic acid bacteria was due to a proteinaceous, heat-stable, inhibitory substance produced by two strains of streptococci (since reclassified as lactococci) found in the original milk sample. This substance was later named nisin (Mattick and Hirsch, 1947). Despite the technological revolution that has occurred in the intervening years, the majority of lantibiotics have been identified using methods that are not extensively dissimilar from those employed in the early years of lantibiotic research and which rely on identifying the ability of one bacterial strain (producer) to inhibit the growth of another (indicator). However, rather than its identification as a consequence of the coincidental observation of antimicrobial activity, as was the case for nisin, the identification of novel antimicrobials using this strategy has most frequently been as a result of purpose-built screens employing specific techniques and numerous bacterial species. These can be performed in a variety of ways. One of the most common of these traditional approaches is the deferred antagonism assay. This involves pipetting a set volume of the producer strain on to the appropriate agar and, following incubation, semi-molten agar seeded with an indicator organism is then overlaid. An alternative is the agar well diffusion assay. In this case, the appropriate molten agar is inoculated with indicator cells. This is allowed to cool before wells are bored. To each well, cell-free supernatant from the producer microorganism or

Table 11.1. The screening method and source employed to discover known lantibiotics.

Lantibiotic	Class/group	Mode of discovery	Strain source	Reference
Nisin A	Type 1, nisin group	Incidental (observed inhibition)	Dairy culture	Whitehead (1933)
Nisin Z	Type 1, nisin group	Not specified	Not specified	Mulders *et al.* (1991)
Nisin F	Type 1, nisin group	Overlay assay	Fresh water catfish faeces	de Kwaadsteniet *et al.* (2008)
Nisin U	Type 1, nisin group	Deferred antagonism assay	Not specified	Wirawan *et al.* (2006)
Nisin U2	Type 1, nisin group	Deferred antagonism assay	Not specified	Wirawan *et al.* (2006)
Nisin Q	Type 1, nisin group	Not specified	Hikosan river water	Zendo *et al.* (2003)
Lacticin NK34	Type 1, nisin group	Lawn spotting	Korean fermented fish (jeotgal)	Lee *et al.* (2008)
Subtilin	Type 1, nisin group	Incidental (observed inhibition)	Not specified	Jansen and Hirschmann (1944)
Ericin (A and S)	Type 1, nisin group	Not specified	Not specified	Stein *et al.* (2002)
Entianin	Type 1, nisin group	Microtitre autoinduction bioassay	Tunisian desert	Fuchs *et al.* (2011)
Microbisporicin	Type 1, nisin group	High-throughput screen	Uncommon environmental Actinomycetes	Castiglione *et al.* (2008)
Planosporicin	Type 1, nisin group	High-throughput screen	Uncommon environmental Actinomycetes	Castiglione *et al.* (2007)
Clausin	Type 1, epidermin group	Not specified	Not specified	Bouhss *et al.* (2009)
Staphylococcin T	Type 1, epidermin group	Not specified	Human throat	Furmanek *et al.* (1999)
Epidermin	Type 1, epidermin group	Not specified	Not specified	Allgaier *et al.* (1986)
Gallidermin	Type 1, epidermin group	Not specified	Chicken crests	Kellner *et al.* (1988)
Mutacin I	Type 1, epidermin group	Stab assay	Several (*Streptococcus mutans*)	Hamada and Ooshima (1975)
Mutacin III	Type 1, epidermin group	Not specified	Caries-active female	Qi *et al.* (1999)
Mutacin 1140	Type 1, epidermin group	Deferred antagonism assay	Not specified	Hillman *et al.* (1998)
Mutacin B-Ny266	Type 1, epidermin group	Deferred antagonism assay	Not specified	Morency *et al.* (1995)
Staphylococcin AU-26	Type 1, epidermin group	Deferred antagonism assay	Vagina	Scott *et al.* (1992)
BSA	Type 1, epidermin group	*in silico*	CA-MRSA isolates	Daly *et al.* (2010)
Streptin	Type 1, streptin group	Molecular	Not specified	Karaya *et al.* (2001)
Pep5	Type 1, Pep5 group	Deferred antagonism assay	Not specified	Kellner *et al.* (1989)
Epicidin 280	Type 1, Pep5 group	Not specified	Not specified	Heidrich *et al.* (1998)
Epilancin K7	Type 1, Pep5 group	Not specified	Human nasal cavity	Pulverer and Jeljaszewicz (1975)
Epilancin 15X	Type 1, Pep5 group	Not specified	Wound infection	Ekkelenkamp *et al.* (2005)
Salivaricin 9	Type 2, lacticin 481 group	*In silico*	Not specified	Wescombe *et al.* (2011)
Lacticin 481	Type 2, lacticin 481 group	Spot assay	Dairy	Picard *et al.* (1990)
Thermophilin 1277	Type 2, lacticin 481 group	Not specified	Raw milk	Kabuki *et al.* (2007)
Bovicin Hj50	Type 2, lacticin 481 group	Agar well diffusion assay	Raw milk	Xiao *et al.* (2004)

Continued

Table 11.1. Continued.

Lantibiotic	Class/group	Mode of discovery	Strain source	Reference
Macedocin	Type 2, lacticin 481 group	Well diffusion/overlay assays	Greek kasseri cheese	Georgalaki *et al.* (2000)
Butyrivibriocin AR10	Type 2, lacticin 481 group	Deferred antagonism assay	Rumen	Kalmokoff and Teather (1997)
Ruminococcin A (RumA/B)	Type 2, lacticin 481 group	Not specified	Male gut flora	Ramare *et al.* (1993)
Variacin	Type 2, lacticin 481 group	Well diffusion method	Salami	Pridmore *et al.* (1996)
Streptococcin A-FF22	Type 2, lacticin 481 group	Deferred and simultaneous antagonism assays	Patient throat cultures	Tagg *et al.* (1973)
Butyrivibriocin OR79A/OR79B	Type 2, lacticin 481 group	Deferred antagonism assay	Dairy cow rumen	Kalmokoff *et al.* (1999)
Mutacin II	Type 2, lacticin 481 group	Deferred antagonism assay	Saliva of healthy children	Novak *et al.* (1994)
Mutacin K8 (mukA123+A′)	Type 2, lacticin 481 group	Deferred antagonism assay	Not specified	Robson *et al.* (2007)
Salivaricin A1	Type 2, lacticin 481 group	Molecular (hybridization)	Oral strain	Simpson *et al.* (1995)
Salivaricin A	Type 2, lacticin 481 group	Deferred antagonism assay	Oral strain	Ross *et al.* (1993)
Salivaricin A2	Type 2, lacticin 481 group	Deferred antagonism assay	Human saliva	Hyink *et al.* (2007)
Salivaricin B	Type 2, lacticin 481 group	Deferred antagonism assay	Human saliva	Hyink *et al.* (2007)
Salivaricin A2/3/4/5	Type 2, lacticin 481 group	Deferred antagonism assay	Human saliva	Wescombe *et al.* (2006)
Nukacin ISK-1	Type 2, lacticin 481 group	Not specified	Nukadoko, fermented rice bran	Kimura *et al.* (1998)
Nukacin 3299	Type 2, lacticin 481 group	Deferred antagonism assay	Bovine mastitis cases	Nascimento *et al.* (2002)
Nukacin KQU-131	Type 2, lacticin 481 group	Not specified	Thai fermented marine fish	Wilaipun *et al.* (2008)
Mersacidin	Type 2, mersacidin group	Not specified	Indian soil sample	Chatterjee *et al.* (1992)
Plantaricin-C	Type 2, mersacidin group	Deferred antagonism/well diffusion assay	Fermentations (without starter cultures)	Gonzalez *et al.* (1994)

Michiganin A	Type 2, mersacidin group	Not specified	Plant pathogen	Holtsmark *et al.* (2006)
Actagardine	Type 2, mersacidin group	Not specified	Indian garden soil	Parenti *et al.* (1976)
Ala(0)-actagardine	Type 2, mersacidin group	Not specified	Not specified	Vertesy *et al.* (1999)
Deoxyactagardine B (DAB)	Type 2, mersacidin group	Molecular (hybridization)	Not specified	Boakes *et al.* (2010)
Smb (SmbA/B)	Type 2, Ltna2/mersacidin	Molecular	Oral strain	Yonezawa and Kuramitsu (2005)
Plantaricin W (Plwa/b)	Type 2, mersacidin/Ltna2	Not specified	Wine (pinot noir)	Holo *et al.* (2001)
Staphylococcin C55 (C55α/β)	Type 2, mersacidin/Ltna2	Lawn spotting/c.f.u. counts	Superficial skin lesions	Dajani and Wannamaker (1969)
Haloduracin (BhaA1/A2)	Type 2, Ltnα	*In silico*	Soil	Lawton *et al.* (2007a); McClerren *et al.* (2006)
Lichenicidin (BliA1/A2)	Type 2, Ltnα	*In silico*	Not specified	Begley *et al.* (2009)
Lacticin 3147 (Ltnα/β)	Type 2, mersacidin/Ltnα	Incidental (observed inhibition)	Cheese culture	Ryan *et al.* (1995)
Cytolysin Ll/Ls	Type 2, cytolysin group	Deferred antagonism assay	Not specified	Brock and Davie (1963)
Lactocin-S	Type 2, lactocin S group	Deferred antagonism assay	Fermented dry sausage	Mortvedt and Nes (1990)
Cinnamycin	Type 2, cinnamycin group	Not specified	Japanese soil	Benedict *et al.* (1952)
Duramycin A	Type 2, cinnamycin group	Not specified	Not specified	Shotwell *et al.* (1958)
Duramycin B	Type 2, cinnamycin group	Phospholipase A inhibitor screen	Not specified	Fredenhagen *et al.* (1990)
Duramycin C	Type 2, cinnamycin group	Phospholipase A inhibitor screen	Not specified	Fredenhagen *et al.* (1990)
Ancovenin	Type 2, cinnamycin group	Enzyme inhibitor screen	Tokyo soil sample	Kido *et al.* (1983)
Carnocin UI49	Not determined	Spot assay	Fresh fish	Stoffels *et al.* (1992)
Paenibacillin	Not determined	Deferred antagonism assay (filter membranes)	Fermented foods	He *et al.* (2007)

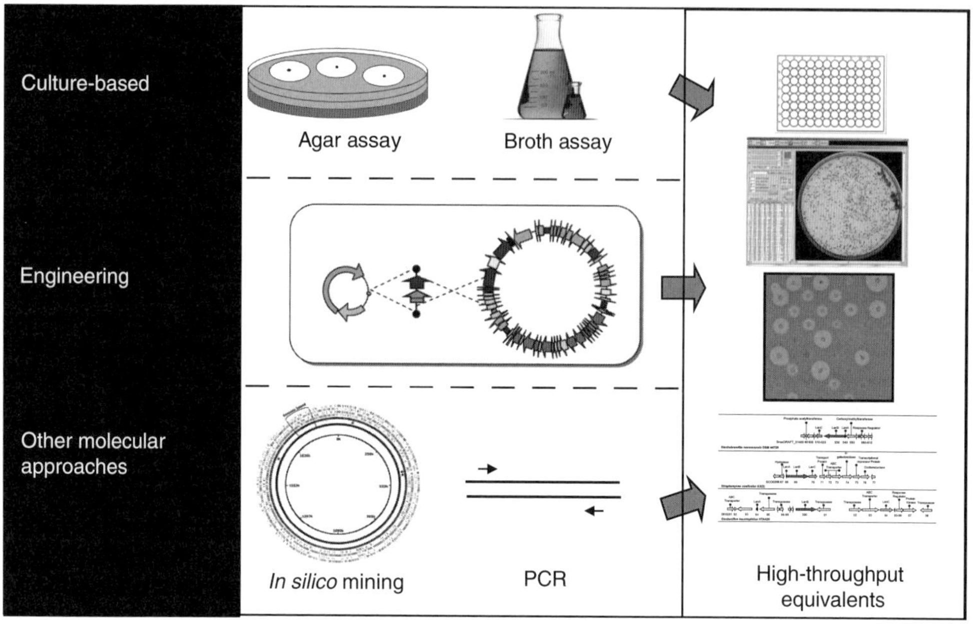

Fig. 11.2. Methods used to screen for novel peptides.

purified peptide is added and, after appropriate incubation (to allow growth of the indicator and diffusion of the antimicrobial), antimicrobial activity can be assessed.

Broth/photometric-based assays can also be employed. Here, the indicator strains are inoculated into broth and cell-free supernatant from the producer organism, or purified peptide is added prior to incubation. After a period of time, cell density is measured using, for example, an absorbance plate reader, revealing whether the growth of the indicator culture has been inhibited. With the exception of standardized assays, such as those recommended by the National Committee for Clinical Laboratory Standards for minimum inhibitory concentration determination (Marshall *et al.*, 1996), the specific details as to how agar and broth-based assays are carried out can vary from laboratory to laboratory. Regardless of these variations, a significant limitation of these functional assays is that novel lantibiotic producers may be overlooked if the parameters employed, such as pH, incubation temperature, time of incubation, carbohydrate source and indicator strain selection, are not optimal. Once antimicrobial activity is detected and revealed, through the use of proteases such as proteinase K, pepsin, trypsin and α-chymotrypsin, to be proteinaceous in nature, the next step generally involves efforts to purify the peptide, most frequently via high-performance liquid chromatography (HPLC) coupled with mass spectrometry. The family of antimicrobials to which the inhibitor belongs can be established definitively through nuclear magnetic resonance (NMR) spectroscopy, although other efforts to elucidate the amino acid sequence of the peptide, through N-terminal peptide sequencing or mass spectrometry, can be valuable. The availability of data with respect to the amino acid sequence (or partial amino acid sequence) of the peptide can in turn also enable identification of the gene cluster of interest through reverse genetics or by genome sequencing of the strain.

Culture-based approaches have facilitated the identification of novel lantibiotic producers from a variety of sources such as milk, fermented foods, oral cavities, the intestine and soil. The frequent use of a starting material that possesses a diverse microbiota stems from the supposition that microbes that need to compete in such environments are most likely to be antimicrobial producers. While here we provide just a few select examples, the source of other lantibiotic-producing bacteria is collated in Table 11.1. Ryan *et al.* (1996) chose to screen lactococci isolated from kefir grains with the intention of finding a *Lactococcus* sp. capable of producing a potent bacteriocin. It was anticipated that such a strain could be used commercially as a starter strain that more successfully controlled spoilage and pathogenic microbes in food fermentations. It was hypothesized that kefir grains could be a rich source of bacteriocin-producing lactococci because, while kefir grains contain a rich microbiota that is chiefly composed of yeast and lactobacilli, lactococci predominate in kefir-fermented milk. Ultimately, a number of antimicrobial-producing lactococci were isolated, including strain DPC3147, which was ultimately found to be the producer of a two-peptide lantibiotic, named lacticin 3147. This lantibiotic has since become one of the most extensively studied lantibiotics (Cotter *et al.*, 2006; Gardiner *et al.*, 2007; Draper *et al.*, 2009; Carroll *et al.*, 2010). The discovery of the lantibiotic butyrivibriocin AR10 stemmed from the study of bacteria isolated from the rumen of cattle (Kalmokoff and Teather, 1997). The rumen is the primary site of microbial fermentation of ingested feed in cattle, and both the rumen and ruminal fluid are known to have an inhibitory effect on non-ruminal bacteria. In total, 49 isolates of *Butyrivibrio fibrisolvens*, and a single isolate of *Butyrivibrio crossotus*, were isolated from the rumen, and their ability to produce antimicrobials was assessed using a deferred antagonism assay, using other *Butyrivibrio* as indicators. Twenty-five isolates were shown to produce inhibitory agents, of which 18 were sensitive to protease digestion. The antimicrobial produced by one such isolate was chosen for purification and further analysis, which culminated in the identification of butyrivibriocin AR10, the first ruminal anaerobe-associated bacteriocin (Kalmokoff and Teather, 1997). Humans can also host many lantibiotic producers. Indeed, staphylococcin Au-26 was characterized from a vaginal isolate of *Staphylococcus aureus* after a study was initiated following the observation that vaginal *S. aureus* associated with toxic-shock syndrome (TSS) were producers of bacteriocins (Scott *et al.*, 1992). It was postulated that this antimicrobial may confer a competitive advantage to the infectious bacteria over the indigenous flora of lactobacilli, and so a deferred antagonism test procedure was carried out using endocervical lactobacilli as indicators, which resulted in the isolation of *S. aureus* strain 26 and the associated lantibiotic, staphylococcin Au26 (Scott *et al.*, 1992). Interestingly, the same lantibiotic was also associated with many community-associated methicillin-resistant *S. aureus* (CA-MRSA) isolates (Daly *et al.*, 2010). Finally, soil has also proven to be a rich repository for producers of lantibiotics, and it is from this source that ancovenin, mersacidin and actagardine (Parenti *et al.*, 1976; Kido *et al.*, 1983; Chatterjee *et al.*, 1992) were identified. Ancovenin was discovered while screening 5200 samples for microbial enzyme inhibitors. Ancovenin was purified from the culture broth of *Streptomyces* sp. no. A647P-2, a strain isolated from a soil sample collected in Tokyo and was initially identified on the basis of its specific inhibitory action against angiotensin I converting enzyme (ACE) rather than as a consequence of possessing antimicrobial activity (Kido *et al.*, 1983).

More recently, efforts have been made to scale up the processes involved in culture-based screening for antimicrobials. The lantibiotics planosporicin and microbisporicin were found as a direct result of a biological-activity-guided, high-throughput screening-based strategy designed to target novel peptidoglycan biosynthesis inhibitors (Castiglione *et al.*, 2007, 2008). This high-throughput screening approach relied on the use of robotics to investigate 40,000 Actinomycetes isolated from the environment, which were then fermented to yield a library of 120,000 broth extracts. The initial step of the antimicrobial activity assay was to assess the ability of the extracts to inhibit the growth of *S. aureus* (in its cell-wall-deficient state) in a liquid microplate assays. The next stage was to disregard those extracts likely to be antimicrobials that had already been characterized i.e. β-lactam antibiotics and glycopeptides. These were eliminated through assays with a β-lactamase cocktail or through use of a D-Ala-D-Ala affinity resin, respectively. This resulted in the identification of five novel lantibiotics, including the aforementioned planosporicin and microbisporicin (Castiglione *et al.*, 2007, 2008). Notably, microbisporicin was subsequently found to have a wide antimicrobial spectrum, being active against many Gram-positive species of medical significance and against some Gram-negative pathogens (Castiglione *et al.*, 2008), making it one of the most potent lantibiotics identified to date.

11.4 Molecular Screening Methods

The second half of the 20th century saw the advent of molecular genetics, which revolutionized many biological fields. Its relevance to the identification and creation of novel peptides lies in its ability to detect and manipulate genes and, consequently, gene products. PCR coupled with gene sequencing have been particularly valuable tools with respect to the detection of novel lantibiotic-encoding operons and will be discussed here. The manipulation of genes using PCR-mediated approaches is also relevant and will be discussed later in this chapter.

A representative example of the use of PCR to identify a novel lantibiotic-encoding cluster was provided during the recent discovery of the type 2 lantibiotic salivaricin 9 (Wescombe *et al.*, 2011). During the course of previous studies, it had been established that *Streptococcus salivarius* strain 9 produces the lantibiotic SalA4 (Wescombe *et al.*, 2006). However, it was soon realized that this was not the only antimicrobial produced by the strain. Using degenerate primers designed to bind to and amplify regions conserved across all *lanM* genes, the *lanM* associated with salivaricin 9 biosynthesis was found to be present on the genome of *S. salivarius* strain 9. Inverse PCR was then used to amplify and sequence the region around *lanM*. Percentage similarities to previously sequenced genes/gene products were determined using the Basic Local Alignment Search Tool (BLAST), an alignment program that compares base-pair similarities of sequences against sequence databases. In this way, the sequenced 6277 bp region was shown to contain genes characteristic of a lantibiotic operon, including a structural gene and regulatory elements. It should be noted, however, that subsequent culture-based approaches were required to confirm that a novel antimicrobial was indeed produced and to determine its antimicrobial spectrum (Wescombe *et al.*, 2011). Similar, degenerate primer-based approaches have been employed to facilitate the identification of the gene clusters associated with the production of Smb (Yonezawa and Kuramitsu, 2005) and BHT-A (Hyink *et al.*, 2005). It is also noteworthy that an alternative set of degenerate *lanM* primers has recently been designed to reflect the availability of an even larger collection of *lanM* sequences (O'Sullivan *et al.*, 2011). A corresponding approach, using *lanB* and *lanC* degenerate primers pairs, led to the identification of the gene cluster associated with the type 1 lantibiotic nisin U (Wirawan *et al.*, 2006). The degenerate primer pairs were designed on the basis of conserved amino acid sequences within the LanBs of streptin, pep5, nisin, epidermin, epicidin and subtilin, while the *lanC* primers were constructed on the basis of conserved regions within the corresponding LanC proteins, as well as that associated with salivaricin A production (Wirawan *et al.*, 2006). Despite the success of these approaches, they have not, to date, been employed as part of high-throughput PCR-based approaches to identify novel lantibiotic-associated clusters from collections of strains.

A quite different molecular tool has been employed in the past to identify novel producers of the lantibiotic nisin from human milk (Beasley and Saris, 2004). This took advantage of the fact that, in addition to being an antimicrobial peptide, nisin is also an autoinducer of its own production (Chandrapati and O'Sullivan, 1999). The milk was initially screened using an agar diffusion test, where milk was spotted on to Luria–Bertani agar and overlaid with a *Micrococcus luteus* indicator. Twenty colonies producing zones of inhibition were selected and their identity was determined by partial 16S rRNA gene sequencing. It was found that the strains isolated were representatives of *Lactococcus lactis* subsp. *lactis* and, as a consequence of the identity of the microbes, it was suspected that they might be producers of nisin. However, characterization of the strains revealed them to be quite different from nisin-producing strains previously isolated from cows' milk. To establish that the antimicrobial activity observed was indeed due to nisin production, a microplate assay designed to detect nisin on the basis of the fusion of a nisin-inducible promoter to a gene encoding a green fluorescent protein reporter (Reunanen and Saris, 2003), was used. Ultimately, these investigations indicated that approximately 30% of human milk contains nisin-producing bacteria.

11.5 Bioinformatic Approaches

As a consequence of the advent of next-generation sequencing technologies, the number of bacterial genome sequences available has increased dramatically. Many of these genome sequences are freely available and accessible via online databases and can be mined for particular genes, including bacteriocin-encoding gene clusters, and their predicted products. The benefits from this approach with respect to lantibiotic discovery have been highlighted on a number of occasions in recent years. Indeed, although approximately 60 lantibiotics have been discovered to date, this number is greatly enhanced when *in silico*-identified lantibiotics are included in the estimate.

Some of the first studies to use a bioinformatic approach to identify novel bacteriocin-associated genes led to the identification of a gene cluster encoding the two-peptide class 2 lantibiotic haloduracin, within the genome of *Bacillus halodurans* C-125. These genes were identified on the basis of the homology between the predicted prepropeptides encoded and those of the prototypical two-peptide lantibiotic lacticin 3147, and the related one-peptide lantibiotic mersacidin (Twomey *et al.*, 2002; McClerren *et al.*, 2006). Analysis of the remainder of the gene cluster revealed the presence of two *lanM* genes, *lanT* (transporter-encodin gene) and two sets of *lanEFG* genes (encoding ABC transporters potentially involved in immunity). The lantibiotic encoded by these genes was accessed through the *in vitro* reconstitution of lantibiotic synthesis (McClerren *et al.*, 2006) and through studies with the C-125 strain and associated cell-free supernatant (Lawton *et al.*, 2007a). This approach has since been used on an even larger scale to reveal additional gene type 2 clusters (Begley *et al.*, 2009). In this case, computational analyses were carried out to search bacterial genome sequences for genes potentially encoding homologues of the lacticin 3147 modification enzyme, LtnM1. This resulted in the generation of a list of 89 relevant genes. Notably, 61 of these were predicted to be produced by strains not previously thought to be lantibiotic producers and five representatives were selected for detailed bioinformatic analysis. One associated strain, *Bacillus licheniformis* ATCC 14580, was selected for wet-lab investigations, which led to the discovery of lichenicidin, a two-peptide lantibiotic that exhibits antimicrobial activity against *Listeria monocytogenes*, MRSA and vancomycin-resistant *Enterococcus*. Inspired by the discovery of lichenicidin, a more recent *in silico* search was undertaken to identify additional novel LanM homologues in DNA databases (O'Sullivan *et al.*, 2011). LtnM1 was again used as a driver sequence to mine publicly available microbial genomes, and by this time the number of LanM-encoding genes had increased to 124. In this instance, nine genes and associated clusters were subjected to an in-depth bioinformatic analysis. In addition, the metagenomic portal CAMERA (Seshadri *et al.*, 2007) was used to search for LtnM1 homologues among all publicly available metagenomic data sets, which revealed a further 11 *lanM* genes associated with lantibiotic gene clusters from a number of diverse environments (O'Sullivan *et al.*, 2011).

A corresponding study has utilized the nisin modification enzymes NisB and NisC as driver sequences to identify novel type 1 lantibiotics (Marsh *et al.*, 2010). In total, 49 previously unrecognized lantibiotics were uncovered in the genomes of microbes isolated from a variety of environments, such as deep-sea hydrothermal vents, the soil, the gastrointestinal tract and skin surfaces. Notably, the microbes in question included those from phyla (Bacteroidetes and Chlamydiae) not previously associated with the production of lantibiotics. The availability of this data has again facilitated the identification of common motifs and residues while also permitting phylogenetic analysis and the construction of evolutionary trees, which have highlighted phylogenetic relatedness and diversity (Marsh *et al.*, 2010).

The mounting interest in the discovery of new bacteriocins utilizing the ever-expanding database of genomic information is also reflected by the development of the web-based bacteriocin genome mining tool BAGEL (de Jong *et al.*, 2006) and the updated BAGEL 2 (de Jong *et al.*, 2010). BAGEL can identify novel bacteriocin clusters using knowledge-based bacteriocin databases and motif databases, and also analyses the sequence surrounding the gene of interest for bacteriocin-associated proteins (e.g. transporters, immunity genes). Importantly, open reading frame detection acts independently of existing annotations and therefore can detect small structural peptides that may otherwise be overlooked. A theoretical drawback is that reliance on motifs will only uncover bacteriocins sharing homology with those already described. It should be noted that the association between gene clusters identified *in silico* and lantibiotic production is putative until such time as antimicrobial activity is confirmed through analysis of the strain in question or through heterologous expression of the relevant genes in an appropriate host (Majchrzykiewicz *et al.*, 2010). However, the studies that have taken place to date indicate the usefulness of these approaches.

It is also notable that the popularity of bacteriocins is such that a database has been generated dedicated to the organization of bacteriocin-related data from the literature. This database, known as BACTIBASE, contains information relating to these bacteriocins, including calculated or predicted structural and physiochemical properties of bacteriocins produced by Gram-positive and Gram-negative bacteria (Hammami *et al.*, 2010).

11.6 Bioengineering of Lantibiotics

An alternative approach to the identification of novel lantibiotics involves the generation of peptides with enhanced antimicrobial activities. The fact that bacteriocins are gene encoded facilitates the use of bioengineering to generate novel derivatives that are, in essence, novel bacteriocins. This contrasts with the majority of 'classical' antibiotics, which are non-ribosomal and are synthesized by multi-enzyme complexes in the absence of a specific structural precursor, thus making genetic manipulation more challenging.

The tolerance of lantibiotics to change is evident from nature in that natural variants of lantibiotics can exist. Nisin is a prime example in that the nisin family includes nisin A, nisin Z, nisin Q, nisin F, nisin U and nisin U2, although in the latter two cases the peptides differ more substantially from nisin A, and their description as nisin variants is debatable (Piper *et al.*, 2010). Over the past 20 years, there have been several efforts to harness this tolerance of change to generate lantibiotic derivatives with enhanced functionalities. Site-directed mutagenesis of lantibiotics was employed for the first time in 1992 (Kuipers *et al.*, 1992; Liu and Hansen, 1992) and has since produced a plethora of information concerning residue function, composition and enzyme activity, which has been invaluable to advancements in lantibiotic engineering and indeed lantibiotic research in general. The first example of the bioengineering of a lantibiotic to enhance activity relates to the nisin-like lantibiotic subtilin (Liu and Hansen, 1992). Subtilin is a type 1 lantibiotic produced by *Bacillus subtilis*, and the bioengineering of this lantibiotic was facilitated by replacement of the *spaS* gene on the chromosome by an engineered version using double cross-over homologous recombination. Using this approach, a mutant in which the fourth residue, glutamate, was replaced with isoleucine displayed enhanced activity with respect to preventing the spore outgrowth of *Bacillus cereus* T spores. Similar strategies have since been employed on a number of occasions, which, although being a relatively time-consuming process, can result in a strain that can be regarded as being non-genetically modified (GM) once used in a contained manner (Sybesma *et al.*, 2006; see http://eur-lex.europa.eu/LexUriServ/LexUriServ.

do?uri=OJ:L:2009:125:0075:0097:EN:PDF). *In trans* complementation and heterologous production approaches have also been frequently employed and can be more rapid but result in the strains losing their non-GM status. While these strategies have been employed to generate a considerable number of lantibiotic derivatives, many of which have been of considerable fundamental value (Field *et al.*, 2010; Cotter *et al.*, 2005a, 2009), here we focus solely on those novel engineered peptides that exhibit enhanced functionalities. In this regard, a number of studies have highlighted the merits of manipulating a three amino acid stretch (Asn20-Met21-Lys22) located at the centre of the nisin propeptide (NisA), which functions as a hinge around which the receptor binding N-terminus and pore-forming C-terminus rotate. Site-specific mutagenesis has shown that this hinge region plays a vital role in affording nisin the conformational plasticity required for antimicrobial activity (Yuan *et al.*, 2004). Changes to this region conferred properties including improved stability at higher temperatures and neutral or alkaline pH, in addition to greater solubility. Furthermore, two peptides with enhanced potency (N20K nisin Z and M21K nisin Z) against the Gram-negative targets *Shigella*, *Pseudomonas* and *Salmonella* were identified. Unfortunately, however, these mutants displayed reduced activity compared with the wild-type peptide against non-pathogenic Gram-positive targets such as *Micrococcus flavus* and *Streptococcus thermophilus* (Yuan *et al.*, 2004) (Fig. 11.3). Although the activity of these peptides is below that required for commercial and clinical use or is against non-pathogenic targets, these findings were none the less of great significance. The importance of the hinge residues has also been highlighted using a non-targeted approach, i.e. from screening of a large bank of producers (8000) of randomly altered nisin peptides (altered to ensure a frequency of one to three mutations within the gene; Field *et al.*, 2008). Although a similar approach had been taken previously (Spee *et al.*, 1993), the bank of strains created on that previous occasion was relatively small. Following extensive randomization (through use of a DNA polymerase that incorrectly incorporated nucleotides during PCR), Field

Nisin a/nisin Z

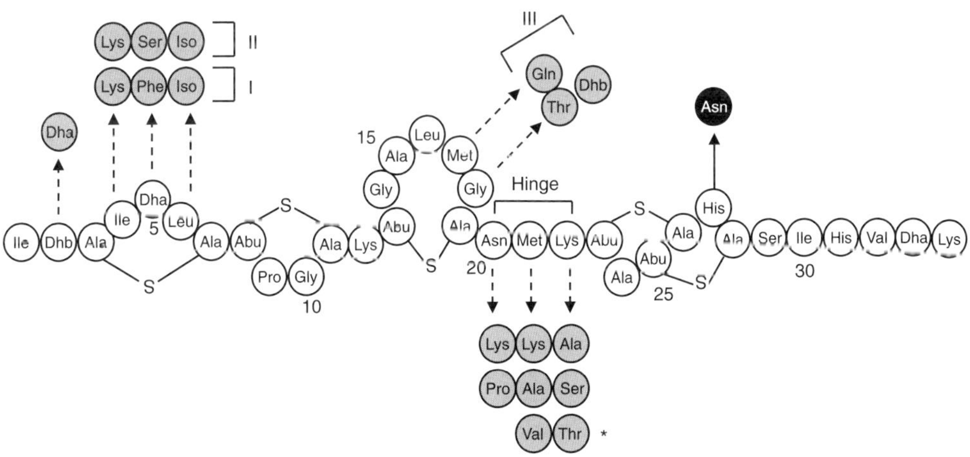

Fig. 11.3. Mutations of nisin A/nisin Z resulting in derivatives with enhanced antimicrobial activity. Nisin A and nisin Z differ by one amino acid, with nisin Z containing an asparagine residue instead of a histidine at position 27. Positions 20–23 are the 'hinge region'. I, Triple mutation: ITL replaced with KFI (Rink *et al.*, 2007b); II, triple mutation: ITL replaced with KSI (Rink *et al.*, 2007b); III, double mutation: MG replaced with QT and Thr also dehydrated to yield Dhb (Kuipers *et al.*, 1996); *, numerous other derivatives showed enhanced activity from mutations in this region, but were not investigated further (Field *et al.*, 2008).

and co-workers specifically looked for producers exhibiting enhanced activity against pathogens, and ultimately coupled this approach with site-directed and site-specific saturation mutagenesis to uncover a number of peptides with improved activity against Gram-positive pathogens of clinical or food relevance. More specifically, initially screening revealed that a strain producing a nisin variant in which a K22T change had occurred in the hinge region displayed increased activity against the mastitic pathogen *Streptococcus agalactiae*. This prompted further site-directed and site-saturation mutagenesis of the three hinge residues. Site-saturation mutagenesis is an approach whereby a bank of derivatives (or producers thereof) is created in which the amino acid located at a particular location in the antimicrobial is changed to each of the other 19 natural amino acids, typically through the use of degenerate PCR primers. The combined use of site-directed and site-saturation mutagenesis led to the identification of a number of additional 'enhanced' peptides including nisin N20P, nisin M21V and nisin K22S (Field *et al.*, 2008) (Fig. 11.1). Similarly, Rink *et al.* (2007b) showed that ring A mutants KFI and KSI were more potent than nisin A against *Lactobacillus johnsonii* and *Leuconostoc mesenteroides*, and *Lactobacillus lactis* and *L. johnsonii*, respectively. Interestingly, Kuipers and co-workers demonstrated how the substitution of threonine in a double mutation simultaneously generated two mutants, G18Thr and a dehydrated form, G18Dhb. The M17Q/G18Thr mutant displayed increased activity against *M. flavus*, while M17Q/G18Dhb showed similar activities to nisin Z. Additionally, it was shown that a T2S mutant had increased activity against *M. flavus* and *S. thermophilus* (Kuipers *et al.*, 1992, 1996).

Site-saturation mutagenesis has also been successfully employed on a number of other occasions. Such an approach was applied to the bioengineering of the *Staphylococcus warneri* ISK-1-produced type 2 lantibiotic nukacin ISK-1 (Islam *et al.*, 2009). During this process of mutagenesis, two variants, D13E and V22I, with twice the potency of the wild type were identified via colony overlay assays, albeit against non-pathogenic strains (such as *Lactobacillus sakei*, *Bacillus coagulans*, *Pediococcus pentococcus* and *Enterococcus faecalis*). Important information regarding the importance of positive charges and ring structures was also obtained during this process. A similar strategy has been utilized in the case of another type 2 lantibiotic, mersacidin (Appleyard *et al.*, 2009). Although a system to facilitate the bioengineering of mersacidin had been identified previously (Szekat *et al.*, 2003), this was improved to facilitate the generation of large numbers of variants (Appleyard *et al.*, 2009). The *trans*-complementation system in question utilizes an inactive *mrsA* (structural peptide-ending gene) mutant of the producing strain, which is complemented through the introduction of a shuttle plasmid carrying the *mrsA* gene or a derivative thereof. A simplified transformation procedure to deliver the plasmid to the host by electroporation of demethylated DNA was developed to facilitate the process. It was noted that, of the 228 mersacidin mutants in the saturation mutagenesis library, more than 80 mutants produced mature mersacidin at acceptable levels. Six variants, G8H, G9S, G10A, G10N, G10V and G10Y, showed increased activity against both MRSA and vancomycin-resistant enterococci (VRE), while another nine, P6H, G7A, G7N, G8N, G8Q, G9A, G9H, L14V and S16A, displayed increased activity against VRE only.

While the 'novel' lantibiotics described above differ quite subtly from the existing antimicrobials, the lantibiotic biosynthetic machinery can also be harnessed *in vivo* or *in vitro* to facilitate the creation of peptides that differ more significantly. In one case, Levengood *et al.* (2009) employed an approach whereby a biosynthetic enzyme was used to modify synthetic substrate analogues via a strategy termed *in vitro* mutasynthesis. More specifically, they showed that LctM, the modification enzyme for the type 2 lantibiotic lacticin 481, continued to modify residues within the lacticin 481 propeptide even when residues (Trp19 and Phe23) were substituted with non-proteinogenic amino acids (naphthylalanine and homophenylalanine, respectively). This resulted in the creation of two analogues with increased biological activity against *L. lactis* HP and *B. subtilis* ATCC 6633, thereby demonstrating the value of this approach. Indeed, it has been established that many lantibiotic biosynthetic proteins can be harnessed (Kuipers *et al.*, 2004; Kluskens *et al.*, 2005; Rink *et al.*, 2005; Chatterjee *et al.*, 2006;

Li *et al.*, 2006; Rink *et al.*, 2007a; Kuipers *et al.*, 2008; van Saparoea *et al.*, 2008), which will undoubtedly facilitate the synthesis of even greater numbers of novel antimicrobials in the future. Indeed, the applications of modification proteins and *in silico* screening have been nicely combined by Majchrzykiewicz *et al.* (2010) who successfully utilized the nisin expression/modification system to produce, modify and secrete entirely unrelated putative lantibiotics identified using BAGEL. The two putative structural peptides of the potentially novel type 2 lantibiotic pneumococcin, A1 and A2, from *Streptocccus pneumoniae* R6, were chosen as the substrates for the nisin enzymes. Their propeptide regions (i.e. mature peptide region) were fused with nisin leader sequences and introduced into a *L. lactis* host that overproduces NisBTC. The peptides produced were shown to be modified and to exhibit biological activity against *M. flavus*. It is thus apparent that the nisin modification and transport machinery can be employed to harness a putative lantibiotic-encoding gene cluster corresponding to a different lantibiotic type and from a different genus, and thus could potentially be employed to access the many other putatively lantibiotic-encoding gene clusters referred to above.

11.7 Non-lantibiotic, Ribosomally Synthesized, Modified Peptides

As noted above, this chapter has focused specifically on lantibiotic-related research with a view to using the developments in this area to highlight the variety of different ways in which modified ribosomally synthesized antimicrobials in general can be identified. However, to highlight the relevance of these approaches to other gene-encoded peptides, a selection of recent examples of note is presented here.

11.7.1 Sactibiotics

Clostridium difficile is the causative agent of nosocomial diarrhoea, and *C. difficile*-associated disease is increasing in both prevalence and severity. The main predisposing factor for this disease is antibiotic therapy, which often eradicates beneficial flora in the gut, allowing *C. difficile* to flourish. To this effect, a bioscreen was devised with the aim of isolating a narrow-spectrum bacteriocin effective against *C. difficile* that would not impact on beneficial microbes in the intestine (Rea *et al.*, 2010). It was hypothesized that spore-forming, anaerobic bacteria would be a probable source of bacteriocins active against a related bacterium such as *C. difficile*. To select for such strains, human faecal samples from healthy and diseased adults were treated with ethanol for 30 min to kill all vegetative cells. These were then plated on Wilkens–Chagrin anaerobic agar (WCAA) and allowed to grow for 5 days at 37°C in an anaerobic chamber. The resulting colonies were overlaid with *C. difficile*-inoculated reinforced *Clostridium* agar and grown for another 18 h to produce a lawn of *C. difficile* growth. The plates were then inspected for zones of clearing, where the initial colony inhibited the growth of *C. difficile*. In total, 30,000 colonies were screened, and only one colony showed potent antimicrobial activity against the overlaid *C. difficile* strain. Interestingly, other faecal bacteria growing in the bottom layer were not inhibited by this antimicrobial, suggesting that it could be a narrow-spectrum antimicrobial. The producing colony in question was removed from the agar using a sterile scalpel and subcultured on to fresh WCAA. Proteinase tests were performed to confirm that the inhibitory substance was proteinaceous in nature and it was ultimately established to be a two-peptide bacteriocin, designated thuricin CD, that underwent post-translational modification resulting in the formation of sulfur to α-carbon linkages (from which the name sactibiotic is derived) (Rea *et al.*, 2010). The thuricin CD gene cluster was identified through reverse genetics and inverse PCR and was found to contain two radical *S*-adenosyl methyltransferase-encoding genes, *trnC* and *trnD* (Rea *et al.*, 2010). An *in silico* screen for novel sactibiotics, using the radical *S*-adenosyl methyltransferase sequences as drivers, uncovered a considerable number of additional gene clusters of note (Murphy *et al.*, 2011).

11.7.2 Labyrinthopeptins

The labyrinthopeptins are a novel family of lantibiotic-like antimicrobials that contain an unprecedented carbacyclic, post-translationally modified amino acid named labionin (Meindl *et al.*, 2010). These were identified when the culture extracts of a newly identified novel actinomycete *Actinomadura namiensis* DSM 6313 (from Namibian desert soil) were shown to have moderate activity against herpes simplex virus. The peptide was isolated using chromatographic methods and shown to have potential applications in the treatment of neuropathic pain.

11.7.3 Thiazole/oxazole-modified microcins

Thiazole/oxazole-modified microcins are a group of post-translationally modified antimicrobial peptides, that includes assorted bacterial products such as microcins, thiopeptides, cyanobactins, putative *Bacillus*-associated thiazole-containing heterocyclic bacteriocins, a nitrile hydrolase and the NifL-1-related precursor family, and which are grouped on the basis of containing thiazole and oxazole structures (Molloy *et al.*, 2011). The culture-, *in silico*- and bioengineering-based approaches described in this review can also be used to identify novel such peptides. By way of example, we will focus on the thiopeptides.

Thiopeptides are another distinct group of ribosomally post-translationally modified antimicrobials (Bagley *et al.*, 2005). Thiopeptides are complex, highly modified sulfur-containing peptides that inhibit the initial steps of protein synthesis in Gram-positive bacteria, including MRSA. They contain a macrocyclic framework consisting of modified heterocyclic residues, including indoles, oxazoles, thiazoles and dehydroamino acids. The development of screening programmes has greatly expanded the number of known thiopeptide antibiotics in recent years. Although micrococcin P_1 was the first thiopeptide antibiotic to be discovered (Su, 1948), thiostrepton has been the most extensively studied. Thiostrepton exhibits activity analogous to that of penicillin but has not yet been developed for clinical use, as bacterial resistance develops before a therapeutic dose can be reached, due to its low solubility (a problem common to many thiopeptide antibiotics). Targeted screening programmes have isolated a number of thiopeptides from a variety of actinomycete sources. The chemical structure of several thiopeptides has been elucidated using X-ray crystallography and NMR techniques, and several, such as promothiocin A, amythiamicin D and thiostreptin, have been synthesized chemically. These results offer a glimpse at a promising future in which chemical thiopeptide structures can be computationally and biologically optimized for antimicrobial activity. A high-throughput screening strategy was employed, using 96- and 384-well microtitre plates, to screen a library of thiopeptide precursor compounds for their ability to inhibit translation or reverse the inhibition of known thiopeptide antibiotics, to identify four distinct classes of precursor peptides (Starosta *et al.*, 2009); an *in silico* screen was used to identify thiocillin, a thiopeptide that undergoes 13 post-translational modifications (Brown *et al.*, 2009); and TP-1161, a thiopeptide antibiotic from a marine *Nocardiopsis* species, was identified by PCR screening (Engelhardt *et al.*, 2010).

11.8 Conclusion

There are numerous strategies available when targeting the identification/creation of novel post-translationally modified antimicrobials. Great advances have been made, and today culture-based methods have evolved to encompass high-throughput screening, molecular tools used to amplify and engineer DNA, and *in silico* databases and search tools enable bioinformatic mining for novel peptides. The continued evolution of these technologies will ensure that the rate of identification of novel modified antimicrobials will continue to increase at a considerable rate.

Acknowledgements

This work was supported by the Science Foundation of Ireland funded Centre for Science, Engineering and Technology (SFI-CSET): the Alimentary Pharmabiotic Centre (APC).

References

Allgaier, H., Jung, G., Werner, R.G., Schneider, U. and Zahner, H. (1986) Epidermin – sequencing of a heterodet tetracyclic 21-peptide amide antibiotic. *European Journal of Biochemistry* 160, 9–22.

Appleyard, A.N., Choi, S., Read, D.M., Lightfoot, A., Boakes, S., Hoffmann, A., Chopra, I., Bierbaum, G., Rudd, B.A.M., Dawson, M.J. and Cortes, J. (2009) Dissecting structural and functional diversity of the lantibiotic mersacidin. *Chemistry and Biology* 16, 490–498.

Bagley, M.C., Dale, J.W., Merritt, E.A. and Xiong, X. (2005) Thiopeptide antibiotics. *Chemical Reviews* 105, 685–714.

Beasley, S.S. and Saris, P.E.J. (2004) Nisin-producing *Lactococcus lactis* strains isolated from human milk. *Applied and Environmental Microbiology* 70, 5051–5053.

Begley, M., Cotter, P.D., Hill, C. and Ross, R.P. (2009) Identification of a novel two-peptide lantibiotic, lichenicidin, following rational genome mining for LanM proteins. *Applied and Environmental Microbiology* 75, 5451–5460.

Benedict, R.G., Dvonch, W., Shotwell, O.L., Pridham, T.G. and Lindenfelser, L.A. (1952) Cinnamycin, an antibiotic from *Streptomyces cinnamoneus* Nov. Sp. *Antibiotics and Chemotherapy* 11, 591–594.

Boakes, S., Appleyard, A.N., Cortes, J. and Dawson, M.J. (2010) Organization of the biosynthetic genes encoding deoxyactagardine B (DAB), a new lantibiotic produced by *Actinoplanes liguriae* NCIMB41362. *Journal of Antibiotics* 63, 351–358.

Bouhss, A., Al-Dabbagh, B., Vincent, M., Odaert, B., Aumont-Nicaise, M., Bressolier, P., Desmadril, M., Mengin-Lecreulx, D., Urdaci, M.C. and Gallay, J. (2009) Specific interactions of clausin, a new lantibiotic, with lipid precursors of the bacterial cell wall. *Biophysical Journal* 97, 1390–1397.

Brock, T.D. and Davie, J.M. (1963) Probable identity of a group D hemolysin with a bacteriocine. *Journal of Bacteriology* 86, 702–712.

Brown, L.C.W., Acker, M.G., Clardy, J., Walsh, C.T. and Fischbach, M.A. (2009) Thirteen posttranslational modifications convert a 14-residue peptide into the antibiotic thiocillin. *Proceedings of the National Academy of Sciences USA* 106, 2549–2553.

Carroll, J., Draper, L.A., O'Connor, P.M., Coffey, A., Hill, C., Ross, R.P., Cotter, P.D. and O'Mahony, J. (2010) Comparison of the activities of the lantibiotics nisin and lacticin 3147 against clinically significant mycobacteria. *International Journal of Antimicrobial Agents* 36, 132–136.

Castiglione, F., Cavaletti, L., Losi, D., Lazzarini, A., Carrano, L., Feroggio, M., Ciciliato, I., Corti, E., Candiani, G., Marinelli, F. and Selva, E. (2007) A novel lantibiotic acting on bacterial cell wall synthesis produced by the uncommon actinomycete *Planomonospora* sp. *Biochemistry* 46, 5884–5895.

Castiglione, F., Lazzarini, A., Carrano, L., Corti, E., Ciciliato, I., Gastaldo, L., Candiani, P., Losi, D., Marinelli, F., Selva, E. and Parenti, F. (2008) Determining the structure and mode of action of microbisporicin, a potent lantibiotic active against multiresistant pathogens. *Chemistry and Biology* 15, 22–31.

Chandrapati, S. and O'Sullivan, D.J. (1999) Nisin independent induction of the *nisA* promoter in *Lactococcus lactis* during growth in lactose or galactose. *FEMS Microbiology Letters* 170, 191–198.

Chatterjee, C., Patton, G.C., Cooper, L., Paul, M. and van der Donk, W.A. (2006) Engineering dehydro amino acids and thioethers into peptides using lacticin 481 synthetase. *Chemistry and Biology* 13, 1109–1117.

Chatterjee, S., Chatterjee, D.K., Jani, R.H., Blumbach, J., Ganguli, B.N., Klesel, N., Limbert, M. and Seibert, G. (1992) Mersacidin, a new antibiotic from *Bacillus*. In vitro and in vivo antibacterial activity. *Journal of Antibiotics* 45, 839–845.

Cotter, P.D., Deegan, L.H., Lawton, E.M., Draper, L.A., O'Connor, P.M., Hill, C. and Ross, R.P. (2006) Complete alanine scanning of the two-component lantibiotic lacticin 3147: generating a blueprint for rational drug design. *Molecular Microbiology* 62, 735–747.

Cotter, P.D., Hill, C. and Ross, R.P. (2005a) Bacterial lantibiotics: strategies to improve therapeutic potential. *Current Protein and Peptide Science* 6, 61–75.

Cotter, P.D., Hill, C. and Ross, R.P. (2005b) Bacteriocins: developing innate immunity for food. *Nature Reviews Microbiology* 3, 777–788.

Dajani, A.S. and Wannamaker, L.W. (1969) Demonstration of a bactericidal substance against β-hemolytic streptococci in supernatant fluids of staphylococcal cultures. *Journal of Bacteriology* 97, 985–991.

Daly, K.M., Upton, M., Sandiford, S.K., Draper, L.A., Wescombe, P.A., Jack, R.W., O'Connor, P.M., Rossney, A., Gotz, F., Hill, C., Cotter, P.D., Ross, R.P. and Tagg, J.R. (2010) Production of the Bsa lantibiotic by community-acquired *Staphylococcus aureus* strains. *Journal of Bacteriology* 192, 1131–1142.

de Jong, A., van Heel, A.J., Kok, J. and Kuipers, O.P. (2010) BAGEL2: mining for bacteriocins

in genomic data. *Nucleic Acids Research* 38, W647–W651.
de Jong, A., van Hijum, S.A.F.T., Bijlsma, J.J.E., Kok, J. and Kuipers, O.P. (2006) BAGEL: a web-based bacteriocin genome mining tool. *Nucleic Acids Research* 34, W273–W279.
de Kwaadsteniet, M., ten Doeschate, K. and Dicks, L.M.T. (2008) Characterization of the structural gene encoding Nisin F, a new lantibiotic produced by a *Lactococcus lactis* subsp *lactis* isolate from freshwater catfish (*Clatias gatiepinus*). *Applied and Environmental Microbiology* 74, 547–549.
Draper, L.A., Grainger, K., Deegan, L.H., Cotter, P.D., Hill, C. and Ross, R.P. (2009) Cross-immunity and immune mimicry as mechanisms of resistance to the lantibiotic lacticin 3147. *Molecular Microbiology* 71, 1043–1054.
Ekkelenkamp, M.B., Hanssen, M., Danny Hsu, S.T., de Jong, A., Milatovic, D., Verhoef, J. and van Nuland, N.A. (2005) Isolation and structural characterization of epilancin 15X, a novel lantibiotic from a clinical strain of *Staphylococcus epidermidis*. *FEBS Letters* 579, 1917–1922.
Engelhardt, K., Degnes, K.F., Kemmler, M., Bredholt, H., Fjaervik, E., Klinkenberg, G., Sletta, H., Ellingsen, T.E. and Zotchev, S.B. (2010) Production of a new thiopeptide antibiotic, TP-1161, by a marine *Nocardiopsis* species. *Applied and Environmental Microbiology* 76, 4969–4976.
Field, D., Connor, P.M.O., Cotter, P.D., Hill, C. and Ross, R.P. (2008) The generation of nisin variants with enhanced activity against specific Gram-positive pathogens. *Molecular Microbiology* 69, 218–230.
Field, D., Hill, C., Cotter, P.D. and Ross, R.P. (2010) The dawning of a 'Golden era' in lantibiotic bioengineering. *Molecular Microbiology* 78, 1077–1087.
Fredenhagen, A., Fendrich, G., Marki, F., Marki, W., Gruner, J., Raschdorf, F. and Peter, H.H. (1990) Duramycins B and C, two new lanthionine containing antibiotics as inhibitors of phospholipase A2. Structural revision of duramycin and cinnamycin. *Journal of Antibiotics* 43, 1403–1412.
Fuchs, S.W., Jaskolla, T.W., Bochmann, S., Kotter, P., Wichelhaus, T., Karas, M., Stein, T. and Entian, K.D. (2011) Entianin, a novel subtilin-like lantibiotic from *Bacillus subtilis* subsp. *spizizenii* DSM 15029(T) with high antimicrobial activity. *Applied and Environmental Microbiology* 77, 1698–1707.
Furmanek, B., Kaczorowski, T., Bugalski, R., Bielawski, K., Bogdanowicz, J. and Podhajska, A.J. (1999) Identification, characterization and purification of the lantibiotic staphylococcin T., a natural gallidermin variant. *Journal of Applied Microbiology* 87, 856–866.
Gardiner, G.E., Rea, M.C., O'Riordan, B., O'Connor, P., Morgan, S.M., Lawlor, P.G., Lynch, P.B., Cronin, M., Ross, R.P. and Hill, C. (2007) Fate of the two-component lantibiotic lacticin 3147 in the gastrointestinal tract. *Applied and Environmental Microbiology* 73, 7103–7109.
Georgalaki, M.D., Sarantinopoulos, P., Ferreira, E.S., De Vuyst, L., Kalantzopoulos, G. and Tsakalidou, E. (2000) Biochemical properties of *Streptococcus macedonicus* strains isolated from Greek Kasseri cheese. *Journal of Applied Microbiology* 88, 817–825.
Gonzalez, B., Arca, P., Mayo, B. and Suarez, J.E. (1994) Detection, purification, and partial characterization of plantaricin C, a bacteriocin produced by a *Lactobacillus plantarum* strain of dairy origin. *Applied and Environmental Microbiology* 60, 2158–2163.
Hamada, S. and Ooshima, T. (1975) Inhibitory spectrum of a bacteriocinlike substance (mutacin) produced by some strains of *Streptococcus mutans*. *Journal of Dental Research* 54, 140–145.
Hammami, R., Zouhir, A., Le Lay, C., Ben Hamida, J. and Fliss, I. (2010) BACTIBASE second release: a database and tool platform for bacteriocin characterization. *BioMed Central Microbiology* 10, 22.
He, Z., Kisla, D., Zhang, L., Yuan, C., Green-Church, K.B. and Yousef, A.E. (2007) Isolation and identification of a *Paenibacillus polymyxa* strain that coproduces a novel lantibiotic and polymyxin. *Applied and Environmental Microbiology* 73, 168–178.
Heidrich, C., Pag, U., Josten, M., Metzger, J., Jack, R.W., Bierbaum, G., Jung, G. and Sahl, H.G. (1998) Isolation, characterization, and heterologous expression of the novel lantibiotic epicidin 280 and analysis of its biosynthetic gene cluster. *Applied and Environmental Microbiology* 64, 3140–3146.
Hillman, J.D., Novak, J., Sagura, E., Gutierrez, J.A., Brooks, T.A., Crowley, P.J., Hess, M., Azizi, A., Leung, K., Cvitkovitch, D. and Bleiweis, A.S. (1998) Genetic and biochemical analysis of mutacin 1140, a lantibiotic from *Streptococcus mutans*. *Infection and Immunity* 66, 2743–2749.
Holo, H., Jeknic, Z., Daeschel, M., Stevanovic, S. and Nes, I.F. (2001) Plantaricin W from *Lactobacillus plantarum* belongs to a new family of two-peptide lantibiotics. *Microbiology* 147, 643–651.
Holtsmark, I., Mantzilas, D., Eijsink, V.G.H. and Brurberg, M.B. (2006) Purification, characterization, and gene sequence of michiganin A, an actagardine-like lantibiotic produced by the tomato pathogen *Clavibacter michiganensis* subsp. *michiganensis*. *Applied and Environmental Microbiology* 72, 5814–5821.

Hsu, S.T.D., Breukink, E., Tischenko, E., Lutters, M.A.G., de Kruijff, B., Kaptein, R., Bonvin, A.M.J.J. and van Nuland, N.A.J. (2004) The nisin–lipid II complex reveals a pyrophosphate cage that provides a blueprint for novel antibiotics. *Nature Structural and Molecular Biology* 11, 963–967.

Hyink, O., Balakrishnan, M. and Tagg, J.R. (2005) *Streptococcus rattus* strain BHT produces both a class I two-component lantibiotic and a class II bacteriocin. *FEMS Microbiology Letters* 252, 235–241.

Hyink, O., Wescombe, P.A., Upton, M., Ragland, N., Burton, J.P. and Tagg, J.R. (2007) Salivaricin A2 and the novel lantibiotic salivaricin B are encoded at adjacent loci on a 190-kilobase transmissible megaplasmid in the oral probiotic strain *Streptococcus salivarius* K12. *Applied and Environmental Microbiology* 73, 1107–1113.

Islam, M.R., Shioya, K., Nagao, J., Nishie, M., Jikuya, H., Zendo, T., Nakayama, J. and Sonomoto, K. (2009) Evaluation of essential and variable residues of nukacin ISK-1 by NNK scanning. *Molecular Microbiology* 72, 1438–1447.

Jansen, E.F. and Hirschmann, D.J. (1944) Subtilin – an antibacterial product of *Bacillus subtilis* culturing conditions and properties. *Archives of Biochemistry* 4, 297–309.

Kabuki, T., Uenishi, H., Watanabe, M., Seto, Y. and Nakajima, H. (2007) Characterization of a bacteriocin, Thermophilin 1277, produced by *Streptococcus thermophilus* SBT1277. *Journal of Applied Microbiology* 102, 971–980.

Kalmokoff, M.L. and Teather, R.M. (1997) Isolation and characterization of a bacteriocin (Butyrivibriocin AR10) from the ruminal anaerobe *Butyrivibrio fibrisolvens* AR10: evidence in support of the widespread occurrence of bacteriocin-like activity among ruminal isolates of *B. fibrisolvens*. *Applied and Environmental Microbiology* 63, 394–402.

Kalmokoff, M.L., Lu, D., Whitford, M.F. and Teather, R.M. (1999) Evidence for production of a new lantibiotic (butyrivibriocin OR79A) by the ruminal anaerobe *Butyrivibrio fibrisolvens* OR79: characterization of the structural gene encoding butyrivibriocin OR79A. *Applied and Environmental Microbiology* 65, 2128–2135.

Karaya, K., Shimizu, T. and Taketo, A. (2001) New gene cluster for lantibiotic streptin possibly involved in streptolysin S formation. *Journal of Biochemistry* 129, 769–775.

Kellner, R., Jung, G., Horner, T., Zahner, H., Schnell, N., Entian, K.D. and Gotz, F. (1988) Gallidermin – a new lanthionine-containing polypeptide antibiotic. *European Journal of Biochemistry* 177, 53–59.

Kellner, R., Jung, G., Josten, M., Kaletta, C., Entian, K.D. and Sahl, H.G. (1989) Pep5 – structure elucidation of a large lantibiotic. *Angewandte Chemie – International Edition* 28, 616–619.

Kido, Y., Hamakado, T., Yoshida, T., Anno, M., Motoki, Y., Wakamiya, T. and Shiba, T. (1983) Isolation and characterization of ancovenin, a new inhibitor of angiotensin-I converting enzyme, produced by Actinomycetes. *Journal of Antibiotics* 36, 1295–1299.

Kimura, H., Sashihara, T., Matsusaki, H., Sonomoto, K. and Ishizaki, A. (1998) Novel bacteriocin of *Pediococcus* sp. ISK-1 isolated from well-aged bed of fermented rice bran. *Enzyme Engineering XIV* 864, 345–348.

Klaenhammer, T.R. (1993) Genetics of bacteriocins produced by lactic acid bacteria. *FEMS Microbiology Reviews* 12, 39–86.

Kluskens, L.D., Kuipers, A., Rink, R., de Boef, E., Fekken, S., Driessen, A.J.M., Kuipers, O.P. and Moll, G.N. (2005) Post-translational modification of therapeutic peptides by NisB, the dehydratase of the lantibiotic nisin. *Biochemistry* 44, 12827–12834.

Kuipers, A., de Boef, E., Rink, R., Fekken, S., Kluskens, L.D., Driessen, A.J.M., Leenhouts, K., Kuipers, O.P. and Moll, G.N. (2004) NisT, the transporter of the lantibiotic nisin, can transport fully modified, dehydrated, and unmodified prenisin and fusions of the leader peptide with non-lantibiotic peptides. *Journal of Biological Chemistry* 279, 22176–22182.

Kuipers, A., Meijer-Wierenga, J., Rink, R., Kluskens, L.D. and Moll, G.N. (2008) Mechanistic dissection of the enzyme complexes involved in biosynthesis of lacticin 3147 and nisin. *Applied and Environmental Microbiology* 74, 6591–6597.

Kuipers, O.P., Rollema, H.S., Yap, W.M.G.J., Boot, H.J., Siezen, R.J. and Devos, W.M. (1992) Engineering dehydrated amino acid residues in the antimicrobial peptide nisin. *Journal of Biological Chemistry* 267, 24340–24346.

Kuipers, O.P., Bierbaum, G., Ottenwalder, B., Dodd, H.M., Horn, N., Metzger, J., Kupke, T., Gnau, V., Bongers, R., van den Bogaard, P., Kosters, H., Rollema, H.S., deVos, W.M., Siezen, R.J., Jung, G., Gotz, F., Sahl, H.G. and Gasson, M.J. (1996) Protein engineering of lantibiotics. *Antonie Van Leeuwenhoek* 69, 161–169.

Lawton, E.M., Cotter, P.D., Hill, C. and Ross, R.P. (2007a) Identification of a novel two-peptide lantibiotic, Haloduracin, produced by the alkaliphile *Bacillus halodurans* C-125. *FEMS Microbiology Letters* 267, 64–71.

Lawton, E.M., Ross, R.P., Hill, C. and Cotter, P.D. (2007b) Two-peptide lantibiotics: a medical perspective. *Mini-Reviews in Medicinal Chemistry* 7, 1236–1247.

Lee, N.K., Park, Y.L., Kim, H.W., Park, Y.H., Rhim, S.L., Kim, J.M., Kim, J.M., Nam, H.M., Jung, S.C. and Paik, H.D. (2008) Purification and characterization of Lacticin NK34 produced by *Lactococcus lactis* NK34 against bovine mastitis. *Korean Journal for Food Science and Animal Science* 28, 457–462.

Levengood, M.R., Kerwood, C.C., Chatterjee, C. and van der Donk, W.A. (2009) Investigation of the substrate specificity of lacticin 481 synthetase by using nonproteinogenic amino acids. *ChemBioChem* 10, 911–919.

Li, B., Yu, J.P.J., Brunzelle, J.S., Moll, G.N., van der Donk, W.A. and Nair, S.K. (2006) Structure and mechanism of the lantibiotic cyclase involved in nisin biosynthesis. *Science* 311, 1464–1467.

Liu, W. and Hansen, J.N. (1992) Enhancement of the chemical and antimicrobial properties of subtilin by site-directed mutagenesis. *Journal of Biological Chemistry* 267, 25078–25085.

Majchrzykiewicz, J.A., Lubelski, J., Moll, G.N., Kuipers, A., Bijlsma, J.J.E., Kuipers, O.P. and Rink, R. (2010) Production of a class II two-component lantibiotic of *Streptococcus pneumoniae* using the class I nisin synthetic machinery and leader sequence. *Antimicrobial Agents and Chemotherapy* 54, 1498–1505.

Marsh, A.J., O'Sullivan, O., Ross, R.P., Cotter, P.D. and Hill, C. (2010) *In silico* analysis highlights the frequency and diversity of type 1 lantibiotic gene clusters in genome sequenced bacteria. *BioMed Central Genomics* 11, 679.

Marshall, S.A., Jones, R.N., Wanger, A., Washington, J.A., Doern, G.V., Leber, A.L. and Haugen, T.H. (1996) Proposed MIC quality control guidelines for National Committee for Clinical Laboratory Standards susceptibility tests using seven veterinary antimicrobial agents: ceftiofur, enrofloxacin, florfenicol, penicillin G-novobiocin, pirlimycin, premafloxacin, and spectinomycin. *Journal of Clinical Microbiology* 34, 2027–2029.

Mattick, A.T. and Hirsch, A. (1947) Further observations on an inhibitory substance (nisin) from lactic streptococci. *Lancet* 250, 5–8.

McClerren, A.L., Cooper, L.E., Quan, C., Thomas, P.M., Kelleher, N.L. and van der Donk, W.A. (2006) Discovery and *in vitro* biosynthesis of haloduracin, a two-component lantibiotic. *Proceedings of the National Academy of Sciences USA* 103, 17243–17248.

Meindl, K., Schmiederer, T., Schneider, K., Reicke, A., Butz, D., Keller, S., Guhring, H., Vertesy, L., Wink, J., Hoffmann, H., Bronstrup, M., Sheldrick, G.M. and Sussmuth, R.D. (2010) Labyrinthopeptins: a new class of carbacyclic lantibiotics. *Angewandte Chemie – International Edition* 49, 1151–1154.

Molloy, E., Cotter, P.D. Hill, C., Mitchell, D.A. and Ross, R.P. (2011) Streptolysin S-like virulence factors: the continuing saga. *Nature Reviews Microbiology* 9, 670–681..

Morency, H., Trahan, L. and Lavoie, M.C. (1995) Preliminary grouping of mutacins. *Canadian Journal of Microbiology* 41, 826–831.

Mortvedt, C.I. and Nes, I.F. (1990) Plasmid-associated bacteriocin production by a *Lactobacillus sake* strain. *Journal of General Microbiology* 136, 1601–1607.

Mulders, J.W., Boerrigter, I.J., Rollema, H.S., Siezen, R.J. and de Vos, W.M. (1991) Identification and characterization of the lantibiotic nisin Z, a natural nisin variant. *European Journal of Biochemistry* 201, 581–584.

Murphy, K., O'Sullivan, O., Rea, M.C., Cotter, P.D., Ross, R.P. and Hill, C. (2011) Genome mining for radical SAM protein determinants reveals multiple sactibiotic-like gene clusters. *PLoS One* 6, e20852.

Nascimento, J.D., dos Santos, K.R.N., Gentilini, E., Sordelli, D. and Bastos, M.D.D. (2002) Phenotypic and genetic characterisation of bacteriocin-producing strains of *Staphylococcus aureus* involved in bovine mastitis. *Veterinary Microbiology* 85, 133–144.

Novak, J., Caufield, P.W. and Miller, E.J. (1994) Isolation and biochemical characterization of a novel lantibiotic mutacin from *Streptococcus mutans. Journal of Bacteriology* 176, 4316–4320.

O'Sullivan, O., Begley, M., Ross, R.P., Cotter, P.D. and Hill, C. (2011) Further identification of novel lantibiotic operons using LanM-based genome mining. *Probiotics and Antimicrobial Proteins* 3, 27–40.

Parenti, F., Pagani, H. and Beretta, G. (1976) Gardimycin, a new antibiotic from Actinoplanes. I. Description of the producer strain and fermentation studies. *Journal of Antibiotics (Tokyo)* 29, 501–506.

Pasteur, L. and Joubert, J. (1877) Charbon et septicemie. *Comptes Rendus Chimie* 85, 101–105.

Picard, J.C., Delorme, F., Giraffa, G., Commissaire, J. and Desmazeaud, M. (1990) Evidence for a bacteriocin produced by *Lactococcus lactis* CNRZ 481. *Netherlands Milk and Diary Journal* 44, 143–158.

Piper, C., Hill, C., Cotter, P.D. and Ross, R.P. (2010) Bioengineering of a nisin A-producing *Lactococcus lactis* to create isogenic strains producing the natural variants nisin F, Q and Z. *Microbial Biotechnology* 4, 375–382.

Pridmore, D., Rekhif, N., Pittet, A.C., Suri, B. and Mollet, B. (1996) Variacin, a new lanthionine-containing bacteriocin produced by *Micrococcus varians*: comparison to lacticin 481 of *Lactococcus lactis*. *Applied and Environmental Microbiology* 62, 1799–1802.

Pulverer, G. and Jeljaszewicz, J. (1975) Staphylococcal micrococcins. I. Isolation of antibiotic-producing strains. *Arzneimittelforschung* 25, 1004–1006.

Qi, F., Chen, P. and Caufield, P.W. (1999) Purification of mutacin III from group III *Streptococcus mutans* UA787 and genetic analyses of mutacin III biosynthesis genes. *Applied and Environmental Microbiology* 65, 3880–3887.

Ramare, F., Nicoli, J., Dabard, J., Corring, T., Ladire, M., Gueugneau, A.M. and Raibaud, P. (1993) Trypsin-dependent production of an antibacterial substance by a human *Peptostreptococcus* strain in gnotobiotic rats and *in vitro*. *Applied and Environmental Microbiology* 59, 2876–2883.

Rea, M.C., Sit, C.S., Clayton, E., O'Connor, P.M., Whittal, R.M., Zheng, J., Vederas, J.C., Ross, R.P. and Hill, C. (2010) Thuricin CD, a post-translationally modified bacteriocin with a narrow spectrum of activity against *Clostridium difficile*. *Proceedings of the National Academy of Sciences USA* 107, 9352–9357.

Rea, M.C. Ross, R.P, Cotter, P.D. and Hill. (2011) Classification of bacteriocins from Gram-positive bacteria. In: Drider, D. and Rebuffat, S. (eds) *Prokaryotic Antimicrobial Peptides*, Part 2, pp. 29–53.

Reunanen, J. and Saris, P.E.J. (2003) Microplate bioassay for nisin in foods, based on nisin-induced green fluorescent protein fluorescence. *Applied and Environmental Microbiology* 69, 4214–4218.

Rink, R., Kuipers, A., de Boef, E., Leenhouts, K.J., Driessen, A.J.M., Moll, G.N. and Kuipers, O.P. (2005) Lantibiotic structures as guidelines for the design of peptides that can be modified by lantibiotic enzymes. *Biochemistry* 44, 8873–8882.

Rink, R., Kluskens, L.D., Kuipers, A., Driessen, A.J.M., Kuipers, O.P. and Moll, G.N. (2007a) NisC, the cyclase of the lantibiotic nisin, can catalyze cyclization of designed nonlantibiotic peptides. *Biochemistry* 46, 13179–13189.

Rink, R., Wierenga, J., Kuipers, A., Kluskens, L.D., Driessen, A.J.M., Kuipers, O.P. and Moll, G.N. (2007b) Dissection and modulation of the four distinct activities of nisin by mutagenesis of rings A and B and by C-terminal truncation. *Applied and Environmental Microbiology* 73, 5809–5816.

Robson, C.L., Wescombe, P.A., Klesse, N.A. and Tagg, J.R. (2007) Isolation and partial characterization of the *Streptococcus mutans* type AII lantibiotic mutacin K8. *Microbiology* 153, 1631–1641.

Ross, K.F., Ronson, C.W. and Tagg, J.R. (1993) Isolation and characterization of the lantibiotic salivaricin A and its structural gene *salA* from *Streptococcus salivarius* 20P3. *Applied and Environmental Microbiology* 59, 2014–2021.

Ryan, M.P., Rea, M.C., Hill, C. and Ross, R.P. (1996) An application in cheddar cheese manufacture for a strain of *Lactococcus lactis* producing a novel broad-spectrum bacteriocin, lacticin 3147. *Applied and Environmental Microbiology* 62, 612–619.

Scott, J.C., Sahl, H.G., Carne, A. and Tagg, J.R. (1992) Lantibiotic-mediated anti-*Lactobacillus* activity of a vaginal *Staphylococcus aureus* isolate. *FEMS Microbiology Letters* 93, 97–102.

Seshadri, R., Kravitz, S.A., Smarr, L., Gilna, P. and Frazier, M. (2007) CAMERA: a community resource for metagenomics. *PLoS Biology* 5, 394–397.

Shotwell, O.L., Stodola, F.H., Michael, W.R., Lindenfelser, L.A., Dworschack, R.G. and Pridham, T.G. (1958) Antibiotics Against Plant Disease. III. Duramycin, a new antibiotic from *Streptomyces cinnamomeus* forma *azacoluta*. *Journal of the American Chemical Society* 80, 3912–3915.

Simpson, W.J., Ragland, N.L., Ronson, C.W. and Tagg, J.R. (1995) A lantibiotic gene family widely distributed in *Streptococcus salivarius* and *Streptococcus pyogenes*. *Developments in Biological Standardization 85, 639–643.*

Spee, J.H., Devos, W.M. and Kuipers, O.P. (1993) Efficient random mutagenesis method with adjustable mutation frequency by use of PCR and dITP. *Nucleic Acids Research* 21, 777–778.

Starosta, A.L., Qin, H.O., Mikolajka, A., Leung, G.Y.C., Schwinghammer, K., Nicolaou, K.C., Chen, D.Y.K., Cooperman, B.S. and Wilson, D.N. (2009) Identification of distinct thiopeptide-antibiotic precursor lead compounds using translation machinery assays. *Chemistry and Biology* 16, 1087–1096.

Stein, T., Borchert, S., Conrad, B., Feesche, J., Hofemeister, B., Hofemeister, J. and Entian, K.D. (2002) Two different lantibiotic-like peptides originate from the ericin gene cluster of *Bacillus subtilis* A1/3. *Journal of Bacteriology* 184, 1703–1711.

Stoffels, G., Nes, I.F. and Guthmundsdottir, A. (1992) Isolation and properties of a bacteriocin-producing *Carnobacterium piscicola* isolated from fish. *Journal of Applied Bacteriology* 73, 309–316.

Su, T.L. (1948) Micrococcin, an antibacterial substance formed by a strain of *Micrococcus*. *British Journal of Experimental Pathology* 29, 473–481.

Suda, S., Westerbeek, A., O'Connor, P.M., Ross, R.P., Hill, C. and Cotter, P.D. (2010) Effect of bioengineering lacticin 3147 lanthionine bridges on specific activity and resistance to heat and proteases. *Chemistry and Biology* 17, 1151–1160.

Sybesma, W., Hugenholtz, J., de Vos, W.M. and Smid, E.J. (2006) Safe use of genetically modified lactic acid bacteria in food. Bridging the gap between consumers, green groups, and industry. *Electronic Journal of Biotechnology* 9, 424–448.

Szekat, C., Jack, R.W., Skutlarek, D., Farber, H. and Bierbaum, G. (2003) Construction of an expression system for site-directed mutagenesis of the lantibiotic mersacidin. *Applied and Environmental Microbiology* 69, 3777–3783.

Tagg, J.R., Read, R.S. and McGiven, A.R. (1973) Bacteriocin of a group A streptococcus: partial purification and properties. *Antimicrobial Agents and Chemotherapy* 4, 214–221.

Twomey, D., Ross, R.P., Ryan, M., Meaney, B. and Hill, C. (2002) Lantibiotics produced by lactic acid bacteria: structure, function and applications. *Antonie Van Leeuwenhoek* 82, 165–185.

van Saparoea, H.B.V., Bakkes, P.J., Moll, G.N. and Driessen, A.J.M. (2008) Distinct contributions of the nisin biosynthesis enzymes NisB and NisC and transporter NisT to prenisin production by *Lactococcus lactis*. *Applied and Environmental Microbiology* 74, 5541–5548.

Vertesy, L., Aretz, W., Bonnefoy, A., Ehlers, E., Kurz, M., Markus, A., Schiell, M., Vogel, M., Wink, J. and Kogler, H. (1999) Ala(0)-actagardine, a new lantibiotic from cultures of *Actinoplanes liguriae* ATCC 31048. *Journal of Antibiotics* 52, 730–741.

Wescombe, P.A., Upton, M., Dierksen, K.P., Ragland, N.L., Sivabalan, S., Wirawan, R.E., Inglis, M.A., Moore, C.J., Walker, G.V., Chilcott, C.N., Jenkinson, H.F. and Tagg, J.R. (2006) Production of the lantibiotic salivaricin A and its variants by oral streptococci and use of a specific induction assay to detect their presence in human saliva. *Applied and Environmental Microbiology* 72, 1459–1466.

Wescombe, P.A., Upton, M., Renault, P., Wirawan, R.E., Power, D., Burton, J.P., Chilcott, C.N. and Tagg, J.R. (2011) Salivaricin 9, a new lantibiotic produced by *Streptococcus salivarius*. *Microbiology* 157, 1290–1299.

Whitehead, H.R. (1933) A substance inhibiting bacterial growth, produced by certain strains of lactic streptococci. *Biochemical Journal* 27, 1793–1800.

Wilaipun, P., Zendo, T., Okuda, K., Nakayama, J. and Sonomoto, K. (2008) Identification of the nukacin KQU-131, a new type-A(II) lantibiotic produced by *Staphylococcus hominis* KQU-131 isolated from Thai fermented fish product (Pla-ra). *Bioscience, Biotechnology and Biochemistry* 72, 2232–2235.

Wirawan, R.E., Kleese, N.A., Jack, R.W. and Tagg, J.R. (2006) Molecular and genetic characterization of a novel nisin variant produced by *Streptococcus uberis*. *Applied and Environmental Microbiology* 72, 1148–1156.

Xiao, H., Chen, X., Chen, M., Tang, S., Zhao, X. and Huan, L. (2004) Bovicin HJ50, a novel lantibiotic produced by *Streptococcus bovis* HJ50. *Microbiology* 150, 103–108.

Yonezawa, H. and Kuramitsu, H.K. (2005) Genetic analysis of a unique bacteriocin, Smb, produced by *Streptococcus mutans* GS5. *Antimicrobial Agents and Chemotherapy* 49, 541–548.

Yuan, J., Zhang, Z.Z., Chen, X.Z., Yang, W. and Huan, L.D. (2004) Site-directed mutagenesis of the hinge region of nisinZ and properties of nisinZ mutants. *Applied Microbiology and Biotechnology* 64, 806–815.

Zendo, T., Fukao, M., Ueda, K., Higuchi, T., Nakayama, J. and Sonomoto, K. (2003) Identification of the lantibiotic nisin Q, a new natural nisin variant produced by *Lactococcus lactis* 61-14 isolated from a river in Japan. *Bioscience, Biotechnology and Biochemistry* 67, 1616–1619.

12 Quantitative Structure–Activity Relationship-based Discovery of Antimicrobial Peptides Active Against Multidrug-resistant Bacteria

Christopher D. Fjell,[1] Håvard Jenssen,[2] Robert E.W. Hancock[1] and Artem Cherkasov[3]

[1]*Centre for Microbial Diseases and Immunity Research, University of British Columbia, Vancouver, British Columbia, Canada;* [2]*Department of Science, Systems and Models, Roskilde University, Roskilde, Denmark;* [3]*Prostate Centre at the Vancouver General Hospital, University of British Columbia, British Columbia, Canada*

12.1 Introduction

Antibiotic resistance among bacterial pathogens is spreading at an alarming rate in hospital environments and more recently in the community (Theuretzbacher and Toney, 2006; Hancock, 2007). Rates of drug resistance in pathogens such as methicillin-resistant *Staphylococcus aureus* (MRSA) now exceed 60% in the hospital environment, and resistance in other pathogens is also increasing rapidly. Furthermore, resistance to vancomycin and fluoroquinolones has jumped from very low incidences to about 30% in the last 10 years. Despite this alarming trend, affecting hundreds of thousands of patients, pharmaceutical companies have largely withdrawn from research into new anti-infectives (Projan, 2003), with only two structurally novel antibiotics entering the market in the last four decades (Spellberg *et al.*, 2004).

Short cationic antimicrobial peptides have drawn significant attention as a promising class of novel antibiotics, with rapid action on a broad range of bacterial strains, infrequent resistance development, and limited toxicity and immunogenicity (Hancock and Sahl, 2006; Yeung *et al.*, 2011). One peptide, MX-226, has demonstrated efficacy in limiting catheter colonization in Phase IIIa clinical trials (Hamill *et al.*, 2008). However, these molecules also have significant costs due to expensive amino acid building blocks and short half-life due to rapid degradation by proteases. In addition, we have only a modest understanding of the structural basis of antimicrobial peptide activity, due in part to one of the most intractable problems in biology: our inability to predict protein structure based on primary sequence, thus limiting rational peptide design. While interaction with cellular membrane appears essential, different peptides can result in either disruption of membrane barriers or translocation across the membrane to attack cytosolic targets (Hancock and Sahl, 2006). Most peptides are now considered 'dirty drugs' that attack multiple targets (Peschel and Sahl, 2006). Interest in peptides as antibiotics follows from the observation of more

 Antimicrobial Drug Discovery: Emerging Strategies (eds G. Tegos and E. Mylonakis)

than 1000 short cationic peptides found throughout nature and involved in antibacterial defences.

Nearly all species of life produce antimicrobial (host defence) peptides. These peptides have a variety of functions, including direct antimicrobial activity and important roles in the orchestration of innate immune and inflammatory responses in mammals, amphibians and insects (Madera *et al.*, 2010). The diversity of natural host defence peptides is indicated in Fig. 12.1 (see also Fjell *et al.*, 2007). Such peptides can possess broad spectra of direct antimicrobial activity that target bacteria, fungi, viruses and parasites (Jenssen *et al.*, 2006).

Cationic antimicrobial peptides always interact with the membrane as part of their mechanism of action (Hancock and Rozek, 2002). Key to their initial interaction with the bacterial cell membrane, these peptides are usually relatively short, from 12 to 50 amino acids, with charges ranging from +2 to +9, that can associate with negatively charged phosphate groups of lipopolysaccharide, anionic phospholipids of Gram-negative bacteria or lipotechoic acids of Gram-positive bacteria, and they contain sufficient hydrophobic amino acids (50% or more) to enable insertion into the interface of phospholipid bilayers (Brogden, 2005; Jenssen *et al.*, 2006). Thus, the initial interaction with the cell surface and contact with the membrane is an important step in the mechanism of action of all antimicrobial peptides (Hancock and Rozek, 2002).

Antimicrobial peptides can form a variety of secondary structure configurations: α-helical, β-sheet, β-turn, loop or extended structures. In the case of extended (unstructured) peptides, these probably form organized structures upon interaction with lipid bilayers. For example, indolicidin is unstructured in solution and takes on a boat-like structure when inserting into a membrane-like environment (Rozek *et al.*, 2000). This flexibility has been proposed as a mechanism that allows a single peptide to interact with

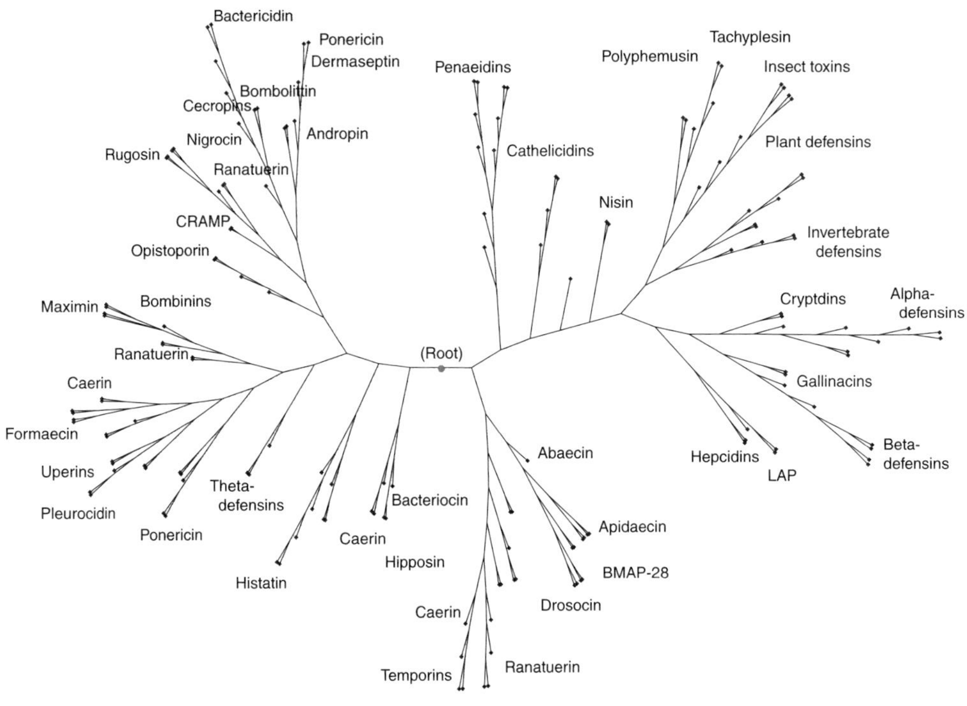

Fig. 12.1. Phylogenetic tree of known antimicrobial peptides.

more than one target such as intracellular DNA, in addition to initial interactions with a membrane (Hsu *et al.*, 2005). Some peptides do not fall into any particular structural classification and can contain a combination of α-helix and β-sheet domains (Uteng *et al.*, 2003). Regardless of specific secondary structure, antimicrobial peptides tend to generate structures with an amphipathic character, with distinct hydrophobic and hydrophilic domains, upon association with a lipid bilayer (Yeaman and Yount, 2003; Brogden, 2005; Jenssen *et al.*, 2006). While the initial interaction relies on electrostatic attraction, subsequent steps are driven by a combination of hydrophobic and electrostatic forces (Jenssen *et al.*, 2006).

The field of cheminformatics involves computer-aided identification of new lead structures and their optimization into drug candidates (Engel, 2006). One of the most broadly used cheminformatics approaches is quantitative structure–activity relationship (QSAR) modelling, which seeks to relate the characteristics of a molecule (through a series of descriptors and mathematical formalism) to its measurable properties, such as biological activity. QSAR analysis has found a broad application in antimicrobial discovery. Early studies of antimicrobial peptides using QSAR modelling focused on variants of three natural peptides (lactoferricin, protegrin and bactenecin) using descriptors including measured properties, such as HPLC retention time and circular dichroism spectroscopy, and calculated properties, such charge and molecular weight (reviewed by Hilpert *et al.*, 2008). In a series of pilot studies, we utilized a variety of chemical descriptors in combination with linear modelling methods such as principal component analysis and partial least-squares projections to successfully predict the antimicrobial activity of limited sets of sequence-specific cationic peptides (Jenssen *et al.*, 2007). These models explicitly relate a series of input descriptors to an output prediction of activity to permit an understanding of structure–activity relationships. However, when we applied these prediction methods separately to two individual libraries of peptides based on templates of the same size and composition but scrambled sequence, we were not able to extrapolate the derived relationships for one library to predict, with any significant accuracy, the activity of peptides in the other library (Jenssen *et al.*, 2008).

Until recently, an insufficient number of peptides with antibacterial activity was available, limiting the ability to relate structure to activity. However the breakthrough application of peptide arrays involving synthesis on cellulose membranes combined with rapid screening technologies has yielded libraries of hundreds of peptides with wide sequence diversity at substantially reduced costs (Hilpert *et al.*, 2005). Such libraries with hundreds of variant peptides have enabled more complex analysis of activity than was possible previously.

Historically, only a few peptide properties have been the focus of antimicrobial peptide design, particularly charge, hydrophobicity and amphipathicity due to their obvious relationship to activity (see above). It has proven impossible, however, to create high-potency small peptides by simple manipulation of the amino acid sequence (Tossi *et al.*, 2000). Structure–activity relationship data for the α-helical peptides (Fig. 12.2 for example) identified at least seven parameters that can influence the potency and spectrum of activity. These include: (i) size; (ii) sequence; (iii) degree of structuring (percentage helical content); (iv) charge; (v) overall hydrophobicity; (vi) amphipathicity; and (vii) respective dimensions of the hydrophobic and hydrophilic faces of the helix. These properties are intimately linked, and therefore modifications intended to enhance one property will necessarily impact on the others. Furthermore, the relative contributions of each of these properties and whether these are the only important design features has never been clear.

12.1.1 QSARs

QSAR-based methodology relates quantitative properties (descriptors) of a given compound, as a surrogate of three-dimensional structure, to a measurable property such as biological activity or toxicity. While

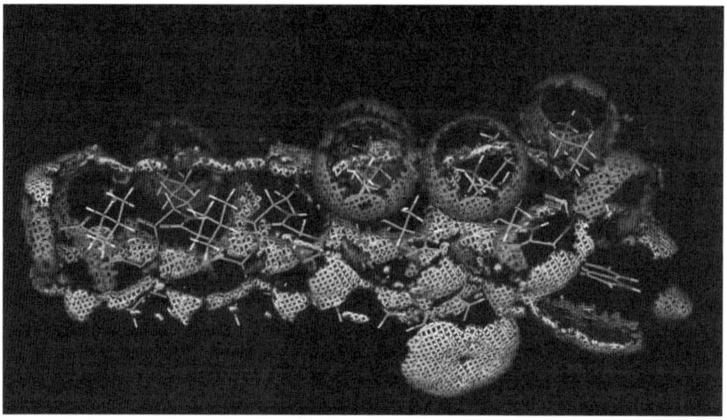

Fig. 12.2. Structure of an α-helical antimicrobial peptide. The peptide IKWLKIFL α-helical structure is shown as an example of separation of charged and hydrophobic regions. Dark grey indicates regions of positive charge and light grey indicates regions of hydrophobicity.

QSAR methods have been used extensively in drug discovery programmes (Perkins *et al.*, 2003), their use for antimicrobial peptides has been reported only relatively recently (Fjell *et al.*, 2009; Cherkasov *et al.*, 2009).

QSAR modelling of cationic antimicrobial peptides involves two major aspects: the selection of QSAR descriptors and the choice of analysis technique to relate descriptor values to antibacterial activity. Descriptors that have been used for QSAR analysis of antibacterial peptides can be divided into two main categories: empirical and computable. A large number of computable QSAR descriptors suitable for small molecules have been reported in the literature and are available within molecular modelling packages (e.g. Molecular Operating Environment, 2005, Chemical Computing Group Inc., Montreal, Canada). Many statistical learning methods are also available to relate descriptors to the detectable activity. Thus, regression models predict the activity of a peptide as a continuous variable such as minimum inhibitory concentration (MIC), while classification models describe peptides as just active or inactive. Primarily, linear regression methods have been used for modelling the activity of antimicrobial peptides in combination with principal component analysis (PCA) and projections to latent structures (PLS) approaches (Jenssen *et al.*, 2008). More complex (non-linear) models such as artificial neural networks (ANNs) give superior predictions but do not clearly relate input descriptors to activity. Some researchers have favoured linear models such as multiple linear regression and PCA because they yield models that explicitly relate the input descriptors to the output prediction of activity; however, they do so at the cost of poorer performance (Weaver, 2004).

12.1.2 'Inductive' QSAR descriptors

The QSAR descriptors originally used for modelling of antimicrobial peptides often required a high degree of similarity between peptides. More general QSAR descriptors have been developed recently that define properties sensitive to the three-dimensional structure of peptides, including 'inductive' QSAR descriptors among others (reviewed by Cherkasov, 2005a). Previously, 'inductive' QSAR descriptors were successfully applied to a number of molecular modelling studies including quantification of the antibacterial activity of organic compounds (Cherkasov, 2005b), prediction of other molecular properties (Cherkasov, 2003) and small-compound lead discovery (Karakoc *et al.*, 2006a). These descriptors were applied to classification of compounds using a variety of different modelling methods, including ANNs, *k*-nearest neighbours, linear discriminative analysis and multiple linear regression. It has been found that ANNs generally result in more accurate predictions, followed closely by *k*-nearest neighbours methods (Karakoc *et al.*, 2006b).

12.2 Modelling of Peptide Activity

The overall process we have used for QSAR modelling of antimicrobial peptides is shown in Fig. 12.3 (Cherkasov *et al.*, 2009; Fjell *et al.*, 2009). The starting point was a set of semi-random peptides with measured activity. For these peptides, the three-dimensional structure of each peptide was approximated through the calculation of QSAR descriptors. Models for peptide activity were built using ANNs based on these descriptors and the known levels of activity. These models were then used to computationally assess the predicted activity a much larger set of virtual peptides that were constructed based on the amino acid preferences of the best peptides in the original test set. We assessed the accuracy of the predictions by synthesizing and testing peptides with various levels of predicted activity.

12.2.1 Effect of control antibacterial peptides on bacteria

The effect of treatment of *Pseudomonas aeruginosa* with the active control peptide

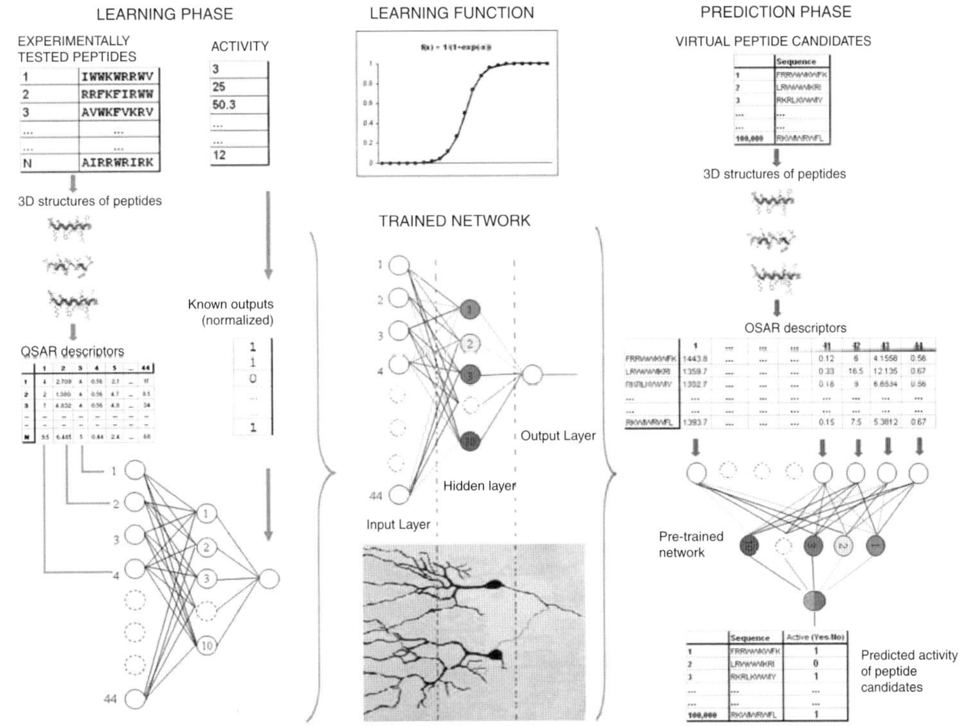

Fig. 12.3. General workflow for QSAR modelling of antimicrobial peptides. (Reproduced from Fjell *et al.*, 2009.)

Bac2A (a synthetic peptide analogue of bovine bactenecin) is shown in transmission electron micrographs of thin sections of *P. aeruginosa* in Fig. 12.4. These electron micrographs showed that Bac2A has a dramatic effect on the morphology of the bacterial cell wall. While the cell wall of control untreated bacteria appears smooth and linear, the Bac2A-treated bacteria had cell walls that were severely damaged, a well-known phenomenon observed when bacterial cells are exposed to cationic peptides (Sawyer *et al.*, 1988). In addition, the periplasmic space between the cell wall and cytoplasmic membrane appeared swollen. The blebs of the cell wall could be better appreciated when the surface of Bac2A-treated bacteria was visualized by scanning electron microscopy (Fjell *et al.*, 2009) (Fig. 12.5).

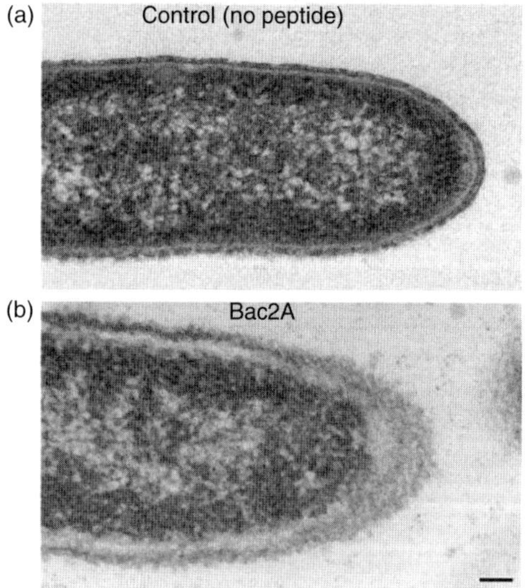

Fig. 12.4. Transmission electron micrographs of cross-sections of *Pseudomonas aeruginosa*. Micrographs are shown for control untreated (a) and Bac2A-treated (b) organisms. Bac2A was used at the MIC. Bacteria were incubated with Bac2A for 1 h at 37°C before fixation and preparation for embedding and thin-section transmission electron microscopy. Bar, 100 nm. (Reproduced from Fjell *et al.*, 2009.)

12.2.2 Peptide data sets for model training

Two initial sets of synthetic peptides of nine amino acids in length were iteratively designed and assayed for antibacterial activity: set A (933 peptides) and set B (500 peptides). The primary sequences of set A were chosen with a bias towards enrichment for the amino acid proportions of the most active peptides found in previous studies (Hilpert *et al.*, 2005). Subsequently, set B peptides were designed with the adjusted amino acid compositions of the initial and set A peptides, as shown in Fig. 12.6. In both sets, there were no constraints on the amino acid proportions found within any particular peptide. The sets were prepared by synthesis on a cellulose support and assayed for activity against *P. aeruginosa* using a luciferase reporter assay, as described previously (Hilpert *et al.*, 2005).

12.2.3 Calculation of peptide activity

Peptide antibacterial activity was measured using a luminescence assay, which assesses the loss of energy generation capacity (required for light production from plasmid-encoded LuxCDABE proteins) and with antimicrobial peptides proportionately reflects lethality (Hilpert *et al.*, 2005). Briefly, peptides were assayed in a dilution series in sets of ten peptides with one control peptide Bac2A per series. Luminescence values for the experimental peptides were fitted to a function describing the expected profile of luminescence for a dilution series (Fig. 12.7). The relative 50% inhibitory concentration (Rel. IC_{50}) values of the experimental peptides were calculated as the ratio of the IC_{50} values for the peptide compared with that of the control peptide Bac2A. The fit of the luminescence experimental values was generally good except for peptides of very low activity for which the plateau at low luminescence (high concentration) was not present. For this reason, inactive peptides were identified as those peptides for which the luminescence at the highest

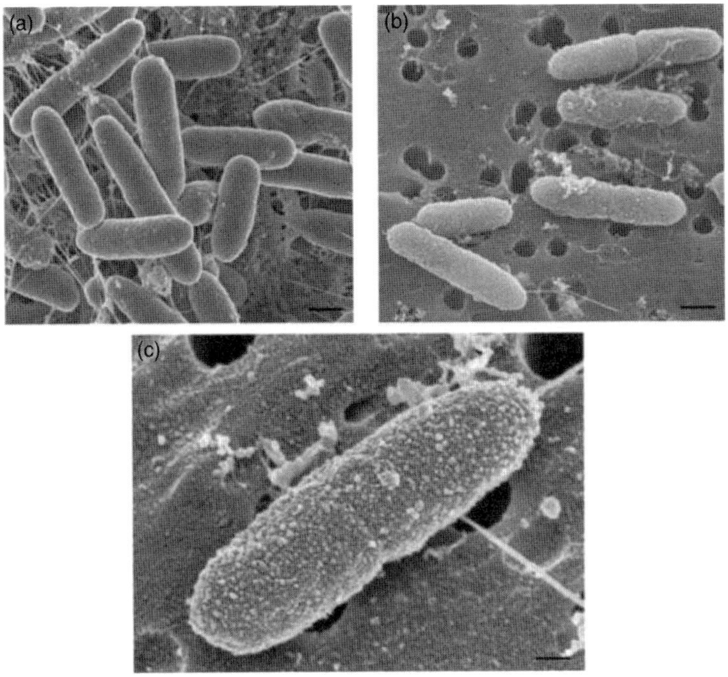

Fig. 12.5. Scanning electron micrographs of *Pseudomonas aeruginosa*. Micrographs are shown for control untreated (a) and Bac2A-treated (b, c) organisms. Bac2A was used at the MIC. Bacteria were incubated with Bac2A for 1 h at 37°C before fixation and preparation for scanning electron microscopy. Bars, 500 nm (a, b); 100 nm (c). (Reproduced from Fjell *et al.*, 2009.)

concentration of peptide was greater than 50% of the luminescence in the absence of peptide; for these peptides, the Rel. IC_{50} value was set to 25 (the approximate lower limit of activity that could be observed). The activity of the two sets is shown in Table 12.1 (Training Set A and B rows) classified into higher activity (Rel. IC_{50} is less than 50% of the control peptide, Bac2A), similar activity (Rel. IC_{50} is between 50 and 150% of control) and lower activity (Rel. IC_{50} greater than 150% of control).

12.2.4 QSAR descriptors and model building

A large number of QSAR descriptors are available to describe the physical chemistry of compounds. A total of 77 descriptors were calculated for each peptide in the two training sets. Some descriptor values were found to be highly correlated with each other, which led to problems in modelling; therefore, a set of 44 descriptors were chosen that showed less than 95% correlation to any other selected descriptor (Cherkasov *et al.*, 2009). We used ANNs to model antibacterial activity, as this had already been successfully demonstrated for small molecules (e.g. Karakoc *et al.*, 2006b). Neural networks typically rank highly among machine-learning techniques in predictive performance and, in addition, they are relatively insensitive to the presence of noise and correlated inputs. We used a network configuration with one hidden layer of ten nodes, 44 input nodes (one for each descriptor) and one output node. A variety of other network configurations were also evaluated and showed no improvement in performance (data not shown).

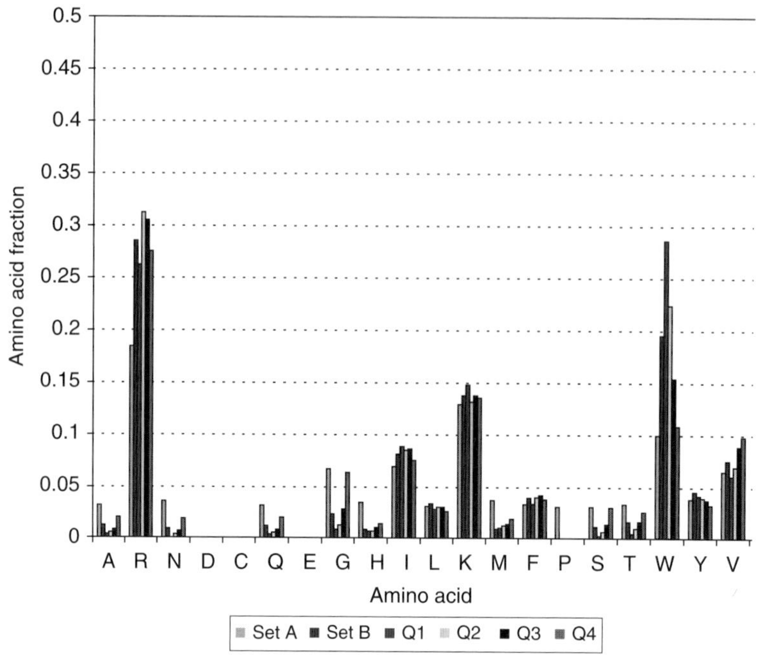

Fig. 12.6. Distribution of amino acids in training and test sets. The quartiles of the activity for the test peptides are indicated as Q1–Q4. (Reproduced from Cherkasov *et al.*, 2009.)

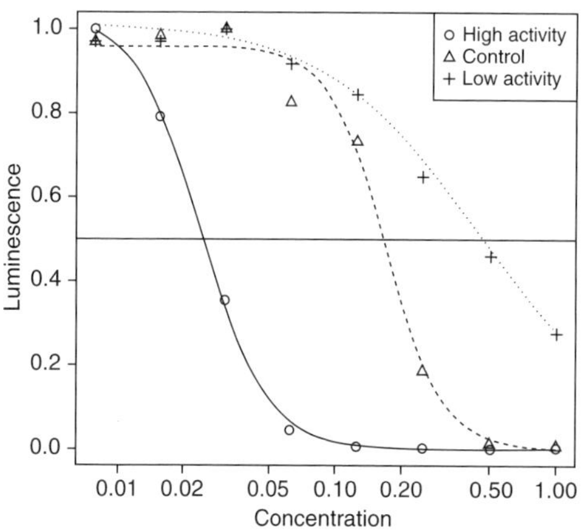

Fig. 12.7. Luminescence profile of a dilution series for three peptides. The luminescence for three peptides having high, medium (control peptide) and low activity are shown. Luminescence and concentration were scaled to a maximum of 1.0. The value at which the horizontal line at luminescence of 0.5 crosses the fitted curves indicates the relative IC_{50} value for each peptide. (Reproduced from Fjell *et al.*, 2009.)

12.2.5 Validation of model performance

The ability of ANN models to predict antibacterial activity was assessed by first classifying the top 5% of the set A and B peptides as active according to the Rel. IC_{50} values – this corresponded to an approximate Rel. IC_{50} threshold of 0.6 (0.56 for set A and 0.61 for set B). A tenfold cross-validation was performed as described below, with 90% of the data allocated to training and 10% to validation (reserving a different 10% for each of the ten validation sets). Sets A and B were synthesized and assayed at different times, and we observed some systematic differences in the luminescence results related to peptides of very low and very high activity. Therefore, we treated sets A and B separately, as well as analysing the pooled set, set A+B. The performance of the three models was assessed using the area under the receiver operating characteristics curves (AROCs). AROC values approaching 1 indicate an increasing ability

Table 12.1. Activities of peptides from training sets and quartiles in the 100,000 test set. (Reproduced from Fjell *et al.*, 2009.)

	Rel. IC_{50}			
Data set	Higher activity (<0.5)	Similar activity (0.5–1.5)	Lower activity (>1.5)	Median
Set A	35 (3.8%)	210 (22.5%)	688 (73.7%)	2.12
Set B	14 (2.8%)	114 (22.8%)	372 (74.4%)	3.33
Q1	47 (94%)	2 (4%)	1 (2%)	0.23
Q2	32 (64%)	15 (30%)	4 (8%)	0.35
Q3	1 (2%)	5 (10%)	44 (88%)	4.38
Q4	0 (0%)	0 (0%)	50 (100%)	8.34

Numbers of peptides with various levels of antibacterial activity are shown. Q1, top of predicted first quartile; Q2, top of second quartile; Q3, bottom of third quartile; Q4, bottom of fourth quartile. Rel. IC_{50} is the relative IC_{50}, the ratio of the IC_{50} for the experimental peptide to the IC_{50} of Bac2A.

to accurately classify data, while AROC values close to 0.5 indicate a poor ability to classify the data. The mean AROC values for sets A, B and A+B were found to be 0.87 ± 0.10, 0.83 ± 0.12 and 0.80 ± 0.09 (means ± SD), respectively. These data showed that the cross-validated performance of the models to predict peptide activity was quite good. We integrated the large number of models generated during the cross-validation in a consensus approach to allow a combined, single prediction for a given peptide. This was done using a 'voting' system where each of the 30 models (ten each for set A, B and A+B) was used to evaluate a test peptide.

12.2.6 Independent model testing

To perform an independent assessment of this approach to identify highly active antibacterial peptides, a random set of approximately 100,000 peptides was created as an independent test set, using the same global amino acid proportions as set B. When the 44 QSAR descriptors were calculated for each peptide, a modest number of peptides (423) fell more than 15% outside the range of descriptor values encountered in sets A and B and were not considered further, as inclusion of such data is believed to lead to a less reliable performance of the models. This left a total of 99,577 test peptides. Each of these peptides was ranked numerically using the voting system described above. As these models were built to classify peptides as active or inactive, rather than to predict actual activity levels, the ranked list of test peptides indicated the relative likelihood that a peptide was highly active.

To independently evaluate these predictions of peptide activity, we selected and synthesized a total of 200 candidate peptides comprising sets of 50 candidate peptides at four positions of ranking. Quartile 1 (Q1) peptides were ranked in the top 50 positions and considered the most likely to be more active than the control. Quartile 2 (Q2) peptides were ranked at the start of the second quartile, positions 24,895–24,944, and thus considered likely to be more active than the control. Quartile 3 (Q3) peptides were ranked at the end of the third quartile, positions 74,633–74,682, and considered likely to be less active than the control. Quartile 4 (Q4) peptides were ranked at the end of the fourth quartile, positions 99,528–99,577, and considered to be most likely to be less active than the control. These 200 predicted peptides were synthesized and assayed for activity using the luminescence assay. As summarized in Table 12.1, the activity was predicted very accurately by the system. Of the 50 peptides in the most likely active set (Q1), 94% were found to be more active than the control. Of the set considered less likely to be active (Q2), 64% were better than the control. Of the peptides predicted to be much less active (Q3), 88% had lower activity than the control. In the set considered least likely to be active (Q4), all peptides (100%)

were less active than the control. Critically, the peptides in Q1 and Q2 far outperformed the peptides synthesized in sets A and B.

Interestingly, despite the very large difference in predicted activities, the peptides in each quartile had rather similar bulk physical properties (charge, hydrophobicity and hydrophobic moment), indicating the importance of using a broad variety of descriptors in neural network modelling. Ten peptides from each quartile are shown in Table 12.2 for discussion. Consistent with the bulk features of the entire library of sequences, for these peptides the charge and hydrophobicity showed a large degree of overlap for most quartiles (Fig. 12.8). Only certain of the peptides from Q4 showed a noticeable difference in these physical properties, specifically in showing a lower charge and hydrophobicity. The importance of charge, hydrophobicity and amphipathicity for antibacterial activity of peptides is well known (Yeaman and Yount, 2003; Jenssen *et al.*, 2006). However, in these groups of peptides, there was a clear difference only between the most active and least active sets (Q1 and Q4) in terms of charge and hydrophobicity, while the differences in activity across all quartiles were quite dramatic. A graphic example that these properties are by themselves insufficient to make predictions can be observed by comparing peptides 10 (KRWWKWIRW) and 74,675 (WRFKVLRQR), which have very similar values for charge (+4), hydrophobicity (0.56 and 0.44, respectively) and hydrophobic moment (a measure of amphipathicity; 4.65 and 4.2, respectively) but have relative IC_{50} values that differ by more than 100-fold (0.04 and 7.1, respectively). This demonstrates that success in predictive modelling is not based on identifying potent peptides using previously known characteristics.

12.2.7 Antibacterial activity of predicted peptides against resistant strains

A selection of 18 of these 200 peptides were synthesized in bulk and tested against a large variety of highly drug-resistant bacterial pathogens (Table 12.3) representing the so-called 'superbugs' plaguing society. A total of 13 peptides from Q1 and Q2 with high activity, and five peptides from Q3 with low activity were evaluated for their *in vitro* effect (measured as MIC) against several multidrug-resistant and problematic pathogens including strains of multidrug-resistant *P. aeruginosa*, MRSA, *Enterobacter cloacae* with derepressed chromosomal β-lactamase, extended-spectrum β-lactamase (ESBL)-producing *Escherichia coli* and *Klebsiella pneumoniae*, and vancomycin-resistant *Enterococcus faecalis* and *Enterococcus faecium*. All 15 peptides belonging to Q1 and Q2 had significant *in vitro* inhibitory activity against antibiotic-resistant bacteria. Moreover, some peptides from Q1, such as peptides 8 and 9, exhibited MICs of 0.3–10 μM against most of the tested superbugs, comparing favourably to the only antimicrobial peptide to show efficacy to date in advanced clinical trials, MX-226 (Hancock and Sahl, 2006), which exhibited MICs of 10–76 μM (Cherkasov *et al.*, 2009). These results characterize the developed peptides as excellent antibiotic candidates for treating some of the most recalcitrant and dangerous human infections. Two other peptides identified from Q1 (ranked 10 and 36) were found to be protective against *S. aureus* infection in animal models (Cherkasov *et al.*, 2009).

It is interesting to note that two of the peptides that had high potency (peptides 45 and 48 in Table 12.3) were active against a large number of the drug-resistant strains but had poor activity against one vancomycin-resistant organism (column R) but were active against another vancomycin-resistant organism (column T). It seems likely that this resistance is due to mechanisms different from those for the conventional antibiotics. For example, β-lactamase would not be expected to inactivate these peptides as they do not contain β-lactam rings.

12.3 Efficient Computational Searching by Genetic Algorithms

A common problem in drug discovery is that an exhaustive search is not possible due to the massive numbers of possible peptide variants (x^{20}, where x is the number of amino acids in

Table 12.2. Predicted activity rank and experimental Rel. IC_{50} values for selected test peptides. (Reproduced from Fjell *et al.*, 2009.)

Peptide number	Quartile	Sequence	Cumulative vote	Average rank	Rel. IC_{50}	Charge	Hydrophobicity	Hydrophobic moment
1	1	RWRWKRWWW	29	2027	0.25	4	0.56	1.48
2	1	RWRRWKVWW	29	2707	0.40	4	0.56	1.96
3	1	RWWRWRKWW	29	2729	0.28	4	0.56	2.11
4	1	RWRRKWWWW	28	2831	0.39	4	0.56	2.75
5	1	RWRWWKRWY	28	3044	0.20	4	0.56	2.86
6	1	RRKRWWWWW	27	2434	0.43	4	0.56	1.22
7	1	RWRIKRWWW	27	2589	0.12	4	0.56	1.84
8	1	KIWWWWRKR	27	2622	0.13	4	0.56	2.06
9	1	RWRRWKWWL	27	3201	0.08	4	0.56	2.12
10	1	KRWWKWIRW	27	3660	0.04	4	0.56	4.65
51	2	IRMWVKRWR	0	13255	0.61	4	0.56	4.24
52	2	RIWYWYKRW	0	13263	0.36	3	0.67	4.06
53	2	FRRWWKWFK	0	13275	0.12	4	0.56	5.40
54	2	RVRWWKKRW	0	13278	0.27	5	0.44	2.27
55	2	RLKKVRWWW	0	13318	0.34	4	0.56	1.16
56	2	RWWLKIRKW	0	13319	0.18	4	0.56	3.85
57	2	LRWWWIKRI	0	13336	0.33	3	0.67	0.99
58	2	TRKVWWWRW	0	13336	0.76	3	0.56	0.78
59	2	KRFWIWFWR	0	13347	3.04	3	0.67	4.11
60	2	KKRWVWVIR	0	13348	0.35	4	0.56	2.92
141	3	KIRRKVRWG	0	67295	10.55	5	0.33	2.02
142	3	AIRRWRIRK	0	67295	4.62	5	0.44	5.94
143	3	WRFKVLRQR	0	67297	7.08	4	0.44	4.20
144	3	RSGKKRWRR	0	67298	6.50	6	0.11	4.66
145	3	FMWVYRYKK	0	67298	1.51	3	0.67	1.81
146	3	RGKYIRWRK	0	67298	3.83	5	0.33	4.94
147	3	WVKVWKYTW	0	67298	5.64	2	0.67	2.41
148	3	VVLKIVRRF	0	67298	25.00	3	0.67	1.86
149	3	GKFYKVWVR	0	67298	1.21	3	0.56	5.39
150	3	SWYRTRKRV	0	67299	6.66	4	0.33	4.24
191	4	GRIGGKNVR	0	98644	9.12	3	0.22	4.30

Continued

Table 12.2. Continued.

Peptide number	Quartile	Sequence	Cumulative vote	Average rank	Rel. IC_{50}	Charge	Hydrophobicity	Hydrophobic moment
192	4	NKTGYRWRN	0	98701	8.33	3	0.22	2.75
193	4	VSGNWRGSR	0	98756	8.54	2	0.22	2.67
194	4	GWGGKRRNF	0	98807	7.38	3	0.22	1.13
195	4	KNNRRWQGR	0	98885	6.45	4	0.11	2.88
196	4	GRTMGNGRW	0	98946	6.93	2	0.22	1.40
197	4	GRQISWGRT	0	98949	8.04	2	0.22	1.94
198	4	GGRGTRWHG	0	99178	8.60	3	0.11	2.63
199	4	GVRSWSQRT	0	99185	8.50	2	0.22	2.56
200	4	GSRRFGWNR	0	99199	8.10	3	0.22	0.58

Forty peptides are shown for discussion, taken from the boundaries of the quartiles of the 200 total test peptides. Hydrophobic moment was assessed according to the Eisenberg scale.

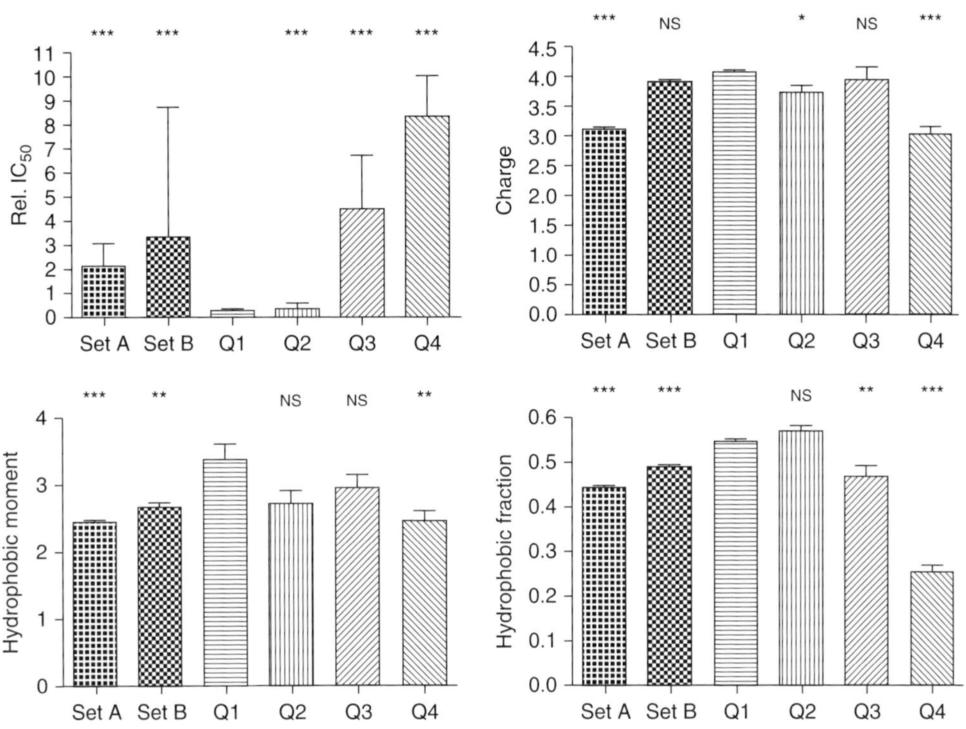

Fig. 12.8. Activity and properties of training and test peptides. Peptide antibacterial activity and physical properties are shown. For Rel. IC_{50} values, these are median values with error bars indicating interquartile range. For all others, these are means with error bars indicating SEM. Top left, median values of Rel. IC_{50} from the training sets A and B and the corresponding median values for 200 experimentally tested peptides separated into activity quartiles, Q1–Q4; top right, median values of formal charge; bottom left, amphipathicity (expressed as hydrophobic moment in Eisenberg units); bottom right, hydrophobic fraction. The statistical significance of difference in means from Q1 values is indicated (NS, not significant; *, $P < 0.05$; **, $P < 0.01$; ***, $P < 0.001$) using a two-tailed Mann–Witney test calculated using GraphPad Prism 4.03. (Reproduced from Fjell *et al.*, 2009.)

the peptide chain) and the time and resources needed for QSAR descriptor calculations. We considered that it would be advantageous to utilize a search strategy that would minimize the number of peptides that need to be evaluated to determine additional highly active peptides. Therefore, genetic algorithms were applied to this problem, as these evolutionary methods have been utilized successfully in other areas of chemoinformatics (Parrill, 1996; Niculescu, 2003; Solmajer and Zupan, 2004; Weaver, 2004). A genetic algorithm is an heuristic method for search and approximation problems and is particularly well suited for problems involving string-like data such as the amino acids in a peptide. Genetic algorithms operate on populations of solutions by iteratively enhancing solutions using operations inspired by natural genetic processes: cross-overs (combining parts of two solutions to suggest another) and mutations (randomly changing one part of a solution to generate another). Each solution ('phenotype' in the jargon of genetic algorithms) is composed of elements ('genes') that are randomly modified ('mutated') or shuffled with other solutions ('crossed over') and evaluated for fitness at each iteration ('generation'). The best solutions are propagated into the next iteration with new solutions added to the population produced based on modifications and combinations of these best peptides. We have demonstrated that a genetic algorithm approach effectively minimizes the number of peptides that must

Table 12.3. Activities against multi-resistant superbugs of selected peptides predicted through the QSAR analysis compared with the peptide Bac2A. (Reproduced from Fjell *et al.*, 2009.)

		MIC (μM)									
Peptide ID	Sequence	A	H	I	J	M	N	O	P	R	T
Bac2A	RLARIVVIRVAR	48	3.0	24	24	192	24	24	12	48	3.0
8	KIWWWWRKR	5.9	3.0	94	12	47	5.9	5.9	24	94	1.5
9	RWRRWKWWL	2.9	0.7	5.8	5.7	11	2.9	2.9	23	92	1.4
10	KRWWKWIRW	0.8	0.4	3.0	1.5	6.2	3.0	1.5	12	49	1.5
20	WRWWKIWKR	5.9	0.8	12	5.9	24	3.0	3.0	24	94	1.5
36	KRWWKWWRR	0.7	1.4	11	5.4	22	2.9	1.4	43	174	1.3
45	WKRWWKKWR	23	1.4	93	23	46	5.8	5.8	93	>186	5.8
48	WKKWWKRRW	23	1.4	23	23	46	1.4	2.9	93	>186	5.8
24,897	FRRWWKWFK	1.5	0.8	24	12	24	1.5	3.0	24	97	6.1
24,901	LRWWWIKRI	13	3.2	50	25	50	6.3	6.3	13	25	1.5
24,910	RKRLKWWIY	25	3.2	13	6.3	50	6.3	6.3	50	202	3.2
24,913	KKRWVWIRY	25	1.6	25	25	51	13	13	25	102	6.4
24,915	KWKIFRRWW	12	1.5	6	24	97	3.1	3.1	24	97	6.1
24,919	RKWIWRWFL	6.1	1.5	3	1.5	3.1	3.1	3.1	6.1	24	3.1
24,921	IWWKWRRWV	6.0	1.5	6	24	12	3.0	3.0	24	48	3.0
24,944	RRFKFIRWW	6.1	0.8	12	12	49	6.1	6.1	12	49	6.1
74,655	AVWKFVKRV	240	60	>240	240	>240	240	240	>240	>240	120
74,658	AWRFKNIRK	>223	>223	>223	>223	>223	>223	>223	>223	>223	223
74,665	KRIMKLKMR	>226	>226	>226	>226	>226	>226	>226	>226	>226	>226
74,674	AIRRWRIRK	>217	108	108	108	>217	54	54	>217	>217	14
74,680	VVLKIVRRF	>241	60	241	>241	>241	241	241	241	>241	60

Peptides from the top quartile (8 to 48) were compared with peptides from the second (24,897 to 24,944) and third (74,655 to 74,680) quartiles. Peptide ID indicates the control Bac2A or the test peptide by rank number. Columns give MIC values (μM) measured in three to five replicates for *Pseudomonas aeruginosa* wild-type strain H103 (A); *Pseudomonas maltophilia* ATCC 13637 (H); constitutive class C chromosomal β-lactamase-expressing *Enterobacter cloacae* 218R (I); Extended-spectrum β-lactamase-producing (ESBL) *Escherichia coli* clinical strain 63103 (J); ESBL-resistant *Klebsiella pneumoniae* clinical strain 63575 (M); *Staphylococcus aureus* ATCC 25923 (N); methicillin-resistant *S. aureus* strain C623 (O); *Enterococcus faecalis* ATCC 29212 (P); vancomycin-resistant *E. faecalis* clinical isolate f43559 (VanB) (R); vancomycin-resistant *Enterococcus faecium* clinical isolate t62764 (VanB) (T).

be evaluated for *in silico* screening of synthetic antimicrobial peptides with high potency (Fjell *et al.*, 2011).

A genetic algorithm solution requires that the problem be described in terms of a genetic representation, and a fitness function must be specified to permit evaluation of each solution. The genetic algorithm then passes high-fitness individuals on to the next generation, removes low-fitness individuals and creates new offspring by cross-over of two existing individuals or by mutation of an existing individual. Examples of mutation and cross-over that showed dramatic changes on peptide fitness are shown in Fig. 12.9, whereby mutation of one amino acid (V to I) increased fitness from 21 to 26, and where cross-over by combining portions of two peptides with fitness 20 yielded a peptide with fitness 0.

12.3.1 Evaluation of peptide fitness score

In our previous studies, described above, we created a software system to predict the activity of 9-amino-acid peptides. This system was constructed to make maximum use of the available experimental data by utilizing models produced by a stratified tenfold cross-validation and consisted of a set of 30 ANN models derived from the two data sets of screened peptides plus the combined set. These represented classification models trained to consider the top 5% as active. Our confidence that a peptide would be active can be judged by the number of models that classified the peptide as active. As reported previously, the accuracy of predicting peptide activity is strongest when the largest

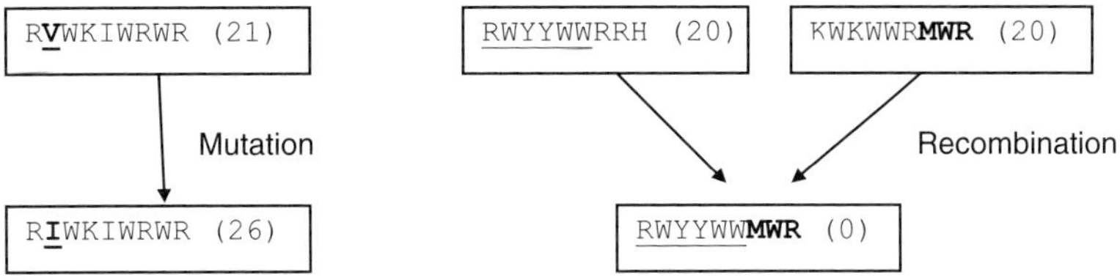

Fig. 12.9. Examples of peptide evolution. Two examples of peptide evolution are shown: mutation of a single amino acid that resulted in an improved peptide, and recombination of two moderate-scoring peptides to form one low-scoring peptide. Values in parentheses are the fitness scores for the peptides. (Reproduced from Fjell *et al.*, 2011.)

Table 12.4. Initial peptide populations for simulations A and B. (Reproduced from Fjell *et al.*, 2011.)

Simulation A		Simulation B	
Sequence	Score	Sequence	Score
KKWWYWWKR	20	ARKWWWRWK	2
KWKRWFKWR	21	AWWRKRKWW	2
KWKWWRMWR	20	FVKRWWRFR	2
MWRKWRRWW	21	IGWWWRKRW	2
RKKWWWLFR	21	IWKRWWRKT	2
RLKWWRWRW	21	KNWKWWRWR	2
RRWRWWWVW	21	KRRSWWKWW	2
RRWWWRLWW	21	KRWRWLRWG	2
RRWWWRRWY	21	KWWRWRRFI	2
RVWKIWRWR	21	QRRRWWWWK	2
RWIRKIWWR	21	RLIRWWIRK	2
RWIWWRRWW	21	RRKRLYWIW	2
RWRWWGWRR	20	RRRWYWKWN	2
RWRWWWKKT	20	RRWRIWWIK	2
RWWRWWKQR	20	RTYKRWYRW	2
RWWWWSRRR	20	RWIRWWRQW	2
RWYYWWRRH	20	RWRHIWWRW	2
RYRWWKWRH	20	RWWKWRWLM	2
TWWWKKWRR	20	RWYKHWRFR	2
		SRWWKRRWY	2
		VKRWWWRRM	2
		WWRKLWRKL	2

Peptides were chosen from a set of biased random sequences that had a score of 20 or 21 in simulation A (moderate confidence in activity) or a fitness score of 2 (low confidence in activity). Peptides were selected to have diverse amino acids populations.

numbers of models predicted activity: for example, for the top 50 peptides predicted out of a set of 100,000 amino-acid-biased semi-random peptides, the number of models indicating high activity ranged from 25 to 29. For these peptides, the accuracy of predicting highly active peptides was 94%. This number of models indicating high activity was therefore taken as the genetic algorithm fitness score.

12.3.2 Initial population of peptides

Genetic algorithm searches were executed, starting from two initial populations of peptides for two purposes (Table 12.4). First, we wished to identify additional peptides with very high fitness scores to evaluate the ability of genetic algorithms to identify novel peptides for screening by antibacterial activity assays. Secondly, we wished to understand the importance of the selected starting population on the composition of later peptide populations within a search. Both sets of peptides were selected from the biased random set of 100,000 peptides described above (Cherkasov *et al.*, 2009) at different levels of fitness score. For the first search (simulation A), we selected peptides that were moderately predicted to be active, having a fitness value of 20 or 21. Peptides were selected to provide a small initial population that maximized the diversity of amino acids present in the peptides with this level of initial fitness score, by ensuring that all amino acids present in the library were present at least to some degree in these peptides. An initial set of 19 peptides was selected that included all of the 12 amino acids present in the 594 peptides of the 100,000 having a fitness value of 20 or 21. As some amino acids had low representation (only one peptide containing each of G, Q and S, and two for H), we decided to use a small population to minimize the effect of the relatively large numbers of certain other amino acids in the population. Similarly, the initial peptides for simulation B were selected to have a fitness score of 2, a low score indicating low confidence that these are highly active peptides.

12.3.3 Iterative improvement in peptides

The two populations were evolved from separate initial starting populations in simulations A and B. For both simulations, there was rapid improvement in scores from the first generation to generation 100, with continued improvement up to generation 600 (Fig. 12.10). In addition, there was a rapid

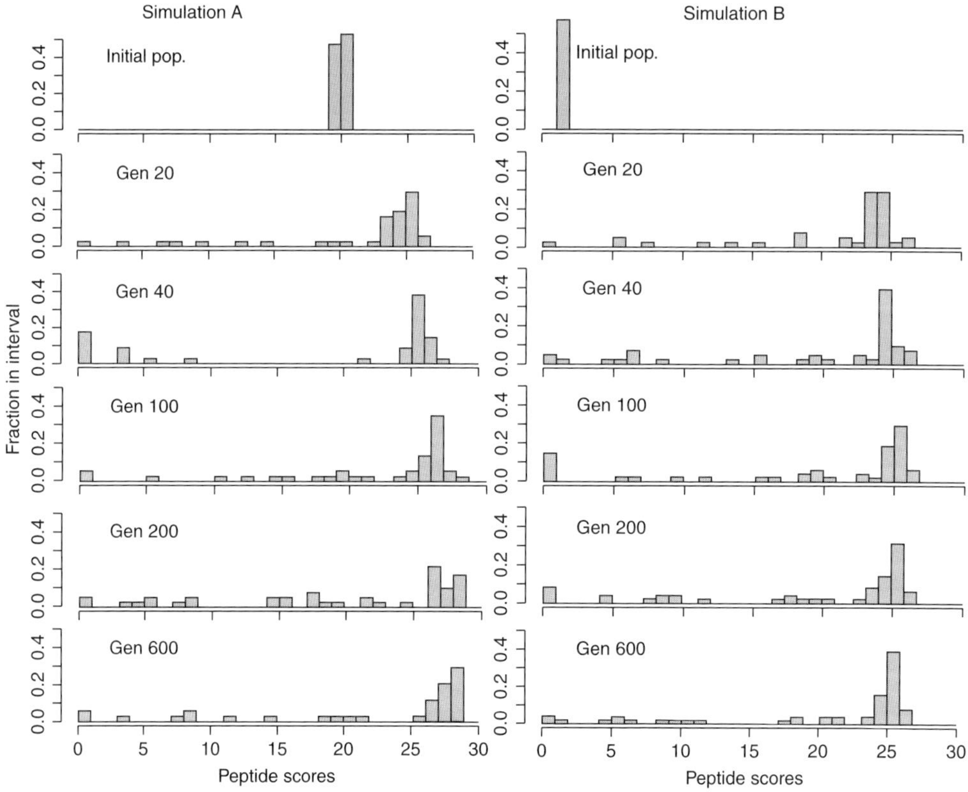

Fig. 12.10. Evolution of peptide scores for simulations A and B. The fraction of peptides in the population at each range of fitness score is shown.

increase in peptide fitness for simulation B, shown from the initial population containing much lower scores, as seen on the right-hand side of Fig. 12.11, showing the first generations in detail, where a dramatic rise in fitness scores could be observed in the first several generations. As expected, throughout the evolution of the population of peptides, the genetic algorithm created a set of peptides with a variety of fitness scores due to the random nature of novel peptide generation. For simulation A, the final generation contained 34 peptides, including ten peptides with a score of 29, and 22 peptides that had scores of 26 or higher (Table 12.5). The highest score observed in any of the peptides studied here or previously (Fjell *et al.*, 2011) was 29 rather than 30. This suggests that this method cannot identify any peptides with a higher score than those already found. Of the ten top-scoring peptides, nine were closely related and started with the sequence RWKRW. This sequence, however, was not sufficient per se for activity, as there were three other peptides starting with this sequence with lower scores: score 28 (**RWKRW**WRIL), 21 (**RWKRW**WKVW) and 1 (**RWKRW**SRLL). The population of peptides always contained a proportion of lower-scoring peptides (as seen on the left-hand side of Fig. 12.11) due to the random nature of how novel peptides are created by the genetic algorithm. The final population of simulation B containing 52 peptides gave similar results (Table 12.5).

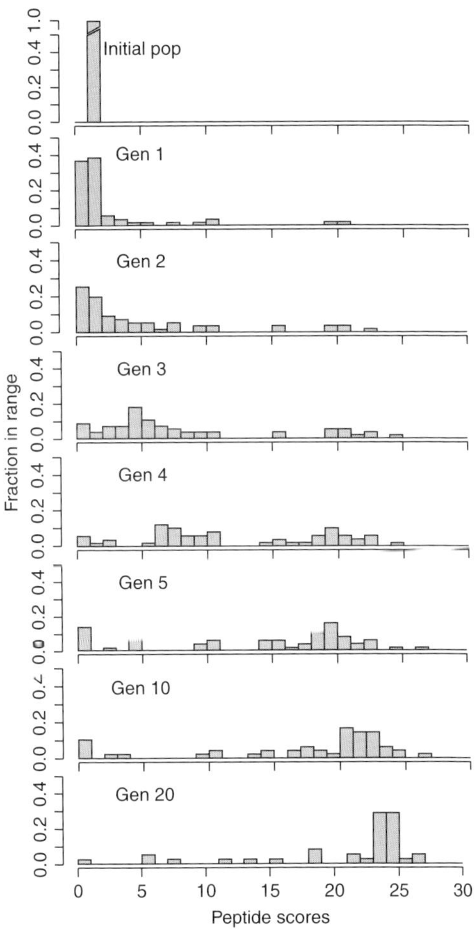

Fig. 12.11. Evolution of peptide scores for simulation B at early generation. The fraction of peptides in the population at each range of fitness score is shown.

There were two peptides in common in the final populations (KWKRWWWWR and KWKRWWWFR) for simulations A and B. Apart from these two peptides, there were no peptides in common between the two final populations, indicating that the processes followed were stochastic. In addition, simulation B had no peptides with fitness scores above 28 but more peptides with high scores, i.e. 25 peptides with a fitness score of ≥26. This indicated that the specific peptides in the final population were largely dependent on the initial population of peptides. This is to be expected, given the nature of the genetic algorithm, as the dominant method of generation of novel sequences is through cross-over from previous peptides, and mutations will affect only a comparatively small number of single amino acids in each generation with the genetic algorithm parameters used here. The number of high-fitness-scoring peptides appeared to be unchanged between generations 400 and 600 (Fig. 12.10) for simulations A and B, suggesting that in each case the genetic algorithm had settled on a local optimal set of sequences from which it was unlikely to escape through continued evolution. Further improvements would probably require the introduction of peptides with dramatically different sequences into the population.

Table 12.5. Final peptide populations for simulations A and B. (Reproduced from Fjell *et al.*, 2011.)

Simulation A			Simulation B	
Sequence	Fitness score	Activity	Sequence	Fitness score
RKRWWWRWW	29	–	IWKRWWWKR	27
RWKRWIRWW	29	–	KWKRWWWIR	27
RWKRWLRWW	29	–	KWKRWWWWR[a]	27
RWKRWWRIW	29	–	RIWKIWWKR	27
RWKRWWRLL	29	0.73	IKKRWWWFR	26
RWKRWWRLW	29	–	IKWKRWWWR	26
RWKRWWRVW	29	–	KLKRWWWFR	26
RWKRWWRWI	29	0.38	KLKRWWWWR	26
RWKRWWRWL	29	–	KWKRWWWFR[b]	26
RWKRWWRWW	29	0.67	KWWKIWRWR	26
KKRWWWWFR	28	–	KWWKRWKWR	26
KRWWWWKFR	28	–	KWWKRWWIR	26
KWWRWRRWW	28	0.37	KWWKRWWKR	26
RKRWWWRWL	28	–	KWWKRWWWR	26
RWKKWWRWL	28	0.38	RFWKIWWKR	26
RWKKWWRWW	28	0.38	RIWKRWWFR	26
RWKRWWRIL	28	–	RLWKIWWRR	26
KKRWWWWWR	27	0.47	RLWKRWWFR	26
KWKRWRRWW	27	–	RLWKRWWIR	26
KWKRWWWWR[a]	27	–	RWWKIWKWR	26
RKRWWWWFR	27	0.41	RWWKIWWKR	26
KWKRWWWFR[b]	26	0.67	RWWKIWWRR	26
RKRWWWRWR	22	–	RWWKRWWFR	26
RWKRWWKVW	21	–	RWWKRWWIR	26
RWKWWWKFR	20	–	RWWKRWWWR	26
RWKKWWRVW	19	–	IKKRWWWWR	25
RWYRWWRIW	15	–	KLKRWWWIR	25
KRWRWWRLL	12	–	KWWKIWWKR	25
KWKKWWRWL	9	–	KWWKRWWFR	25
KWKRWWWWL	9	–	RIWKRWWWR	25
KKKRWRRWW	8	–	RLKRWWWFR	25
RWKYWWRII	4	–	**RWKRW**WWFR	25
RKRWWWRGL	1	–	KLWKRWWWR	24
RWKRWSRLL	1	–	RWWKIWRWR	24
			KWWKIWKWR	22
			RWWKWWWIR	22
			CWKRWWWKR	21
			RFWKIWRWR	21
			KWKRIWWKR	19
			RWWKRWAIR	19
			RTWKRWWIR	18
			RTWKIWKWR	12
			KWWKRWWIH	11
			KWWKRWSWR	10
			RLWTRWWFR	9
			RIWARWWFR	7
			KWWKDWWKR	6
			RFEKIWWKR	6
			RIDKIWLKR	5

Continued

Table 12.5. Continued.

Simulation A			Simulation B	
Sequence	Fitness score	Activity	Sequence	Fitness score
			RLWKNWWRR	2
			RFWQIWRWR	0
			RWSKRWWWV	0

The final generation (generation 600) of peptides is sorted by score. The common subsequence RWKRW is shown in bold and discussed in the text. Activity values for nine peptide sequences were determined using a bioluminescence assay against *Pseudomonas aeruginosa*; units are IC_{50} relative to the Bac2A control peptide; '–' indicates activity not determined. Two peptides appeared in both final populations, KWKRWWWWR and KWKRWWWFR (indicated by [a] and [b], respectively).

12.3.4 Evolution of amino acid composition

The amino acid distribution of the peptide populations varied during the peptide sequence evolution. As described above, the number of amino acid types was maximized when selecting the initial population to include 14 amino acid types for simulation A and 16 amino acids for simulation B. During evolution over the 600 generations, the number of amino acid types was reduced to seven (in decreasing proportions: W, R, K, L, I, F and V) for the high-scoring peptides in simulation A and six (in decreasing proportions: W, R, K, I, F and L) for the high-scoring peptides in simulation B. This proportion of amino acids for high-scoring peptides was similar to the proportions we found previously for high-scoring peptides based on neural network modelling of a biased random library of 100,000 peptides.

12.3.5 Assessment of genetic algorithm performance

In our previous study (Fjell *et al.*, 2009), we examined 100,000 peptides from a biased random library of sequences. We empirically tested the activity of the 50 peptides ranked highest by fitness score. As reported previously, 94% of these peptides were found to be highly active. This group of highly active peptides included all peptides with fitness scores of 29 to 26, and some peptides scoring 25 (although some peptides scoring 25 were also found outside this group). Therefore, for comparison, we considered here that peptides receiving a fitness score of 26 or higher could be relatively confidently predicted to have high antibacterial activity. When we performed a computational search using 99,576 peptides in the random library (the 100,000 random peptides minus duplicates), we found only 22 peptides scoring 26 or higher, or 0.026% highly active peptides of these evaluated. In contrast, using genetic algorithms we identified, over all generations of the simulated evolution of the peptide populations, there was a combined efficiency of 0.50% highly active peptides identified per peptide evaluated, with 22 of the 4492 evaluated peptides scoring ≥26 or above in simulation A (0.49% highly active) and 25 out of 5067 peptides evaluated in simulation B (0.51% highly active). Taking these two values as representative of the two methods (0.026% for searching a large random library and 0.50% for a genetic algorithm search), we observed a 19-fold enhancement in discovery of highly active peptides. In addition, the progressive clustering of peptides' scores in the high-scoring region was much slower after the first 100 generations. This suggests that stopping the genetic algorithm at approximately generation 100 will be more efficient, as further peptides will not be identified efficiently after this point.

The antibacterial activity for a selection of peptides was performed using a luminescence assay, as described previously

(Hilpert *et al.*, 2005). In this classification work, we considered a peptide to be highly active if its IC_{50} value was less than half that of the control peptide, Bac2A. The Rel. IC_{50} values shown in Table 12.5 indicated that six of the nine peptides (66%) assayed were highly active (Rel. IC_{50} <0.5), with the remainder more active than the control, but lower than this threshold, with a result accuracy (66%) lower than the 94% accuracy of prediction found through neural network modelling. We believe that this discrepancy arose because of the small sample size of nine peptides tested and/or variability in the relative performance of the luminescence assay for antibacterial activity. It is important to note that there was also substantial variability of individual peptides derived from the neural network model.

12.4 Conclusions

With the availability of large numbers of synthetic peptides created using peptide array synthesis methods and a rapid luminescence-based assay to determine their antibacterial activity, larger sets of data on peptide sequence and activity can now be created. Based on two random libraries containing a total of more than 1400 peptides, we developed ANN models that predicted and ranked the relative activities of novel antimicrobial peptides with remarkable accuracy: in an independent test set of 100,000 virtual peptides, 94% of the 50 highest-ranked peptides that were predicted to be highly active were indeed found to be highly active. In addition to creating more complex models that utilize the 'inductive' QSAR methodology, the availability of a high quantity and quality of peptide activity data also allows more rigorous training and evaluation of the machine-learning techniques.

However, a serious constraint on the use of QSAR descriptors utilizing three-dimensional atomic resolution information is the computational expense in terms of time and resources. The use of a genetic algorithm allowed us to efficiently create and evaluate novel peptides computationally that have a high likelihood of being strongly antibacterial. By using a genetic algorithm, we were able to identify additional active peptides with greater efficiency: 0.50% of evaluated peptides compared with 0.026% of evaluated peptides, although evaluation of relative performance awaits more rigorous and higher-throughput testing of the predicted peptides. Nevertheless, there are indicators that genetic algorithm methods offer increased efficiency, allowing a dramatically increased capability to identify novel antimicrobial peptide candidates.

References

Brogden, K.A. (2005) Antimicrobial peptides: pore formers or metabolic inhibitors in bacteria? *Nature Reviews Microbiology* 3, 238–250.

Cherkasov, A. (2003) Inductive electronegativity scale. Iterative calculation of inductive partial charges. *Journal of Chemical Information and Computer Science* 43, 2039–2047.

Cherkasov, A. (2005a) 'Inductive' descriptors. 10 successful years in QSAR. *Current Computer-aided Drug Design* 1, 21–42.

Cherkasov, A. (2005b) Inductive QSAR Descriptors. Distinguishing compounds with antibacterial activity by artificial neural networks. *International Journal of Molecular Sciences* 6, 63–86.

Cherkasov, A., Hilpert, K., Jenssen, H., Fjell, C.D., Waldbrook, M., Mullaly, S.C., Volkmer, R. and Hancock, R.E. (2009) Use of artificial intelligence in the design of small peptide antibiotics effective against a broad spectrum of highly antibiotic-resistant superbugs. *ACS Chemical Biology* 4, 65–74.

Engel, T. (2006) Basic overview of chemoinformatics. *Journal of Chemical Information and Modeling* 46, 2267–2277.

Fjell, C.D., Hancock, R.E. and Cherkasov, A. (2007) AMPer: a database and an automated discovery tool for antimicrobial peptides. *Bioinformatics* 23, 1148–1155.

Fjell, C.D., Jenssen, H., Hilpert, K., Cheung, W.A., Panté, N., Hancock, R.E. and Cherkasov, A. (2009) Identification of novel antibacterial peptides by chemoinformatics and machine learning. *Journal of Medicinal Chemistry* 52, 2006–2015.

Fjell, C.D., Jenssen, H., Cheung, W.A., Hancock, R.E. and Cherkasov, A. (2011) Optimization of antibacterial peptides by genetic algorithms and cheminformatics. *Chemical Biology & Drug Design* 77, 48–56.

Hamill, P., Brown, K., Jenssen, H. and Hancock, R.E. (2008) Novel anti-infectives: is host defence the answer? *Current Opinion in Biotechnology* 19, 628–636.

Hancock, R.E. (2007) The end of an era? *Nature Reviews Drug Discovery* 6(28).

Hancock, R.E. and A. Rozek (2002) Role of membranes in the activities of antimicrobial cationic peptides. *FEMS Microbiology Letters* 206, 143–149.

Hancock, R.E.W. and Sahl, H.G. (2006) Antimicrobial and host-defense peptides as new anti-infective therapeutic strategies. *Nature Biotechnology* 24, 1551–1557.

Hilpert, K., Fjell, C.D. and Cherkasov, A. (2008) Short linear cationic antimicrobial peptides: screening, optimizing, and prediction. *Methods in Molecular Biology* 494, 127–159.

Hilpert, K., Volkmer-Engert R., Walter, T. and Hancock, R.E. (2005) High-throughput generation of small antibacterial peptides with improved activity. *Nature Biotechnology* 23, 1008–1012.

Hsu, C.H., Chen, C., Jou, M.L., Lee, A.Y., Lin, Y.C., Yu Y.P., Huang, W.T. and Wu, S.H. (2005) Structural and DNA-binding studies on the bovine antimicrobial peptide, indolicidin: evidence for multiple conformations involved in binding to membranes and DNA. *Nucleic Acids Research* 33, 4053–4064.

Jenssen, H., Fjell, C.D., Cherkasov, A. and Hancock, R.E. (2008) QSAR modeling and computer-aided design of antimicrobial peptides. *Journal of Peptide Science* 14, 110–114.

Jenssen, H., Hamill, P. and Hancock, R.E. (2006) Peptide antimicrobial agents. *Clinical Microbiology Reviews* 19, 491–511.

Jenssen, H., Lejon, T., Hilpert, K., Fjell, C.D., Cherkasov, A. and Hancock, R.E. (2007) Evaluating different descriptors for model design of antimicrobial peptides with enhanced activity toward P. aeruginosa. *Chemical Biology & Drug Design* 70, 134–142.

Karakoc, E., Sahinalp, S.C. and Cherkasov, A. (2006a) Comparative QSAR- and fragments distribution analysis of drugs, druglikes, metabolic substances, and antimicrobial compounds. *Journal of Chemical Information and Modeling* 46, 2167–2182.

Karakoc, E., Cherkasov, A. and Sahinalp, S.C. (2006b) Distance based algorithms for small biomolecule classification and structural similarity search. *Bioinformatics* 15, e243–e251.

Madera, L., Ma, S. and Hancock, R.E.W. (2010) Host defence (antimicrobial) peptides and proteins. In: Kaufmann, S.H.E., Rouse B. and Sacks, D. (eds) *The Immune Response to Infection.* ASM Press, Washington, DC, pp. 57–68.

Niculescu, S.P. (2003) Artificial neural networks and genetic algorithms in QSAR. *Journal of Molecular Structure –THEOCHEM* 622, 71–83.

Parrill, A.L. (1996) Evolutionary and genetic methods in drug design. *Drug Discovery Today* 1, 514–521.

Perkins, R., Fang, H., Tong, W. and Welsh, W.J. (2003) Quantitative structure-activity relationship methods: perspectives on drug discovery and toxicology. *Environmental Toxicology and Chemistry* 22, 1666–1679.

Peschel, A. and Sahl, H.G. (2006) The co-evolution of host cationic antimicrobial peptides and microbial resistance. *Nature Reviews Microbiology* 4, 529–536.

Projan, S.J. (2003) Why is big Pharma getting out of antibacterial drug discovery? *Current Opinion in Microbiology* 6, 427–430.

Rozek, A., Friedrich, C.L. and Hancock, R.E. (2000) Structure of the bovine antimicrobial peptide indolicidin bound to dodecylphosphocholine and sodium dodecyl sulfate micelles. *Biochemistry* 39, 15765–15774.

Sawyer, J.G., Martin, N.L. and Hancock, R.E. (1988) Interaction of macrophage cationic proteins with the outer membrane of *Pseudomonas aeruginosa. Infection and Immunity* 56, 693–698.

Solmajer, T. and Zupan, J., (2004) Optimization algorithms and natural computing in drug discovery. *Drug Discovery Today* 1, 247–252.

Spellberg, B., Powers, J.H., Brass, E.P., Miller, L.G. and Edwards, J.E. Jr (2004) Trends in antimicrobial drug development: implications for the future. *Clinical Infectious Diseases* 38, 1279–1286.

Theuretzbacher, U. and Toney, J.H. (2006) Nature's clarion call of antibacterial resistance: are we listening? *Current Opinion in Investigational Drugs* 7, 158–166.

Tossi, A., Sandri, L. and Giangaspero, A. (2000) Amphipathic, α-helical antimicrobial peptides. *Biopolymers* 55, 4–30.

Uteng, M., Hauge, H.H., Markwick, P.R., Fimland, G., Mantzilas, D., Nissen-Meyer J. and Muhle-Goll C. (2003) Three-dimensional structure in lipid micelles of the pediocin-like antimicrobial peptide sakacin P and a sakacin P variant that is structurally stabilized by an inserted C-terminal disulfide bridge. *Biochemistry* 42, 11417–11426.

Weaver, D.C. (2004) Applying data mining techniques to library design, lead generation and lead optimization. *Current Opinion in Chemical Biology* 8, 264–270.

Yeaman, M.R. and Yount, N.Y. (2003) Mechanisms of antimicrobial peptide action and resistance. *Pharmacological Reviews* 55, 27–55.

Yeung, A.T., Gellatly, S.L. and Hancock, R.E. (2011) Multifunctional cationic host-defence peptides and clinical applications. *Cellular and Molecular Life Sciences* 68, 2161–2176.

13 Acetyl-CoA Carboxylase as a Target for Antibacterial Development

Grover L. Waldrop
Division of Biochemistry and Molecular Biology, Louisiana State University, Baton Rouge, Louisiana, USA

13.1 Fatty Acid Synthesis and Acetyl-CoA Carboxylase

The never-ending struggle between man and microorganisms has created an alarming increase in the number of antibiotic-resistant bacteria (Boucher *et al.*, 2009). Antibiotic resistance is observed in both Gram-positive (e.g. methicillin-resistant *Staphylococcus aureus* (MRSA)) and Gram-negative pathogens such as *Klebsiella pneumonia*, *Acinetobacter baumannii* and *Pseudomonas aeruginosa* (Peleg and Hooper, 2010). The increase in antibiotic resistance may be due in part to the limited number of proteins (<30–40) used as targets for the current arsenal of antibiotics. Thus, there is a pressing need for new antibacterials directed at new targets. In this chapter, the potential and current developments of using acetyl-CoA carboxylase as a novel target for antibacterial discovery are presented.

Acetyl-CoA carboxylase catalyses the first committed step in fatty acid biosynthesis and, with a few exceptions, the enzymes of fatty acid synthesis have remained largely unexplored for antibacterial development. As fatty acids are used primarily for membrane biogenesis in bacteria, inhibition of any of the enzymes in the fatty acid synthetic pathway would be bactericidal (Campbell and Cronan, 2001; Heath *et al.*, 2001; Zhang *et al.*, 2006). In fact, there are two notable antibacterial agents that inhibit fatty acid synthesis and provide a strong precedent that inhibiting enzymes in this essential pathway would be bactericidal. Triclosan is widely used as the active ingredient in antibacterial soap, while isoniazid is a frontline antitubercular agent. Both of these compounds inhibit enoyl-acyl carrier protein reductase (encoded by *FabI*) (Lu and Tonge, 2008). Moreover, scientists at Merck discovered that the natural product platensimycin produced by *Streptomyces platensis* has antibacterial activity by inhibiting the condensing enzymes encoded by the *FabF/B* genes (Wang *et al.*, 2006).

It should be pointed out that Brinster *et al.* (2009) have questioned targeting fatty acid biosynthesis in Gram-positive bacteria for antibacterial development because the organisms can scavenge fatty acids from human serum. However, the generality of this conclusion is suspect, as only one pathogen, *Streptococcus agalactiae*, was studied. In fact, Balemans *et al.* (2010) questioned the findings of Brinster *et al.* (2009) with respect to the Gram-positive pathogen *S. aureus*.

Fatty acid synthesis in bacteria is commonly referred to as fatty acid synthesis II (FAS II) to distinguish it from the eukaryotic pathway, which is called fatty acid synthesis I (FAS I). FAS II is distinguished from FAS I by the fact that all of the enzymes in the pathway are separate proteins, whereas in FAS I the enzymes constitute domains on a single polypeptide. Acetyl-CoA carboxylase catalyses the first committed step in both FAS I and FAS II and is a multifunctional enzyme that catalyses the two-step reaction shown in Fig. 13.1. In *Escherichia coli*, acetyl-CoA carboxylase consists of three different proteins: biotin carboxylase, biotin carboxyl carrier protein (BCCP) and carboxyltransferase (Cronan and Waldrop, 2002). Both biotin carboxylase and carboxyltransferase retain their activity in the absence of the other components. Biotin carboxylase is a homodimer that catalyses the first half-reaction in Fig. 13.1, which involves the ATP-dependent phosphorylation of bicarbonate to form a reactive carboxyphosphate intermediate, followed by transfer of the carboxyl group to the vitamin biotin. *In vivo*, biotin is covalently attached to BCCP. The second half-reaction, catalysed by carboxyltransferase (an $\alpha_2\beta_2$ heterotetramer), transfers the carboxyl group from carboxybiotin to acetyl-CoA to make malonyl-CoA. The malonyl-CoA is then transferred to the acyl carrier protein where it undergoes iterative condensation reactions with acetyl-CoA to make fatty acids.

Both the biotin carboxylase and the carboxyltransferase components of acetyl-CoA carboxylase can serve as targets for antibacterial agents. However, it was initially thought that biotin carboxylase was not an ideal target for antibacterials because of the potential for inhibition of other biotin-dependent enzymes and therefore the increased likelihood of toxicity. The reason for the concern was because, in addition to acetyl-CoA carboxylase, humans utilize three other biotin-dependent enzymes in their metabolism: pyruvate carboxylase, propionyl-CoA carboxylase and methylmalonyl-CoA carboxylase. All four biotin-dependent enzymes follow the same two-step pathway outlined in Fig. 13.1 with the only difference being the carboxyl group acceptor, which varies depending on the enzyme. For instance, pyruvate carboxylase utilizes pyruvate as an acceptor, while acetyl-CoA carboxylase utilizes acetyl-CoA. Thus, the biotin carboxylase reaction of acetyl-CoA carboxylase is identical to the reaction in the other three biotin-dependent enzymes and any inhibitor of the biotin carboxylase of acetyl-CoA carboxylase was thought to inhibit the other three enzymes as well. Fortunately, this concern was unfounded, and 2 years ago, bacterial biotin carboxylase was validated as a target for antibacterial development (Miller *et al.*, 2009). In fact, biotin carboxylase is now the target for three different types of antibacterial compounds: pyridopyrimidines, amino-oxazoles and benzimidazole carboxyamides, while the carboxyltransferase component of

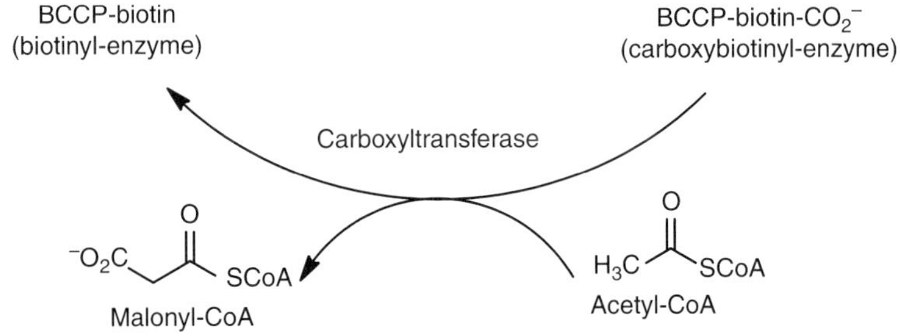

Fig. 13.1. Schematic of the reaction catalysed by acetyl-CoA carboxylase.

acetyl-CoA carboxylase is the target of the antibacterial natural product pyrrolidinediones. So far, while the pyridopyrimidines have been the only compounds tested *in vivo*, they have not shown any toxicity to the host (Miller *et al.*, 2009), which suggests that it is possible to selectively target the bacterial enzyme over the mammalian enzyme.

13.2 Biotin Carboxylase as a Target for Antibacterial Development

13.2.1 Pyridopyrimidines

The first antibacterial compounds found to inhibit biotin carboxylase were discovered by scientists at Pfizer quite unexpectedly (Miller *et al.*, 2009; Walsh and Fischbach, 2009). The Pfizer group screened whole bacterial cells against an existing 1.6 million compound anticancer library directed against tyrosine protein kinases. Several pyridopyrimidines were found to exhibit antibacterial activity against certain types of Gram-negative bacteria. An example of the pyridopyrimidines is compound 1 in Fig. 13.2(a). The target of the pyridopyrimidines was identified by making resistant mutants of *Haemophilus influenzae* and mapping the resistance-conferring gene. Resistance to the pyridopyrimidines was conferred by mutations in the gene encoding biotin carboxylase. The Pfizer team coined the name Compound Driven Target Identification (CDTI) to describe their approach for identification of novel antibacterial compounds and targets.

The pyridopyrimidine compound 1 exhibited slow, tight binding inhibition of biotin carboxylase, and binding studies using surface plasmon resonance determined a dissociation constant (K_d) of 0.8nM. Moreover, compound 1 was more selective for biotin carboxylase as it did not significantly inhibit 28 other eukaryotic protein kinases. The product from the *Src* gene was the only kinase that was inhibited by compound 1; however, the inhibition was 70-fold weaker than with biotin carboxylase. Most importantly, compound 1 did not inhibit rat liver acetyl-CoA carboxylase.

The pyridopyrimidines inhibited biotin carboxylase by binding in the ATP-binding site, which is not surprising given that the screening library was composed of protein kinase inhibitors. Structural analyses of co-crystals of biotin carboxylase and compound 1 showed unequivocally that the inhibitor bound in the ATP site of the biotin carboxylase active site. Comparison of the inhibitor-enzyme structure with the structure of ATP (compound 2, Fig. 2c) bound to biotin carboxylase (Mochalkin *et al.*, 2008) revealed that many of the same active site residues are utilized to bind both substrate and inhibitor (Fig. 13.2b and d).

The pyridopyrimidines were found to be bactericidal against Gram-negative organisms such as *E. coli*, *H. influenzae* and *Moraxella catarrhalis* and the Gram-positive *S. aureus*. However, the minimum inhibitory concentration (MIC) values for the Gram-negative organisms were lower than for *S. aureus* indicating a much greater selectivity for biotin carboxylase from Gram-negative organisms (Table 13.1).

In fact, compound 1 was found to have *in vivo* antibacterial activity in murine models of both tissue-localized (thigh) and systemic infections of *H. influenzae*. In the tissue-localized infection, after oral dosing, the plasma concentration of compound 1 needed to give 50% of the maximal effect was 5.6 ± 1.8 μg/ml. In the systemic infection model, animals that were dosed at 200 mg/kg twice a day showed 50% survival. Most importantly, toxicity was not observed with compound 1 at any of the doses tested.

The difference in activity of pyridopyrimidines between Gram-negative and Gram-positive organisms can be traced to the resistant mutants used to identify the target of the pyridopyrimidines. The mutation in the biotin carboxylase gene imparting resistance to the pyridopyrimidines resulted in the replacement of isoleucine at position 437 with threonine. It turns out that, in biotin carboxylase from Gram-positive bacteria, the amino acid at the position equivalent to 437 is threonine. Structural analysis of the I437T mutant of *E. coli* biotin carboxylase and compound 1 revealed the loss of shape

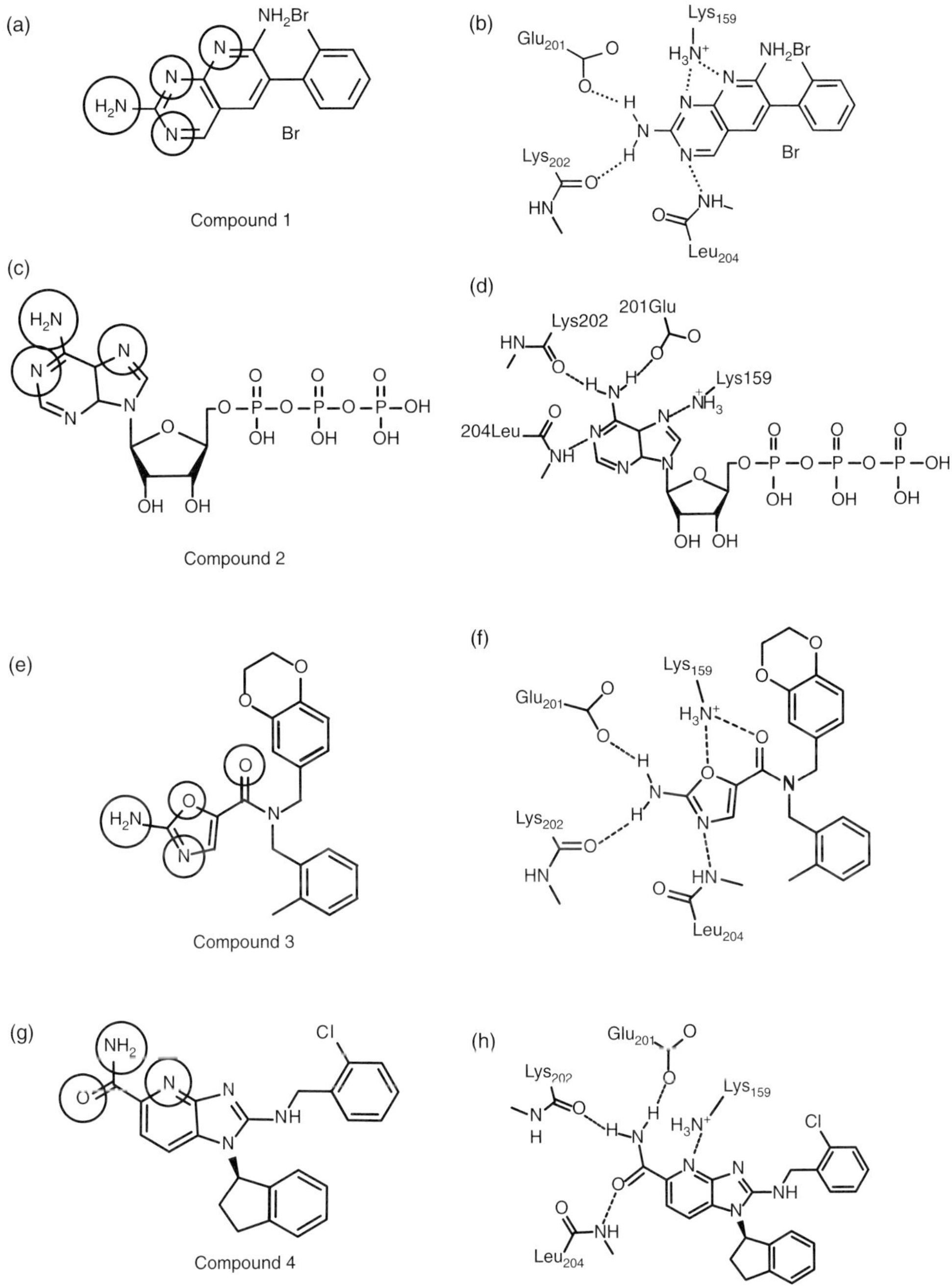

Fig. 13.2. Inhibitors of biotin carboxylase. (a) Pyridopyrimidine; (b) active-site interactions with the pyridopyrimidine; (c) biotin carboxylase substrate ATP; (d) active-site interactions with ATP; (e) amino-oxazole; (f) active-site interactions with the amino-oxazole; (g) benzimidazole carboxamide; (h) active-site interactions with the benzimidazole carboxamide. The pharmacophore features that compounds 1–4 have in common are highlighted with a circle.

Table 13.1. Microbiological data for acetyl-CoA carboxylase inhibitors.

Drug candidate	Target enzyme	Bacterial spectrum	MIC (μg/ml)
Pyridopyrimidine	Biotin carboxylase	*Escherichia coli*	16
		Haemophilus influenzae	0.125
		Moraxella catarrhalis	1
		Staphylococcus aureus (MRSA)	32
		Streptococcus pneumoniae	>64
		Enterococcus faecalis	>64
		Pseudomonas aeruginosa	>64
Amino-oxazole	Biotin carboxylase	*E. coli*	>64
		H. influenzae	>64
		M. catarrhalis	16
Benzimidazole carboxamide	Biotin carboxylase	*E. coli*	0.8
Pyrrolidinedione	Carboxyltransferase	*E. coli*	32
		S. aureus	8
		S. pneumoniae	32
		Bacillus subtilis	1
		P. aeruginosa	>64

complementarity between the enzyme and inhibitor, as well as a loss of hydrophobic contacts between the enzyme and phenyl ring. These structural differences may explain the significant decrease in affinity of pyridopyrimidines for biotin carboxylase with threonine at position 437.

While the pyridopyrimidines did not have broad-spectrum antibacterial activity, they none the less firmly established that biotin carboxylase is a legitimate target for antibacterial development. They also served as a starting point for a virtual screening programme to discover different types of biotin carboxylase inhibitors.

13.2.2 Amino-oxazole derivatives

The discovery of the pyridopyrimidine inhibitors of biotin carboxylase served as a springboard for the Pfizer group to identify novel chemical matter that inhibited biotin carboxylase using a combination of virtual and fragment screening (Mochalkin *et al.*, 2009; Waldrop, 2009). Starting from a virtual screen of 2.2 million compounds, 48 compounds were eventually found to have 50% inhibitory concentration (IC_{50}) values of less than 10 μM. Interestingly, the hit rate in the virtual screen was about 200-fold higher than in a conventional high-throughput screen. At the same time, the biochemical screening of 5200 fragments ultimately yielded 142 compounds that exhibited significant inhibition of biotin carboxylase. Examination of the compounds obtained from both the virtual and fragment screening revealed that they had many pharmacophore features in common. These features are highlighted in the amino-oxazole derivative compound 3 (Fig. 13.2e). Moreover, the same arrangement of hydrogen bond acceptors and donors found in compound 3 are also shared in the pyridopyrimidine compound 1.

While fragment screening has the advantage of being able to screen a larger expanse of chemical space than conventional high-throughput screening methods, the major disadvantage is that the compounds usually bind to the target with low affinity. This was certainly the case with the fragments that inhibited biotin carboxylase. However, unlike compounds in a high-throughput screening library, the compounds in a fragment library are very amenable to synthetic elaboration. Thus, the Pfizer team utilized fragment growing, merging and morphing of the compounds discovered by virtual and fragment screening to generate compounds with a much higher affinity for biotin carboxylase. One example of this approach is compound 3 (Fig. 13.2e). In this case, the amino-oxazole fragment was used as an anchor for binding to the ATP site on the enzyme, while the carboxyl group was easily modified with amide derivatives. The chemical moieties linked to the amino-oxazole were chosen based on their 'drug likeliness' or adherence to Lipinski's rules. The other criterion was their similarity to the pyridopyrimidine compound 1. Using these guidelines, the IC_{50} went from 21.5 μM for the parent compound to 0.007 μM for compound 3 in only three steps.

Characterization of the molecular and antibacterial properties of compound 3 showed a striking similarity to the pyridopyrimidine compound 1. First, structural analysis of compound 3 bound to biotin carboxylase showed that the amino-oxazole fragment interacted with the same active-site residues as the pyridopyrimidine compound 1 (Fig. 13.2f). Secondly, when testing the selectivity of compound 3, it was shown not to inhibit 40 different protein kinases or eukaryotic acetyl-CoA carboxylase. Thirdly, like the pyridopyrimidine compound 1, the amino-oxazoles only exhibited significant activity against Gram-negative bacteria and were not effective against bacteria in which biotin carboxylase contained threonine at position 437 (i.e. Gram-positive bacteria). The bacteria tested against the amino-oxazole compound 3 and the MIC values are given in Table 13.1. The antibacterial properties of the amino-oxazoles were not tested in an *in vivo* model.

While the amino-oxazole derivatives display many similarities to the pyridopyrimidines, there is one significant difference. The amino-oxazoles possess the flexibility to be easily modified so they can be made effective against Gram-positive bacteria. Moreover, if fragments that bind in the biotin-binding site could be discovered, then fragment linking with the amino-oxazole derivatives, which bind in the ATP-binding site, could lead to a very potent antibacterial agent inhibiting biotin carboxylase.

13.2.3 Benzimidazole carboxamide derivatives

At the same time, Pfizer was discovering the pyridopyrimidines and amino-oxazoles Schering-Plough was developing another class of antibacterials that target biotin carboxylase (Cheng *et al.*, 2009). The Schering-Plough group employed high-throughput screening using affinity-selection mass spectrometry (Annis *et al.*, 2007) to identify benzimidazole carboxamides as inhibitors of biotin carboxylase. The hits from the initial screen were subjected to structure-based drug design and computer-aided modelling to develop a series of benzimidazole carboxamides that bound biotin carboxylase with high affinity and exhibited antibacterial activity. An example of one of the most potent benzimidazole carboxamides, compound 4, is shown in Fig. 13.2(g).

The benzimidazole carboxamides exhibit competitive inhibition with respect to ATP, and structure analyses by X-ray crystallography have confirmed inhibitor binding in the ATP site, as well as showing how the active-site residues interact with the inhibitor. The interactions of compound 4 with the active-site amino acids are shown in Fig. 2(h). If the interactions of compound 4 with biotin carboxylase are compared with the active-site interactions of the pyridopyrimidines and amino-oxazoles, several similarities become apparent (Fig. 2b, f and h). For instance, Lys202 and Glu201 hydrogen bond to the amide nitrogen similar to the way those residues interact with the amino group of the pyridopyrimidines and amino-oxazoles. Moreover, the main-chain NH group of Leu204 hydrogen bonds with the carbonyl oxygen and the carboxamide, while Lys159 binds to one of the nitrogens in the benzimidazole ring.

The benzimidazole carboxamide derivatives inhibited acetyl-CoA carboxylase from a broad spectrum of pathogenic bacteria and were found to selectively inhibit fatty acid biosynthesis with no effect on DNA, RNA or protein biosynthesis. In addition, like the pyridopyrimidines and amino-oxazoles, the benzimidazole carboxamide derivatives did not inhibit human kinases or eukaryotic acetyl-CoA carboxylase. The bacterial strains tested against the benzimidazole carboxamide compound 4 and the MIC values are listed in Table 13.1. No *in vivo* testing was reported. As the benzimidazole carboxamide derivatives inhibit a broad spectrum of biotin carboxylases, it may be a worthwhile exercise to incorporate the chemical features of the benzimidazole carboxamide derivatives with the amino-oxazoles (which are only effective against Gram-negative organisms) to develop amino-oxazoles with broad-spectrum activity.

In summary, the work by the Pfizer and Schering-Plough groups have firmly established the biotin carboxylase component of acetyl-CoA carboxylase as a viable target for antibacterial development and provided three very promising lead compounds that, following further development, could lead to clinically useful antibacterial agents.

13.3 Carboxyltransferase as a Target for Antibacterial Development

13.3.1 Pyrrolidinediones

In contrast to biotin carboxylase, there is only one class of molecules that inhibit the carboxyltransferase component of acetyl-CoA carboxylase and that also possess antibacterial activity. Also, unlike all the biotin carboxylase inhibitors, which are synthetic in origin, the carboxyltransferase inhibitor is a natural product. This natural product, andrimid (Fig. 13.3), was first isolated from the culture broth of an *Enterobacter* sp. that is found in the eggs of the insect *Nilparvata lugens* (brown plant hopper; Fredenhagen *et al.*, 1987). It showed potent activity against *Xanthomonas campestris*, which causes bacterial blight in rice plants. Seven years later, andrimid as well as three new related natural products with antibacterial activity, were isolated from the extract of a strain of *Pseudomonas fluorescens* collected at Prince of Wales Island in Moira Sound, Alaska (Needham *et al.*, 1994). One of the new metabolites, moiramide B (Fig. 13.3), exhibited very potent activity against a broad spectrum of organisms. Andrimid and moiramide B have

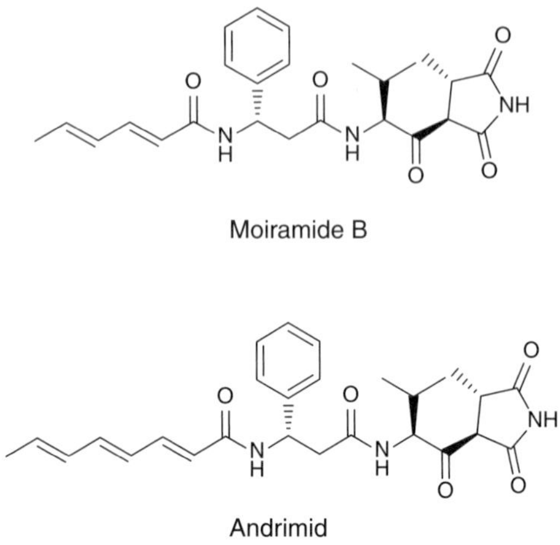

Fig. 13.3. Structure of andrimid and moiramide B.

a polypeptide scaffold where the N terminus is acylated, and the C terminus contains a pyrrolidinedione ring (Fig. 13.3).

Ten years after the discovery of the antibacterial potential of moiramide B, scientists at Bayer determined that carboxyltransferase was the target (Freiberg *et al.*, 2004). Using *E. coli*, moiramide B was found to inhibit the incorporation of radiolabelled acetate into phospholipids, suggesting that an enzyme in fatty acid synthesis was affected. Subsequently, using *E. coli* extracts, moiramide B did not affect the incorporation of [^{14}C]malonyl-CoA into fatty acids, indicating that the target was acetyl-CoA carboxylase. Inhibition studies with the isolated biotin carboxylase and carboxyltransferase revealed that the latter was the target of moiramide B and andrimid.

While co-crystallization of andrimid and moiramide B with carboxyltransferase has so far not been successful, the inhibition of carboxyltransferase by moiramide B was competitive with respect to malonyl-CoA (dissociation constant (K_i) 5 nM) and non-competitive with respect to biocytin. These inhibition patterns suggest that moiramide B binds in both the malonyl-CoA and biocytin sites. If moiramide B only bound to the malonyl-CoA site, then the inhibition pattern with respect to biocytin would be uncompetitive because carboxyltransferase has an ordered addition of substrates, with malonyl-CoA binding before biocytin (Blanchard and Waldrop, 1998; Levert and Waldrop, 2002).

Carboxyltransferase from *E. coli* is routinely assayed in the non-physiological direction because of the availability of a spectrophotometric continuous assay that couples the production of acetyl-CoA with the reduction of NAD^+ by the combined reactions of citrate synthase and malate dehydrogenase (Blanchard and Waldrop, 1998). Biocytin is biotin with a lysine attached to the carboxyl group of the valeric acid side chain via an amide linkage with the ε-amino group. Biocytin is used instead of biotin because it gives maximal velocities three orders of magnitude higher than biotin (Blanchard and Waldrop, 1998).

Information on which active-site residues the inhibitor might be interacting with can be gleaned from resistant mutants. The Bayer team made resistant mutants to help identify the target of moiramide B and found that a single mutation in the β-subunit of *E. coli* carboxyltransferase rendered the bacterium less sensitive to the inhibitor. The mutation S207Y is not far from two conserved glycine residues at positions 204 and 205 where the peptidic NH groups form an oxyanion hole to stabilize the enolate anion formed in acetyl-CoA during catalysis. In an analogous study, Liu *et al.* (2008) examined the genes encoding the two subunits of carboxyltransferase in an andrimid-producing bacterium (*Pantoea agglomerans*) and found that the organism is resistant because of a mutation in the active site of the β-subunit. The mutation corresponds to M203L in *E. coli* carboxyltransferase, which rendered bacteria harbouring this mutation more resistant to andrimid. M203L is adjacent to one (residue 204) of the conserved glycine residues that forms part of the oxyanion hole. Presumably, these two mutations, S207Y and M203L, cause local conformational changes that decrease the affinity of the inhibitor for the enzyme. Based on these observations, it is tempting to speculate that one of the carbonyl oxygens of the pyrrolidinedione moiety of andrimid and moiramide B hydrogen bonds to the peptidic NH groups of the oxyanion hole. Evidence in support of this notion is that structure–activity relationship studies of andrimid and moiramide B have shown that alterations to the pyrrolidinedione moiety dramatically decrease the efficacy of these compounds as antibacterial agents, whereas variations in the fatty acid side chain had no effect on activity (McWhorter *et al.*, 1989; Pohlmann *et al.*, 2005).

Lastly, moiramide B was found to inhibit carboxyltransferase from both Gram-negative and Gram-positive organisms, which is consistent with its broad-spectrum activity, and, like the biotin carboxylase inhibitors, moiramide B did not inhibit eukaryotic acetyl-CoA carboxylase. The bacterial strains tested against moiramide B and the MIC values are given in Table 13.1. No studies on the activity of moiramide B *in vivo* have been reported, suggesting that it may not be useful clinically. None the less, the pyrrolidinediones provide an excellent framework from which modifications can be made to improve the physicochemical parameters to make them clinically viable.

13.3.2 The zinc-finger domain as a potential target

When the three-dimensional structure of carboxyltransferase from *E. coli* and *S. aureus* was determined by X-ray crystallography, it was found, quite unexpectedly, that on the N terminus of the β-subunit was a Cys4 zinc-finger domain (Bilder *et al.*, 2006). The physiological function of the zinc-finger domain appears to be that it allows carboxyltransferase to bind to the mRNA coding for the α- and β-subunits, which in turn leads to inhibition of translation (Meades *et al.*, 2010). However, the substrate acetyl-CoA relieves the inhibition. In a reciprocal manner, the binding of mRNA to the enzyme inhibited catalysis while acetyl-CoA relieved the inhibition. All of these observations taken together suggested that the role of the zinc-finger domain on carboxyltransferase was to bind to the mRNA coding for the α- and β-subunits in order to regulate carboxyltransferase activity and gene expression (Meades *et al.*, 2010).

The most important aspect of this type of enzyme regulation with respect to antibacterial development is that mRNA binding and catalysis are not separate functions as in most dual-function enzymes. Instead, mRNA binding and catalysis are inextricably linked such that they are mutually exclusive of one another. Equally important is that the zinc-finger domain is only found on carboxyltransferase from Gram-positive and Gram-negative bacteria (Bilder *et al.*, 2006). Thus, this provides a unique target with very little chance of cross-reactivity with the human enzyme. In addition, the cysteines in the zinc-finger domain are intolerant to mutation. Mutation of two or more of the cysteines results in an inactive enzyme (Meades *et al.*, 2010). This would help mitigate the development of resistance to any compound that binds to the zinc-finger domain.

There are two possible strategies for targeting the zinc-finger domain. First, as DNA and heparin (Benson *et al.*, 2008) as well as RNA were found to interact with the zinc-finger domain and inhibit catalysis, small molecules that bind to the zinc-finger domain and inhibit catalysis could be developed. Secondly, molecules that bind to the zinc-finger domain and eject the zinc atom would collapse the structure of the zinc domain, thereby inactivating the enzyme. There is a precedent for using both of these approaches in the treatment of AIDS (Rice *et al.*, 1995; Tummino *et al.*, 1996) and cancer (Beerheide *et al.*, 1999).

13.4 Holo-acetyl-CoA Carboxylase as a Target for Antibacterial Development

The discussion so far has focused on targeting the individual enzymes that comprise acetyl-CoA carboxylase. This is because it is commonly thought that biotin–BCCP is carboxylated at the active site of biotin carboxylase and then dissociates from the enzyme and by diffusion then binds to carboxyltransferase. Instead, there is evidence that catalysis takes place only when all three components, biotin carboxylase, biotin–BCCP and carboxyltransferase, form a multifunctional enzyme complex (T.C. Broussard and G.L. Waldrop, unpublished observations). The fact that activity is dependent on protein–protein interactions greatly expands the number of potential target sites beyond just the traditional active sites. Furthermore, the formation of a multienzyme complex suggests relatively close proximity of the active sites of biotin carboxylase and carboxyltransferase. The proximity of the active sites provides the opportunity to make a multiligand inhibitor that incorporates both biotin carboxylase and carboxyltransferase inhibitors. Multiligand inhibitors are usually much more potent than either one of the individual ligands and a multiligand antibacterial agent would lessen the chance of developing resistance (Morphy and Rankovic, 2005; Silver, 2007; Corson *et al.*, 2008; Le Calvez, 2009).

What is needed in order to target the protein–protein interactions in acetyl-CoA carboxylase for antibacterial development is a robust assay for high-throughput screening. While a high-throughput screening assay for just the carboxyltransferase component was available (Santoro *et al.*, 2006), an assay for the holoenzyme was lacking until scientists at Schering-Plough developed an assay following cleavage of [γ-^{32}P]ATP by the biotin carboxylase component (Soriano *et al.*, 2006). After stopping the reaction, the amount of $^{32}P_i$ was quantified using a spectrophotometric technique. The major drawbacks to this assay are the precautions and waste that accompany any assay involving radioactivity. The Pfizer group made a slight variation on the Schering-Plough assay that eliminated the radioactivity by using a continuous coupled enzyme phosphate detection assay (Miller *et al.*, 2009). The shortcoming for both of these assays is that, if a reduction in activity is detected (i.e. a 'hit'), it is not known which half-reaction is inhibited. Therefore, in order for high-throughput screening of acetyl-CoA carboxylase to really come to fruition, an assay that monitors the progress of both half-reactions simultaneously needs to be developed.

13.5 Summary

There is a pressing need to expand the repertoire of antibacterial targets beyond those currently in use such as in DNA, RNA and protein biosynthesis. The enzymes of fatty acid biosynthesis for the most part remain an untapped reservoir of antibacterial targets. The above discussion has made it abundantly clear that acetyl-CoA carboxylase is a very attractive target for antibacterial development. There are three different classes of molecules that inhibit the biotin carboxylase component and also exhibit antibacterial activity: pyridopyrimidines, amino-oxazoles and benzimidazole carboxamides. In contrast, the carboxyltransferase component has only one type of molecule that inhibits and has antibacterial activity: the natural product pyrrolidinediones. The inhibitors for both biotin carboxylase and carboxyltransferase provide a solid foundation from which to build clinically useful compounds. Other potential targets on acetyl-CoA carboxylase are the zinc-finger domain on carboxyltransferase and the protein–protein interactions between biotin–BCCP and either biotin carboxylase or carboxyltransferase. As the need for more antibacterial agents continues to grow, acetyl-CoA carboxylase will hopefully play an important role in satisfying that need.

Acknowledgement

The author would like to thank Ms Molly Hughes for constructive comments on the manuscript and for preparing the figures.

References

Annis, D.A., Nickbarg, E., Yang, X., Ziebell, M.R. and Whitehurst, C.E. (2007) Affinity selection-mass spectrometry screening techniques for small molecule drug discovery. *Current Opinion in Chemical Biology* 11, 518–526.

Balemans, W., Lounis, N., Gilissen, R., Guillemont, J., Simmen, K., Andries, K. and Koul, A. (2010) Essentiality of FASII pathway for *Staphylococcus aureus*. *Nature* 463, E3; discussion E4.

Beerheide, W., Bernard, H.U., Tan, Y.J., Ganesan, A., Rice, W.G. and Ting, A.E. (1999) Potential drugs against cervical cancer: zinc-ejecting inhibitors of the human papillomavirus type 16 E6 oncoprotein. *Journal of the National Cancer Institute* 91, 1211–1220.

Benson, B.K., Meades G. Jr, Grove, A. and Waldrop, G.L. (2008) DNA inhibits catalysis by the carboxyltransferase subunit of acetyl-CoA carboxylase: implications for active site communication. *Protein Science* 17, 34–42.

Bilder, P., Lightle, S., Bainbridge, G., Ohren, J., Finzel, B., Sun, F., Holley, S., Al-Kassim L., Spessard, C., Melnick, M., Newcomer, M. and Waldrop, G.L. (2006) The structure of the carboxyltransferase component of acetyl-CoA carboxylase reveals a zinc-binding motif unique to the bacterial enzyme. *Biochemistry* 45, 1712–1722.

Blanchard, C.Z. and Waldrop, G.L. (1998) Overexpression and kinetic characterization of the carboxyltransferase component of acetyl-CoA carboxylase. *Journal of Biological Chemistry* 273, 19140–19145.

Boucher, H.W., Talbot, G.H., Bradley, J.S., Edwards, J.E. Jr, Gilbert, D., Rice, L.B., Scheld, M., Spellberg, B. and Bartlett, J. (2009) Bad bugs, no drugs: no ESKAPE! An update from the Infectious Diseases Society of America. *Clinical Infectious Diseases* 48, 1–12.

Brinster, S., Lamberet, G., Staels, B., Trieu-Cuot, P., Gruss, A. and Poyart, C. (2009) Type II fatty acid synthesis is not a suitable antibiotic target for Gram-positive pathogens. *Nature* 458, 83–86.

Campbell, J.W. and Cronan, J.E. Jr (2001) Bacterial fatty acid biosynthesis: targets for antibacterial drug discovery. *Annual Reviews of Microbiology* 55, 305–332.

Cheng, C.C., Shipps, G.W. Jr, Yang, Z., Sun, B., Kawahata, N., Soucy, K.A., Soriano, A., Orth, P., Xiao, L., Mann, P. and Black, T. (2009) Discovery and optimization of antibacterial *AccC* inhibitors. *Bioorganic and Medicinal Chemistry Letters* 19, 6507–6574.

Corson, T.W., Aberle, N. and Crews, C.M. (2008) Design and applications of bifunctional small molecules: why two heads are better than one. *ACS Chemical Biology* 3, 677–692.

Cronan, J.E. Jr and Waldrop, G.L. (2002) Multi-subunit acetyl-CoA carboxylases. *Progress in Lipid Research* 41, 407–435.

Fredenhagen, A., Tamura, S.Y., Kenny, P.T.M., Komura, H., Naya, Y., Nakanishi, K., Nishiyama, K., Sugiura, M. and Kita, H. (1987) Andrimid, a new peptide antibiotic produced by an intracellular bacterial symbiont isolated from a brown planthopper. *Journal of the American Chemical Society* 109, 4409–4411.

Freiberg, C., Brunner, N.A., Schiffer, G., Lampe, T., Pohlmann, J., Brands, M., Raabe, M., Häbich, D. and Ziegelbauer, K.J. (2004) Identification and characterization of the first class of potent bacterial acetyl-CoA carboxylase inhibitors

with antibacterial activity. *Journal of Biological Chemistry* 279, 26066–26073.
Heath, R.J., White, S.W. and Rock, C.O. (2001) Lipid biosynthesis as a target for antibacterial agents. *Progress in Lipid Research* 40, 467–497.
Le Calvez, P.B. (2009) Multisubstrate adduct inhibitors: drug design and biological tools. *Journal of Enzyme Inhibition and Medicinal Chemistry* 24, 1291–1318.
Levert, K.L. and Waldrop, G.L. (2002) A bisubstrate analog inhibitor of the carboxyltransferase component of acetyl-CoA carboxylase. *Biochemical and Biophysical Research Communications* 291, 1213–1217.
Liu, X., Fortin, P.D. and Walsh, C.T. (2008) Andrimid producers encode an acetyl-CoA carboxyltransferase subunit resistant to the action of the antibiotic. *Proceedings of the National Academy of Sciences USA* 105, 13321–13326.
Lu, H. and Tonge, P.J. (2008) Inhibitors of FabI, an enzyme drug target in the bacterial fatty acid biosynthesis pathway. *Accounts of Chemical Research* 41, 11–20.
Meades, G. Jr, Benson, B.K., Grove, A. and Waldrop, G.L. (2010) A tale of two functions: enzymatic activity and translational repression by carboxyltransferase. *Nucleic Acids Research* 38, 1217–1227.
Miller, J.R., Dunham, S., Mochalkin, I., Banotai, C., Bowman, M., Buist, S., Dunkle, B., Hanna, D., Harwood, H.J., Huband, M.D., Karnovsky, A., Kuhn, M., Limberakis, C., Liu, J.Y., Mehrens, S., Mueller, W.T., Narasimhan, L., Ogden, A., Ohren, J., Prasad, J.V.N.V., Shelly, J.A., Skerlos, L., Sulavik, M., Thomas, V.H., VanderRoest, S., Wang, L., Wang, Z., Whitton, A., Zhu, T. and Stover, C.K. (2009) A class of selective antibacterials derived from a protein kinase inhibitor pharmacophore. *Proceedings of the National Academy of Sciences USA* 106, 1737–1742.
Mochalkin, I., Miller, J. R., Evdokimov, A., Lightle, S., Yan, C., Stover, C.K. and Waldrop, G.L. (2008) Structural evidence for substrate-induced synergism and half-sites reactivity in biotin carboxylase. *Protein Science* 17, 1706–1718.
Mochalkin, I., Miller, J.R., Narasimhan, L., Venkataraman, T., Erdman, P., Cox, P.B., Vara Prasad, J.V.N., Lightle, S., Huband, M.D. and Stover, C.K. (2009) Discovery of antibacterial biotin carboxylase inhibitors by virtual screening and fragment-based approaches. *ACS Chemical Biology* 4, 473- 483.
Morphy, R. and Rankovic, Z. (2005) Designed multiple ligands. An emerging drug discovery paradigm. *Journal of Medicinal Chemistry* 48, 6523–6543.
McWhorter, W., Fredenhagen, A., Nakanishi, K. and Komura, H. (1989) Stereocontrolled synthesis of andrimid and a structural requirement for activity. *Journal of Chemical Society, Chemical Communications* 299–301.
Needham, J., Kelly, M.T., Ishige, M. and Andersen, R.J. (1994) Andrimid and moiramides A–C, metabolites produced in culture by a marine isolate of the bacterium *Pseudomonas fluorescens*: structure elucidation and biosynthesis. *Journal of Organic Chemistry* 59, 2058–2063.
Peleg, A.Y. and Hooper, D.C. (2010) Hospital-acquired infections due to Gram-negative bacteria. *New England Journal of Medicine* 362, 1804–1813.
Pohlmann, J., Lampe, T., Shimada, M., Nell, P.G., Pernerstorfer, J., Svenstrup, N., Brunner, N.A., Schiffer, G. and Freiberg, C. (2005) Pyrrolidinedione derivatives as antibacterial agents with a novel mode of action. *Bioorganic and Medicinal Chemistry Letters* 15, 1189–192.
Rice, W.G., Supko, J.G., Malspeis, L., Buckheit, R.W., Clanton, D., Bu, M., Graham, L., Schaeffer, C.A., Turpin, J.A., Domagala, J., Gogliotti, R., Bader, J.P., Halliday, S.M., Coren, L., Sowder, R.C., Arthur, L.O. and Henderson, L.E. (1995) Inhibitors of HIV nucleocapsid protein zinc fingers as candidates for the treatment of AIDS. *Science* 270, 1194–1197.
Santoro, N., Brtva, T., Vander Roest, S., Siegel, K. and Waldrop, G.L. (2006) A high-throughput screening assay for the carboxyltransferase subunit of acetyl-CoA carboxylase. *Analytical Biochemistry* 354, 70–77.
Silver, L.L. (2007) Multi-targeting by monotherapeutic antibacterials. *Nature Reviews Drug Discovery* 6, 41–55.
Soriano, A., Radice, A.D., Herbitter, A.H., Langsdorf, E.F., Stafford, J.M., Chan, S., Wang, S., Liu, Y. and Black, T. (2006) *Escherichia coli* acetyl-coenzyme A carboxylase: characterization and development of a high-throughput assay. *Analytical Biochemistry* 349, 268–276.
Tummino, P.J., Scholten, J.D., Harvey, P.J., Holler, T.P., Maloney, L., Gogliotti, R., Domagala, J. and Hupe, D. (1996) The *in vitro* ejection of zinc from human immunodeficiency virus (HIV) type 1 nucleocapsid protein by disulfide benzamides with cellular anti-HIV activity. *Proceedings of the National Academy of Sciences USA* 93, 969–973.
Waldrop, G.L. (2009) Smaller is better for antibiotic discovery. *ACS Chemical Biology* 4, 397- 399.
Walsh, C.T. and Fischbach, M.A. (2009) Repurposing libraries of eukaryotic protein kinase inhibitors for antibiotic discovery. *Proceedings of the National Academy of Sciences USA* 106, 1689–1690.

Wang, J., Soisson, S.M., Young, K., Shoop, W., Kodali, S., Galgoci, A., Painter, R., Parthasarathy, G., Tang, Y.S., Cummings, R., Ha, S., Dorso, K., Motyl, M., Jayasuriya, H., Ondeyka, J., Herath, K., Zhang, C., Hernandez, L., Allocco, J., Basilio, A., Tormo, J.R., Genilloud, O., Vicente, F., Pelaez, F., Colwell, L., Lee, L.H., Michael, B., Felcetto, T., Gill, C., Silver, L.L., Hermes, J.D., Bartizal, K., Barrett, J., Schmatz, D., Becker, J.W., Cully, D. and Singh, S.B. (2006) Platensimycin is a selective FabF inhibitor with potent antibiotic properties. *Nature* 44, 358–361.

Zhang, Y., White, S.W. and Rock, C.O. (2006) Inhibiting bacterial fatty acid synthesis. *Journal of Biological Chemistry* 281, 17541–17544.

14 Underexploited Targets in Lipopolysaccharide Biogenesis for the Design of Antibacterials

Laura Cipolla, Luca Gabrielli, Davide Bini and Laura Russo
Department of Biotechnology and Biosciences, University of Milano-Bicocca, Milan, Italy

14.1 Introduction

Lipopolysaccharides (LPSs), also known as endotoxins (Raetz and Whitfield, 2002; Raetz *et al.*, 2009; Reid and Szymanski, 2009; Wang and Quinn, 2010), are amphiphilic macromolecules including three distinct regions (Fig. 14.1), usually referred to as lipid A, the core region and the polysaccharide region. Lipid A constitutes the hydrophobic moiety of LPS located in the outer leaflet of the outer membrane, while the core and polysaccharide regions are exposed on the bacterial cell surface.

Lipid A is a diphosphorylated β(1→6) *N*-acetylglucosamine dimer, with four to seven fatty acids acylating – either symmetrically or asymmetrically – the hydroxyl and amino groups of the two units (Raetz *et al.*, 2007).

The core region is an oligosaccharide portion, containing up to 15 sugars (Holst and Brade, 1992; Holst, 2002, 2007) inserted between lipid A and the structurally diverse polysaccharide region. Although the polysaccharides of LPSs are composed of a wide range of different monosaccharides, 2-keto-3-deoxy-D-manno-octulosonic acid (Kdo) is universally present (Unger, 1983; Angata and Varki, 2002). The breakdown of Kdo biosynthesis may result in an accumulation of lipid A precursor (Raetz, 1990), with consequences for bacterial viability (Reynolds and Raetz, 2009), and thus Kdo is a promising target for antibacterial design. The number of Kdo molecules linked to lipid A can vary from one up to four for different species (Rick and Osborn, 1977; Belunis *et al.*, 1992; White *et al.*, 1997; Vinogradov *et al.*, 1998; Isobe *et al.*, 1999; Holst, 2007; Mamat *et al.*, 2009).

The polysaccharide region most often comprises the so-called O-specific polysaccharide, also known as O-antigen, but may also be the enterobacterial common antigen (ECA) or a capsular polysaccharide (Whitfield, 2006). The O-antigens of LPS show high structural diversity and determine the antigenic specificity of bacterial strains (Vinogradov *et al.*, 2002; Knirel *et al.*, 2006).

14.2 Kdo: a Fundamental Monosaccharide in LPS Biogenesis

Kdo (Figs 14.1 and 14.2) is an acidic monosaccharide included in the large family of 2-keto-3-deoxy-sugar acids, which are relevant constituents of complex carbohydrates (Angata and Varki, 2002; Schauer, 2004), with considerable roles in biological systems. Among

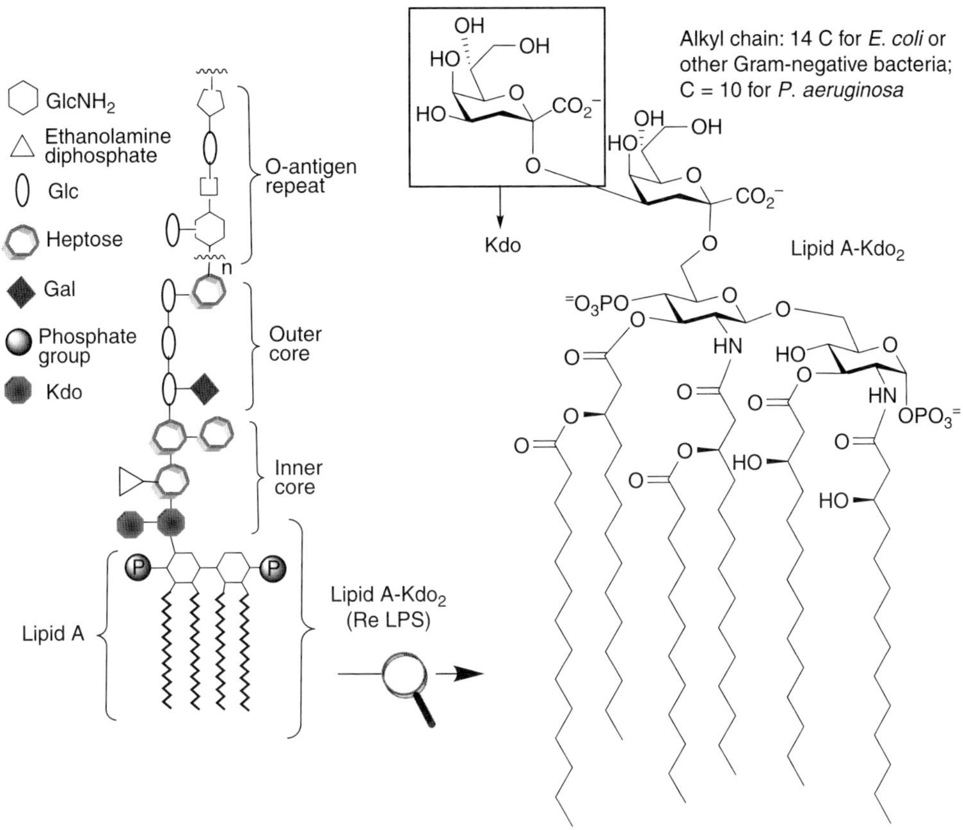

Fig. 14.1. General structure of bacterial LPSs.

this family, Kdo is an essential component of LPSs in Gram-negative bacteria, but it is also expressed in higher plants and green algae (as a component of cell-wall polysaccharides).

Kdo was first isolated in 1959 (Levin and Racker, 1959) and in the 1960s it was recognized as a glycosidic component of *Escherichia coli* O111:B4 LPS (Ghalambomr *et al.*, 1966). Since then, it has been reported in the LPSs of all members of the Enterobacteriaceae (Holst, 2007).

In this chapter, we will discuss Kdo, its role in bacterial LPSs biosynthesis and its potential as a target for antibacterial design. As the Kdo structure is the only recurrent structural element in all bacterial LPSs, its biosynthesis is a promising target for the design of novel and wide-ranging antibacterials.

14.3 Kdo Metabolism Leading to Kdo Glycosides

The presence of Kdo in all LPS structures has prompted investigations into the enzymes involved in its biosynthesis and their biocatalytic mechanisms. Four sequential enzymatic steps (Fig. 14.2) are involved in the Kdo biosynthetic pathway, starting from D-ribulose-5-phosphate (Ru5P):

1. Isomerization of Ru5P to D-arabinose 5-phosphate (A5P) mediated by A5P isomerase (API, KdsD/GutQ, EC: 5.3.1.31; Ray *et al.*, 1983).

2. Condensation of phosphoenolpyruvate (PEP) and A5P to Kdo-8-phosphate (Kdo8P) catalysed by Kdo8P synthase (Kdo8PS or KdsA, EC: 2.5.1.55; Dotson *et al.*, 1995).

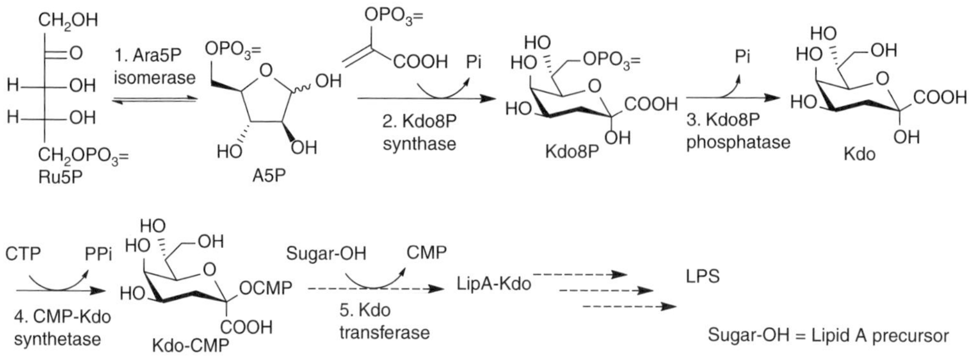

Fig. 14.2. Biosynthetic steps in the production of Kdo.

3. Hydrolysis of the Kdo8P phosphate ester leading to catalysis of Kdo by Kdo8P phosphatase (KdsC, EC: 3.1.3.45; Wu and Woodard, 2003).
4. Kdo activation as a cytidine monophosphate (CMP) glycoside (Kdo-CMP) by the action of CMP-Kdo synthetase (CKS, or KdsB, EC: 2.7.7.38; Goldman and Kohlbrenner, 1985).

At this point, biosynthetic intermediates $LipIV_A$ and activated CMP-Kdo converge by the action of a specific membrane-bound Kdo transferase (Fig. 14.2). Thus, transferase Waa in *E. coli* and in most bacteria catalyses the addition of Kdo units to lipid A, prior to its full acylation, while in *Pseudomonas aeruginosa* Kdo is transferred to fully acylated lipid A (Goldman *et al.*, 1988b; Mohan and Raetz, 1994; Rocchetta *et al.*, 1999; King *et al.*, 2009).

These enzymes are all essential for *E. coli* survival, but when gene redundancy exists (for example, KdsD and GutQ sharing the same API activity, see below), both the isozyme genes need to be knocked out to arrest cell growth (Meredith and Woodard, 2005).

14.3.1 API: structure and catalytic mechanism

A5P is the first intermediate, unique to the Kdo biosynthetic pathway, that is not readily available via glycolysis. A5P is synthesized by a reversible aldo–keto isomerization of a ketose sugar (Ru5P) to an aldose sugar (A5P), via a *cis*-enediol intermediate (Rose, 1975; Walsh, 1979). In *E. coli*, there are two APIs, KdsD (formerly known as YrbH; Meredith and Woodard, 2003) and GutQ (Meredith and Woodard, 2005), that have been characterized and shown to have nearly identical biochemical properties. After sequencing of the genomes of Gram-negative bacteria, KdsD has been always identified, while only a small number of Enterobacteriaceae express GutQ. The biological significance of this API redundancy in *E. coli* is not yet clear (Sperandeo *et al.*, 2006). In addition, a third paralogous gene, *kpsF*, has been found in pathogenic *E. coli* strains such as CFT073, K1 and K5.

Domain analysis of KdsD showed a core N-terminal sugar isomerase (SIS) domain (Bateman, 1999) of 210 amino acids, followed by a pair of C-terminal cystathionine β-synthase (CBS) domains of 50–60 amino acids each (Meredith and Woodard, 2003). The structure of *E. coli* KdsD has recently been predicted by homology modelling (Sommaruga *et al.*, 2009), but the catalytic and structural details are still limited. It is a tetrameric protein, presenting a Rossmann fold in each monomer. Residues postulated to be involved in the catalysis have estimated dissociation constant (pK_a) values of 6.55 and 10.34 (Dotson *et al.*, 1995), suggesting the presence of a histidine or possibly a carboxylate along with a lysine or arginine, similar to other sugar isomerases (Straus *et al.*, 1985; Lolis and Petsko, 1990; Jeffery *et al.*, 2001; Taylor *et al.*, 2008; Tello *et al.*, 2008).

Furthermore, homology modelling studies together with point-mutation experiments (Sommaruga *et al.*, 2009) suggest that Lys59, Glu111 and Glu152 are confined close to the presumed active site and are required for enzyme activity. KdsD from *E. coli* (Airoldi *et al.*, 2010) and *P. aeruginosa* (Airoldi *et al.*, 2011) was also characterized by nuclear magnetic resonance (NMR) studies, which highlighted key features needed for enzyme recognition and catalytic activity. The acidic phosphate group at carbon 5 and the 3-OH with the correct stereochemistry are needed for enzyme recognition. However, the substituents at positions 2 and 4 do not seem to be crucial for the interaction with the enzyme. A 4-OH (involved in the hemi-acetal ring formation) is not needed for recognition or catalysis. Kinetics data indicate that aldo–keto isomerization is faster on open-chain substrates (i.e. 4-deoxy-A5P), suggesting that the presence of the free carbonyl function speeds up the reaction, provided that the remaining functional groups are in place (i.e. phosphate and 3-OH). These data might be used for the rational design of substrate analogues with inhibitory activity.

14.3.2 Kdo8PS: structure and catalytic mechanism

Kdo8PS (or KdsA, EC: 4.1.2.16) mediates the condensation of A5P and PEP to Kdo8P (Ray, 1980; Hedstrom and Abeles, 1988). Two different classes of Kdo8PS have been identified based on their necessity for metal ions (Duewel and Woodard, 2000; Krosky *et al.*, 2002). *E. coli* Kdo8PS is the best-characterized member of the metal-ion-independent class (Radaev *et al.*, 2000; Wagner *et al.*, 2000; Asojo *et al.*, 2001). Kdo8PS from the hyperthermophilic microorganism *Aquifex aeolicus* is the best studied among the metal-dependent class (Duewel *et al.*, 2001; J. Wang *et al.*, 2001, 2002; Birck and Woodard, 2001). A divalent cation is needed for activity, probably Fe^{2+} or Zn^{2+}. All known bacterial Kdo8PSs possess a tetrameric quaternary structure (e.g. *E. coli* Kdo8PS, PDB code 1X8F) (Wu *et al.*, 2004). The *E. coli* enzyme active site was identified by crystallographic studies of binary complexes (PDB codes 1Q3N, 1PHW and 1X6U) of the synthase with PEP, Kdo8P and a cyclic analogue of A5P, 1-deoxy-A5P, and by solid-state rotational-echo double resonance (REDOR) NMR (Kaustov *et al.*, 2000; Vainer *et al.*, 2005).

Like the *E. coli* enzyme, Kdo8PS from *A. aeolicus* (PDB codes 1FX6, 1FXP, 1FWN, 1FY6 and 1FXQ) (Duewel *et al.*, 2001; J. Wang *et al.*, 2001, 2002; Birck and Woodard, 2001) is a tetramer with an optimal activity at 95°C. Two reciprocal single mutants of Kdo8PS from *Aquifex pyrophilus* and *E. coli* were prepared (Shulami *et al.*, 2004) to clarify the role of the metal. It was shown that the metal ion has a structural role, without any involvement in the reaction mechanism catalysed by metal-dependent Kdo8PS; the structural function of the metal may be equally maintained by a conserved asparagine residue in the metal-independent enzymes.

Different studies by rapid chemical quench flow (Liang *et al.*, 1997), mass spectrometry (Li *et al.*, 2003) and NMR (Kaustov *et al.*, 2003a; Vainer *et al.*, 2005) have been performed with various analogues of PEP, A5P and putative transient intermediates (Du *et al.*, 1999; Baasov and Belakov, 2000; Baasov *et al.*, 2001; Furdui *et al.*, 2005) to elucidate the catalytic mechanism. Kdo8P synthesis is a sequential process in which PEP binding precedes the binding of A5P, and the release of inorganic phosphate comes before the dissociation of the product Kdo8P. The mechanism is common to both metal-dependent and metal-independent enzymes. The condensation is stereospecific, with the *si* face of PEP attacking the *re* face of the carbonyl group of A5P, affording an unstable, acyclic bisphosphate intermediate through a transient oxocarbenium ion (compound 1, Fig. 14.3) at C-2 of PEP, which is subsequently captured by bulk water, producing an acyclic hemiketal phosphate

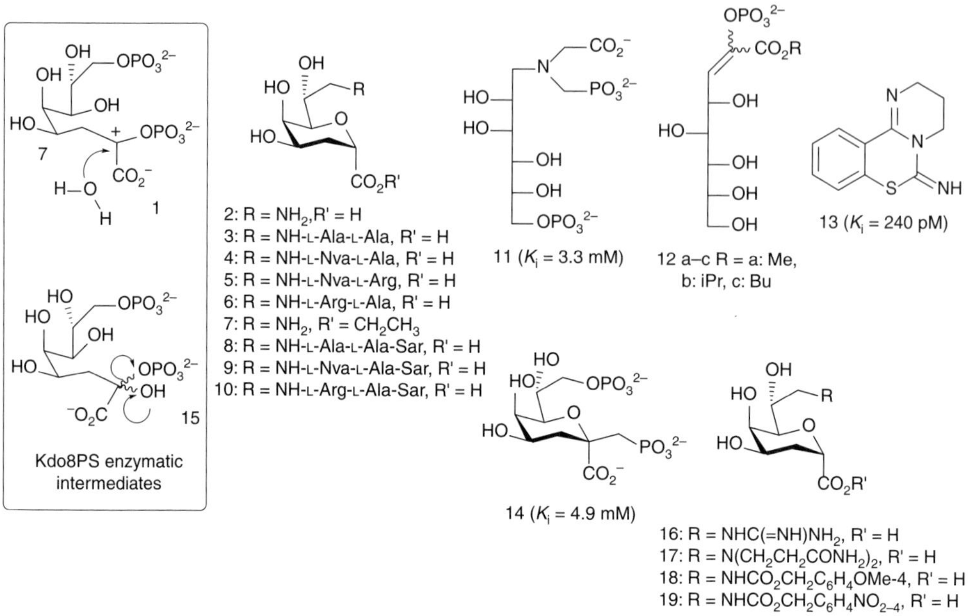

Fig. 14.3. Compounds 1 and 15, Kdo8PS postulated enzymatic intermediates; compounds 2–10, CKS inhibitors used as 'antibiotic adjuvants'; compounds 11–14, Kdo8PS inhibitors and their K_i values (where available); compounds 16–19, recently proposed inhibitors for CKS.

(compound 15, Fig. 14.3) that rapidly decomposes to Kdo8P and inorganic phosphate.

of non-polar and polar interactions with surrounding amino acids.

14.3.3 KdsC: structure and catalytic mechanism

KdsC cleaves Kdo8P producing Kdo and a molecule of inorganic phosphate. Only the *E. coli* (Wu and Woodard, 2003) enzyme structure has been determined solved (PDB code 2R8E) (Biswas *et al.*, 2009).

The cloned enzyme KdsC is a tetramer, requiring a divalent metal cofactor for activity, and has an optimal pH of 5.5 for activity. It is highly specific for Kdo8P and possesses elevated catalytic efficiency (Kuznetsova *et al.*, 2006). The active site of one monomer seems to be covered by a neighbouring monomer (Allen and Dunaway-Mariano, 2004). The crystal structure locates the active site at the interface between adjacent monomers, where Kdo is fitted into place by a network

14.3.4 CKS: structure and catalytic mechanism

CMP-Kdo synthetase or Kdo cytidyltransferase (CKS or KdsB in *E. coli*, EC: 2.7.7.38) catalyses the activation of Kdo by the addition of CMP to the anomeric position (Ray *et al.*, 1981; Goldman *et al.*, 1986).

CMP-Kdo is essential and its formation is the rate-limiting step in LPS biosynthesis (Goldman *et al.*, 1986). The sugar is activated in a single step, by direct introduction of the nucleotide on to the free anomeric hydroxyl group.

In *E. coli*, two isoenzymes have been found. The first, known as L-CKS, is involved in the biosynthesis of LPSs; the second, named capsule-specific CKS or K-CKS, has been identified in pathogenic strains whose CKS activity increases above 20°C (Finke *et al.*, 1989; Jann and Jann, 1992). Investigations of the *E. coli* enzyme catalytic mechanism have been performed (Jelakovic *et al.*, 1996; Jelakovic and Schulz, 2001; Jelakovic and Schulz, 2002) taking advantage of the known X-ray structure of CKS isoenzymes (PDB codes 1VH1 and 1H6J) (Badger *et al.*, 2005), while preliminary X-ray crystallographic studies were presented in the case of CKS from *Haemophilus influenzae* (Ku *et al.*, 2003), also complexed with its substrate, 3-deoxy-*manno*-octulosonate in the β configuration (Yoon *et al.*, 2008).

A ternary complex KdsB-CTP-2β-deoxy-Kdo crystal structure was recently obtained, providing details of the catalytic mechanism (Heyes *et al.*, 2009). 2β-Deoxy-Kdo is a substrate analogue lacking the β-anomeric hydroxyl substituent that was found to be a potent *in vitro* competitive inhibitor (Claesson *et al.*, 1987b), although it is ineffective *in vivo* due to its inability to cross the inner membrane (Goldman *et al.*, 1987; Hammond *et al.*, 1987). Both CTP and the Kdo analogue are positioned such that an SN_2 substitution can occur by attack of the anomeric hydroxyl group of Kdo to the β-phosphate of CTP. Two magnesium ions support the correct placing of the substrates and activation of CTP β-phosphate, while only one of them is responsible for activation of the Kdo anomeric hydroxyl group.

14.4 Analogues of Kdo Biosynthetic Intermediates: Underexploited Targets for Enzyme Inhibition

The Kdo biosynthetic pathway appears to be an ideal target for the development of novel antibacterials, as Kdo enzymes and biosynthetic intermediates are typical of these species with no counterparts in humans, thus allowing drug selectivity. In addition, as Kdo is a critical building block for LPS, disruption of its biosynthesis can critically threaten bacterial viability.

Thus, the development of new potential drugs targeting the enzymes of the Kdo pathway will provide novel molecules that can act as enzyme inhibitors (antibiotic properties), resulting in bacterial killing as a result of the loss of the outer-membrane assembly processes, or that can provoke the formation of a highly permeable outer membrane (antibiotic adjuvants) as a consequence of an incomplete LPS structure.

Over the years a number of analogues of biosynthetic intermediates have been proposed as inhibitors of Kdo biosynthesis: some have shown potent activity *in vitro* but none has been effective *in vivo*, mainly because they were not able to permeate the outer membrane (Cipolla *et al.*, 2008, 2009). A recent example showed the synergistic effect *in vitro* of CKS inhibitors (Fig. 14.3) with the antibiotics kanamycin and fosfomycin on enterohaemorrhagic *E. coli* O157:H7 (Kondo *et al.*, 2004).

Kdo analogues have been derivatized with short peptides at C-8 (Fig. 14.3, compounds 2–10) in order to facilitate cell uptake through the oligopeptide permease system. Once inside the cell, the peptide can subsequently be cleaved by endogenous bacterial aminopeptidases in the cytoplasm, releasing the active form of the inhibitor. Among compounds 2–10, alanylalanyl, norvalylalanyl and arginylnorvalyl derivatives (compounds 3–5) showed good antibacterial activity *in vitro* against *Salmonella* and *E. coli* strains (Claesson *et al.*, 1987a; Goldman and Devine, 1987; Goldman *et al.*, 1988a). However, this mechanism of uptake and processing allowed a route to resistance (e.g. transporter mutations), and these compounds have not found clinical application.

In parallel with the studies of the catalytic mechanism of Kdo8PS (Kaustov *et al.*, 2000; Vainer *et al.*, 2005), a few potential inhibitors of this enzyme have been synthesized (compounds 11–14, Fig. 14.3) (Baasov and Belakov, 2000; W. Wang *et al.*, 2001). The amino phosphonate compound 11 mimicking the structural and electrostatic properties of the biocatalytic intermediate compound 15 actually resulted in a potent competitive inhibitor (dissociation constant (K_i) 3.3 μM) (Baasov *et al.*, 2001; Kaustov *et al.*, 2003b; Belakhov *et al.*, 2004). The most active compound (compound 13, K_i 240 pM) (Birck *et al.*, 2000) was very effective *in vitro*, but it poorly affected bacterial growth, suggesting scarce bioavailability or that the compound is rapidly exported from the cell or metabolized. In addition, phosphonate compound 14 inhibited the enzyme with a K_i of 4.9 μM (Sheffer-Dee-Noor *et al.*, 1993).

It is reasonable to speculate that inhibition of API might have similar cellular effects as direct Kdo synthase inhibition, thus providing a good antibiotic target. Based on the postulated isomerization mechanism, a number of inhibitors have been synthesized in the 1980s, but none of them showed interesting activity (Bigham *et al.*, 1984). However, in the last few years, a more detailed knowledge of APIs has been gained (Airoldi *et al.*, 2010), thus invoking new efforts on this interesting target.

KdsC is the third attractive target for the design of inhibitors as new-generation antibiotics. However, to the best of our knowledge, no inhibitors have been developed against this enzyme to date.

CKS has been suggested as possible drug target since the 1980s, and a series of powerful *in vitro* inhibitors based on the structure of 2-β-deoxy-Kdo was synthesized (the most recent ones are shown in Fig. 14.3; see also Cipolla *et al.*, 2008, 2009, for more details). Compounds 16–19 (Fig. 14.3) (Adachi *et al.*, 2006), 2-deoxy-β-Kdo modified at position 8, are moderate enzyme inhibitors *in vitro*.

None of the 2-deoxy-β-Kdo analogues developed recently has shown *in vivo* activity because of their inability to cross the inner membrane, with the exception of compounds 3–5 (Fig. 14.3); however, these have developed resistance.

14.5 Future Perspectives

A detailed understanding of structural and catalytic features of enzymes involved in Kdo biosynthesis has been gained. However, this pathway has been underexploited in terms of the design of inhibitors as potent antibacterial and/or antibiotic adjuvants. Thanks to the deeper knowledge at our disposal, we believe that this field will rapidly move forward, with the design and synthesis of new molecules giving new impulse to research in this area.

References

Adachi, H., Kondo, K.-I., Kojima, F., Umezawa, Y., Ishino, K., Hotta, K. and Nishimura, Y. (2006) Synthesis and inhibitory activity of 8-substituted 2-deoxy-β-KDO against CMP-KDO synthetase. *Natural Product Research B: Bioactive Natural Products* 20, 361–370.

Airoldi, C., Sommaruga, S., Merlo, S., Sperandeo, P., Cipolla, L., Polissi, A. and Nicotra, F. (2010) Targeting bacterial membranes: NMR characterization of substrate recognition and binding requirements of D-arabinose 5P isomerase, a key enzyme in the biosynthesis of LPS. *Chemistry – A European Journal* 16, 1897–1902.

Airoldi, C., Merlo, S., Cipolla, L., Polissi, A. and Nicotra, F. (2011) Targeting bacterial membranes: identification of *Pseudomonas aeruginosa* D-Arabinose-5P Isomerase and NMR characterization of its substrate recognition and binding properties. *ChemBioChem* DOI: 10.1002/cbic.200.

Allen, K.N. and Dunaway-Mariano, D. (2004) Phosphoryl group transfer: evolution of a catalytic scaffold. *Trends in Biochemical Sciences* 29, 495–503.

Angata, T. and Varki, A. (2002) Chemical diversity in the sialic acids and related α-keto acids: an evolutionary perspective. *Chemical Reviews* 102, 439–470.

Asojo, O., Friedman, J., Adir, N., Belakhov, V., Shoham, Y. and Baasov, T. (2001) Crystal structures of KDOP synthase in its binary complexes with the substrate phosphoenolpyruvate and with a mechanism-based inhibitor. *Biochemistry* 40, 6326–6334.

Baasov, T. and Belakov, V. (2000) Towards a new class of synthetic antibacterials acting on lipopolysaccharide biosynthesis. *Drug Development Research* 50, 416–424.

Baasov, T., Tkacz, R., Sheffer-Dee-Noor, S. and Belakhov, V. (2001) Catalytic mechanism of 3-deoxy-D-manno-2-octulosonate-8-phosphate synthase. *Current Organic Chemistry* 5, 127–138.

Badger, J., Sauder, J.M., Adams, J.M., Antonysamy, S., Bain, K., Bergseid, M.G., Buchanan, S.G., Buchanan, M.D., Batiyenko, Y., Christopher, J.A., Emtage, S., Eroshkina, A., Feil, I., Furlong, E.B., Gajiwala, K.S., Gao, X., He, D., Hendle, J., Huber, A., Hoda, K., Kearins, P., Kissinger, C., Laubert, B., Lewis, H.A., Lin, J., Loomis, K., Lorimer, D., Louie, G., Maletic, M., Marsh, C.D., Miller, I., Molinari, J., Muller-Dieckmann, H.J., Newman, J.M., Noland, B.W., Pagarigan, B., Park, F., Peat, T.S., Post, K.W., Radojicic,

S., Ramos, A., Romero, R., Rutter, M.E., Sanderson, W.E., Schwinn, K.D., Tresser, J., Winhoven, J., Wright, T.A., Wu, L., Xu, J. and Harris, T.J.R. (2005) Structural analysis of a set of proteins resulting from a bacterial genomics project. *Proteins* 60, 787–796.

Bateman, A. (1999) The SIS domain: a phosphosugar-binding domain. *Trends Biochemical Sciences* 24, 94–95.

Belakhov, V., Dovgolevsky, E., Rabkin, E., Shulami, S., Shohamb, Y. and Baasov, T. (2004) Synthesis and evaluation of a mechanism-based inhibitor of KDO8P synthase. *Carbohydrate Research.* 339, 385–392.

Belunis, C.J., Mdluli, K.E., Raetz, C.R. and Nano, F.E. (1992) A novel 3-deoxy-D-manno-octulosonic acid transferase from *Chlamydia trachomatis* required for expression of the genus-specific epitope. *Journal of Biological Chemistry* 267, 18702 - 18707.

Bigham, E.C., Gragg, C.E., Hall, W.R., Kelsey, J.E., Mallory, W.R., Richardson, D.C., Benedict, C. and Ray, P.H. (1984) Inhibition of arabinose 5-phosphate isomerase. An approach to the inhibition of bacterial lipopolysaccharide biosynthesis. *Journal of Medicinal Chemistry* 27, 717–726.

Birck, M.R. and Woodard, R.W. (2001) *Aquifex aeolicus* 3-deoxy-D-manno-2-octulosonic acid 8-phosphate synthase: a new class of KDO 8-P synthase? *Journal of Molecular Evolution* 52, 205–214.

Birck, M.R., Holler, T.P. and Woodard, R.V. (2000) Identification of a slow tight binding inhibitor of 3-deoxy-D-manno-octulosonic acid 8-phosphate synthase. *Journal of the American Chemical Society* 122, 9334–9335.

Biswas, T., Yi, L., Aggarwal, P., Wu, J., Rubin, J.R., Stuckey, J.A., Woodard, R.W. and Tsodikov, O.V. (2009) The tail of KdsC: conformational changes control the activity of a haloacid dehalogenase superfamily phosphatase. *Journal of Biological Chemistry* 284, 30594–603.

Cipolla, L., Airoldi, C., Galliani, P., Polissi, A. and Nicotra, F. (2008) LPS biogenetic pathway: enzyme characterisation and synthetic efforts towards inhibitors. *Current Organic Chemistry* 12, 576–600.

Cipolla, L., Polissi, A., Airoldi, C., Galliani, P., Sperandeo, P. and Nicotra, F. (2009) The Kdo biosynthetic pathway toward OM biogenesis as target in antibacterial drug design and development. *Current Drug Discovery Technologies* 6, 19–33.

Claesson, A., Jansson, A.M., Pring, B.G., Hammond, S.M. and Ekstroem, B. (1987a) Design and synthesis of peptide derivatives of a 3-deoxy-D-manno-2-octulosonic acid (KDO) analogue as novel antibacterial agents acting upon lipopolysaccharide biosynthesis. *Journal of Medicinal Chemistry* 30, 2309–2313.

Claesson, A., Luthman, K., Gustafsson, K. and Bondesson, G. (1987b) A 2-deoxy analogue of KDO as the first inhibitor of the enzyme CMP-KDO synthetase. *Biochemical and Biophysical Research Communications* 143, 1063–1068.

Dotson, G.D., Dua, R.K., Clemens, J.C., Wooten, E.W. and Woodard, R.W. (1995) Overproduction and one-step purification of *Escherichia coli* 3-deoxy-D-manno-octulosonic acid 8-phosphate synthase and oxygen transfer studies during catalysis using isotopic-shifted heteronuclear NMR. *Journal of Biological Chemistry* 270, 13698–705.

Du, S., Faiger, H., Belakhov, V. and Baasov, T. (1999) Towards the development of novel antibiotics: synthesis and evaluation of a mechanism-based inhibitor of Kdo8P synthase. *Bioorganic & Medicinal Chemistry Letters* 7, 2671–2682.

Duewel, H.S. and Woodard, R.W. (2000) A metal bridge between two enzyme families. 3-Deoxy-D-manno-octulosonate-8-phosphate synthase from *Aquifex aeolicus* requires a divalent metal for activity. *Journal of Bacteriology* 275, 22824–22831.

Duewel, H.S., Radaev, S., Wang, J., Woodard, R.W. and Gatti, D.L. (2001) Substrate and metal complexes of 3-deoxy-D-*manno*-octulosonate-8-phosphate synthase from *Aquifex aeolicus* at 1.9-Å resolution. *Journal of Biological Chemistry* 276, 8393–8402.

Finke, A., Roberts, I., Boulnois, G., Pazzani, C. and Jann, K.J. (1989) Activity of CMP-2-keto-3-deoxyoctulosonic acid synthetase in *Escherichia coli* strains expressing the capsular K5 polysaccharide: implication for K5 polysaccharide biosynthesis. *Journal of Bacteriology* 171, 3074–3079.

Furdui, C.M., Sau, A.K., Yaniv, O., Belakhov, V., Woodard, R.W., Baasov, T. and Anderson, K.S. (2005) The use of (E)- and (Z)-phosphoenol-3-fluoropyruvate as mechanistic probes reveals significant differences between the active sites of KDO8P and DAHP synthases. *Biochemistry* 44, 7326–35.

Ghalambomr, A., Levinee, M. and Heathe, C. (1966) The biosynthesis of cell wall lipopolysaccharide in *Escherichia coli*. IV. Purification and properties of cytidine-monophosphate-3-deoxy-D-*manno*-octulosonate synthetase. *Journal of Biological Chemistry* 241, 3207–3215.

Goldman, R.C. and Devine, E.M. (1987) Isolation of *Salmonella typhimurium* strains that utilize exogenous 3-deoxy-D-manno-octulosonate for synthesis of lipopolysaccharide. *Journal of Bacteriology* 169, 5060–5065.

Goldman, R.C. and Kohlbrenner, W.E. (1985) Molecular cloning of the structural gene coding for CTP:CMP-3-deoxy-manno-octulosonate cytidylyltransferase from *Escherichia coli* K-12. *Journal of Bacteriology* 163, 256–261.

Goldman, R.C., Bolling, T.J., Kohlbrenner, W.E., Kim, Y. and Fox, J.L. (1986) Primary structure of CTP:CMP-3-deoxy-D-manno-octulosonate cytidylyltransferase (CMP-KDO synthetase) from *Escherichia coli*. *Journal of Biological Chemistry*. 261, 15831–5.

Goldman, R., Kohlbrenner, W., Lartey, P. and Pernet, A. (1987) Antibacterial agents specifically inhibiting lipopolysaccharide synthesis. *Nature* 329, 162–164.

Goldman, R.C., Doran, C.C. and Capobianco, J.O. (1988a) Analysis of lipopolysaccharide biosynthesis in Salmonella typhimurium and *Escherichia coli* by using agents which specifically block incorporation of 3-deoxy-D-manno-octulosonate. *Journal of Bacteriology* 170, 2185–2191.

Goldman, R.C., Doran, C.C., Kadam, S.K. and Capobianco, J.O. (1988b) Lipid A precursor from *Pseudomonas aeruginosa* is completely acylated prior to addition of 3-deoxy-D-manno-octulosonic acid. *Journal of Biological Chemistry* 263, 5217–5223.

Hammond, S.M., Claesson, A., Jansson, A.M., Larsson, L.G., Pring, B.G., Town, C.M. and Ekström, B. (1987) A new class of synthetic antibacterials acting on lipopolysaccharide biosynthesis. *Nature* 327, 730–732.

Hedstrom, L. and Abeles, R. (1988) 3-Deoxy-manno-octulonate 8-phosphate synthase catalyzes the C-O bond cleavage of phosphoenolpyruvate. *Biochemical and Biophysical Research Communications* 157, 816–820.

Heyes, D.J., Levy, C., Lafite, P., Roberts, I.S., Goldrick, M., Stachulski, A.V., Rossington, S.B., Stanford, D., Rigby, S.E.J., Scrutton, N.S. and Leys, D. (2009) Structure-based mechanism of CMP-2-keto-3-deoxymanno-octulonic acid synthetase: convergent evolution of a sugar-activating enzyme with DNA/RNA polymerases. *Journal of Biological Chemistry* 284, 35514–23.

Holst, O. (2002) Chemical structure of the core region of lipopolysaccharides. *Trends in Glycoscience and Glycotechnology* 14, 87–103.

Holst, O. (2007) The structures of core regions from enterobacterial lipopolysaccharides *FEMS Microbiology Letters* 271, 3–11

Holst, O. and Brade, H. (1992) Chemical structure of the core region of lipopolysaccharides. In: Morrison, D.C. and Ryan, J.L. (eds) *Bacterial Endotoxic Lipopolysaccharides*, Vol. I. CRC Press, Boca Raton, Florida, pp. 135–170.

Isobe, T., White, K.A., Allen, A.G., Peacock, M., Raetz, C.R. and Maskell, D.J. (1999) *Bordetella pertussis waaA* encodes a monofunctional 2-keto-3-deoxy-D-*manno*-octulosonic acid transferase that can complement an *Escherichia coli waaA* mutation. *Journal of Bacteriology* 181, 2648–2651.

Jann, K. and Jann, B. (1992) Capsules of *Escherichia coli*, expression and biological significance. *Canadian Journal of Microbiology* 38, 705–710.

Jeffery, C.J., Hardre, R. and Salmon, L. (2001) Crystal structure of rabbit phosphoglucose isomerase complexed with 5-phospho-D-arabinonate identifies the role of Glu357 in catalysis. *Biochemistry* 4, 1560–1566.

Jelakovic, S. and Schulz, G.E. (2001) The structure of CMP:2-keto-3-deoxy-manno-octonic acid synthetase and of its complexes with substrates and substrate analogs. *Journal of Molecular Biology* 312, 143–155.

Jelakovic, S. and Schulz, G.E. (2002) Catalytic mechanism of CMP:2-keto-3-deoxy-manno-octonic acid synthetase as derived from complexes with reaction educt and product. *Biochemistry* 41, 1174–1181.

Jelakovic, S., Jann, K. and Schulz, G.E. (1996) The three-dimensional structure of capsule-specific CMP: 2-keto-3-deoxy-*manno*-octonic acid synthetase from *Escherichia coli*. *FEBS Letters* 391, 157–161.

Kaustov, L., Kababya, S., Du, S., Baasov, T., Gropper, S., Shoham, Y. and Schmidt, A. (2000) Structural and mechanistic investigation of 3-deoxy-D-manno-octulosonate-8-phosphate synthase by solid-state REDOR NMR. *Biochemistry* 39, 14865–14876.

Kaustov, L., Baasov, T. and Schmidt, A. (2003a) Binding of the natural substrates and products to KDO8P synthase: ^{31}P and ^{13}C solution NMR characterization. *Bioorganic Chemistry*. 31, 306–321.

Kaustov, L., Kababya, S., Belakhov, V., Baasov, T., Shoham, Y. and Schmidt, A. (2003b) Inhibition mode of a bisubstrate inhibitor of KDO8P synthase: a frequency-selective REDOR solid-state and solution NMR characterization. *Journal of the American Chemical Society* 125, 4662–4669.

King, J.D., Kocíncová, D., Westman, E.L. and Lam, J.S. (2009) Lipopolysaccharide biosynthesis in *Pseudomonas aeruginosa*. *Innate Immunity* 15, 261–312.

Knirel, Y.A., Dentovskaya, S.V., Senchenkova, S.N., Shaikhutdinova, R.Z., Kocharova, N.A. and Anisimov, A.P. (2006) Conserved and variable structural features in the lipopolysaccharide of

Pseudomonas aeruginosa. *Journal of Endotoxin Research*. 12, 324–336.
Kondo, K.-I., Doi, H., Adachi, H. and Nishimura, Y. (2004) Synergistic effect of CMP/KDO synthase inhibitors with antimicrobial agents on inhibition of production and release of Vero toxin by enterohaemorrhagic *Escherichia coli* O157:H7. *Bioorganic and Medicinal Chemistry Letters* 14, 467–470.
Krosky, D.J., Alm, R., Berg, M., Carmel, G., Tummino, P.J., Xu, B. and Yang, W. (2002) *Helicobacter pylori* 3-deoxy-D-manno-octulosonate-8-phosphate (KDO-8-P) synthase is a zinc-metalloenzyme. *Biochimica Biophysica Acta* 1594, 297–306.
Ku, M.-J., Yoon, H.-J., Ahn, H.J., Kim, H.-W., Baek, S.-H. and Suh, S.W. (2003) *Acta Crystallographica* 59, 180.
Kuznetsova, E., Proudfoot, M., Gonzalez, C.F., Brown, G., Omelchenko, M.V., Borozan, I., Carmel, L., Wolf, Y.I., Mori, H., Savchenko, A.V., Arrowsmith, C.H., Koonin, E.V., Edwards, A.M. and Yakunin, A.F. (2006) Genome-wide analysis of substrate specificities of the *Escherichia coli* haloacid dehalogenase-like phosphatase family. *Journal of Biological Chemistry* 281, 36149–36161.
Levin, D.H. and Racker, E. (1959) Condensation of arabinose 5-phosphate and phosphorylenol pyruvate by 2-keto-3-deoxy-8-phosphooctonic acid synthetase. *Journal of Biological Chemistry* 234, 2532–2539.
Li, Z., Sau, A.K., Shen, S., Whitehouse, C., Baasov, T. and Anderson, K.S. (2003) A snapshot of enzyme catalysis using electrospray ionization mass spectrometry. *Journal of American Chemical Society* 125, 9938–9939.
Liang, P.-H., Kohen, A., Baasov, T. and Anderson, K.S (1997) Catalytic mechanism of Kdo8P synthase. Pre-steady-state kinetic analysis using rapid chemical quench flow methods. *Bioorganic and Medicinal Chemistry Letters* 7, 2463–2468.
Lolis, E. and Petsko, G.A. (1990) Crystallographic analysis of the complex between triosephosphate isomerase and 2-phosphoglycolate at 2.5Å resolution: implications for catalysis. *Biochemistry* 29, 6619–6625.
Mamat, U., Schmidt, H., Munoz, E., Lindner, B., Fukase, K., Hanuszkiewicz, A., Wu, J., Meredith, T.C., Woodart, R.W., Hilgenfeld, R., Mesters, J.R. and Holst, O. (2009) WaaA of the hyperthermophilic bacterium *Aquifex aeolicus* is a monofunctional 3-deoxy-D-manno-oct-2-ulosonic acid transferase involved in lipopolysaccharide biosynthesis. *Journal of Biological Chemistry* 284, 22248–22262.
Meredith, T.C. and Woodard, R.W. (2003) *Escherichia coli* YrbH Is a D-arabinose 5-phosphate isomerase. *Journal of Biological Chem*istry 278, 3271–3277.
Meredith, T.C. and Woodard, R.W. (2005) Identification of GutQ from *Escherichia coli* as a D-arabinose 5-phosphate isomerase. *Journal of Bacteriology* 187, 6936–6942.
Mohan, S. and Raetz, C.R.H. (1994) Endotoxin biosynthesis in *Pseudomonas aeruginosa*: enzymatic incorporation of laurate before 3-deoxy-D-manno-octulosonate. *Journal of Bacteriology* 176, 6944–6951.
Radaev, S., Dastidar, P., Patel, M., Woodard, R.W. and Gatti, D.L. (2000) Structure and mechanism of 3-deoxy-D-*manno*-octulosonate 8-phosphate synthase. *Journal of Biological Chem*istry 275, 9476–9484.
Raetz, C.R. (1990) Biochemistry of endotoxins. *Annual Review of Biochemistry* 59, 129–170.
Raetz, C.R.H. and Whitfield, C. (2002) Lipopolysaccharide endotoxins. *Annual Review of Biochemistry* 71, 635–700.
Raetz, C.R.H., Reynolds, C.M., Stephen Trent, M. and Bishop, R.E. (2007) Lipid A modification systems in Gram-negative bacteria. *Annual Review of Biochemistry* 76, 295–329.
Raetz, C.R.H., Guan, Z., Ingram, B.O., Six, D.A., Song, F., Wang, X. and Zhao, J. (2009) Discovery of new biosynthetic pathways: the lipid A story. *Journal of Lipid Research* 50, 103–108.
Ray, P.H. (1980) Purification and characterization of 3-deoxy-D-manno-octulosonate 8-phosphate synthetase from *Escherichia coli. Journal of Bacteriology* 141, 635–644.
Ray, P.H., Benedict, C.D. and Grasmuk, H.J. (1981) Purification and characterization of cytidine 5′-triphosphate:cytidine 5′-monophosphate-3-deoxy-D-manno-octulosonate cytidylyltransferase. *Journal of Bacteriology* 145, 1273–1280.
Ray, P.H., Kelsey, J.F., Bigham, E.C., Benedict, C.D. and Miller, T.A. (1983) Synthesis and use of 3-deoxy-d-manno-2-octulosonate (KDO). In: Anderson, L., and Unger, F.M. (eds) Escherichia coli: Potential Sites of Inhibition. ACS Symposium Series 231. American Chemical Society, Washington, DC, pp.141–169.
Reid, A.N. and Szymanski, C.M. (2009) Biosynthesis and assembly of capsular polysaccharides. In: Moran, A., Holst, O., Brennan, P. and von Itzstein, M. (eds) *Microbial Glycobiology: Structures, Relevance and Applications*. Academic Press, London, pp. 351–373.
Reynolds, C.M. and Raetz, C.R.H. (2009) Replacement of lipopolysaccharide with free lipid A molecules in *Escherichia coli* mutants

lacking all core sugars. *Biochemistry* 48, 9627–9640.

Rick, P.D. and Osborn, M.J. (1977) Lipid A mutants of *Salmonella typhimurium. Journal of Biological Chemistry* 252, 4895–4903.

Rocchetta, H.L., Burrows, L.L. and Lam, J.S. (1999) Genetics of O-antigen biosynthesis in *Pseudomonas aeruginosa. Microbiology and Molecular Biology Reviews* 63, 523–553.

Rose, I. (1975) Mechanism of the aldose–ketose isomerase reactions. *Advances in Enzymology and Related Areas of Molecular Biology* 43, 491–517.

Schauer, R. (2004) Sialic acids: fascinating sugars in higher animals and man. *Zoology* 107, 49–64.

Sheffer-Dee-Noor, S., Belakhov, V. and Baasov, T. (1993) Insight into the catalytic mechanism of KDO8P synthase. *Bioorganic & Medicinal Chemistry Letters* 3, 1583–1588.

Shulami, S., Furdui, C., Adir, N., Shoham, Y., Anderson, K.S. and Baasov, T. (2004) A reciprocal single mutation affects the metal requirement of 3-deoxy-D-manno-2-octulosonate-8-phosphate (KDO8P) synthases from *Aquifex pyrophilus* and *Escherichia coli. Journal of Biological. Chemistry* 43, 45110–45120.

Sommaruga, S., De Gioia, L., Tortora, P. and Polissi, A. (2009) Structure prediction and functional analysis of KdsD, an enzyme involved in lipopolysaccharide biosynthesis. *Biochemical and Biophysical Research Communications* 388, 222–227.

Sperandeo, P., Pozzi, C., Dehò, G. and Polissi, A. (2006) Non-essential KDO biosynthesis and new essential cell envelope biogenesis genes in the *Escherichia coli* yrbG–yhbG locus. *Research in Microbiol*ogy 157, 547–558.

Straus, D., Raines, R., Kawashima, E., Knowles, J.R. and Gilbert, W. (1985) Active site of triosephosphate isomerase: in vitro mutagenesis and characterization of an altered enzyme. *Proceedings of the National Academy of Sciences USA* 82, 2272–2276.

Taylor, P.L., Blakely, K.M., de Leon, G.P., Walker, J.R., McArthur, F., Evdokimova, E., Zhang, K., Valvano, M.A., Wright, G.D. and Junop, M.S. (2008) Structure and function of sedoheptulose-7-phosphate isomerase, a critical enzyme for lipopolysaccharide biosynthesis and a target for antibiotic adjuvants. *Journal of Biological Chemistry* 283, 2835–2845.

Tello, M., Rejzek, M., Wilkinson, B., Lawson, D.M. and Field, R.A. (2008) Tyl1a, a TDP-6-deoxy-D-*xylo*-4-hexulose 3,4-isomerase from *Streptomyces fradiae*: structure prediction, mutagenesis and solvent isotope incorporation experiments to investigate reaction mechanism. *ChemBioChem* 9, 1295–1302.

Unger, F.M. (1983) The chemistry and biological significance of 3-deoxy-D-manno-2-octulosonic acid (Kdo). *Advances in Carbohydrate Chemistry and Biochemistry* 348, 323–347.

Vainer, R., Belakhov, V., Rabkin, E., Baasov, T. and Adir, N. (2005) Crystal structures of *Escherichia coli* KDO8P synthase complexes reveal the source of catalytic irreversibility. *Journal of Molecular Biology* 351, 641–652.

Vinogradov, E.V., Petersen, B.O. and Thomas-Oates, J.E. (1998) Characterization of a novel branched tetrasaccharide of 3-deoxy-D-*manno*-oct-2-ulopyranosonic acid. The structure of the carbohydrate backbone of the lipopolysaccharide from *Acinetobacter baumanii* strain NCTC 10303 (ATCC 17904). *Journal of Biological Chemistry* 273, 28122–28131.

Vinogradov, E., Sidorczyk, Z. and Knirel, Y.A. (2002) Structure of the lipopolysaccharide core region of the bacteria of the genus *Proteus. Australian Journal of Chemistry* 55, 61–67.

Wagner, T., Kretsinger, R.H., Bauerle, R. and Tolbert, W.D. (2000) 3-Deoxy-D-*manno*-octulosonate-8-phosphate synthase from *Escherichia coli.* Model of binding of phosphoenolpyruvate and D-arabinose-5-phosphate. *Journal of Molecular Biology* 301, 233–238.

Walsh, C. (1979) *Enzymatic Reaction Mechanisms.* W.H. Freeman & Co., San Francisco, California, pp. 585–599.

Wang, J., Duewel, H.S., Woodard, R.W. and Gatti, D.L. (2001) Structures of *Aquifex aeolicus* KDO8P synthase in complex with R5P and PEP and with a bisubstrate inhibitor: role of active site water in catalysis. *Biochemistry* 40, 15676–15683.

Wang, J., Duewel, H.S., Stuckey, J.A., Woodard, R.W. and Gatti, D.L. (2002) Function of His185 in *Aquifex aeolicus* 3-deoxy-D-manno-octulosonate 8-phosphate synthase. *Journal of Molecular Biology* 324, 205–214.

Wang, W., Kim, R., Jancarik, J., Yokota, H. and Kim, S.H. (2001) Crystal structure of phosphoserine phosphatase from *Methanococcus jannaschii*, a hyperthermophile, at 1.8 A resolution. *Structure* 9, 65–71.

Wang, X. and Quinn, P.J. (2010) Lipopolysaccharide: biosynthetic pathway and structure modification. *Progress in Lipid Res*earch 49, 97–107.

White, K.A., Kaltashov, I.A., Cotter, R.J. and Raetz, C.R. (1997) A mono-functional 3-deoxy-D-manno-octulosonic acid (Kdo) transferase and a Kdo kinase in extracts of *Haemophilus influenzae. Journal of Biological Chemistry* 272, 16555–16563.

Whitfield, C. (2006) Biosynthesis and assembly of capsular polysaccharides in *Escherichia coli*. *Annual Review of Biochemistry* 75, 39–68.

Wu, J. and Woodard, R.W. (2003) *Escherichia coli* YrbI is 3-deoxy-D-manno-octulosonate 8-phosphate phosphatase. *Journal of Biological Chemistry* 278, 18117–18123.

Wu, J., Patel, M.A., Sundaram, A.K. and Woodard, R.W. (2004) Functional and biochemical characterization of a recombinant *Arabidopsis thaliana* 3-deoxy-D-manno-octulosonate 8-phosphate synthase. *Biochemical Journal* 381, 185–193.

Yoon, H.-J., Ku, M.-J., Mikami, B. and Suh, S.W. (2008) Structure of 3-deoxy-*manno*-octulosonate cytidylyltransferase from *Haemophilus influenzae* complexed with the substrate 3-deoxy-manno-octulosonate in the β-configuration. *Acta Crystallographica Section D* 64, 1292–1294.

15 Predicting and Dissecting High-order Molecular Complexity by Information-driven Biomolecular Docking

Panagiotis L. Kastritis and Alexandre M.J.J. Bonvin
Bijvoet Center for Biomolecular Research, Science Faculty, Utrecht University, Utrecht, The Netherlands

15.1 Increased Molecular Flexibility and Complexity in Antimicrobial Drug Design

Drug discovery today is moving towards the development of more complicated agents, especially in the field of antimicrobial drug design. In order to enhance lead compounds potency and optimize the design of more successful lead molecules, the incorporation of structural knowledge is deemed necessary (Hajduk and Greer, 2007). This process is called structure-based drug design (SBDD), the process of finding new medications based on the knowledge of the structure and function of the biological target of interest, generally by using computer modelling (docking).

Molecular docking is a computational method used to predict the preferred binding mode of one molecule to another, starting from their unbound conformations. In protein–ligand docking, the candidate target is usually a protein with medical relevance, and the lead compound is (usually) an organic compound that can inhibit the activity of the protein (see Chapters 3–5, this volume). SBDD has already demonstrated its power through the discovery of novel therapeutics over the years (Simmons *et al.*, 2010). For example, knowledge of the human immunodeficiency virus (HIV) protease three-dimensional structure enabled the design and optimization of five inhibitors that are now commercially available antiretroviral drugs (Erickson *et al.*, 1990; Roberts *et al.*, 1990; Dorsey *et al.*, 1994). SBDD has been successfully applied to the development of other drugs, including zanamivir for influenza (GlaxoSmithKline; McCauley, 1999) and several non-steroidal anti-inflammatory agents targeting cyclooxygenase 2 (e.g. celecoxib, Pfizer; Stratton and Alberts, 2002). New approaches in SBDD, such as fragment-based drug design (FBDD) continue to flourish, opening the route to the *ab initio* design of agents with increased ligand potency (Murray and Blundell, 2010). FBDD is based on the idea that the use of small inhibitors as building blocks can lead to the development of larger compounds with higher affinity. FBDD is moving towards the design of more complex and affine biomolecules. Analysis and understanding of the increased complexity and flexibility of such ligands is deemed necessary for success in drug design. Current developments in antimicrobial agents are not limited to SBDD/FBDD methods; there has also been special interest in the discovery, development and application of (natural) complex organic compounds (Cowan, 1999; Hann *et al.*, 2001), hybrid molecules derived from click chemistry (Kolb and Sharpless, 2003) and peptide antimicrobial agents (Jenssen *et al.*, 2006) (see Fig. 15.1). Click chemistry encompasses all chemical procedures tailored to generate molecules quickly and reliably by joining small units together. The latter is inspired by the fact that nature also generates substances by joining small modular units, such as proteins, sugars, nucleic acids and lipids.

A novel approach in modern drug discovery, which challenges the traditional concept of inhibiting enzymes, is to design inhibitors that specifically target protein–protein complexes, blocking or modulating their underlying interactions (Arkin and Wells, 2004). Indeed, protein–protein interactions should also form an important class of therapeutic targets (Patel and Player, 2008) as they are involved in nearly all normal and pathological pathways, including signal transduction, cell adhesion, proliferation, growth, differentiation, structure of cellular cytoskeleton, programmed cell death and virus self-assembly (Toogood, 2002). Inhibitors designed for this category of targets are usually larger and more complex compared with traditional ligands that target enzymes. The interface that these ligands have to inhibit is also larger compared with an enzymatic active site. A collection of crystallographically determined protein–protein complexes with known inhibitors has been compiled in the 2P2I protein–protein inhibition database (http://2p2idb.cnrs-mrs.fr/; Bourgeas *et al.*, 2010). As of February 2012, we have calculated that the mean molecular weight of all 45 ligands present in the database, targeting two classes of protein–protein interactions and 10 different protein–protein complexes, is 535±156 Da.

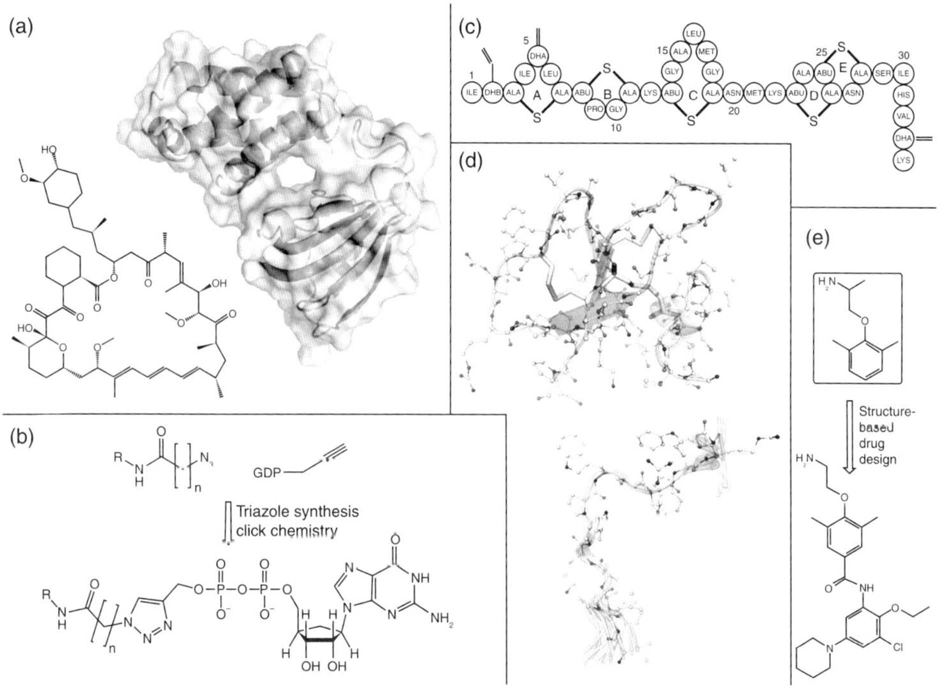

Fig. 15.1. Complexity of molecules used to inhibit protein molecules. (a) The protein–protein complex of immunophilin–immunosuppressant FKBP12 is inhibited by rapamycin (PDB ID: 1FAP). (b) Triazole synthesis used in click chemistry in order to derive molecules of higher-order molecular complexity. Azide fragments are coupled with an alkyne GDP core. (c) The nisin A molecule composed of natural and unnatural amino acids, such as didehydroalanine (DHA), didehydroaminobutyric acid (DHB) and α-aminobutyric acid (ABU). (d) Natural peptide inhibitors, human β-defensin-2 (PDB ID: 1FQQ) and indolicidin, an unstructured peptide (PDB ID: 1G89). (e) Process of structure-based drug design, where a new, larger urokinase inhibitor with higher potency is synthesized (50% inhibitory concentration (IC_{50}) = 0.003 μM) based on the initial inhibitor (IC_{50} = 0.91 μM).

All newly emerging methods for designing potential antimicrobial agents (Fig. 15.1) have to deal with a common challenge: the increased complexity of the complexes that involve larger and rather complicated molecules. These are typically rather flexible systems, behaving more like fluids than rigid bodies, in contrast to what is usually assumed in SBDD, where proteins are treated as rigid entities (mostly due to the computational cost, as very large libraries of compounds have to be screened against a target receptor molecule). For a recent review on protein flexibility and its role in drug design, see Fuentes *et al.* (2011).

Since the discovery of the importance of flexibility in biomolecular association, for example with the flexible protein recognition model of Grunberg *et al.* (2004) where recognition is proposed to occur in sequential steps involving: (i) diffusion; (ii) conformer selection from a pool of conformers; and (iii) induced fit, some progress has been achieved in the inclusion of flexibility in SBDD (Meagher and Carlson, 2004). Nevertheless, these are rather limited, as tackling both receptor and ligand flexibility simultaneously with conventional methods remains very challenging due to the explosion in the number of degrees of freedom of the system under study, which can translate into exorbitant computational costs.

A multipurpose docking program that can be used to address this type of challenge is HADDOCK (high-ambiguity-driven biomolecular docking) (Dominguez *et al.*, 2003; de Vries *et al.*, 2007). In this chapter, we will describe this program and its successful applications to protein–small ligand docking, with specific emphasis on antimicrobial agents, and will consider this with regard to the treatment of flexibility and its associated challenges. In Section 15.2, the key idea fundamental to data-driven biomolecular docking is introduced: how can a wide variety of experimental and/or predicted information be used to drive the modelling process, thereby restricting the interaction space to be searched? Relevant technical and theoretical aspects are discussed in this section, where treatment of molecular complexity and flexibility is introduced. In this way, the reader should be able to understand better the subsequent sections of this chapter, where applications of data-driven docking in small-molecule design are described. Specifically, in Section 15.3, different examples from recent literature are portrayed in which data-driven docking has been successful in providing structural insights for the design of small-molecule inhibitors that can act as antimicrobial agents.

15.2 Data-driven Docking

X-ray crystallography and nuclear magnetic resonance (NMR) are widely used experimental techniques to obtain atomic resolution structures of protein–ligand complexes and unravel the structural details of the recognition process. However, their traditional use often implies high costs in terms of time, resources and maintenance, whereas their applicability to protein–ligand complexes is strongly case dependent (Jahnke, 2007). On the other hand, advances in X-ray crystallography and NMR have expanded the range of tractable targets along with improving the overall throughput (Blundell *et al.*, 2002; Betz *et al.*, 2006). For example, if the X-ray structure of the target is known, a simple crystallographic screening may be used. Ideally, the active site of the target macromolecule should be open to solvent channels in the crystal to allow complex formation by the ligand-soaking method: the crystal is soaked in a solution containing a mixture of compounds; from this, the most potent ligand will bind in the active site of the crystalline macromolecule by diffusion into the crystal. X-ray crystallography might, however, fail to yield a protein–ligand structure for various reasons, often because some proteins simply do not crystallize. Other possible reasons for failure include the fact that the ligand molecule might occupy the active site of the enzyme within the crystal insufficiently or in a disordered manner that makes the electron density much less defined, or because crystal packing might prevent binding by the fragments. A case representing the abovementioned crystallographic artefact can be found in the structure of the homodimeric enzyme malate dehydrogenase, which was crystallized as a tetramer (Protein Data Bank (PDB) ID: 4MDH; http://www.rcsb.org/pdb/). In 4MDH, the chains building the homodimer are involved in different crystal contacts: Chain A has crystal contacts near the catalytic site, whereas chain B does not show such contacts. As a consequence, the conformation of loop 89–104 close to the active site is extensively affected. In one of the monomers, this loop is surrounded by solvent while in the other it contacts another chain in the crystal. This results in a different conformation of the loop, which in turn affects the conformation of the active site. Another possible problem with crystallographic studies is that ligand binding is often achieved by soaking crystals of the protein into a solution containing the ligand. For large and flexible ligands, this soaking procedure might disrupt the crystal.

NMR can provide a powerful alternative to X-ray crystallography as it allows studying of the binding and behaviour of molecules in solution and can provide three-dimensional structural information about the complex. Developments in the field of NMR are therefore of particular interest, as a vast amount of experimental data relevant to the protein–ligand system can be extracted, provided that the structure of the target is known. For example, depending on the size of the target, the labelling schemes and the binding regime, a variety of NMR data can be obtained relevant to the ligand and/or the protein sides, such as chemical shift perturbation (CSP) data, nuclear Overhauser effects (NOEs), residual dipolar couplings and cross-correlation rates. Data sources that can provide information about a complex are, however, not restricted to NMR. For example, even simple mutagenesis experiments can provide valuable information that can assist a modelling procedure. All these data can be used in sophisticated algorithms to model protein–ligand complexes *in silico*. Such algorithms are referred to as information-driven (data-driven) and rely on such data to derive three-dimensional models of the systems in atomistic detail. A unique computational method falling under this category is HADDOCK (Dominguez *et al.*, 2003).

HADDOCK is an information-driven flexible docking approach for the modelling of biomolecular complexes (Dominguez *et al.*, 2003). Compared with other docking methods, HADDOCK is unique in the sense that it can handle a wide variety of experimental and/or bioinformatics data to drive the modelling process (Melquiond and Bonvin, 2010). The method allows for a rather sophisticated treatment of flexibility by limiting the search to the relevant interaction space of the biomolecules that are being docked. The program incorporates information about the interface regions of the binding molecules (a binding pocket/active site of an enzyme is also considered an interface). The latter can be identified by several experimental methods/techniques, including mutagenesis in combination with a binding assay, chemical modifications (e.g. by cross-linkers or oxidative agents) detected by mass spectrometry (MS), hydrogen/deuterium exchange detected by either MS or NMR, and a variety of valuable NMR data such as CSP, cross-saturation transfer, INPHARMA (protein-mediated interligand NOEs for pharmacophore mapping; Sanchez-Pedregal *et al.*, 2005) and structure–activity relationships by interligand NOEs (Becattini and Pellecchia, 2006). Bioinformatics predictions, for example based on evolutionary information, can also be used when experimental data are scarce or unavailable (de Vries and Bonvin, 2008). As well as being able to deal with such a large variety of experimental and/or predicted information, HADDOCK also supports classical NMR restraints such as distances from NOEs and paramagnetic relaxation enhancement measurements, dihedral angles, residual dipolar couplings, diffusion anisotropy restraints and pseudo-contact shifts, the latter three providing valuable information about the relative orientation of the components in a complex. For more information about useful sources for restraining the docking, see Melquiond and Bonvin (2010), Schmitz *et al.* (2012) and van Dijk *et al.* (2005).

Most of the information sources described in the previous paragraph typically only identify or predict interfacial regions, and do not define the contacts across an interface. In HADDOCK, these are implemented as ambiguous interaction restraints (AIRs) that will force the interfaces to come together without imposing a particular orientation. AIRs are entered as a list of active and passive residues. The active residues correspond to the (experimentally) identified interface residues, whereas passive residues correspond to their solvent-accessible neighbouring residues. The latter ensure that residues located in the interface but not detected can satisfy the AIRs. Note that this terminology is not restricted to amino acid residues of proteins, despite the fact that the algorithm was originally developed for protein–protein docking; for example, a residue can also be a non-standard amino acid, a nucleotide base, a sugar or any organic compound. An AIR corresponds to an ambiguous intermolecular distance (d_{iAB}^{eff}) with a maximum value of typically 2 Å between any atom m of an active residue i of protein A (m_{iA}) and any atom n of both active and passive residues k (N_{resB} in total) of protein B (n_{kB}) (and inversely for protein A). The effective distance, corresponding to each restraint is calculated using the following equation:

$$d_{iAB}^{eff} = \left(\sum_{m_{iA}=1}^{N_{Aatoms}} \sum_{k=1}^{N_{resB}} \sum_{n_{kB}=1}^{N_{Batoms}} \frac{1}{d_{m_{iA}n_{kB}}^{6}} \right)^{-1/6} \qquad (15.1)$$

where $\frac{1}{d_{m_{iA}n_{kB}}^{6}}$ denotes a potential that resembles the Lennard–Jones attractive term.

The function has the property that all d_{iAB}^{eff} will always be smaller than the shorter distance $d_{m_{iA}n_{kB}}$ entering the sum. The AIRs effectively enforce the defined interfaces to come together without imposing any restraint on their relative orientation. The AIRs can be further fine-tuned manually to restrict them to specific atoms or groups of atoms (for example, pharmacophore groups).

15.2.1 Dealing with molecular flexibility

HADDOCK deals with molecular flexibility at different levels, both implicitly and explicitly, starting from the initial coordinate files of the biomolecules until the final flexible refinement in explicit water with subsequent energy minimization.

First level – implicit (as starting point for the docking)

ENSEMBLE DOCKING. The HADDOCK program supports ensemble docking, meaning that it can handle as input more than one configuration of any of the partners, such as, for example, an ensemble of NMR structures or different crystal structures of the same enzyme. Other methods can also be used to produce ensemble of structures for docking, such as molecular dynamics simulation, normal modes analysis and principal components analysis; however, these will not be covered in this chapter.

In such cases, HADDOCK performs a cross-docking of all possible combinations of starting structures. Ideally, the number of initial rigid-body docking poses generated should be a multiple of the number of all combinations, with each combination sampled multiple times (e.g. at least 100). Ensembles that are too large might result in a dilution effect, meaning by that, if only a few structures have a proper conformation for binding, only a small fraction of all sampled combinations might lead to a successful docking.

FRAGMENT-BASED DOCKING. If the target protein molecule undergoes significant conformational changes, a multibody docking protocol can be used (Karaca *et al.*, 2011). The protein target is then treated as a collection of separate domains (Karaca and Bonvin, 2011).

TREATMENT OF ENZYME FLEXIBILITY IN HADDOCK. A good example of flexibility treatment is the case of the enzyme dihydrofolate reductase (DHFR). The enzyme catalyses the reduction of 5,6-dihydrofolate to 5,6,7,8-tetrahydrofolate, utilizing NADPH as a cofactor (Sawaya and Kraut, 1997). DHFR is important in drug discovery, as blockade of its enzymatic activity leads to irreversible cell death. A large number of crystal structures of the enzyme complexed with different compounds and substrates have been deposited in the PDB. For example, if docking of a specific compound and *Escherichia coli* DHFR is performed, one can use all 55 experimental structures of the *E. coli* enzyme in the PDB (as of February 2012) (a requisite is, however, that they are all consistent with each other and contain the same atoms – missing fragments/side chains should thus be added prior to docking). The ensemble docking method allows simultaneous docking of the compound to all chains, implicitly treating the receptor flexibility in the initial rigid-body stage of the docking by the collection of different conformers. Similarly, different conformations of the second molecule can be introduced (for example, one more), leading to 2 × 55 different combinations of starting structures for the docking.

The catalytic mechanism of the *E. coli* DHFR enzyme was deciphered by Sawaya and Kraut (1997), who concluded that the M20 loop adopts different configurations when the substrate and the cofactor of the enzyme are bound. Therefore, DHFR can be treated as a collection of two domains, one corresponding to the enzyme without the loop and a second corresponding to the M20 loop. During a docking run with a lead compound, a simultaneous three-body docking protocol can be applied, connecting the M20 loop at the hinge regions with the rest of the molecule by defining additional distance restraints. Such treatment of the system might allow discovery of a possible low-energy orientation of both the M20 loop and the lead compound in the active site of the enzyme simultaneously.

Second level – explicit (during docking)

The docking protocol in HADDOCK, which makes use of the crystallography and NMR system package (Brunger *et al.*, 1998) as computational engine, consists of three successive steps.

1. Rigid-body energy minimization. At this step, called *it0*, the molecules are brought together as rigid units by energy minimization, using the effective distance criterion (see above) and non-bonded energies (electrostatic and van der Waals energies) that become effective once the molecules are within the non-bonded cut-off (typically 8.5 Å).

2. Semi-flexible refinement in torsion angle space. Typically, the top 10–20% of the models in *it0* are subsequently subjected to flexible refinement in torsion angle space (the *it1* step). Selection of the structures to be subjected to this refinement stage is based on the HADDOCK score, which is a weighted sum of various terms (buried surface area, empirical desolvation term, electrostatic, van der Waals and restraint violation energies) (see de Vries *et al.*, 2007 for details). The flexible regions are by default automatically defined as all residues within 5 Å of the partner molecule plus their preceding sequential neighbour. A manual definition of flexible segments is also possible. The flexible refinement stage consists of three simulated annealing refinements and a final steepest-descent energy minimization:

- In the first simulated annealing stage, the molecules are treated as rigid entities and their relative orientation is optimized.
- In the second stage, side chains at the interface are allowed to move to optimize the packing. In the case of protein–ligand docking, the ligand molecule can be treated as fully flexible (see below).
- In the third stage, both side chains and backbone at the interface are allowed to move to allow for small conformational rearrangements.
- A final energy minimization is applied in order to optimize the derived complexes and calculate the underlying energetics for each docked solution that derived from *it1*.

3. Final refinement in explicit solvent. The final stage consists of a gentle refinement in explicit water, or in DMSO for hydrophobic molecules (e.g. transmembrane proteins). The system is first heated to 300 K with position restraints on all atoms except for the flexible side chains at the interface. Short molecular dynamics simulation steps are then performed at 300 K with position restraints only on non-interface backbone-heavy atoms. During the final cooling stage (reaching finally 100 K), the position restraints are limited to backbone atoms outside the interface. A final energy minimization step is again applied and the final energy of each derived complex is calculated.

Only by an explicit treatment of flexibility during the refinement stages of the docking can well-packed biomolecular models be obtained. These typically do not contain intermolecular clashes, resembling in this aspect structures deposited in the PDB.

Note that one can define *fully flexible segments* that are treated as fully flexible throughout the entire docking run (except the initial rigid-body minimization). This is, for example, one way of increasing the sampling of conformations in case of very flexible ligands or unstructured peptides.

15.2.2 Ways of addressing molecular complexity within data-driven docking

HADDOCK was developed initially for the prediction of protein–protein complexes (Dominguez *et al.*, 2003). Since its initial implementation, HADDOCK has extended its functionalities to account for a variety of molecules, including nucleic acids, sugars and small molecules. The program also supports a number of modified amino acid residues and inorganic elements. With its solvated docking implementation (Kastritis *et al.*, 2012; van Dijk and Bonvin, 2006), docking of fully solvated molecules can be performed. The HADDOCK web server (http://haddock.chem.uu.nl/services/HADDOCK/; further information on manuals and tutorials is given at the end of the chapter; de Vries *et al.*, 2010b) offers a user-friendly interface. When a PDB file of a small molecule is uploaded, topology and parameter files of the ligand are automatically retrieved from the PRODRG server (http://davapc1.bioch.dundee.ac.uk/prodrg/; Schuttelkopf and van Aalten, 2004). Additionally, protonation states of histidine residues are also considered by the program, and when not supplied by the user, these are assigned automatically using the WHAT IF web server (http://swift.cmbi.ru.nl/servers/html/; Vriend, 1990).

Another important feature is that the code is not restricted to bivalent molecular docking. The program supports up to six-body docking, meaning that up to six (bio)molecules can be docked simultaneously, independent of their molecular type. HADDOCK is therefore suitable for drug design targeting biomolecular complexes, as these systems might be composed of more than two molecules or domains.

15.3 Applications of Data-driven Docking in Antimicrobial Drug Discovery and Beyond: When Flexibility Matters

Data-driven docking has been applied extensively to a large variety of systems and has shown a very strong performance in the blind critical assessment of the prediction of interactions (see CAPRI (critical assessment of predicted interactions), a community-wide experiment on the comparative evaluation of protein–protein docking for structure prediction: http://www.ebi.ac.uk/msd-srv/capri/; de Vries *et al.*, 2010a; Lensink and Wodak, 2010). A considerable number of experimental structures of complexes calculated using HADDOCK have been deposited into the PDB, including structures of proteins with antibacterial activity, such as hydramycin-1 (Jung *et al.*, 2009).

Data-driven docking can also be used to model protein–ligand interactions and give structural insights and details of enzymatic or inhibitory mechanisms. For this, however, a modified version of the default HADDOCK protocol should preferably be used: during all docking steps, the ligand must be kept fully flexible while the residues within the protein-binding site are only defined as active for the rigid-body docking stage (*it0*) and considered as passive for the subsequent semi-flexible refinement stage (*it1*). This strategy effectively pulls the ligand within the binding site during rigid-body docking while allowing a more thorough exploration of the binding pocket during the refinement stage.

At the end of the protocol, clustering based on pairwise root mean square deviation criteria is performed and the lowest energy structure of the lowest energy cluster is usually taken as the best solution, depending on the quality of the experimental data available. Clustering is automatically performed by HADDOCK and is an integral part of the docking and scoring procedure. It is, however, recommended to check a number of (top) clusters and their statistics and also inspect their three-dimensional structures to comprehend the docking predictions. If possible, additional information might be used, if available, to guide the selection. For clustering of protein–ligand solutions, it is recommended to lower the clustering cut-off from the default value of 7.5 Å to a small value (e.g. 2.0 Å). Protein–ligand docking options are easily accessible via the web server version of HADDOCK (de Vries *et al.*, 2010b), under the guru interface. Note that this interface is meant for experienced users only (for details on the HADDOCK protocol and its web server, see de Vries *et al.*, 2010b; Melquiond and Bonvin, 2010; Schmitz *et al.*, 2012). In the future, a specific protein–ligand interface will be made available, but at this time a ligand should be entered as 'protein' in the web interface using the HETATM fields in the PDB file.

Applications of data-driven docking on protein–ligand systems are extensive (Rutten *et al.*, 2006; Song *et al.*, 2007; Tomaselli *et al.*, 2007; Wu *et al.*, 2007; Arnusch *et al.*, 2008; Rutten *et al.*, 2009; Krzeminski *et al.*, 2010; Schneider *et al.*, 2010; Fiamegos *et al.*, 2011), including the dissection of catalytic mechanisms concerning several membrane and soluble enzymes, as well as the characterization of inhibitors/antimicrobial agents for targets of medical relevance. Rather flexible ligands have also been studied, skipping the initial rigid-body search step and performing the docking in a fully flexible manner during the refinement stage. This has been applied successfully to decipher structure–activity relationships between lectins and oligosaccharides (Wu *et al.*, 2007). Animation movies corresponding to applications of the two different protein–ligand docking protocols, illustrating the docking procedure and the interaction between lectins and oligosaccharides can be found in the following links:

- standard protein–ligand protocol (Krzeminski *et al.*, 2010): http://www.nmr.chem.uu.nl/haddock/movies/hgal3.html.
- fully flexible docking, skipping the initial rigid-body docking (Wu *et al.*, 2007): http://www.nmr.chem.uu.nl/haddock/movies/cg1.html.

15.3.1 Unveiling substrate specificity and catalytic mechanisms of outer-membrane proteins from pathogenic Gram-negative bacteria using HADDOCK

The lipid A portion of lipopolysaccharide is the major component of the outer leaflet of the outer membrane of Gram-negative bacteria, which is toxic to humans. The toxicity of lipid A can be reduced by modifications, often accomplished by specific enzymes located in the same cellular compartment. For these enzymes, data-driven docking has provided useful insights into their catalytic mechanisms (Rutten *et al.*, 2006, 2009), thereby opening the route for the SBDD of novel antimicrobial agents for these targets.

PagL from *Pseudomonas aeruginosa* is an outer-membrane lipid A deacylase located in the bacterial cell wall. PagL hydrolyses the ester bond at the 3-position of lipid A, thereby releasing the primary 3-OH C14 moiety. Due to the protein's localization and because lipid A is modified by PagL, this protein can help bacteria to finally evade the host immune system. Therefore, PagL is a suitable target for antimicrobial agents; however, its structure and catalytic mechanisms, which were still unknown at the time, were unveiled in this study (Rutten *et al.*, 2006). Interaction restraints between lipid A and PagL were derived based on the following information: (i) the crystallized protein is active; (ii) some residues in the interface affected the activity of the protein *in vitro* (demonstrated through mutagenesis studies); and (iii) the structure shares structural homology with the dimeric form of outer-membrane phospholipase A (although PagL is a monomer). Modelling of the substrate lipid A on to the active site by data-driven docking reveals that the 3-*O*-acyl chain is accommodated in a hydrophobic groove perpendicular to the membrane plane. In addition, an aspartate makes a hydrogen bond with the hydroxyl group of the 3-*O*-acyl chain, probably providing specificity of PagL towards lipid A (Fig. 15.2a).

Another illustration of data-driven docking with HADDOCK is provided by the outer-membrane protein LpxR from *Salmonella typhimurium*, a Gram-negative bacterium. LpxR is a lipid A-modifying

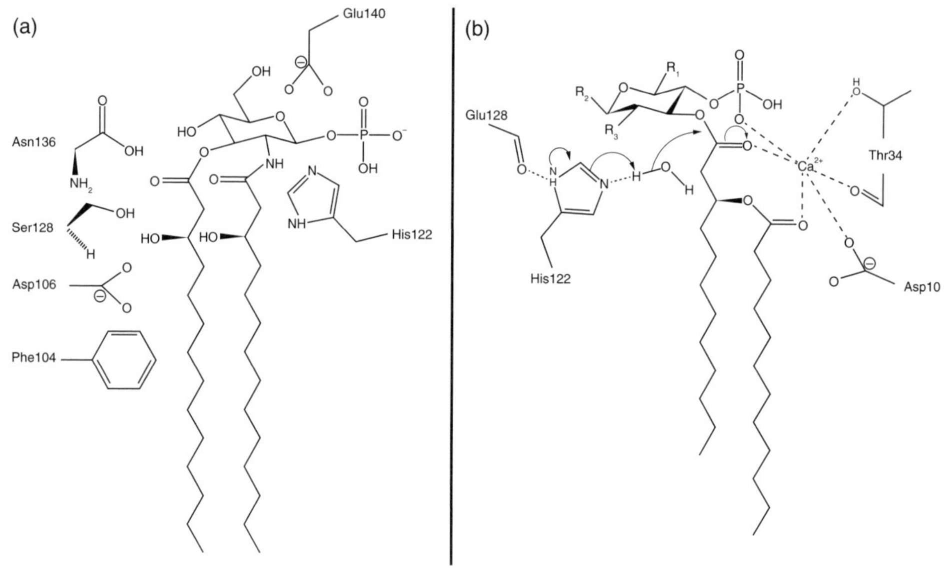

Fig. 15.2. Two-dimensional representations of docking results for lipid X molecules in outer-membrane proteins. (a) Critical interactions of lipid X and residues in the hydrophobic cleft of PagL. (b) Catalysis of lipid A by LpxR as deciphered by data-driven docking (see text).

enzyme (Rutten *et al.*, 2009) that removes the 3′-acyloxyacyl moiety of the lipid A portion of lipopolysaccharide, utilizing Ca^{2+} as a cofactor. In order to decipher its catalytic mechanism, the crystal structure of the apoenzyme of the 32kDa *S. typhimurium* LpxR was used as the receptor molecule. By having experimental data about residues located in the active site through mutagenesis experiments and knowing that the structure shares structural homology with phospholipase A2 (of which the catalytic mechanism is known), insight into the catalytic mechanism of LpxR could be provided. Data-driven docking was used to model the catalytic mechanism by docking lipid A to the active site of the protein, providing structural details about the recognition mechanism. Based on the derived models, the catalytic mechanism of the enzyme was established: briefly, Ca^{2+} forms the oxyanion hole and a histidine activates a water molecule (or a cascade of two water molecules) that subsequently attacks the carbonyl oxygen of the scissile bond (Fig. 15.2b).

Such detailed results for catalytic mechanisms derived for both outer-membrane proteins are unique in a sense that data-driven docking was successful in modelling the flexibility of the lipid A, a complex substrate consisting of a glucosamine (carbohydrate/sugar) unit with attached acyl chains ('fatty acids'), and one phosphate group on each carbohydrate. The resulting structural models allowed rationalization of the catalytic mechanism of these transmembrane enzymes.

15.3.2 Targeting the bacterial Achilles' heel, lipid II, using data-driven docking

The bacterial cell wall is composed of a polymerized peptidoglycan matrix that resists the high osmotic pressure of the cytoplasm, shielding the bacterium from stress. Its vital role for bacteria is also reflected by its very high conservation throughout evolution and therefore it is a prominent target for many antibiotics (Breukink and de Kruijff, 2006). The building block of the peptidoglycan matrix is the monomeric peptidoglycan unit. The latter consists of two amino sugars (*N*-acetylglycosamine and *N*-acetylmuramic acid) and a pentapeptide (commonly L-Ala-D-γ-Glu-L-Lys-D-Ala-D-Ala) attached to the carboxyl group of *N*-acetylmuramic acid. In the cellular cytosol, the membrane-anchoring carrier undecaprenyl phosphate assembles the peptidoglycan unit parts, yielding lipid II (Fig. 15.3a). Lipid II is thereafter transported to the extracellular environment for polymerization of the peptidoglycan moiety. Many antimicrobial peptides target lipid II because of its essential role in cell-wall biosynthesis. One of the most potent inhibitors of lipid II is nisin, which interacts with lipid II through a sequence of events. First, nisin binds to the lipid II-containing membrane and forms a complex with lipid II by targeting its pyrophosphate group. It then assembles into a pore, thereby inducing leakage of cytosolic contents.

HADDOCK was used as a structure-determination program to determine the solution structure of the complex of nisin and lipid II (PDB ID: 1UZT). A wealth of distance and dihedral restraints (e.g. 619 NOEs in total) was introduced to derive the three-dimensional structure of the complex of nisin and lipid II. The structure revealed a novel lipid II-binding motif (Fig. 15.3b) in which the pyrophosphate moiety of lipid II is primarily coordinated by the N-terminal backbone amides of nisin via intermolecular hydrogen bonds and strong van der Waals interactions. Side-chain interactions thus only play a minor role in the interaction of nisin with lipid II (Hsu *et al.*, 2004), which makes it less susceptible to mutations in the peptidic region of lipid II. This cage structure offers a template for structure-based design of novel antibiotics targeting the cell-wall biosynthesis of bacteria.

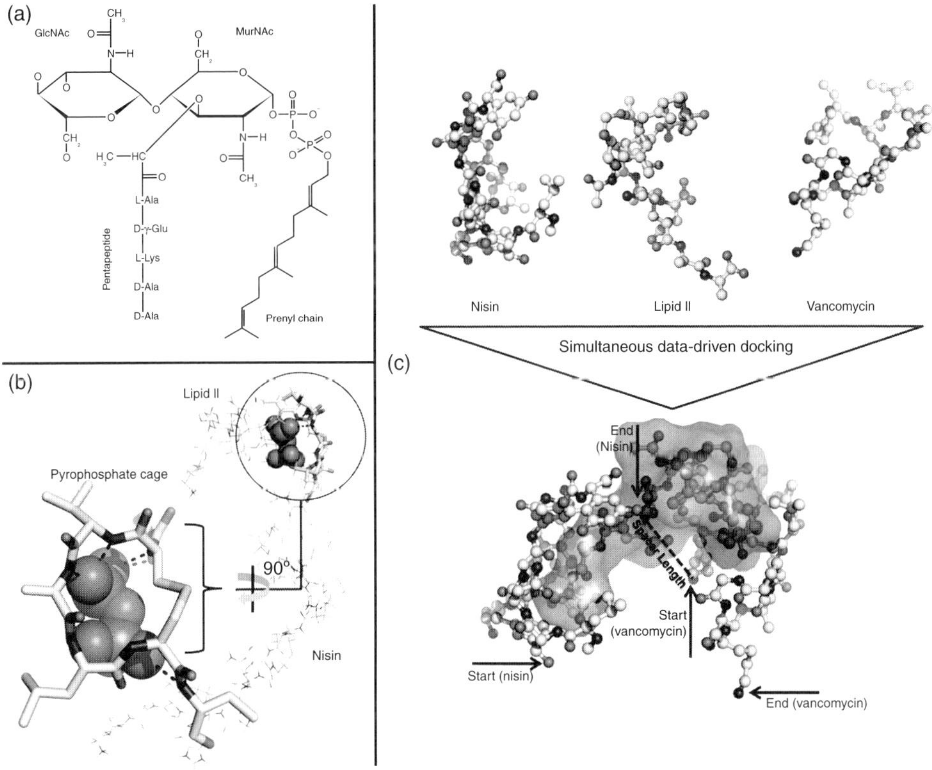

Fig. 15.3. (a) Chemical structure of the lipid II molecule. (b) Lipid II–nisin complex and the pyrophosphate cage as deciphered by HADDOCK (see text). (c) Data-driven docking of three molecules in order to derive the hybrid nisin–vancomysin molecule with click chemistry. HADDOCK was used to predict complexes and calculate spacer lengths between nisin and vancomycin (ball-and-stick representations), using lipid II as scaffold (ball-and-stick and surface representation).

Based on the structural findings for the nisin–lipid II complex, and the information for the interaction of vancomycin with the tripeptide part (Lys-D-Ala-D -Ala) of lipid II (Barna and Williams, 1984), three-body data-driven docking was applied to derive a model of the complex of both inhibitors and lipid II (Arnusch *et al.*, 2008). The model revealed that, due to the different binding modes of vancomycin and nisin, lipid II was able to bind both molecules simultaneously. The resulting models were analysed to derive distance distributions between potential linkage points between nisin (N and C termini) and vancomycin (N and C termini) (Fig. 15. 3c). Using click chemistry, nisin and vancomycin were connected with either an alkyne or an azide group, and hybrid molecules were synthesized, one of which exhibited an antimicrobial activity superior to that of the individual agents. Data-driven docking was used in the sense that, by overcoming the obstacles of the highly sophisticated structures of the antimicrobial agents, it produced models from which spacer lengths were derived for the design of novel hybrid inhibitors of lipid II by click chemistry.

In another recent application (Schneider *et al.*, 2010), data-driven docking with HADDOCK provided a model for the interaction between a fungal defensin (plectasin) and lipid II. This defensin can target the bacterial cell-wall precursor lipid II in a similar way to the vancomycin–nisin hybrid molecule that was designed with the aid of data-driven docking. CSP data obtained from the titration of lipid II with defensin were used to define AIRs to drive the modelling process. The model reveals that the 40 amino acid amphipathic defensin molecule binds to the solvent-exposed part of lipid II, and in particular to the pyrophosphate group. Plectasin seems thus to bind lipid II in a similar way to nisin.

15.3.3 Interactions between bile acid-binding protein (BABP) and bile acids decrypted by NMR, MS and computational modelling

Although not a potential target for antimicrobial agents, BABP is a key element in cholesterol homeostasis as it controls the physiological balance of the bile salts and the bile acids in the liver cytosol. Therefore, in the light of its biological function, it can be a suitable target for SBDD. In order to determine the ternary complex of BABP with two bile salt molecules, a hybrid computational/experimental approach was followed (Tomaselli *et al.*, 2007). To drive the modelling process, MS and NMR data for the protein were obtained and were translated into distance restraints in HADDOCK. In this venture, a wealth of experimental information was available, including CSP, NOE and ^{15}N relaxation experiment data from NMR and limited proteolysis data from MS. During these calculations, three-body docking was performed, meaning that the two identical bile acid molecules plus the protein were docked simultaneously, making use of HADDOCK's ability to deal with multicomponent systems. A larger number of models were generated at every docking step compared with the default settings to deal with the complexity of the simultaneous three-body docking and allow a more thorough sampling of the interaction space. The resulting models revealed that residues involved in binding are mainly located in two loops at the C terminus of the protein; their orientation plays a major role in binding of the small molecules to the protein. It was also observed that polar residues pointing towards the protein interior are involved in motion communication, highlighting their prominent role in ligand interactions (Tomaselli *et al.*, 2007).

This work emphasizes that, in such a highly demanding system where one protein can interact with two ligands simultaneously, HADDOCK can model the ternary complex, irrespective of the degree of flexibility and complexity of the system, provided enough experimental data can be used to drive the modelling process.

15.3.4 Scoring in HADDOCK as an estimate of binding energies of peptide inhibitors for the treatment of HIV-1 viral infections

HIV-1 attachment to $CD4^+$ target T cells and subsequent fusion of viral and cellular membranes resulting in release of the viral core into the cell is accomplished by the HIV-1 envelope glycoprotein complex (Env), a class I viral fusion protein. HIV-1 Env is a trimer, with each monomer consisting of two subunits, proteins gp120 and gp41. Whereas gp120 is responsible for adhesion and (partially) fusion, gp41 induces fusion of the viral envelope with the plasma membrane, thereby initiating infection. Each gp41 molecule contains an N-terminal leucine/isoleucine heptad repeat (HR) segment that has been crystallographically shown to form a central triple-stranded α-helical coiled-coil core (Weissenhorn *et al.*, 1997). Peptides based on the second heptad repeat (HR2) of viral class I fusion proteins are effective inhibitors of virus entry. For example, a fusion inhibitor has been approved for treatment of HIV infections (T20, or enfuvirtide).

For this kind of system, only the water refinement part of the HADDOCK protocol was used to extract the energetics of protein–peptide complexes of modelled wild-type and mutant gp41 proteins, in complex with three different inhibitors (including enfuvirtide).

The derived modelled complexes were constructed based on homology with existing crystallographic structures (Caffrey *et al.*, 1998), in light of mutational experiments that were mapped on to the models. The intermolecular energies of the complexes were obtained and compared with experimental knowledge about the resistance of mutant gp41 proteins to the inhibitory peptides. This allowed the proposition of four different mechanisms of resistance to fusion inhibitors. Although scoring should not be interpreted in terms of affinity (Kastritis and Bonvin, 2010), the modelling data suggested that the presence of exposed charges on the peptide at the drug–target interface, unless involved in an intramolecular salt bridge, is not desirable. Exposed charges may provide the virus with an easy possibility to generate the most powerful mechanism of resistance – electrostatic repulsion. Such findings may guide the design of novel fusion inhibitors targeting viruses with class I fusion proteins.

15.4 Conclusions

As the antimicrobial drug discovery community moves towards more complicated systems, in terms of both the ligands and the targets, relevant computational methods are needed to tackle the challenges in modelling their three-dimensional structures and interaction mode. The trend towards increased molecular weight of the designed agents goes together with an increase in degrees of freedom and underlying flexibility of the biomolecules. In addition, molecules are becoming more and more complicated, being built of different chemical groups from different classes of chemical molecules such as, for example, those targeting lipid II biosynthesis. On the receptor side, the targets are getting also more complex. For example, protein–protein interactions and their interfaces are becoming relevant for the development of novel therapeutics. The plasticity and flexibility of some interfaces can be a challenge, even for the most sophisticated docking programs. Recognition events mediated by local folding or unfolding of biomolecules, large loop rearrangements and binding-affinity prediction of the modelled interactions still represent three major bottlenecks that docking programs have to face in the years to come.

Despite its limitations, data-driven docking offers a good solution to tackle some of these challenges, as highlighted by the various applications described in the previous sections. Provided enough experimental data are available, HADDOCK can work as a structure-determination program, able to generate three-dimensional structures of biomolecular complexes, acting as a catalyst for deciphering biomolecular interactions. This is illustrated by the fact that, as of February 2012, 85 macromolecular complexes have been deposited into the PDB for which HADDOCK has been used as a structure-determination package.

Manuals and Tutorials on Data-driven Docking

Further information on the use of HADDOCK can be found as follows:

1. HADDOCK: http://www.wenmr.eu/wenmr/tutorials/nmr-tutorials/haddock. In this website, several tutorials related to data-driven docking can be found:

- A case study: preparing input files for a manual HADDOCK run
- Generating the necessary restraint files for running HADDOCK manually
- How to prepare PDB files for running HADDOCK manually
- HADDOCK web server tutorial

2. A demo web form for the easy interface with pre-loaded parameters: http://haddock.science.uu.nl/enmr/services/HADDOCK/haddockserver-demo.html.

3. Tutorial movie on data-driven docking: http://haddock.science.uu.nl/Files/e2a-hpr-demo.swf.

Acknowledgements

The authors thank all members of the Computational Structural Biology Laboratory in Utrecht University, past and present, whose support contributed to the development of data-driven HADDOCKing. This work was supported by the Netherlands Organization for Scientific Research (VICI grant #700.56.442 to A.M.J.J.B.) and by the European Community FP7 e-Infrastructure WeNMR project (grant number 261572).

References

Arkin, M.R. and Wells, J.A. (2004) Small-molecule inhibitors of protein–protein interactions: progressing towards the dream. *Nature Reviews Drug Discovery* 3, 301–317.

Arnusch, C.J., Bonvin, A.M., Verel, A.M., Jansen, W.T., Liskamp, R.M., de Kruijff, B., Pieters, R.J. and Breukink, E. (2008) The vancomycin–nisin(1–12) hybrid restores activity against vancomycin resistant enterococci. *Biochemistry* 47, 12661–12663.

Barna, J.C. and Williams, D.H. (1984) The structure and mode of action of glycopeptide antibiotics of the vancomycin group. *Annual Reviews in Microbiology* 38, 339–357.

Becattini, B. and Pellecchia, M. (2006) SAR by ILOEs: an NMR-based approach to reverse chemical genetics. *Chemistry* 12, 2658–2662.

Betz, M., Saxena, K. and Schwalbe, H. (2006) Biomolecular NMR: a chaperone to drug discovery. *Current Opinion in Chemical Biology* 10, 219–225.

Blundell, T.L., Jhoti, H. and Abell, C. (2002) High-throughput crystallography for lead discovery in drug design. *Nature Reviews Drug Discovery* 1, 45–54.

Bourgeas, R., Basse, M.J., Morelli, X. and Roche, P. (2010) Atomic analysis of protein–protein interfaces with known inhibitors: the 2P2I database. *PLoS One* 5, e9598.

Breukink, E. and de Kruijff, B. (2006) Lipid II as a target for antibiotics. *Nature Reviews Drug Discovery* 5, 321–332.

Brunger, A.T., Adams, P.D., Clore, G.M., DeLano, W.L., Gros, P., Grosse-Kunstleve, R.W., Jiang, J.S., Kuszewski, J., Nilges, M., Pannu, N.S., Read, R.J., Rice, L.M., Simonson, T. and Warren, G.L. (1998) Crystallography and NMR system: a new software suite for macromolecular structure determination. *Acta Crystallographica D: Biological Crystallography* 54, 905–921.

Caffrey, M., Cai, M., Kaufman, J., Stahl, S.J., Wingfield, P.T., Covell, D.G., Gronenborn, A.M. and Clore, G.M. (1998) Three-dimensional solution structure of the 44 kDa ectodomain of SIV gp41. *EMBO Journal* 17, 4572–4584.

Cowan, M.M. (1999) Plant products as antimicrobial agents. *Clinical Microbiology Reviews* 12, 564–582.

de Vries, S.J. and Bonvin, A.M. (2008) How proteins get in touch: interface prediction in the study of biomolecular complexes. *Current Protein and Peptide Science* 9, 394–406.

de Vries, S.J., van Dijk, A.D., Krzeminski, M., van Dijk, M., Thureau, A., Hsu, V., Wassenaar, T. and Bonvin, A.M. (2007) HADDOCK versus HADDOCK: new features and performance of HADDOCK2.0 on the CAPRI targets. *Proteins* 69, 726–733.

de Vries, S.J., Melquiond, A.S., Kastritis, P.L., Karaca, E., Bordogna, A., van Dijk, M., Rodrigues, J.P. and Bonvin, A.M. (2010a) Strengths and weaknesses of data-driven docking in critical assessment of prediction of interactions. *Proteins: Structure, Function and Bioinformatics* 78, 3242–3249.

de Vries, S.J., van Dijk, M. and Bonvin, A.M. (2010b) The HADDOCK web server for data-driven biomolecular docking. *Nature Protocols* 5, 883–897.

Dominguez, C., Boelens, R. and Bonvin, A.M. (2003) HADDOCK: a protein–protein docking approach based on biochemical or biophysical information. *Journal of the American Chemical Society* 125, 1731–1737.

Dorsey, B.D., Levin, R.B., McDaniel, S.L., Vacca, J.P., Guare, J.P., Darke, P.L., Zugay, J.A., Emini,

E.A., Schleif, W.A., Quintero, J.C., Quintero, J.C., Linn, J.H., Chen, I.W., Holloway, M.K., Fitzgerald, P.M.D., Axel, M.G., Ostovic, D., Anderson, P.S. and Huff, J.R. (1994) L-735,524: the design of a potent and orally bioavailable HIV protease inhibitor. *Journal of Medicinal Chemistry* 37, 3443–3451.

Erickson, J., Neidhart, D.J., VanDrie, J., Kempf, D.J., Wang, X.C., Norbeck, D.W., Plattner, J.J., Rittenhouse, J.W., Turon, M., Wideburg, N., Kohlbrenner, W.E., Simmer, R., Helfrich, R., Paul, D.A. and Knigge, M. (1990) Design, activity, and 2.8 Å crystal structure of a C2 symmetric inhibitor complexed to HIV-1 protease. *Science* 249, 527–533.

Fiamegos, Y.C., Kastritis, P.L., Exarchou, V., Han, H., Bonvin, A.M.J. J., Vervoort, J., Lewis, K., Hamblin, M.R. and Tegos, G.P. (2011) Antimicrobial and efflux pump inhibitory activity of caffeoylquinic acids from *Artemisia absinthium* against Gram-positive pathogenic bacteria. *PLoS One*, 6, e18127.

Fuentes, G., Dastidar, S.H., Madhumalar, A. and Verma, C.S. (2011) Role of protein flexibility in the discovery of new drugs. *Drug Development Research* 72, 26–35.

Grunberg, R., Leckner, J. and Nilges, M. (2004) Complementarity of structure ensembles in protein–protein binding. *Structure* 12, 2125–2136.

Hajduk, P.J. and Greer, J. (2007) A decade of fragment-based drug design: strategic advances and lessons learned. *Nature Reviews Drug Discovery* 6, 211–219.

Hann, M.M., Leach, A.R. and Harper, G. (2001) Molecular complexity and its impact on the probability of finding leads for drug discovery. *Journal of Chemical Information in Computer Sciences* 41, 856–864.

Hsu, S.T., Breukink, E., Tischenko, E., Lutters, M.A., de Kruijff, B., Kaptein, R., Bonvin, A.M. and van Nuland, N.A. (2004) The nisin–lipid II complex reveals a pyrophosphate cage that provides a blueprint for novel antibiotics. *Nature Structure and Molecular Biology* 11, 963–967.

Jahnke, W. (2007) Perspectives of biomolecular NMR in drug discovery: the blessing and curse of versatility. *Journal of Biomolecular NMR* 39, 87–90.

Jenssen, H., Hamill, P. and Hancock, R.E. (2006) Peptide antimicrobial agents. *Clinical Microbiology Reviews* 19, 491–511.

Jung, S., Dingley, A.J., Augustin, R., Anton-Erxleben, F., Stanisak, M., Gelhaus, C., Gutsmann, T., Hammer, M.U., Podschun, R., Bonvin, A.M., Leippe, M., Bosch, T.C. and Grotzinger, J. (2009) Hydramacin-1, structure and antibacterial activity of a protein from the basal metazoan Hydra. *Journal of Biological Chemistry* 284, 1896–1905.

Karaca, E. and Bonvin, A.M. (2011) A multi-domain flexible docking approach to deal with large conformational changes in the modeling of biomolecular complexes. *Structure* 19, 555–565.

Karaca, E., Melquiond, A.S., de Vries, S.J., Kastritis, P.L. and Bonvin, A.M. (2011) Building macromolecular assemblies by information-driven docking: introducing the HADDOCK multibody docking server. *Molecular and Cellular Proteomics* 9, 1784–1794.

Kastritis, P.L. and Bonvin, A.M. (2010) Are scoring functions in protein–protein docking ready to predict interactomes? Clues from a novel binding affinity benchmark. *Journal of Proteome Research* 9, 2216–2225.

Kastritis, P.L., van Dijk, A.-J. and Bonvin, A.M.J.J. (2012) Explicit treatment of water molecules in data-driven docking: the Solvated HADdocking approach. *Methods in Molecular Biology* 819, 5–374.

Kolb, H.C. and Sharpless, K.B. (2003) The growing impact of click chemistry on drug discovery. *Drug Discovery Today* 8, 1128–1137.

Krzeminski, M., Singh, T., Andre, S., Lensch, M., Wu, A.M., Bonvin, A.M. and Gabius, H.J. (2010) Human galectin-3 (Mac-2 antigen): defining molecular switches of affinity to natural glycoproteins, structural and dynamic aspects of glycan binding by flexible ligand docking and putative regulatory sequences in the proximal promoter region. *Biochimica et Biophysica Acta* 1810, 150–161.

Lensink, M.F. and Wodak, S.J. (2010) Blind predictions of protein interfaces by docking calculations in CAPRI. *Proteins: Structure, Function and Bioinformatics* 78, 3085–3095.

McCauley, J. (1999) Relenza. *Current Biology* 9, R796.

Meagher, K.L. and Carlson, H.A. (2004) Incorporating protein flexibility in structure-based drug discovery: using HIV-1 protease as a test case. *Journal of the American Chemical Society* 126, 13276–13281.

Melquiond, A.S.J. and Bonvin, A.M.J.J. (2010) Data-driven docking: using external information to spark the biomolecular rendez-vous. In: Zacharias, M. (ed.) *Protein–Protein Complexes: Analysis, Modelling and Drug Design*. Imperial College Press, Munich, Germany, pp. 183–209.

Murray, C.W. and Blundell, T.L. (2010) Structural biology in fragment-based drug design. *Current Opinion in Structural Biology* 20, 497–507.

Patel, S. and Player, M.R. (2008) Small-molecule inhibitors of the p53–HDM2 interaction for the treatment of cancer. *Expert Opinion on Investigational Drugs* 17, 1865–1882.

Roberts, N.A., Martin, J.A., Kinchington, D., Broadhurst, A.V., Craig, J.C., Duncan, I.B.,

Galpin, S.A., Handa, B.K., Kay, J., Krohn, A., Lambert, R., Merrett, J., Mills, J, Parks, K., Redshaw, S., Taylor, D., Thomas, G. and Machin, P. (1990) Rational design of peptide-based HIV proteinase inhibitors. *Science* 248, 358–361.

Rutten, L., Geurtsen, J., Lambert, W., Smolenaers, J.J., Bonvin, A.M., de Haan, A., van der Ley, P., Egmond, M.R., Gros, P. and Tommassen, J. (2006) Crystal structure and catalytic mechanism of the LPS 3-O-deacylase PagL from *Pseudomonas aeruginosa*. *Proceedings of the National Academy of Sciences USA* 103, 7071–7076.

Rutten, L., Mannie, J.P., Stead, C.M., Raetz, C.R., Reynolds, C.M., Bonvin, A.M., Tommassen, J.P., Egmond, M.R., Trent, M.S. and Gros, P. (2009) Active-site architecture and catalytic mechanism of the lipid A deacylase LpxR of *Salmonella typhimurium*. *Proceedings of the National Academy of Sciences USA* 106, 1960–1964.

Sanchez-Pedregal, V.M., Reese, M., Meiler, J., Blommers, M.J., Griesinger, C. and Carlomagno, T. (2005) The INPHARMA method: protein-mediated interligand NOEs for pharmacophore mapping. *Angewandte Chemie International Edition* 44, 4172–4175.

Sawaya, M.R. and Kraut, J. (1997) Loop and subdomain movements in the mechanism of *Escherichia coli* dihydrofolate reductase: crystallographic evidence. *Biochemistry* 36, 586–603.

Schmitz, C., Melquiond, A.S.J., de Vries, S.J., Karaca, E., van Dijk, M., Kastritis, P.L. and Bonvin, A.M.J.J. (2012) Chapter 9.2. HADDOCK. In: Bertini, I., McGreevy, K.S. and Parigi, G. (eds) *NMR of Biomolecules: Towards Mechanistic Systems Biology*. Wiley, Chichester, UK (in press).

Schneider, T., Kruse, T., Wimmer, R., Wiedemann, I., Sass, V., Pag, U., Jansen, A., Nielsen, A.K., Mygind, P.H., Raventos, D.S., Neve, S., Ravn, B., Bonvin, A.M., De Maria, L., Andersen, A.S., Gammelgaard, L.K., Sahl, H.G. and Kristensen, H.H. (2010) Plectasin, a fungal defensin, targets the bacterial cell wall precursor Lipid II. *Science* 328, 1168–1172.

Schuttelkopf, A.W. and van Aalten, D.M. (2004) PRODRG: a tool for high-throughput crystallography of protein–ligand complexes. *Acta Crystallographica D Biological Crystallography* 60, 1355–1363.

Simmons, K.J., Chopra, I. and Fishwick, C.W. (2010) Structure-based discovery of antibacterial drugs. *Nature Reviews Microbiology* 8, 501–510.

Song, J., Zhao, K.Q., Newman, C.L., Vinarov, D.A. and Markley, J.L. (2007) Solution structure of human sorting nexin 22. *Protein Science* 16, 807–814.

Stratton, M.S. and Alberts, D.S. (2002) Current application of selective COX-2 inhibitors in cancer prevention and treatment. *Oncology (Williston Park)* 16 (Suppl. 4), 37–51.

Tomaselli, S., Ragona, L., Zetta, L., Assfalg, M., Ferranti, P., Longhi, R., Bonvin, A.M. and Molinari, H. (2007) NMR-based modeling and binding studies of a ternary complex between chicken liver bile acid binding protein and bile acids. *Proteins: Structure, Function and Bioinformatics* 69, 177–191.

Toogood, P.L. (2002) Inhibition of protein–protein association by small molecules: approaches and progress. *Journal of Medicinal Chemistry* 45, 1543–1558.

van Dijk, A.D. and Bonvin, A.M. (2006) Solvated docking: introducing water into the modelling of biomolecular complexes. *Bioinformatics* 22, 2340–2347.

van Dijk, A.D., Boelens, R. and Bonvin, A.M. (2005) Data-driven docking for the study of biomolecular complexes. *FEBS Journal* 272, 293–312.

Vriend, G. (1990) WHAT IF: a molecular modeling and drug design program. *Journal of Molecular Graphics* 8, 52–56.

Weissenhorn, W., Dessen, A., Harrison, S.C., Skehel, J.J. and Wiley, D.C. (1997) Atomic structure of the ectodomain from HIV-1 gp41. *Nature* 387, 426–430.

Wu, A.M., Singh, T., Liu, J.H., Krzeminski, M., Russwurm, R., Siebert, H.C., Bonvin, A.M., Andre, S. and Gabius, H.J. (2007) Activity–structure correlations in divergent lectin evolution: fine specificity of chicken galectin CG-14 and computational analysis of flexible ligand docking for CG-14 and the closely related CG-16. *Glycobiology* 17, 165–184.

16 Antifungals and Antifungal Drug Discovery

Richard Calderone, William Fonzi, Francoise Gay-Andrieu, Nuo Sun, Dongmei Li, Hui Chen and Deepu Alex
Department of Microbiology and Immunology, Georgetown University Medical Center, Washington, DC, USA

16.1 Introduction

Fungi are common agents of disease in both immunocompetent and immunocompromised patient populations. The types of diseases include cutaneous and subcutaneous infection, mucosal invasion and commonly bloodstream infections (BSIs) that may be life-threatening (Groll *et al.*, 1996; Boechk and Marr, 2002; Gavalda *et al.*, 2005; Sobel, 2007; Caston-Osorio *et al.*, 2008; Ameen and Arenas, 2009; Neofytos *et al.*, 2009; Pappas *et al.*, 2009, 2010; Horn *et al.*, 2009; Bonifaz *et al.*, 2010; Kontoyiannis *et al.*, 2010; Lehrnbecher *et al.*, 2010). Of all fungal diseases, dermatophytosis is probably the most prevalent but also least studied in regard to host–fungus interactions. Fungal diseases are endemic (e.g. histoplasmosis, blastomycosis, coccidioidomycosis, penicilliosis and paracoccidiomycosis) or pandemic (e.g. invasive candidiasis (IC), aspergillosis including invasive aspergillosis (IA), cryptococcosis, fusariosis, mucormycosis and dermatophytosis). It is probable that the greatest threat to life includes those pathogens that cause BSIs, yet with IA and IC, diagnosis is not easy and often these diseases are treated empirically when blood cultures are negative for bacterial pathogens. In the case of IC, there can be numerous risk factors that, for the most part, are non-specific. BSI and invasive pathogens are acquired through inhalation of fungal-laden aerosols (in IA, for example) or reside as normal microbiota of mucosal tissues and gain advantage in the patient populations described below (in IC, endogenous disease). The lack of rapid diagnostic tests for IA and IC complicates therapeutic intervention, i.e. when to start and end treatment. Biomarkers are unavailable, symptoms are non-specific, vaccines are not yet in clinical trial and diagnosis is often decided following exclusion of bacterial BSI, as stated above.

We will use IC as a fungal disease to illustrate the complexity described above. IC is caused by several species of the genus *Candida*. The frequency of various species that cause this disease has changed over the last (at least) two to three decades, and this change has coincided with the introduction of triazole antifungal drugs to the patient population (Pfaller *et al.*, 2004, 2009, 2010a,b; Pfaller and Diekema, 2007; Hachem *et al.*, 2008; Trofa *et al.*, 2008; Lass-Florl, 2009; Pappas *et al.*, 2009, 2010; Niimi *et al.*, 2010; Lortholary *et al.*, 2011). Thus, *Candida albicans* was the leading cause of IC and BSIs prior to the use of fluconazole, far outdistancing other species in the clinical setting. As other *Candida* spp. such as *Candida glabrata*, *Candida krusei* and *Candida parapsilosis* are inherently more resistant to triazoles such as fluconazole, clinicians and the supporting diagnostic laboratories now have to contend with species identification and minimum inhibitory concentration (MIC) assays to determine levels of resistance to triazole antifungals. Standardized drug susceptibility assays are now more routinely carried out when implementing antifungal therapy. The heightened frequency of drug resistance among clinical isolates has been noted in publications; however, the clinical impact of resistance remains understudied.

Candidiasis of humans is really a spectrum of diseases at various body sites. Generally, the cutaneous and mucosal infections are relatively easy to identify compared with BSIs, as mentioned above. Immune protection against candidiasis is only partially understood but is thought to be dependent on the location of the disease, implying site-specific host immunity. As examples, oral and oropharyngeal (OPC; mucosal) candidiasis are frequent in human immunodeficiency virus/acquired immunodeficiency syndrome (HIV/AIDS) patients, with invasion rarely encountered. One can therefore ask why vaginal and recurrent vulvovaginal diseases are not more common in HIV/AIDS patients, especially as both OPC and vaginitis are mucosal diseases. The answer is not known for certain, but the risk factors for both types of mucosal diseases appear to be dissimilar.

For oral candidiasis and OPC, the prevailing paradigm is that a deficiency in $CD4^{+}$ T cells leads to mucosal candidiasis but rarely BSI and IC, as HIV/AIDS patients have significant numbers of protective innate immune cells. Invasive disease and BSI are seen in patients undergoing allogeneic bone-marrow transplantation or immunosuppression associated with cancer chemotherapy In both situations, neutropenia is thought to be the contributing risk factor. However, surgery, premature infants, indwelling urinary tract catheters and lung ventilators are also high risk factors, among others (Walsh, *et al.*, 1994; Bougnoux *et al.*, 2008; Bennett, 2009; Pappas *et al.*, 2009, 2010).

16.2 Candidiasis as a Global Infectious Disease

Candidiasis is found throughout the world (e.g. Harbarth *et al.*, 1999 Okome-Nkoumou *et al.*, 2000; Jabra-Rizk *et al.*, 2001; Blignaut, 2007; Chakrabarti *et al.*, 2008; Chakraborty *et al.*, 2008; Hamza, *et al.*, 2008; Nadagir *et al.*, 2008; Lass-Florl, 2009; Zhang *et al.*, 2009; Nishikaku *et al.*, 2010; Sampaio-Camargo, *et al.*, 2010). The global nature of candidiasis is associated with its presence as part of the normal microbiota of humans. However, the type of candidiasis often reflects predisposing factors or other diseases prevalent in that country. HIV/AIDS remains very high in some countries for many reasons, not least of which is inadequate health care and social disorder. Does candidiasis commonly occur in this clinical setting? In Gabon, Africa, of the opportunistic infections in HIV/AIDS patients, the rate of OPC (37%) exceeded that of tuberculosis (14.5%) (Okome-Nkoumou *et al.*, 2000). The same correlations were noted in China where the frequency of candidiasis is higher than all other infectious diseases in the HIV/AIDS patient population (Zhang *et al.*, 2009). In India, the top two opportunistic gastrointestinal diseases are candidiasis (88%) and tuberculosis (Chakrabarti *et al.*, 2008). Thus, these types of candidiasis have not gone away, in spite of therapeutic efforts.

Likewise, invasive fungal infections such as IC and IA occur globally in situations where medical advances have lengthened lives in developed countries. A brief look at the incidence of IA and IC demonstrates this. Fungal infections have risen sharply over the past few decades. From 1980 to 1997, mortality due to invasive mycotic disease increased from the tenth most common cause of death due to infectious disease to the seventh most common. The five leading mycoses during this change in demographics were candidiasis (including IC), IA, histoplasmosis, cryptococcosis and coccidioidomycosis (Pfaller and Diekema, 2007). For candidiasis and cryptococcosis, the increase was at least partially due to the rapid emergence of the HIV/AIDS pandemic, but other comorbidities such as immunosuppressive cancer chemotherapy and immunosuppression following bone-marrow transplantation, surgery, and the use of ventilators and indwelling central-line catheters were also responsible, especially in patients that developed IC and IA infections. This increase has levelled out more recently in the case of IC and in fact has decreased somewhat for IA (Pfaller and Diekema, 2007). Nevertheless, *Candida* spp. rank among the top three or four causes of bacterial/fungal nosocomial infectious diseases, and *Aspergillus fumigatus* is the most deadly and frequent mould infection of humans.

Are there data to indicate that IC and IA are a public health concern? Here, the verdict is too often, but importantly, determined by the cost of treating these infections. There are several studies that convincingly establish their importance. The lack of rapid diagnostic tests, delayed treatment and failure to diagnose fungal BSI results in an increased length of hospital stay. Thus, IC results in a considerable increase in length of hospital stay compared with the rapidly developing, more easily diagnosed bacterial BSIs. This unfortunate situation means that the cost of treating IC and IA patients is about the same as that of the most common bacterial BSIs such as coagulase-negative staphylococci, despite fewer IC disease cases but rather due to the longer length of hospital stay and high cost of treatment (Rentz *et al.*, 1998; Miller *et al.*, 2001; van Gool, 2001; Wilson *et al.*, 2002; Olaechea, *et al.*, 2004; Fleming, 2006; Nomura *et al.*, 2006; Gagne and Goldfarb, 2007; Zilberberg *et al.*, 2010; see also http://www.doctorfungus.org/thedrugs/cost1.php). Similar studies have been done for cryptococcosis (Micol *et al.*, 2010). What is the actual cost investment in treating IC? The type of study that is meaningful in this regard should be one that compares multiple sites. For example, Miller *et al* (2001) compared patient data from two sites in the USA. The median total hospital charge was US$44,696–77,534 per patient. The projection is that, for IC, the total financial burden is about US$1.7 billion. When added to the costs of treating all fungal infections in the USA, the estimate is approximately US$2.6 billion per year, or about 0.24% of the total US health expenditure (Wilson *et al.*, 2002).

16.3 Current Therapeutics for Treating Fungal Diseases, Especially IC and IA

It seems that the inability to demonstrate mycotic infections as a public health concern is perhaps one of the more important reasons for the stagnant development of new antifungal drugs. Furthermore, the current economic situation also means that decisions have to be made for investment, and the perceived infrequency of fungal infections generally means less commitment to the development of new antifungal compounds. There is no question that new rapid diagnostics for IC and IA are critical yet underdeveloped. If available, such assays may certainly be useful in terms of when to start/stop antifungal therapeutics. Is investment in new drug discovery required? Several daunting factors need mentioning. First, and this speaks to the need for rapid diagnostic tests, there is a narrow window of opportunity for effective therapy once a blood culture becomes positive (Knaus *et al.*, 1991). Not surprisingly, a delay in treatment means increased patient mortality. Secondly, current therapies are few in number. Thirdly, safety issues exist with azoles and polyenes. Fourthly, current therapies target about 0.0004% of the *C. albicans* genome, and this percentage does not include the human orthologues of *C. albicans* genes that account for about 30% of the *C. albicans* genome. The utilization of genomic data bases that are available among many fungal pathogens provides advantages that have not been extensively used. Broadly conserved targets can be identified and, if needed, the function of those targets determined. Several laboratories have focused on methods of constructing mutant libraries across the entire *C. albicans* genome that can be used in drug screens (discussed below). However, while genome databases are available for most fungal pathogens, much of these genomes remain functionally unknown. Attempts to increase functional annotation have employed bar-coding methods to identify mutants with interesting phenotypes, along with gene replacement and conditionally expressed strains (Roemer *et al.*, 2003; Rodriguez-Suarez *et al.*, 2007; Xu *et al.*, 2007; Oh *et al.*, 2010). Of these, the more recent construction of a 4238 mutant library has been described, representing about two-thirds of the *C. albicans* genome (Oh *et al.*, 2010).

The current antifungals and their targets are summarized in Fig. 16.1 (see also Odds *et al.*, 2003; Espinel-Ingroff, 2009).

The target of azoles is Erg11p, which is a fungal cytochrome P450-dependent lanosterol 14-α-demethylase that converts lanosterol to ergosterol (Fig. 16.1). The so-called toxic sterols that form as a consequence of azole treatment result in a membrane that does not function as well as with ergosterol, which leads to growth inhibition. The newer class of antifungals is the echinocandins, which inhibit the synthesis of cell-wall β-1,3 glucan. 5-Flucytosine was used in treatment with amphotericin B but now is used rarely. By itself, high levels of resistance in patient isolates were observed. Finally, the original 'gold standard' to which all new drugs are compared is the polyene amphotericin B, although nystatin is occasionally used in the treatment of mucosal candidiasis. The toxicity of amphotericin B has been mentioned above, and its lipid-encapsulated derivatives have been shown to be more efficacious in treatment but very costly. Polyenes (amphotericin B and nystatin) are amphoteric and bind to plasma membrane ergosterol forming channels. Consequently, disruption of membrane function occurs, leading to cell death. Toxicity is associated with the binding of polyenes to cholesterol and disruption, although not to the same magnitude, of mammalian cell membranes. Thus, there are instances when discontinuation of amphotericin B treatment is required; if toxicity is observed, damage to the patient is reversible. Of the classes of antifungals, with some exceptions (see below), all can be used in the treatment of invasive diseases, while fluconazole is often used in treating mucosal candidiasis infections such as OPC and primary and recurrent vaginitis (Sobel, 2007). Triazoles are grouped into two classes, the imidazoles such as miconazole or ketoconazole, which are used almost exclusively for topical treatment of superficial infections, and the triazoles, which include fluconazole, itraconazole, posaconazole and voriconazole. With the triazoles, the substitution of a triazole pharmacore to replace the imidazole pharmacore enhances its specificity for the fungal cytochrome P450 cofactor and also slows down the metabolism of triazoles (Ostrosky-Zeichner *et al.*, 2010). The most recent of the triazoles offer improvements over the initial compounds such as fluconazole.

The most important questions in determining the adequacy of existing antifungal compounds include the following: are the

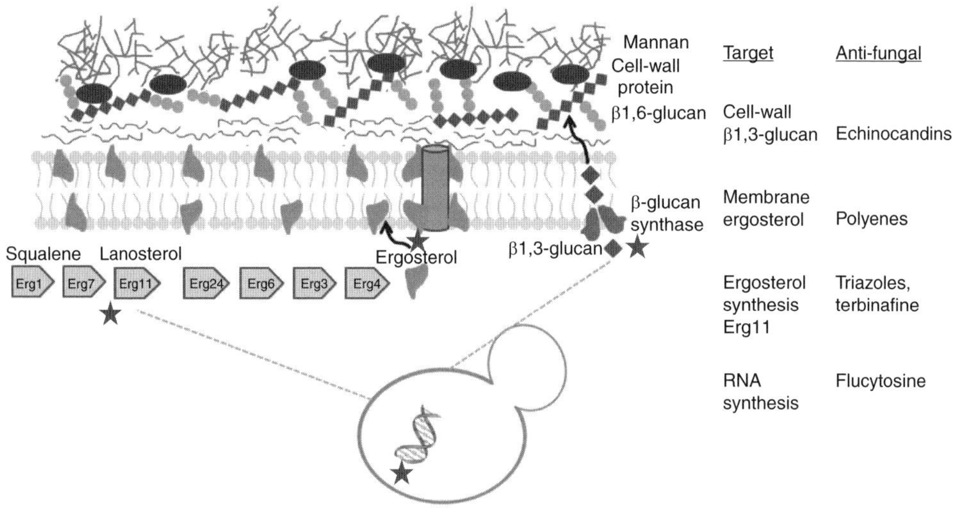

Fig. 16.1. The major types of antifungal drugs are shown along with representative targets of each (right). The triazoles and terbinafine inhibit ergosterol synthesis. Polyenes bind to ergosterol, perturbing membrane function (polyenes). 5-Flucytosine is included (right) but is seldom used in treating patients unless combined with amphotericin B.

compounds broad in specificity, non-toxic, fungicidal and stable, and do they yield little resistance? The answers to these questions are dependent on the drug. Thus, amphotericin B is toxic but fungicidal and is usually broadly specific. The triazoles can induce drug–drug interactions, are fungistatic and, because of the latter property, often result in drug-resistant fungal pathogens. The echinocandins are relatively broad spectrum and have no safety issues, but resistance is now appearing in clinical isolates (Perlin, 2011).

The list of choices is relatively small and is confounded by the underlying problems exhibited by the patient, including neutropenia or not, prior use of triazoles, which usually implies that another antifungal may be required due to the selection of resistant strains, nephrotoxicity-associated drug therapy and pharmaco-economic considerations. Candidiasis is a global problem, and in some countries acquisition of antifungals is not possible due to cost. Ostrosky-Zeichner *et al.* (2010) have given a concise review of the antifungal pipeline and the new compounds that offer some hope for eradication of fungal diseases. Their conclusions were as follows:

1. The echinocandins represent the first class of antifungals that act against a specific component of fungal pathogens. As such, their safety profile is quite good, unlike triazoles, which are notorious for causing drug–drug interactions and toxicity.
2. The formulation of amphotericin B was changed to achieve better absorption and this drug is now available as a lipid formulation (encapsulation). This modification has reduced toxicity due to binding of the compound but has increased cost (Cagnoni *et al.*, 2000).
3. Enhanced activity has been observed with two of the newer triazoles, posaconazole and voriconazole.
4. New triazoles are in development (abaconazole and ravuconazole).
5. Echinocandins are slow in development and are ineffective against *C. neoformans.* While β-1,3-glucan is present in the cell wall of this pathogen, caspofungin may have reduced activity against the β-1,3-glucan synthase (Feldmesser *et al.*, 2000).
6. Drug resistance to triazoles is a common feature of several species of *Candida*, and an increase in resistance to echinocandins is frequently reported.
7. Importantly, the authors encourage the development of new antifungals. Because of the impressive number of publications of resistance to triazoles, we will discuss this in more detail. Readers are directed to a number of reviews, especially the more recent ones by Pfaller *et al.* (2010c).

16.4 Antifungal Drug Resistance

To identify drug resistance, susceptibility testing of strains has been developed. Two protocols have been developed, by the Clinical and Laboratory Standards Institute (CLSI) and the European Committee on Antimicrobial Susceptibility Testing (EUCAST) to determine the 50% MIC (MIC_{50}). Isolates are classified as susceptible (S), susceptible dose dependent (SDD) or resistant (R). Both methods are similar except for the inoculum density, with the EUCAST method using a density 2 logs higher than the CLSI method. Both provide clinical breakpoints (CBPs) for fluconazole and *Candida* spp., although the range of species classified is smaller with the EUCAST method. Recent attempts to establish common CBPs appear complete; the current data now establish MICs of S ≤ 2 μg/ml, SDD 4 μg/ml and R ≥ 8 μg/ml for *C. albicans*, *Candida tropicalis* and *C. parapsilosis*, and SDD ≤ 32 μg/ml and R ≥ 64 μg/ml for *C. glabrata*. Decreased patient response rates were seen with > 4 μg/ml for the first three species and > 16 μg/ml for *C. glabrata* (Pfaller *et al.*, 2010c). Adjusted CLSI CBPs should allow the detection of fluconazole resistance and consistency in CBP determinations by both methods.

Data suggest that the efficacy of fluconazole may be improved if optimal dosing and adjustments of critical MIC values are considered (Pfaller *et al.*, 2010c). Among their suggestions are the following:

1. Underdosing of fluconazole remains a serious problem. The recommendation is to emphasize the total amount of drug administrated. Thus, the ratio of the area under the serum concentration curve (AUC, or total amount of drug exposure) to MIC (AUC/MIC) needs to be around 25. When this is achieved, greater efficacy is seen in treatment (Louie *et al.*, 1998; Andes, 2003; Andes, 2006). **2.** CBPs for *C. glabrata* versus other *Candida* spp. such as *C. albicans* are critically different, a fact that needs to be emphasized in treatment (Pfaller *et al.*, 2006, 2010a,b). Thus, as stated above, the CBP for fluconazole and *C. glabrata* is 32 μg/ml (for both the CLSI and EUCAST methods), reflecting its greater resistance. Eradication of BSIs by *C. glabrata* was 91% if doses of >400 mg/day were achieved, compared with 50% if doses were ≤ 400 mg/day.

Among the current antifungal drugs, resistance to fluconazole as well as other triazoles among the species of *Candida* listed above and in *Candida dubiniensis* reveals common mechanisms, including overexpression of efflux pumps, overexpression or mutations of the Erg11p target and mutations in *ERG3* in *C. albicans*. *C. glabrata* fluconazole resistance has also been established in strains that have respiratory deficiencies associated with mutations relating to mitochondrial DNA (Bouchara *et al.*, 2000). Mutations in the transcription factors Tac1p and Mrr1p result in overexpression of the CDR and MDR efflux pumps, respectively (Coste *et al.*, 2004; Dunkel *et al.*, 2008). Echinocandin resistance in *C. albicans* and especially *C. glabrata* is associated with hot-spot point mutations in the *FKS1* and *FKS2* genes encoding the subunits of β-1,3-glucan synthase, presumably reducing binding of the drug to the target enzyme (Garcia-Effron *et al.*, 2008; Canton *et al.*, 2009; Perlin, 2011). Resistance to triazoles is not limited to *Candida* spp., and over the past decade now includes *A. fumigatus* (Howard *et al.*, 2009; Howard and Arendrup, 2011). In fact, fluconazole is not used in the treatment of aspergillosis, as the pathogen is inherently resistant so other triazoles such as itraconazole are used. Of critical importance is the observation that biofilm formation in fungal pathogens interferes with therapeutic intervention, presumably by preventing or reducing penetration of an antifungal. In this regard, regulators of β-1,3-glucan synthesis may be important targets to prevent biofilm formation and its inherent contribution to drug resistance (Nett *et al.*, 2011).

In spite of this extensive body of information on the resistance of clinical isolates, two points require brief mention. First, the clinical correlate of fluconazole resistance and patient response remains uncertain and in need of more extensive investigation. Secondly, the antifungal pipeline has slowed down considerably. New antifungals are remodelled older versions, a situation that is similar to that of antibacterial drug discovery, especially against drug-resistant bacteria (Boucher *et al.*, 2009). With this concept in mind, we will discuss approaches to new antifungal drug discovery.

16.5 Antifungal Drug Discovery

There are two general approaches to antifungal drug discovery that are quite different with regard to starting point but are in fact highly interrelated. It should be stated that neither approach is unique to antifungal discovery. The traditional or classical approach seeks first to identify active compounds, generally from large compound libraries, using a panel of fungal pathogens in standardized assays, when possible. The second approach is referred to as genetic, genomic or bioinformatic, in which the objective is initially to identify broadly represented targets in fungal pathogens and even non-pathogens (Weig and Brown, 2007). The targets may be essential for growth or proven to be required for virulence. The so-called 'antivirulence' drugs (Cegelski *et al.*, 2008) have gained a conceptual foothold in the antibacterial drug discovery paradigm but are underappreciated in the fungal literature. The genomics approach implies functional annotation that may not as yet be achieved in some fungal pathogens. These two approaches are discussed below.

The traditional approach described above in the context of the entire drug discovery process is shown in Fig. 16.2 (from 'hits' to market). The requirements for the traditional approach include the availability of compound libraries and a panel of reference species to test, most importantly (but not exclusively) clinical isolates. Achieving the first requirement is the most difficult. The second requirement is rather easy to address as strains are available for purchase or from other laboratories. Along with pathogens, the use of non-pathogenic *Saccharomyces cerevisiae* in compound screens is also important; this will be explained below. The following benchmarks are essential to the traditional approach. First, potency should reflect or be superior to those of current therapeutics. The CLSI or EUCAST assays were described briefly above; they provide information (MIC_{50}) about compound potency, but the method is not standardized for a number of other pathogens such as the dermatophytic or ringworm fungi. Secondly, a compound that is fungicidal is much better than one which is fungistatic. Minimal fungicidal concentration (MFC) is defined as a compound whose activity is less than or equal to fourfold greater than its MIC. MFC determinations can be made by plating the test organism on standard growth medium after treatment with a compound at or above the MIC_{50} value. Thirdly, at least preliminary *in vitro* compound toxicity testing should be done using mammalian or human cell cultures that are incubated with each compound at variable concentrations to identify the 50% cell cytotoxicity (CC_{50}). These assays are cheap, rapid and offer some promise, although much more extensive testing is required. The two that we use in our laboratory utilize the cell viability stains neutral red and 3-(4,5-dimethylthiazol-2-yl)-2,5-diphenyltetrazolium bromide (MTT). Fourthly, active compounds may need to be

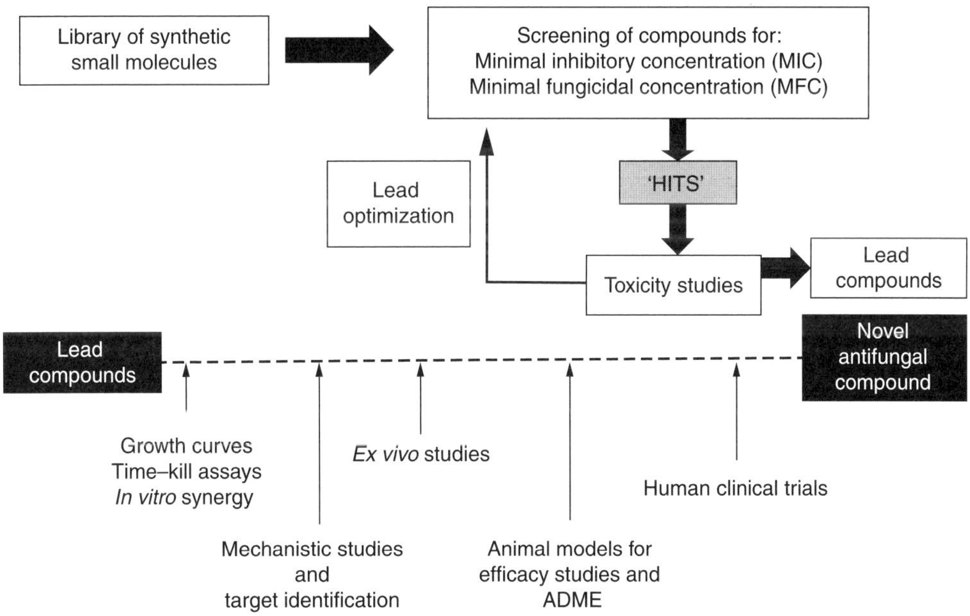

Fig. 16.2. An antifungal drug discovery flow chart. A library of small molecules is screened against a panel of test organisms, most often clinical isolates of fungal pathogens. Compound 'hits' are identified using the CLSI standard methodology and recycled through structural modifications, referred to as lead optimization. Active compounds are screened *in vitro* for toxicity in human cell lines. If toxicity is not displayed, lead compounds are then evaluated further by the assays indicated, followed by mechanism-of-action, *ex vivo* and animal infection studies to evaluate compound activity *in vivo*. *Ex vivo* assays (reconstituted tissues that are infected) may also be used to minimize the costs of *in vivo* testing. A critical step in the development pipeline is the absorption, distribution, metabolism and excretion (ADME) toxicity testing. The entire discovery process including clinical trials is a long-term and costly investment.

further altered structurally to be improved, a process called lead optimization. This statement means recycling of active compounds to achieve absolute maximum potency.

At this stage in the identification of active compounds, *in vivo* efficacy should be established. One of the problems in the early stages of the drug discovery pipeline is the cost of development. Conventional animal models require extensive numbers of animals and a great deal of time, involve ethical issues and require extensive technical support to establish the *in vivo* efficacy of test compounds. A solution to this problem, especially when a number of compounds are to be evaluated, is the use of invertebrate models (Anastassopoulou *et al.*, 2011). In this regard, the nematode *Caenorhabditis elegans* model offers an attractive alternative as a screening tool in early drug discovery. Of several candidate compounds, further testing with those efficacious in the invertebrate model will be needed in conventional models.

Mechanism-of-action (MOA) studies are presumably next in development and are of a huge benefit for at least two reasons: they ensure that the active compound inhibits a unique target and not targets of existing market drugs. Furthermore, with the target in hand, molecular modelling studies may be possible that could lead to increased compound potency. One way to verify that a 'hit' compound is against a unique target is to use a screen against a panel of triazole-, amphotericin B- and micafungin-resistant strains of *C. albicans* and *C. glabrata* and other pathogens (which can be obtained from a more than willing community). Sensitivity of resistant strains to the test compound is likely to indicate a target that is different from current therapeutics. MOA studies can follow two or more approaches. Macromolecular synthesis using radiolabelled precursors with treated or non-treated cells is useful but may only define a pathway and not the target itself. Nevertheless, this approach offers some predictive value of compound specificity.

Compounds that indicate sensitivity and specificity by MOA identification also can be gleaned using *S. cerevisiae* libraries of diploid homozygotic, heterozygotic (haploinsufficiency) or overexpression mutants. These assays, referred to as Hip-Hop profiling (haploinsufficiency/homozygosity profiling), are useful in attempts to decipher MOA (Baetz *et al.*, 2004; Bredel and Jacoby, 2004; Giaever *et al.*, 2004; Arita *et al.*, 2009; Batova *et al.*, 2010; Smith *et al.*, 2010). Each method has drawbacks but also offers opportunities for target discovery, as summarized in Fig. 16.3(a). Mutant libraries can be screened against compounds and compared with untreated control strains in large Petri dishes against 96 mutants per plate or in batch culture as each mutant is bar-coded. Each of these libraries is available through the European *Saccharomyces cerevisiae* archive for functional analysis (EUROSCARF: http://web.uni-frankfurt.de/fb15/mikro/euroscarf/index.html). Thus: (i) null strains lacking both copies of genes may be hypersensitive or resistant to test compounds; resistant mutants may define a target, as the lack of the target could confer resistance; (ii) strains that are hemizygotic and display haploinsufficiency reveal sensitivity to compounds because of reduced gene dosage; in this case, a lack of 'fitness' to a compound reflects reduced gene dosage; and (iii) strains that overexpress targets may exhibit a resistance phenotype; thus, increased target expression is displayed as resistance to the compound. With all screens, it is common to identify multiple hypersensitive or resistant mutants. For this outcome, algorithms for clustering genes to cell location and function include Funspec (http://funspec.med.utoronto.ca/) and Gene Ontology (http://www.geneontology.org/). To use the *S. cerevisiae* libraries requires that this species is sensitive to the 'hit' compound(s). None the less, the road to MOA using this genetic approach does have inherent problems. Homozygotic null libraries do not contain mutants in growth-essential genes, and so about 25% of the genome cannot be evaluated for sensitivity or resistance. Haploinsufficient mutants may not have a phenotype if a single gene copy provides fitness. Overexpression libraries are known to have mutants that are growth impaired, as overexpression of some genes leads to cell toxicity. In *S. cerevisiae*, about 15% of such strains are at least partially defective in growth. From all the libraries mentioned, a pathway, function and cell location of the

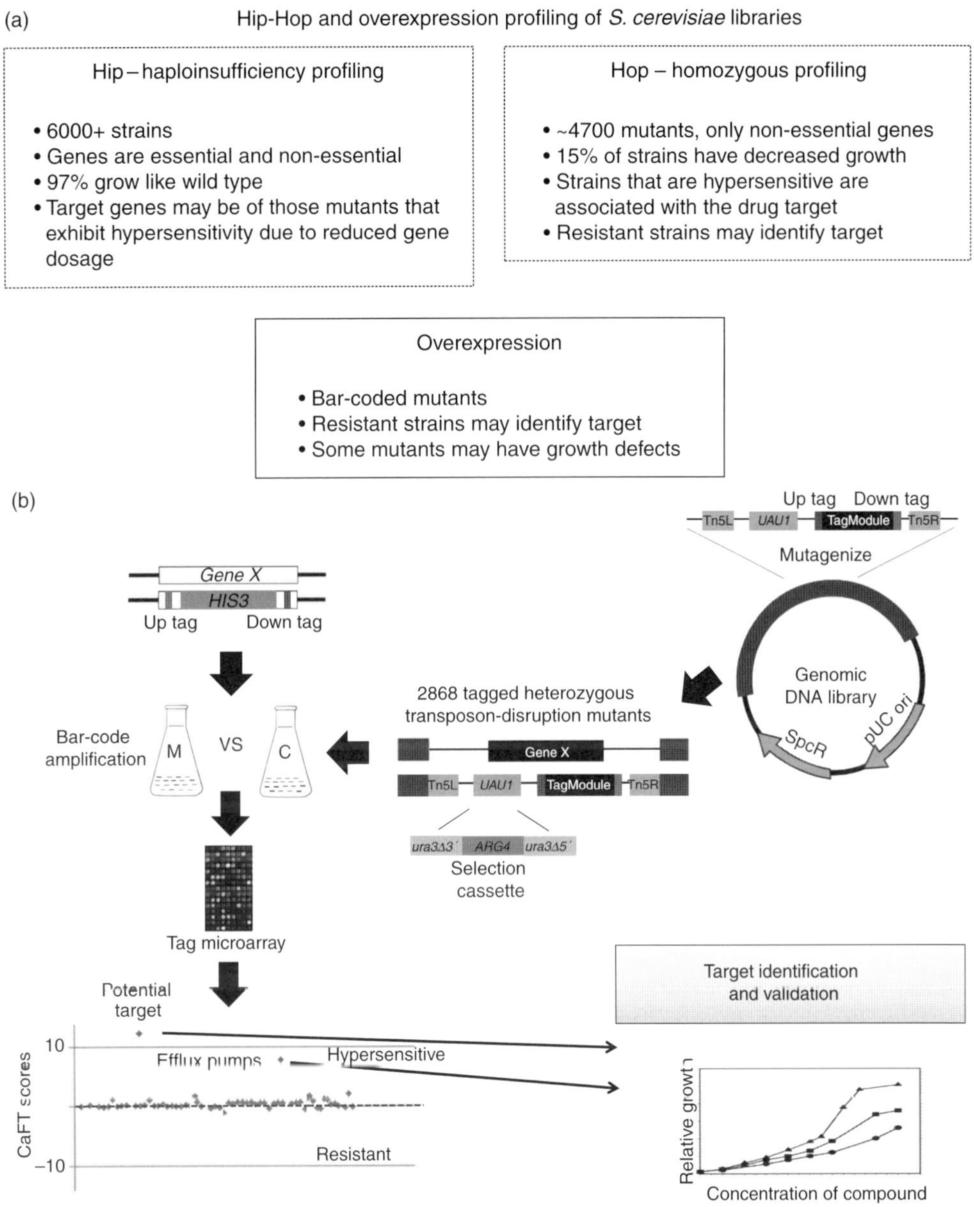

Fig. 16.3. Target identification. (a) Hip-Hop profiling of *S. cerevisiae* homozygous null mutants (upper left), heterozygous haploinsufficient mutants (upper right) or overexpression (lower) libraries. For each library, the advantages and disadvantages are listed. (b) Genome-wide fitness testing in *C. albicans*. Left: for each mutant, one allele of a selected gene was replaced with a cassette of *HIS3* flanked by different upstream and downstream bar codes to identify each of 2868 mutants (Xu *et al.*, 2007). Genes were selected for disruption based on the known essential genes of *S. cerevisiae* or conserved in other pathogens such as *A. fumigatus*. Mixed cultures were grown in the absence (M, mock) or presence (C) of compounds and then subjected to microarray analysis of PCR-amplified tags to determine fitness using PCR of up and down tags. Shown at the bottom are the fitness scores of two mutants, where loss of that gene resulted in hypersensitive growth. On the right, a similar approach, but using transposon mutagenesis, resulted in the construction of 3600+ mutants that could similarly be screened for fitness against compounds (Oh *et al.*, 2010).

target can be determined, but one is still left with many gene candidates. The latter problem can be remedied somewhat with extensive phenotyping of drug-treated parental strains. Thus, compound profiling that may indicate a cell-wall target, for example, can be demonstrated more specifically by biochemical analysis to determine whether a wild-type strain has impaired synthesis of a cell-wall component in treated cells. Microarray analysis may also be helpful in verifying mutant screens (Batova *et al.*, 2010). Finally, data showing efficacy in an animal model is highly advantageous. Animal testing is, however, time-consuming and costly, and is better served by collaboration with a testing service. The National Institutes of Health/National Institute of Allergy and Infectious Diseases does provide this service to investigators.

As mentioned above, these two approaches intersect. For example, a *C. albicans* mutant lacking a gene that is functionally important to that organism and broadly conserved among only fungi can be screened for resistance to compound libraries in traditional screening assays (see below). Again, the paradigm is that a strain lacking a gene product should be resistant to a compound, but target verification is still needed. Another way of intersecting both approaches is to design a strain in which the target gene contains a reporter gene cassette. That strain can be then assayed against a compound library and active compound(s) identified by reduced reporter activity. In spite of all these approaches, the determination of MOA for a compound is probably the most challenging part of the discovery process. Most of what has been described above applies only to *S. cerevisiae* libraries, and, in fact, this approach would miss about 30% of the *C. albicans* genes of which the former organism lacks orthologues.

For pathogens such as *C. albicans*, only mutant libraries that cover a portion of the genome have been constructed (Roemer, *et al.*, 2003; Rodriguez-Suarez, *et al.*, 2007; Xu *et al.*, 2007; Oh *et al.*, 2010). However, proof of principle has been established in that specific mutants (Erg11, for example) are sensitive to drugs that target those genes (fluconazole, for instance). Thus, large mutant libraries are useful in compound screens of genes including those that are growth essential. Heterozygous, bar-coded libraries of mutants have been constructed to detect haploinsufficiency (referred to as fitness) following treatment with compound libraries (Xu *et al.*, 2007; Oh *et al.*, 2010) (Fig. 16.3b). For *A. fumigatus*, a small library of essential gene mutants was identified using a conditional promoter replacement with the nitrogen-regulated *NiiA* promoter (p*NiiA*; Hu *et al.*, 2007). This strategy allowed phenotypic analyses *in vitro* (cidal terminal growth phenotype) or *in vivo* (virulence). The authors suggest that conditional promoter replacement may be useful in examining target-specific chemical hypersensitivity.

16.6 Current Examples of Antifungal Compound Discovery and Target Identification

It is unlikely that a magic (antifungal) bullet exists that will inhibit all fungal pathogens. Fungal pathogens are quite different in many respects, not least of which is their variable expression of key targets. A case in point is the cell wall of pathogens, in regard to both the absolute quantity and even the absence/presence of wall components from fungus to fungus. *C. neoformans* has β-1,3-glucan in its cell wall, but the echinocandins may not have as much activity against this synthase as with other pathogens (Feldmesser *et al.*, 2000). *A. fumigatus* lacks β-1,6-glucan, and consequently a drug to this target would not be of use in treating patients with aspergillosis. Furthermore, the quantity of a cell-wall component may differ among pathogens. Here, we contrast *Candida* spp. (low chitin content) with *Coccidioides immitis* (high chitin content); nikkomycin, a chitin synthesis inhibitor, is not used in treating candidiasis but may be useful in treating coccidioidomycosis (Hector *et al.*, 1990; Ostrosky-Zeichner *et al.*, 2010). Therefore, it might be better to focus on conserved signal pathways as potential targets among fungi. Recent data have shown that membrane sensor proteins of signal pathways and downstream transcription factors for that pathway and especially the proteins that link sensors and transcription factors in pathways are broadly conserved among pathogenic and non-pathogenic fungi (Nikolaou *et al.*, 2009). The point is that these types of proteins are conserved among numerous pathogenic fungi, and, importantly, not found in mammalian cells. We offer an example of this below.

16.6.1 Two-component histidine kinases

Histidine kinases (HKs) are found in numerous bacteria, fungi and plants. Their important role in drug resistance, and other functions related to disease development among bacterial pathogens has led to the search for anti-HK antibiotics (Qin *et al.*, 2006). Below, we discuss only the HKs of human fungal pathogens. For a broad perspective of HKs in fungi, readers are directed to several reviews (Santos and Shiozaki, 2001; Catlett *et al.*, 2003; Li *et al.*, 2009; Lavin *et al.*, 2010).

Conservation of HKs is evident when one searches the genomes of pathogens. Thus, *Candida* spp., *Blastomyces dermatitidis*, *Histoplasma capsulatum*, *C. immitis*, *Cryptococcus neoformans*, *A. fumigatus*, *Paracoccidioides brasiliensis* and *Penicillium marneffei* all have one or more HK. For the majority of these organisms, functional annotation has been done to indicate their requirement for virulence, morphogenesis, growth, conidia formation, cell-wall synthesis, adaptation to stress, antifungal drug activity and/or sexual reproduction (Srikantha *et al.*, 1998; Balın *et al.*, 2006; Nemecek *et al.*, 2009; Chapeland-Leclerc *et al.*, 2007; Wang *et al.*, 2009).

All of the fungal HK proteins have an N-terminal H-box and C-terminal receiver domains, the former containing a key histidine residue and the latter an aspartate residue that are each involved in phosphotransfer. Hence, they are referred to as hybrid HKs. This is in comparison with most bacterial HKs, which have an H-box domain but not a receiver domain. Phosphotransfer is thought to occur on these residues based on data from other fungal and bacterial HK proteins. Most fungal HKs have other domains that may indicate cell location or function. Sln1p, for example, is a transmembrane protein, but Nik1p and Chk1p are thought to be located in the cytoplasm and not to be membrane bound. Sln1p is phosphorylated in the absence of stress. Subsequent phosphotransfer to proteins Ypd1p and then Ssk1p occurs, but phosphorylated Ssk1p cannot activate the HOG1 mitogen-activated protein kinase (MAPK) pathway. When osmotic stress occurs, Sln1p is not phosphorylated, allowing Ssk1p to activate the HOG1 MAPK, resulting in adaptation of cells to this stress. Nik1p may be part of this pathway, but Chk1p is not. The proteins Sln1p, Ypd1p and Ssk1p thus are sometimes referred to as three-component signal transduction, in deference to most bacteria which have an HK protein that is used to directly phosphorylate a response regulator protein that acts as a transcription factor. In bacteria, this pathway is referred to as two-component signalling.

Candida spp. have three HKs, CHK1, SLN1 and NIK1, each of which is required for virulence in murine models of IC caused by *C. albicans* (Yamada-Okabe *et al.*, 1999; Li *et al.*, 2010). Sln1p appears to be solely associated with the HOG MAPK pathway and provides adaptive functions to stress (Yamada-Okabe *et al.*, 1999). Nik1p may also be related to the HOG MAPK pathway and in *C. albicans* is at least partially required for the opaque–white switch, which is critical to virulence and variability (Srikantha *et al.*, 1998). The Nik1p (FOS-1) of *A. fumigatus* is also required for virulence (Clemons *et al.*, 2002). There are several interesting functions associated with CHK1, although alignment to a specific MAP pathway has not been shown. However, there is data to indicate that Chk1p is part of a pathway parallel to that of the CEK1 MAPK (Li *et al.*, 2009). Mention was made of its requirement for virulence in *C. albicans*. The protein is also linked to a functional role in cell-wall synthesis by regulating β-glucan and mannan synthesis (Kruppa *et al.*, 2003; Li *et al.*, 2009). Strains lacking a CHK1 have hypersensitivity to fluconazole and voriconazole, implying that Chk1p is part of a regulatory pathway for transport of at least fluconazole, as much greater uptake of [^{14}C]fluconazole was noted in the null strain compared with the parental and a *CHK1*-reintegrated strain (Chauhan *et al.*, 2007). More recently, it has been shown that the reduction in cell-wall mannan in the *chk1* null strain exposes underlying β-1, 3-glucan, which results in a greater recognition by phagocytes (Klippel *et al.*, 2010). Thus, a compound that inhibits this HK can also impact positively on immune responses to *C. albicans*.

Ongoing research in our laboratory now utilizes our screens of a wild-type, *CHK1* null, reintegrant strain, as well as other HK mutants with compound libraries. Our objective is to identify compounds to which the null strain is resistant, with the hypothesis being that no gene target (Chk1p) could indicate an active compound that affects the activity of this protein. Additional experiments will be needed to verify this hypothesis. For example, synergy with known cell-wall inhibitors may indicate a common target. A Chk1p promoter-reporter strain can be used to screen compound libraries or a compound to which the mutant but not the reconstituted strain is less resistant (Li *et al.*, 2004). If proven, the application of genomics to select targets along with traditional compound screens of specific mutants will be a promising approach to drug discovery.

16.6.2 Defining MOA using a *S. cerevisiae* deletion mutant library by the application of chemogenetics: two examples

Using chemogenetics (Bredel and Jacoby, 2004), recent investigations established a role for 7-chlorotetrazolo (5,1-c) benzo (1,2,4) triazine (CTBT) in strongly inhibiting several fungi, including *C. albicans*, when used in combination with other antifungals (Batova *et al.*, 2010). However, CTBT was weakly antifungal when used alone. To understand the MOA of CTBT, a *S. cerevisiae* library of homozygous deletion mutants was screened with CTBT (Batova *et al.*, 2010). For CTBT to be inhibitory, drug-sensitivity assays required molecular oxygen. A total of 169 CTBT hypersensitive mutants were identified from agar cultures containing 2 or 4 μg/ml of compound. Gene ontology clustering revealed that the most prominent gene ontology assignment included those functions related to mitochondria, DNA repair and the stress response. Of these, the largest group of hypersensitive mutants corresponded to those with mitochondrial biogenesis defects. To support the mutant analysis data, transcriptional profiling of treated versus untreated cells was done. Temporal changes showed that antioxidants were induced most rapidly after treatment with CTBT. Equally suggestive was a stress response associated with mitochondrial functions. Oxidant stress response factors such as Yap1 and Skn7 were part of the early (2–4 min) response to CTBT, and growth reduction in the presence of CTBT was greater in strains lacking *SOD1*. Thus, the use of multiple approaches to MOA determination of CTBT, i.e. null mutant and transcriptional profiling as well as standard-type assays, yield valuable information on MOA.

A second example (and proof of principle) of the same nature was a report that defined the MOA of nickel sulfate. Arita *et al* (2009) identified a total of 149 haploid, sensitive strains of *S. cerevisiae* when cells were treated with nickel sulfate, representing about 3.1% of all strains tested. Clustering indicated a significant number of gene knockout strains with deficiencies in the homeostasis of metal ions.

A significant problem with these types of analysis is that no single target is identified. Rather, pathways define the initial observations of MOA, and additional experimentation is needed before more direct data establishes a specific MOA.

16.7 Conclusions

If we accept the paradigm that there are adequate antifungals, then the current antifungal therapeutics used in the clinic should be fungicidal, specific for fungal pathogens and safe. Yet what is used has inherent problems of toxicity, either as defined for amphotericin B or as drug–drug toxicity such as with triazoles. Furthermore, fungistatic triazole antifungals select for drug-resistant strains. The change in the landscape of *Candida* spp. among pathogens since the introduction of fluconazole has been described. In such cases, the further development of compounds is compromised. Identifying active compounds is a straightforward task. Compounds usually fall out of the process for their toxicity, but the entire process of discovery also requires a clear mandate that antifungal development is needed. Our reason for the issues raised in this chapter on the importance of fungal diseases was done solely to project such a need. Drug discovery is fraught with speed bumps other than toxicity, MOA determinations being another. For this reason, we have summarized current approaches to the identification of compound MOAs. Both approaches – random screening (traditional) as well as target-based hunting – have advantages and disadvantages, suggesting that multiple approaches to new drug discovery are better.

References

Ameen, M. and Arenas, R. (2009) Developments in the management of mycetomas. *Clinical Experimental Dermatology* 32, 1–7.

Anastassopoulou, C., Fuchs, B. and Mylonakis, E. (2011) *Caenorhabditis elegans*-based model systems for antifungal drug discovery. *Current Pharmacological Design* 17, 1225–1233.

Andes, D. (2003) *In vivo* pharmacodynamics of antifungal drugs in treatment of candidiasis. *Antimicrobial Agents and Chemotherapy* 47, 1179–1185.

Andes, D. (2006) Pharmacokinetics and pharmacodynamics of antifungals. *Infectious Disease Clinics of North America* 20, 679–697.

Arita, A., Zhou, X., Ellen, T.P., Liu, X., Bai, J., Rooney, J., Kurtz, A., Klein, C., Dai, W., Begley, T. and Costa, M. (2009) A genome-wide deletion mutant screen identifies pathways affected by nickel sulfate in *Saccharomyces cerevisiae*. *BMC Genomics* 10, 524.

Baetz, K., McHardy, L., Gable, K., Tarling, T., Reberioux, D., Bryan, J., Andersen, R., Dunn, T., Hieter, P. and Roberge, M. (2004) Yeast genome-wide drug-induced haploinsufficiency screen to determine drug mode of action. *Proceedings National Academy Science USA* 101, 4525–4530.

Bahn, Y.S., Kojima, K., Cox, G. and Heitman, J. (2006) A unique two-component system regulates stress responses, drug sensitivity, sexual development, and virulence of *Cryptococcus neoformans*. *Molecular Biology of the Cell* 17, 3122–3135.

Batova, M., Klobucnikova, V., Oblasova, Z., Gregan, J., Zahradnik, P., Hapala, I., Subik, J. and Schuller, C. (2010) Chemogenomic and transcriptome analysis identifies mode of action of the chemosensitizing agent CTBT (7-chlorotetrazolo[5,1-c]benzo[1,2,4]triazine). *BMC Genomics* 11, 153–169.

Bennett, J.E. (2009) The changing face of febrile neutropenia – from monotherapy to moulds to mucositis. Management of mycoses in neutropenic patients: a brief history, 1960–2008. *Journal of Antimicrobial Chemotherapy* 63 (Suppl. 1), i23–i26.

Blignaut, E. (2007) Oral candidiasis and oral yeast carriage among institutionalized South African paediatric HIV/AIDS patients. *Mycopathologia* 163, 67–73.

Boechk, M. and Marr, K. (2002). Infection in hematopoietic stem cell transplantation,. In: Rubin, E and Young, L (eds) *Clinical Approach to Infection in the Compromised Host*. Kluwer Academic/Plenum, New York, pp. 527–571.

Bonifaz, A., Vazquez-Gonzalex, D. and Perusquia-Ortiz, A. (2010) Subcutaneous mycoses: chromoblastomycosis, sporotrichosis, and mycetoma. *Journal of the German Society of Dermatology* 8, 619–627.

Bouchara, J., Zouhair, R., Le Boudouil, S., Reiner, G., Filmong, R., Chabasse, D., Hallet, J. and Defontaine, A. (2000). *In vivo* selection of an azole resistant petite mutant of *Candida albicans*. *Journal of Medical Microbiology* 49, 977–984.

Boucher, H.W., Talbot, G., Bradley, J., Edwards, J., Gilbert, D., Rice, L., Scheld, M., Spellberg, B. and Bartlett, J. (2009) Bad bugs, no drugs: no ESKAPE! An update from the Infectious Diseases Society of America. *Clinical Infectious Diseases* 48, 1–12.

Bougnoux, M.E., Kac, G., Aegerter, P., d'Enfert, C., Fagon, J. and CandiRea Study Group. (2008) Candidemia and candiduria in critically ill patients admitted to intensive care units in France: incidence, molecular diversity, management and outcome. *Intensive Care Medicine* 34, 292–299.

Bredel, M., and Jacoby, E. (2004) Chemogenomics: an emerging strategy for rapid target and drug discovery. *Nature Reviews Genetics* 5, 262–275.

Cagnoni, P.J., Walsh, T., Prendergast, M., Bodensteiner, D., Hiemenz, S., Greenberg, R., Arndt, C., Schuster, M., Seibel, N., Yeldandi, V. and Tong, K. (2000) Pharmacoeconomic analysis of liposomal amphotericin B versus conventional amphotericin B in the empirical treatment of persistently febrile neutropenic patients. *Journal of Clinical Oncology* 18, 2476–2483.

Canton, E., Peman, J., Valentin, A., Espinel-Ingroff, A. and Gobernado, M. (2009) *In vitro* activities of echinocandins against *Candida krusei* determined by three methods: MIC and minimal fungicidal concentration measurements and time-kill studies. *Antimicrobial Agents and Chemotherapy* 53, 3108–3111.

Caston-Osorio, J.A. Rivero, A. and Torre-Cisneros, J. (2008) Epidemiology of invasive fungal infection. *International Journal of Antimicrobial Agents* 32 (Suppl. 2), S103–S109.

Catlett, N., Yoder, O. and Turgeon, B. (2003) Whole-genome analysis of two-component signal transduction genes in fungal pathogens. *Eucaryotic Cell* 2, 1151–1161.

Cegelski, L., Marshall, G., Eldridge, R. and Hultgren, S. (2008) The biology and future prospects of antivirulence therapies. *Nature Reviews Microbiology* 6,17–27.

Chakrabarti, A., Chatterjee, S. and Shivaprakash, M. (2008) Overview of opportunistic fungal infections in India. *Japanese Journal of Medical Mycology* 49, 165–172.

Chakraborty, N., Mukherjee, A., Santra, S., Sarkar, R., Banerjee, D., Guha, S., Chakraborty, S. and Bhattacharyya, S. (2008) Current trends of opportunistic infections among HIV-seropositive patients from Eastern India. *Japanese Journal of Infectious Disease* 61, 49–53.

Chapeland-Leclerc, F., Paccallet, P., Ruprich-Robert, G., Reboutier, D., Chastin, C. and Papon, N. (2007) Differential involvement of histidine kinase receptors in pseudohyphal development, stress adaptation, and drug sensitivity of the opportunistic yeast *Candida lusitaniae. Eukaryotic Cell* 6, 1782–1794.

Chauhan, N., Kruppa, M. and Calderone, R. (2007) The Ssk1p response regulator and Chk1p histidine kinase mutants of *Candida albicans* are hypersensitive to fluconazole and voriconazole. *Antimicrobial Agents and Chemotherapy* 51, 3747–3751.

Clemons, K., Miller, T., Selitrenikoff, C and Stevens, D. (2002) *fos-1*, a putative histidine kinase as a virulence factor for systemic aspergillosis. *Medical Mycology* 40, 259–262.

Coste, A., Karababa, M., Ischer, F., Bille, J. and Sanglard, D. (2004) *TAC1*, transcriptional activator of CDR genes, is a new transcription factor involved in the regulation of *Candida albicans* ABC transporters *CDR1* and *CDR2. Eukaryotic Cell* 3, 1639–1652.

Dunkel, N., Blas, J., Rogers, P. and Morschhauser, J. (2008) Mutations in the multidrug resistance regulator *MRR1*, followed by loss of heterozygosity, are the main cause of *MDR1* overexpression in fluconazole-resistant *Candida albicans* strains. *Molecular Microbiology* 69, 827–840.

Espinel-Ingroff, A. (2009) Novel antifungal agents, targets or therapeutic strategies for the treatment of invasive fungal diseases: a review of the literature (2005–2009). *Revista Iberoamericana de Micología* 26, 15–22.

Feldmesser, M., Kress, Y., Mednick, A. and Casadevall, A. (2000) The effect of the echinocandin analogue caspofungin on cell wall glucan synthesis by *Cryptococcus neoformans. Journal of Infectious Diseases* 182, 1791–1795.

Fleming, T. (ed.) (2006) *Red Book: Pharmacy's Fundamental Reference.* Thomson PDR, Montvale, New Jersey.

Gagne, J. and Goldfarb, N. (2007) Candidemia in the in-patient setting: treatment options and economics. *Expert Opinion in Pharmacotherapy* 8, 1643–1650.

Garcia-Effron, G., Katiyar, S., Park, S., Edlind, T. and Perlin, D. (2008) A naturally occurring proline-to-alanine amino acid change in Fks1p in *Candida parapsilosis, Candida orthopsilosis,* and *Candida metapsilosis* accounts for reduced echinocandin susceptibility. *Antimicrobial Agents and Chemotherapy* 52, 2305–2312.

Gavalda, J., Len, O., San Juan, R., Aguado, J., Fortun, J., Lumbreras, C., Moreno, A., Munoz, P., Blanes, M., Ramos, A., Rufi, G., Gurgui, M., Torre-Cisneros, T., Montejo, M., Cuenca-Estrella, M., Rodriguez-Tudela, J., Pahissa, A. and RESITRA (Spanish Network for Research on Infection in Transplantation) (2005) Risk factors for invasive aspergillosis in solid-organ transplant recipients: a case–control study. *Clinical Infectious Diseases* 41, 52–59.

Giaever, G., Flaherty, P., Kumm, J., Proctor, M., Nislow, C., Jaramillo, D., Chu, A., Jordan, M., Arkin, A. and Davis, R. (2004) Chemogenomic profiling: identifying the functional interactions of small molecules in yeast. *Proceedings of the National Academy Science USA* 101, 793–798.

Groll, A., Shah, P., Mentzel, C., Schneider, M., Just-Nuebling, G. and Huebner, K. (1996) Trends in the postmortem epidemiology of invasive fungal infections at a university hospital. *Journal of Infection* 33, 23–32.

Hachem, R., Hanna, H., Kontoyiannis, D., Jiang, Y. and Raad, I. (2008) The changing epidemiology of invasive candidiasis: *Candida glabrata* and *Candida krusei* as the leading causes of candidemia in hematologic malignancy. *Cancer* 112, 2493–2499.

Hamza, O., Matee, M., Moshi, M., Simon, E., Mugusi, F., Mikx, F., Helderman, W., Rijs, A., van der Ven, A. and Verweij, P. (2008) Species distribution and *in vitro* antifungal susceptibility of oral yeast isolates from Tanzanian HIV-infected patients with primary and recurrent oropharyngeal candidiasis. *BMC Microbiology* 8, 135.

Harbarth, S., Ruef, C., Francioli, P., Widmer, A. and Pittet, D. (1999) Nosocomial infections in Swiss university hospitals: a multi-centre survey and review of the published experience. Swiss-Noso Network. *Schweizerische Medizinische Wochenschrift* 129, 1521–1528.

Hector, R., Zimmer, B. and Pappagianis, D. (1990) Evaluation of nikkomycins X and Z in murine models of coccidioidomycosis, histoplasmosis, and blastomycosis. *Antimicrobial Agents and Chemotherapy* 34, 587–593.

Horn, D., Neofytos, D., Anaissie, E., Fishman, J., Steinbach, W., Olyaei, A., Marr, K., Pfaller, M., Chang, C. and Webster, K. (2009) Epidemiology and outcomes of candidemia in 2019 patients: data from the prospective antifungal therapy alliance registry. *Clinical Infectious Diseases* 48, 1695–1703.

Howard, S. and Arendrup, M. (2011) Acquired antifungal drug resistance in *Aspergillus fumigatus*: epidemiology and detection. *Medical Mycology* 48 (Suppl. 1), S90–S95.

Howard, S., Cerar, D., Anderson, M., Albarrag, A., Fisher, M., Pasquqlotto, A., Laverdiere, M., Arendrup, M., Perlin, D. and Denning, D. (2009) Frequency and evolution of azole resistance in *Aspergillus fumigatus* associated with treatment failure. *Emerging Infectious Diseases* 15, 1068–1076.

Hu, W., Sillaots, S., Lemieux, S., Davison, J., Kauffman, S., Breton, A., Linteau, A., Xin, C., Bowman, J., Becker, J., Jiang, B. and Roemer, T. (2007) Essential gene identification and drug target prioritization in *Aspergillus fumigatus*. *PLoS Pathogens* 3, e24.

Jabra-Rizk, M., Falkler, W. Jr, Enwonwu, C., Onwujekwe, D. Jr, Merz, W. and Meiller, T. (2001) Prevalence of yeast among children in Nigeria and the United States. *Oral Microbiology and Immunology* 16, 383–385.

Klippel, S., Cui, S., Groebe, L. and Bilitewski, U. (2010) Deletion of the *Candida albicans* histidine kinase gene *CHK1* improves recognition by phagocytes through an increased exposure of cell wall β-1,3-glucan. *Microbiology* 156, 3432–3444.

Knaus, W., Wagner, D., Draper, E., Zimmerman, J., Bergner, M., Bastos, P., Sirio, C., Murphy, D., Lotring, T. and Damiano, A. (1991) The APACHE III prognostic system. Risk prediction of hospital mortality for critically ill hospitalized adults. *Chest* 100, 1619–1636.

Kontoyiannis, D., Marr, K., Park, B., Alexander, B., Anaissie, E., Walsh, T., Ito, J., Andes, D., Baddley, J., Brown, J., Brumble, L., Freifeld, A., Hadley, S., Herwaldt, L., Kauffman, C., Knapp, K., Lyon, G., Morrison, V., Papanicolaou, G., Patterson, T., Perl, T., Schuster, M., Walker, R., Wannemuehler, K., Wingard, J., Chiller, T. and Pappas, P. (2010) Prospective surveillance for invasive fungal infections in hematopoietic stem cell transplant recipients, 2001–2006: overview of the transplant-associated infection surveillance network (TRANSNET) database. *Clinical Infectious Diseases* 50, 1091–1100.

Kruppa, M., Goins, T., Cutler, J., Lowman, D., Williams, D., Chauhan, N., Menon, V., Singh, P., Li, D. and Calderone, R. (2003). The role of the *Candida albicans* histidine kinase (*CHK1*) gene in the regulation of cell wall mannan and glucan biosynthesis. *FEMS Yeast Research* 3, 289–299.

Lass-Florl, C. (2009) The changing face of epidemiology of invasive fungal disease in Europe. *Mycoses* 52, 197–205.

Lavin, J., Ramirez, L., Ussery, D., Pisabarro, A. and Oquiza, J. (2010) Genomic analysis of two-component signal transduction proteins in Basidiomycetes. *Journal of Molecular Microbiology Biotechnology* 18, 63–73.

Lehrnbecher, T., Frank, C., Engels, K., Kriener, S., Groll, A. and Schwabe, D. (2010) Trends in the postmortem epidemiology of invasive fungal infections at a university hospital. *Journal of Infection* 61, 259–265.

Li, D., Gurkovska, V., Sheridan, M., Calderone, R., and Chauhan, N. (2004) Studies on the regulation of the two-component histidine kinase gene *CHK1* in *Candida albicans* using the heterologous *lacZ* reporter gene. *Microbiology* 150, 3305–3313.

Li, D., Williams, D., Lowman, D., Monteiro, A., Tan X,. Kruppa, M., Fonzi, W., Roman, W., Pla, J. and Calderone, R. (2009) The *Candida albicans* histidine kinase Shk1p: signaling and cell wall mannan. *Fungal Biology Genetics* 46, 731–741.

Li, D., Agrellos, O. and Calderone, R. (2010) Histidine kinases keep fungi safe and vigorous. *Current Opinion in Microbiology* 13, 424–430.

Lortholary, O., Desnos-Ollivier, M., Sitbon, K., Fontanet, A., Bretagne, S., Dromer, F. and the French Mycosis Study Group (2011) Recent exposure to caspofungin or fluconazole influences the epidemiology of candidemia: a prospective multicenter study involving 2,441 patients. *Antimicrobial Agents and Chemotherapy* 55, 532–538.

Louie, A., Drusano, G., Banerjee, P., Liu, W., Kaw, M., Shayegoniz, H., Tuber, H. and Miller, M. (1998) Pharmacodynamics of fluconazole in a murine model of systemic candidiasis. *Antimicrobial Agents and Chemotherapy* 42, 1105–1109.

Micol, R., Tajahmady, A., Lortholary, O., Balkan, S., Quillet, C., Dousset, J., Chanroeun, H., Madec, Y., Fontanet, A. and Yazdanpanah, Y. (2010) Cost-effectiveness of primary prophylaxis of AIDS associated cryptococcosis in Cambodia. *PLoS One* 5, e13856.

Miller, L., Hajjeh, R. and Edwards, J. Jr (2001) Estimating the cost of nosocomial candidemia in the United States. *Clinical Infectious Diseases* 32, 1110.

Nadagir, S., Chunchanur, S., Halesh, L., Yasmeen, K., Chandrasekhar, M. and Patil, B. (2008) Significance of isolation and drug susceptibility testing of non-*Candida albicans* species causing oropharyngeal candidiasis in HIV patients. *Southeast Asian Journal of Tropical Medicine and Public Health* 39, 492–495.

Nemecek, J., Wüthrich, M. and Klein, B. (2009) Global control of virulence and dimorphism in fungi. *Science* 312, 583–588.

Neofytos, D., Horn, D., Anaissie, E., Steinbach, W., Olyaei, A., Fishman, J., Pfaller, M., Chang, C., Webster, K. and Marr, K. (2009) Epidemiology and outcome of invasive fungal infection in adult hematopoietic stem cell transplant recipients: analysis of Multicenter Prospective Antifungal Therapy (PATH) Alliance registry. *Clinical Infectious Disease* 48, 265–273.

Nett, J., Sanchez, H., Cain, M., Ross, K. and Andes, D. (2011) Interface of *Candida albicans* biofilm matrix-associated drug resistance and cell wall Integrity regulation. *Eukaryotic Cell* 10, 1660–1669.

Niimi, M., Firth, N. and Cannon, R. (2010) Antifungal drug resistance of oral fungi. *Odontology* 98, 15–25.

Nikolaou, E., Agrafioti, I., Stumph, M., Quinn, J., Stansfield, I. and Brown, A.J. (2009) Phylogenetic diversity of stress signaling pathways in fungi. *BMC Evolutionary Biology* 9, 44.

Nishikaku, A., Melo, A. and Colombo, A. (2010) Geographic trends in invasive candidiasis. *Current Fungal Infections* 4, 210–218.

Nomura, K., Kawasugi, K. and Morimoto, T. (2006) Cost-effectiveness analysis of antifungal treatment for patients on chemotherapy. *European Journal of Cancer Care* 15, 44–50.

Odds, F.C., Brown, A. and Gow, N.A. (2003) Antifungal agents: mechanisms of action. *Trends in Microbiology* 11, 272–279.

Oh, J., Fung, E., Schlecht, U., Davis, R., Giaever, G., St Onge, R., Deutschbauer, A. and Nislow, C. (2010) Gene annotation and drug target discovery in *Candida albicans* with a tagged transposon mutant collection. *PLoS Pathogens* 6, e1001140.

Okome-Nkoumou, M., Mbounja-Loclo, M. and Kombila, M. (2000) Spectrum of opportunistic infections in subjects infected with HIV at Libreville. *Gabon Sante* 10, 329–337 (in French).

Olaechea, P., Palomar, M., Leon-Gil, C., Alvarez-Lerma, F., Jorda, R., Nolla-Salas, J., Leon-Regidor, M. and EPCAN Study Group. (2004) Economic impact of *Candida* colonization and *Candida* infection in the critically ill patient. *European Journal of Clinical Microbiology and Infectious Disease* 23, 323–330.

Ostrosky-Zeichner, L., Casadevall, A., Galgiani, J., Odds, F. and Rex, J. (2010) An insight into the antifungal pipeline: selected new molecules and beyond. *Nature Reviews Drug Discovery* 9, 719–727.

Pappas, P., Kauffman, C., Andes, D., Benjamin, D. Jr, Calandra, T., Edwards, J. Jr, Filler, S., Fisher, J., Kullberg, B., Ostrosky-Zeichner, L., Reboli, A., Rex, J., Walsh, T., Sobel, J. and the Infectious Diseases Society of America (2009) Clinical practice guidelines for the management of candidiasis: 2009 update by the Infectious Diseases Society of America. *Clinical Infectious Diseases* 48, 503–535.

Pappas, P., Alexander, B., Andes, D., Hadley, S., Kauffman, C., Freifeld, A., Anaissie, E., Brumble, L., Herwaldt, L., Ito, J., Kontoyiannis, D., Lyon, G., Marr, K., Morrison, V., Park, B., Patterson, T., Perl, T., Oster, R. Schuster, M., Walker, R., Walsh, T., Wannemuehler, K. and Chiller, T. (2010) Invasive fungal infections among organ transplant recipients: results of the Transplant-Associated Infection Surveillance Network (TRANSNET). *Clinical Infectious Diseases* 50, 1101–1111.

Perlin, D. (2011) Current perspectives on echinocandin class drugs. *Future Microbiology* 6, 441–457.

Pfaller, M. and Diekema, D. (2007) Epidemiology of invasive candidiasis: a persistent public health problem. *Clinical Microbiology Reviews* 20, 133–163.

Pfaller, M., Diekema, D. and the International Fungal Surveillance Participant Group (2004) Twelve years of fluconazole in clinical practice: global trends in species distribution and fluconazole susceptibility of bloodstream isolates of *Candida. Clinical Microbiology Infection* 10 (Suppl. 1), 11–23.

Pfaller, M., Boyken, L., Hollis, R., Messer, S., Tendolkar, S. and Diekema, D. (2006) *In vitro* susceptibilities of *Candida spp.* to caspofungin:

four years of global surveillance. *Journal Clinical Microbiology* 44, 760–763.

Pfaller, M., Diekema, D., Gibbs, D., Newell, V., Bijie, H., Dzierzanowska, D., Klimko, N., Letscher-Bru, V., Lisalova, M., Muehlethaler, K., Rennison, C., Zaidi, M. and Global Antifungal Surveillance Group (2009) Results from the ARTEMIS DISK Global Antifungal Surveillance Study, 1997 to 2007: 10.5-year analysis of susceptibilities of noncandidal yeast species to fluconazole and voriconazole determined by CLSI standardized disk diffusion testing. *Journal of Clinical Microbiology* 47, 117–123.

Pfaller, M., Castanheira, M., Messer, S., Moet, G. and Jones, R. (2010a) Variation in *Candida* spp. distribution and antifungal resistance rates among bloodstream infection isolates by patient age: report from the SENTRY Antimicrobial Surveillance Program (2008–2009). *Diagnostic Microbiology and Infectious Disease* 68, 278–283.

Pfaller, M., Diekema, D., Gibbs, D., Newell, V., Ellis, D., Tullio, V., Rodloff, A., Fu, W., Ling, T. and the Global Antifungal Surveillance Group (2010b) Results from the ARTEMIS DISK Global Antifungal Surveillance Study, 1997 to 2007: a 10.5-year analysis of susceptibilities of *Candida* species to fluconazole and voriconazole as determined by CLSI standardized disk diffusion. *Journal of Clinical Microbiology* 48, 1366–1377.

Pfaller, M., Andes, D., Diekema, D., Espinel-Ingroff, A., Sheehan, D. and the CLSI Subcommittee for Antifungal Susceptibility Testing (2010c) Wild-type MIC distributions, epidemiological cutoff values and species-specific clinical breakpoints for fluconazole and *Candida*: time for harmonization of CLSI and EUCAST broth microdilution methods. *Drug Resistance Updates* 13, 180–195.

Qin, Z., Zhang, J., Xu, B., Chen, L., Wu, Y., Yang, X., Shen, X., Molin, S., Danchin, A., Jiang, H. and Qu, D. (2006) Structure-based discovery of inhibitors of the YycG histidine kinase: new chemical leads to combat *Staphylococcus epidermidis* infections. *BMC Microbiology* 6, 96.

Rentz, A., Halpern, M. and Bowden, R. (1998) The impact of candidemia on length of hospital stay, outcome, and overall cost of illness. *Clinical Infectious Diseases* 27, 781–788.

Rodriguez-Suarez, R., Xu, D., Veillette, K., Davison, J., Sillaots, S., Kauffman, S., Hu, W., Bowman, J., Martel, N., Trosok, S., Wang, H., Zhang, L., Huang, L., Li, Y., Rahkhoodaee, F., Ransom, T., Gauvin, D., Douglas, C., Youngman, P., Becker, J., Jiang, B. and Roemer, T. (2007) Mechanism-of-action determination of GMP synthase inhibitors and target validation in *Candida albicans* and *Aspergillus fumigatus*. *Chemical Biology* 14, 1163–1175.

Roemer, T., Jiang, B., Davison, J., Ketela, T., Veillette, K., Breton, A., Tandia, F., Linteau, A., Sillaots, S., Marta, C., Martel, N., Veronneau, S., Lemieux, S., Kauffman, S., Becker, J., Storms, R., Boone, C. and Bussey, H. (2003) Large-scale essential gene identification in *Candida albicans* and applications to antifungal drug discovery. *Molecular Microbiology* 50, 167–181.

Sampaio-Camargo, T., Marra, A., Silva, C., Cardoso, M., Martino, M., Camargo, L. and Correa, L. (2010) Secular trends of candidemia in a tertiary care hospital. *American Journal of Infection Control* 38, 546–551.

Santos, J. and Shiozaki, K., (2001) Fungal histidine kinases. *Science STKE* 2001, re1.

Smith, A., Ammar, R., Nislow, C. and Giaever, G. (2010) A survey of yeast genomic assays for drug and target discovery. *Pharmacology Therapeutics* 127, 156–164.

Sobel, J. (2007) Vulvovaginal candidosis. *Lancet* 369, 1961–1971.

Srikantha, T., Tsai, L., Daniels, K., Enger, L., Highley, K. and Soll, D. 1998. The two-component histidine kinase regulator *CaNik1* of *Candida albicans. Microbiology* 144, 2715–2719.

Trofa, D., Gacser, A. and Nosanchuk, J. (2008) *Candida parapsilosis*, an emerging fungal pathogen. *Clinical Microbiology Reviews* 21, 606–625.

van Gool, R. (2001).The cost of treating systemic fungal infections. *Drugs* 61 (Suppl. 1), 49–56.

Walsh, T., Hiemenz, J. and Pizzo, P. (1994) Evolving risk factors for invasive fungal infections – all neutropenic patients are not the same. *Clinical Infectious Diseases* 18, 793–798.

Wang, F., Tao, J., Qian, Z., You, S., Dong, H., Shen, H., Chen, X., Tang, S. and Ren, S. (2009) A histidine kinase *PmHHK1* regulates polar growth, sporulation and cell wall composition in the dimorphic fungus *Penicillium marneffei. British Mycological Journal* 113, 915–923.

Weig, M. and Brown, A.J. (2007) Genomics and the development of new diagnostics and anti-*Candida* drugs. *Trends in Microbiology* 15, 310–317.

Wilson, L., Reyes, C., Stolpman, M., Speckman, J., Allen, K. and Beney, J. (2002) The direct cost and incidence of systemic fungal infections. *Value in Health* 5, 26–34.

Xu, D., Jiang, B., Ketela, T., Lemieux, S., Veillette, K., Martel, N., Davison, J., Sillaots, S., Trosok, S., Bachewich, C., Bussey, H., Youngman, P. and Roemer, T. (2007) Genome-wide fitness test and mechanism-of-action studies of inhibitory compounds in *Candida albicans*. *PLoS Pathogens* 3, e92.

Yamada-Okabe, T., Mio, T., Ono, N., Kashima, Y., Matsui, M., Arisawa, M. and Yamada-Okabe, H. (1999) Roles of three histidine kinases in hyphal growth and virulence of the pathogenic fungus *Candida albicans*. *Journal of Bacteriology* 181, 7243–7247.

Zhang, X., Reichart, P. and Song, T. (2009) Oral manifestations of HIV/AIDS in China: a review. *Oral Maxillofacial Surgery* 13, 63–68.

Zilberberg, M., Kollef, M., Arnold, H., Labelle, L., Micek, S., Kothari, S. and Shorr, A. (2010) Inappropriate empiric antifungal therapy for candidemia in the ICU and hospital resource utilization: a retrospective cohort study. *BMC Infectious Disease* 10, 150.

17 Pathosystematic Studies and the Rational Design of Antifungal Interventions

Elaine M. Bignell and Darius Armstrong-James
Division of Infectious Diseases, Faculty of Medicine, Imperial College London, London, UK

17.1 Introduction

17.1.1 Overview

The emergence of novel therapeutic entities and new developments in drug delivery place a heightened emphasis on knowledge-based discovery, which is becoming a major driving force for rational design of biological therapeutics.

Our understanding of pathogenic microorganisms has been revolutionized by the availability of whole-genome sequences, comparative genomics and bioinformatics. Similar advances in the field of immunology, and host responses to disease, present new opportunities to consider disease from a holistic perspective (Zak and Aderem, 2009). Such considerations are intrinsic to developing an understanding of the modulatory hubs of host and pathogen regulatory networks, which represent 'weak links' in terms of therapeutic intervention, thereby revealing novel strategies that might target aspects of both host and pathogen physiology.

Fungal pathogenesis is the result of successfully integrating sensory and niche-adapting cellular processes via coordinated transcriptional and post-translational mechanisms with the appropriate spatial and temporal resolution. The complexity of eukaryotic pathogens and their similarity, at the molecular level, to the human hosts they sometimes colonize demands an equally sophisticated understanding of the temporal host response for rational interventions to be revealed. Host factors are undeniably important when it comes to opportunistic pathogens. It therefore follows that a precise understanding of the immune deficits that predispose to disease is fundamentally important. In many instances, the immune environment, which normally defends adequately against pathogen attack, has become dysfunctional. This can occur through qualitative and quantitative means, or both, neither of which has (for fungal diseases) thus far been accurately quantified in a whole-animal context. A better understanding of the relative potency of immune effectors in specific disease states, and of the interactivity between innate and adaptive immunity, is still required.

In the absence of an adequate immune response, an unchallenged fungal pathogen can prosper. This requires the ability to source nutrients and trace elements vital for fungal growth. Despite the apparent ease with which many fungal pathogens achieve this aim, the stress endured by the pathogen during such infective growth is immense. This is evidenced by the catastrophic impact of disabling key stress adaptation mechanisms

 Antimicrobial Drug Discovery: Emerging Strategies (eds G. Tegos and E. Mylonakis)

such as alkaline adaptation (Davis *et al.*, 2000; Bignell *et al.*, 2005) or iron acquisition (Schrettl *et al.*, 2004, 2007) on fungal survival. The therapeutic potential of targeting host adaptation mechanisms is further evidenced by the finding that iron-chelation therapy has utility in the treatment of zygomycete infections. Therapeutic interventions can, therefore, capitalize on the negative impact of host-imposed stress if the regulatory circuitry is understood well enough, and the action or design of novel drugs should always be considered within the context of the stresses imposed by the host environment.

Given our specialist knowledge of *Aspergillus* spp., the weight of discussion in this chapter rests upon advances in our understanding of disease caused by *Aspergillus fumigatus*. However, the principles we will explore are extendable to most other fungal pathogens of humans and, wherever relevant, we refer the reader to literary sources that address similar principles in other fungi. It also noteworthy that this commentary is derived from combined academic and clinical perspectives. The commercial and financial implications of drug discovery and development are not extensively addressed here, although it is our firm belief that the discovery of novel knowledge-based interventions is well within the capabilities of most laboratory scientists. Indeed, such endeavour will become pivotal to future drug development, as reductions in commercial research funding shift the onus of research and development further into the academic realm.

A fully pathosystematic view of disease processes requires a number of data types, which crucially includes genomics, functional genomics and transcriptomics, derived from both host and pathogen sources. In each of these cases, this chapter will explore the currently available data, the context within which their use has led to new insight on fungal pathogenesis and therapeutics, and the areas in which more progress is required. The additional insight afforded by proteomic and metabolic analyses in whole-animal infections has yet to be interrogated on a global scale, mainly due to the technical challenges associated with sample acquisition. None the less, where relevant studies offer an insight, we include an appraisal of their value.

17.1.2 A theoretical framework for describing disease processes

Severely immunocompromised hosts are at the highest risk for invasive fungal diseases, which are caused primarily by opportunistic pathogens (Odds *et al.*, 2001), thereby implicating host factors as major determinants of pathogenicity. However, early searches for virulence factors in such fungal pathogens were prohibitively dismissive of the host component of disease (Casadevall and Pirofski, 2003, 2009). A much broader definition of microbial virulence emerges if one defines disease as the product of both host and microbial factors, and a more unified approach to the study of microbial pathogenicity is therefore demanded. Crucially, if virulence is viewed as the product of an *interaction* between microbe and host, a measure of host-mediated damage (such as that invoked by, or directly attributable to, excessive inflammation), as well as pathogen-mediated damage, is required. It therefore follows that a holistic approach to studying infection is required, and a primary focus of this chapter is to embed such principles firmly into our current and future views of pathosystematic study.

In the context of fungal disease, which includes both infections and allergic or inflammatory responses to fungal exposure, a remarkably wide spectrum of outcomes exists (Zmeili and Soubani, 2007). This multifaceted ability to cause disease has been particularly well described for *Aspergillus* spp. and is consistent with the damage-response framework described by Casadevall and co-workers (Casadevall and Pirofski, 2003; Casadevall and Pirofski, 2009). The most aggressive form of angioinvasive aspergillosis is seen in patients with severe and prolonged neutropenia, and consists of hyperacute disease characterized by direct, and seemingly unimpeded, hyphal invasion of host tissue. In patients on steroid therapy, a more indolent and granulomatous form of disease is seen, with stunted hyphal invasion (Walsh *et al.*, 1994).

Over the last decade, there have been major clinical advances in defining a group of seemingly non-immunocompromised individuals who develop chronic cavitatory pulmonary aspergillosis in the absence of exogenous immunosuppression. To date, no clear immunogenetic cause for this disease has been established, although associations with certain mannose-binding lectin (MBL), surfactant protein A, interleukin (IL)-10 and transforming growth factor (TGF)-β1 polymorphisms (Sambatakou *et al.*, 2006; Vaid *et al.*, 2007; Lambourne *et al.*, 2009) have been uncovered. On the opposing side of the immune spectrum underlying *Aspergillus*-related disease lie allergic bronchopulmonary aspergillosis (ABPA), severe asthma with fungal sensitization, and fungal immune response inflammatory syndrome. All of these diseases may be considered a consequence of an overexuberant immune response. ABPA is characterized by wheeze, pulmonary infiltrates, proximal bronchiectasis and fibrosis. This is associated with heightened T-helper 2 (Th2) responses to a number of *A. fumigatus* antigens (Moss, 2010), and consequently the primary therapy for this condition is corticosteroid immunosuppression. Thus, some patients with heightened immune responses and *Aspergillus*-dependent disease require steroid immunosuppression to alleviate pathology, whereas others, such as those with invasive aspergillosis, develop pathology as a consequence of steroid therapy. These examples demonstrate clearly how the use of steroids to modulate the damage-response framework can have either beneficial or deleterious consequences.

17.1.3 Whole-animal models of infection

Clearly, an integrated understanding of disease demands a whole-animal host. In terms of a better understanding the biology of disease, the validity of extracting information from the isolated study of a distinct pathophysiological feature, such as adhesion, hyphal growth or tissue invasion, and recreating it *in vitro* or *ex vivo* provides important insights. However, functional predictions having therapeutic value at the level of an intact host are not possible from such experimentation, and, moreover, host status can be a key determinant of a pathogen's virulence capacity. A case in point is provided by the secondary metabolite gliotoxin, which has potent immunomodulatory activity *in vitro* (Orciuolo *et al.*, 2007; Ben-Ami *et al.*, 2009) and is detectable in infected host tissues of mice and humans (Lewis *et al.*, 2005). Despite the potent immunotoxigenic activities of this toxin, the relevance of gliotoxin as a virulence factor in the clinical setting has been hotly debated, as gliotoxin non-producing isolates can be isolated in the clinic (Lewis *et al.*, 2005), and mutants that lack the ability to synthesize gliotoxin are fully virulent in neutropenic mice (Kwon-Chung and Sugui, 2009). However, subsequent investigations of the same mutants in corticosteroid-treated animals have identified decreased virulence of gliotoxin mutants (Sugui *et al.*, 2007), thereby supporting the conclusion that neutrophils (which are largely absent in neutropenic mice) are the major target of gliotoxin activity in the host. Indeed, in subsequent experimentation, the physiological relevance of this claim was further substantiated and the anti-apoptotic mitochondrial protein Bak was identified as a modulator of gliotoxin-mediated neutrophil apoptosis (Pardo *et al.*, 2006). Furthermore, in hydrocortisone-treated Bak knockout mice, the virulence of a wild-type *A. fumigatus* strain was attenuated, although the precise mechanism by which Bak activity promotes gliotoxin-mediated fungal virulence remains unknown.

The vast majority of whole-animal fungal disease studies are conducted in mice (de Repentigny, 2004, Clemons and Stevens, 2005; Capilla *et al.*, 2007; Szabo and MacCallum, 2011). For each of the fungal pathogens, the modes of immunosuppression (if required), routes and methods of inoculation, and sampling regimes are highly varied. In most instances, such variation has become incorporated to reflect clinically relevant facets of disease, to circumvent barriers to effective reconstruction of the clinical situation or to establish reproducibility.

For modelling of *A. fumigatus* diseases (Clemons and Stevens, 2005), two immunosuppressive regimens are widely adopted and have been compared extensively in the recent literature (Balloy *et al.*, 2005; Lewis and

Wiederhold, 2005). For pathogenicity studies, an intranasal route of infection is most often utilized to mimic the natural route of acquisition of infectious particles and establish primary infectious lesions in the lungs, bronchioles and alveoli (Clemons and Stevens, 2005). A less physiologically relevant but more reproducible means of administering infectious particles is via the tail vein, providing a systemic model of aspergillosis favoured for drug-efficacy studies (Clemons and Stevens, 2005). Chemotherapeutic and corticosteroid immunosuppressive regimens are most often used for establishing murine aspergillosis (Balloy *et al.*, 2005). These treatment regimens are considered to reproduce most accurately the immune environment in patients receiving myelotoxic chemotherapy for cancer or corticosteroids for prevention or treatment of rejection after allogeneic transplantation. In mice, the corticosteroid regimen is recapitulated using intraperitoneal or subcutaneous administrations of cortisone acetate at regular intervals throughout disease (every 2 days on average), commencing 3 days prior to infection (Balloy *et al.*, 2005). Chemotherapeutic regimens employ intravenous administration of vinblastine (Balloy *et al.*, 2005), cyclophosphamide (Lewis and Wiederhold, 2005) or neutrophil-specific antibodies such as RB6-8C5, anti-Ly6G (Morrison *et al.*, 2003) or Gr-1 (Bruns *et al.*, 2010), with optional incorporation of a single corticosteroid dose the day prior to disease. In such murine hosts, an intranasal dose of 10^7 spores leads to fatal disease with 100% mortality by day 6 in corticosteroid-treated hosts and 2–3 days in neutropenic hosts.

The kinetics of host-cell infiltration differs substantially between regimens, commencing at 3h in immunocompetent animals and peaking at 48h (Balloy *et al.*, 2005). In contrast, polymorphonuclear leukocyte concentrations in corticosteroid-treated hosts increase rapidly to 24h and remain high throughout the course of disease. In neutropenic hosts, no polymorphonuclear leukocyte recruitment is observed. Concordant with these observations, the levels of pro-inflammatory cytokines also differs between models of disease. Tumour necrosis factor (TNF)-α peaks at 48h in immunocompetent animals, is not detected in corticosteroid-treated animals and is highest at 48h in neutropenic animals where disease cannot be cleared (Balloy *et al.*, 2005). Lung samples collected at 48 and 72h after disease identify exudative bronchiolitis as the defining feature of corticosteroid diseases, with destruction of bronchioles and alveoli. In neutropenic animals, inflammatory exudates were not evident, and alveoli were invaded by numerous hyphae of *A. fumigatus* (Balloy *et al.*, 2005). Further animal models have been developed to accurately represent the pathobiology of invasive aspergillosis in the context of chronic granulomatous disorder and stem-cell transplantation (Mencacci *et al.*, 2001; Lambourne *et al.*, 2009). In the stem-cell transplant model of pulmonary aspergillosis, there is severe necrosis and bronchial wall damage but minimal inflammatory-cell recruitment 3 days after infection, consistent with the standard neutropenic model (Romani *et al.*, 2006). In contrast, mice with X-linked chronic granulomatous disorder ($gp91^{-/-}$) develop a necrotizing bronchoalveolar pneumonia with severe inflammatory-cell infiltrates, microabscess formation and hyphal invasion (Pollock *et al.*, 1995). These diverse immunopathological observations further underscore the requirement for clinically representative murine models of fungal infection that enable rational and systematic identification of the key pathogen and host determinants of outcome from infection in different human disease states.

17.2 Host and Pathogen Genome Analyses and Novel Therapeutic Targets

Interrogation of host and pathogen genomes can yield significant clinical and biological insight when comparative analyses of susceptible and resistant hosts, and pathogenic versus non-pathogenic fungal species are performed (Fig. 17.1).

17.2.1 Host genomes and genetic susceptibility to fungal disease

Genetic susceptibility to fungal diseases is becoming increasingly well characterized

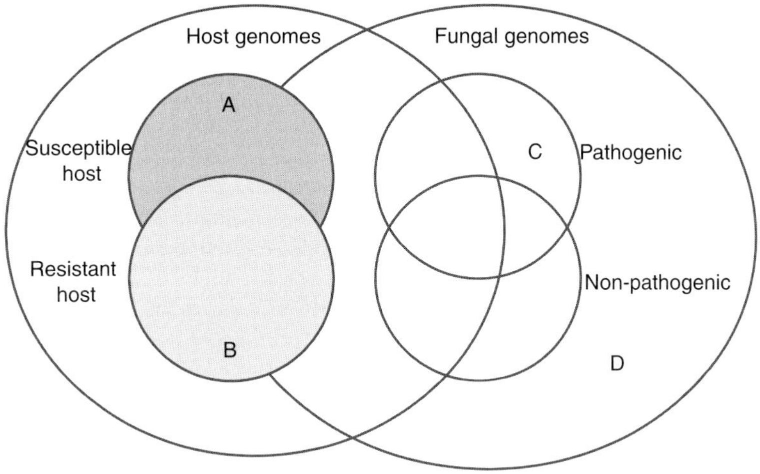

Fig. 17.1. Utility of comparative genome analyses for target prioritization. Comparative analysis of the genomes of susceptible and resistant hosts can provide information on host genes (A and B) where polymorphism leads, respectively, to susceptibility or resistance to disease, while comparative analysis of the genomes of pathogenic and non-pathogenic fungal species *may* identify genes or genomic traits (C) that affect virulence. Comparative analysis of host and pathogen genomes can identify genes (D) restricted to the pathogen genome and therefore encoding functions with potential as drug targets.

among human patient populations (Carvalho *et al.*, 2010; Mezger *et al.*, 2010; Romani, 2011). A number of clinical studies have linked polymorphic genetic loci to increased susceptibility to fungal disease in humans. For the most part, such analyses have identified components of host immunity as carrying the variant loci, including MBL (*MBL2*), Dectin-1 (*DECTIN1*), *IL4* and Toll-like receptor 4 (*TLR4*) where polymorphism leads to broad-range susceptibility to fungal pathogens (Romani, 2011).

MBL is a plasma protein of the collectin family, which contain a C-terminal carbohydrate recognition domain. Multimeric MBL complexes recognize carbohydrate moieties displayed at the surfaces of microbial cells (Jack *et al.*, 2001), including those of *A. fumigatus* and *Candida albicans* (Cross and Bancroft, 1995; Neth *et al.*, 2000). MBL binding leads to activation, via the MBL-associated proteases MASP1/3 and MASP2/MAPp19, of the complement system, prompting opsonization of microbes and/or direct microbial killing. MBL polymorphisms affect oligomerization of MBL subunits (single-nucleotide polymorphisms (SNPs) at codons 52, 54 and 57, collectively known as O variants) and (via differential promoter haplotypes) serum MBL levels (Steffensen *et al.*, 2000; Garred *et al.*, 2003). Granell *et al.* (2006) analysed MBL and MASP2 sequences in 106 donor–recipient pairs undergoing HLA-identical sibling allogeneic stem-cell transplantation. Individuals were genotyped for the presence of SNPs in the promoter and exon 1 of the *MBL2* gene, as well as in exon 3 of *MASP2*. After a median follow-up period of 24 months, overall survival in the group was 52%. There were 16 cases of invasive fungal infection (IFI). Of 11 recipients where donors had an *MBL*-low genotype, four (36%) experienced an IFI, whereas among 95 patients having *MBL*-sufficient donors, 11 (12%) experienced IFIs. Of the three recipients with Asp105Gly MASP2 variants, two (67%) experienced IFIs compared with 13% of the remaining 95 recipients. The study therefore concluded that donor and/or recipient genetic variants of *MBL2* and *MASP2* are independent risk factors for developing IFIs after allogeneic stem-cell transplantation.

Based on multiple reports that the codon 54 *MBL* polymorphism is associated with recurrent vaginal candidiasis (RVC) (Babovic-Vuksanovic *et al.*, 1999; Babula *et al.*, 2003; Giraldo *et al.*, 2007; Donders *et al.*, 2008), Donders *et al.* (2008) examined *MBL2* codon 54 polymorphisms in 109 women suffering from the condition. Control women were found to be more likely to be homozygous for the wild-type *MBL2* allele (87 versus 63%), and the RVC patients were almost three times more likely to have a heterozygous phenotype (3 versus 13%). Moreover, homozygosity for the *MBL2* variant allele ($n = 4$) was observed only among RVC sufferers, and the presence of the variant allele was also found to correlate with poor responses to fluconazole maintenance therapy compared with homozygotic wild-type RVC sufferer controls. Vaid *et al.* (2007) examined the association of SNPs in the collagen region of *MBL2* with respiratory allergy, including sufferers of allergic rhinitis ($n = 49$), and ABPA ($n = 11$) compared with unrelated age-matched controls. Among five SNPs identified in exon 1 and intron 1 of *MBL2*, two novel polymorphisms (A816G in exon 1 and G1011A in intron 1) were identified by this study. Among the two patient cohorts, the G1011A polymorphism was found to occur significantly more frequently in patients with bronchial asthma, allergic rhinitis and ABPA than in controls. The previously identified polymorphisms did not exhibit any biased distribution among patient cohorts. To evaluate the functional impact of SNP G1011A, MBL levels and complement activity were examined in 60 patients and 40 controls, identifying a significantly higher mean MBL level and mean MBL-induced complement activity than in individuals homozygous for the wild-type G allele. Allergic patients homozygous for the variant A allele were found have significantly higher peripheral blood eosinophilia than those with the G/G phenotype.

Chronic mucocutaneous candidiasis consists of persistent colonization and/or disease of the skin and mucosa with (predominantly) *C. albicans*, which results from impaired clearance of fungal diseases (Kirkpatrick, 2001). Although this condition is associated with human immunodeficiency virus (HIV) diseases and corticosteroid use, the fact that familial patterns of susceptibility occasionally occur (Kirkpatrick, 2001) indicates that primary genetic immunodeficiencies are also an underlying risk factor.

Mucocutaneous fungal diseases are typically found in patients who have no known immune defects. In a study of four related women who were affected by recurrent vulvovaginal candidiasis or onychomycosis, an early stop codon mutation, Tyr238X, was identified in the β-glucan receptor Dectin-1 (Ferwerda *et al.*, 2009). Dectin-1 is a C-type lectin receptor, which recognizes 1,3-linked β-glucans to amplify TLR2- and TLR4-induced cytokine induction, in a Syk kinase-dependent manner (Dennehy *et al.*, 2008). The Tyr238X mutation leads to loss of the last nine amino acids of the Dectin-1 carbohydrate-binding domain (Ferwerda *et al.*, 2009). Monocytes and macrophages from patients carrying the Tyr238X mutation were non-responsive to challenge with either β-glucan or heat-killed *C. albicans* hyphae (as measured by IL-6 production). Interestingly, monocytes and macrophages from patients homozygous for this mutation were not defective in killing *C. albicans*, thereby demonstrating an important role for Dectin-1-mediated cytokine induction in protection against mucocutaneous disease and onychomycosis. A further phenotype associated with Dectin-1 polymorphisms is reduced IL-17 production. A subsequent investigation of Dectin-1 polymorphism identified a significant association of the Tyr238X mutation with invasive aspergillosis in haematopoietic stem-cell transplant (HSCT) patients (Cunha *et al.*, 2010). Similar to responses reported in Tyr238X peripheral blood mononuclear cells challenged with *C. albicans*, Dectin-1 polymorphism resulted in a reduction of IL-1b and IL-6 levels following *A. fumigatus* challenge.

Genetic studies performed in 36 members of a five-generation family also examined the basis of genetic predisposition to chronic mucocutaneous candidiasis (Glocker *et al.*, 2009), identifying an autosomal-recessive form of susceptibility to such disease linked with homozygous mutations in *CARD9*, encoding the adaptor protein for Dectin-1. To identify the genetic basis for susceptibility to chronic mucocutaneous candidiasis, Glocker *et al.* (2009) examined genotypes among a large Iranian family with multiple cases of the condition. The index patient was a 19-year-old man who had suffered from oral candidiasis since the age of 3. The other individuals studied had suffered intermittent thrush leading to *Candida* meningitis and death, chronic vaginal candidiasis, dermatophytoses and *Candida* meningoencephalitis. Analysis of the SNP genotypes, compared with unaffected family members, identified a region of perfect segregation on linkage group 9, within which 121 gene candidates were examined for putative functional significance. On the strength of the observation that $CARD9^{-/-}$ mice are susceptible to fungal diseases (Gross *et al.*, 2006) the authors sequenced *CARD9* in the affected patients and 18 other relatives, identifying a single homozygous point mutation in exon 6 that resulted in a premature stop codon. The affected site was also examined in 50 unrelated healthy Iranians and 180 unrelated healthy white subjects among whom there were no incidences of polymorphism identified. Analysis of CARD9 expression by Western blotting using peripheral blood mononuclear cells from patients identified a complete absence of CARD9 protein in cells from patients homozygous for the Gln295X mutation (albeit determined using a C-terminally targeted polyclonal antibody that would not have identified the truncated CARD9 protein). Moreover, when primary bone marrow cells from CARD9-deficient mice were transfected with human wild-type and variant *CARD9*, derivative macrophages were restored in Dectin-1-triggered TNF-α production following expression of full-length human CARD9. Additionally, the mean proportion of Th17 cells in the affected patients was found to be significantly lower than in healthy controls.

The availability of increasingly detailed genome data from individual inbred mouse strains over the last decade presents the opportunity to identify disease-susceptible genotypes for mammalian diseases. Observing that invasive aspergillosis affects only a subset of at-risk HSCT recipients, Zaas *et al.* (2008) hypothesized that genetic variation within key innate or adaptive immune genes could influence susceptibility to, or outcome of, invasive aspergillosis in the human patient population. Initially, the authors studied the outcome of murine *Aspergillus* diseases following transient immunosuppression with cyclophosphamide and cortisone acetate. Among the ten inbred mouse strains utilized, susceptible (A/J and C3H/HcJ), intermediate (MRL/MJP and NZW/LacJ) and resistant (AKR/J, C57/Bl6J, 129/SvJ, Balb/CJ and BalbCByJ) strains were identified. While susceptible murine hosts demonstrated 100% mortality at 6 days post-infection, resistant hosts demonstrated 30–60% survival at 14 days after disease. Haplotype-based computational analysis was used to identify murine genetic factors affecting survival following *A. fumigatus* challenge. Following construction of a haplotype block map of the murine genome, haplotype blocks that correlated strongly with observed phenotypic data (in this instance, area under survival curve for each of the infected murine strains, based on 10–30 mice per strain) were observed. This identified two genetic loci, plasminogen (*PLG*) and UDP-glucose ceramide glucosyltransferase-like 1 (*Ugcgl1*) where strong correlations with murine survival were observed. The onward analysis focused on *PLG*. Among 423 SNPs identified by sequencing the *PLG* alleles of 20 murine inbred strains, a single non-synonymous SNP (G110S) was identified, the presence of which correlated with murine susceptibility to disease. The glycine residue in question, which is conserved among mouse and human plasminogen alleles, was noted to occur within a protein domain critical for binding of plasminogen to fibrin and for regulation of plasmin-induced cell detachment. An investigation of 20 human HSCT donor–recipient pairs similarly identified a non synonymous SNP (Asp472Asn) having a minor allele frequency of 25%. Extending this analysis to examine the genotypes of 236 allogeneic HSCT recipients, the authors revealed a significant risk for invasive aspergillosis among patients carrying this SNP. The identification of plasminogen as a significant modulator of outcome from aspergillosis is biologically plausible given the known relationship between angioinvasive aspergillosis and fibrinolysis. Furthermore, the authors were able to demonstrate that plasminogen allelles also influenced susceptibility to aspergillosis in HSCT patients and that plasminogen directly binds swollen conidia. These observations demonstrated proof of principle for multispecies genetic mapping for identification of genetic susceptibility to invasive fungal diseases.

SNPs that protect against fungal infection have also been unearthed. Plantinga *et al.* (2010) looked for variants of *Dectin1*, *TLR2*, *TLR4*, *TIRAP* or *CAPSASE-12* among 223 East African, HIV-infected patients to ascertain whether SNPs led to heightened susceptibility to oropharyngeal candidiasis. An unexpected finding was a protective effect against oropharyngeal candidiasis of the *DECTIN-1* SNP Ile223Ser. Looking for factors that predispose to oral carriage of *Candida* spp., Jurevic *et al.* (2003) examined the role of human β-defensin gene variants among diabetic (n = 43) and non-diabetic (n = 50) individuals. The authors found a higher level of *Candida* carriage in diabetic subjects and a significant association between a C-to-G SNP at position –44 and lower *Candida* burden.

17.2.2 Fungal genomes and comparative genomics

Among the most significant fungal pathogens of humans, lifestyles and physiology differ dramatically. At the time of writing, the National Centre for Biotechnology Information (NCBI) genome projects (http://www.ncbi.nlm.nih.gov/) include sequencing projects, in progress or completed, for multiple pathogenic fungal species including *Aspergilli* (n = 16), *Candida* (n = 8), *Cryptococcus* (n = 5), *Coccidioides* (n = 15), *Fusarium* (n = 2) and *Paracoccidioides* (n = 3). The insight afforded by scrutiny of such data has been valuable in terms of deriving a better understanding of fungal pathogenicity and is therefore important for the design of future therapeutic strategy. Rather than highlighting groups of highly selected pathogenicity genes in pathogenic versus non-pathogenic species, comparative genome analyses have largely concluded that metabolic versatility, contingent with the various lifestyles and corresponding dietary constraints of pathogenic fungi, are a major contributing factor (Tekaia and Latge, 2005; Moran *et al.*, 2011). For example, a comparative analysis (Tekaia and Latge, 2005) of 9925 *A. fumigatus* protein sequences against those encoded by 102 other eukaryotic, archeal and bacterial species detected concordance among predicted *A. fumigatus* glycosyl hydrolases and those of the phytopathogens *Magnaporthe grisea* and *Fusarium graminearum* fungi, while the model yeasts *Saccharomyces cerevisiae* and *Schizosaccharomyces pombe* lack the capacity to produce such enzymes. *A. fumigatus* is a saprophytic mould and abundant spore producer (Latge, 1999) whose reliance, in ecological niches, on organic and plant-derived macromolecular nutrients requires a battery of catabolic and polysaccharide-degrading enzymes. Scrutiny of the *A. fumigatus* genome, therefore, provides significant clues regarding modes of nutrition, which in turn reflect the demands imposed by the organisms' natural environment, which is understood to be soil and compost.

Candida spp. cause a range of mucosal and invasive diseases of varying severity, the most common manifestation being superficial and referred to as 'thrush'. Unlike *Aspergillus*, *Candida* spp. often colonize human niches and thus participate in extended interactions with human hosts. Under normal circumstances such interactions would not be detrimental to the host; however, immune dysfunction at mucosal surfaces, surgery, exogenous immunosuppression or intubation may lead to disease of varying severities (van der Meer *et al.*, 2010). A striking feature of the *C. albicans* genome, relative to that of *S. cerevisiae*, is expansion of gene families having nutrient acquisition functionality such as lipases, secreted aspartyl proteases and transporters (Braun *et al.*, 2005; van Het *et al.*, 2007). Certain of these gene families were subsequently found to be enriched among pathogenic species members in broader genome comparison studies (Butler *et al.*, 2009; Moran *et al.*, 2011). Importantly, comparative genome analyses involving the very closely related but differentially virulent species *C. albicans* and *Candida dubliniensis* (Moran *et al.*, 2011) reveal very subtle differences at the level of gene conservation but include the absence of the hypha-specific *ALS3* protein and two hypha-specific secreted aspartyl proteases.

In terms of identifying virulence factors, the resolving power of comparative genomics is still challenged by a paucity of available fungal genomes, the limiting factor among genera occupied by both pathogenic and non-pathogenic species being evolutionary distance between differentially virulent species. At first glance, comparison of very closely related, differentially virulent species might seem to be promising; however, a crucial consideration is the certain, in some instances well-characterized (Lavoie *et al.*, 2010), differences in transcriptional circuitry between strains and species. Given that a tiny fraction of known fungal species are able to colonize human niches, it must follow that some aspect of the physiology or genetic make-up of these pathogenic species also endows pathogenicity. However, the view that acquisition of an individual gene could promote the emergence of virulence in a previously non-pathogenic species is probably an oversimplification. An example of acquired, effector-mediated fungal pathogenicity has been reported among *Fusarium* spp. where, from comparative genome analysis of three differently virulent *Fusarium* spp., a pathogenicity chromosome has been defined and moved between species (Ma *et al.*, 2010).

Comparative genomics has been utilized to impressive effect within the genus *Aspergillus* where the sequences of two very closely related but differing virulent *Aspergillus* spp. (*Neosartorya fischeri* and *Aspergillus clavatus*) have been compared to that of *A. fumigatus*. The three species have collectively been referred to as the Affc lineage (Fedorova *et al.*, 2008). Important comparators for this analysis included a further four *Aspergillus* spp., again of differing virulence, but from an evolutionary perspective much further removed from the Affc lineage. The power of such an analysis lies with the ability to identify cohorts of genes that are conserved among all species, regardless of pathogenicity, and therefore unlikely to include functions that have evolved to promote virulence. Among the three Affc lineage species, a high degree of identity, including more than 7500 orthologous core genes, is observable (Fedorova *et al.*, 2008). In contrast to non-pathogenic *Aspergillus nidulans* and *Aspergillus oryzae* spp., genomes of the Affc lineage species are enriched for genes involved in carbohydrate metabolism, transport and secondary metabolism, whereas 8.5, 13.5 and 12.6%, respectively, of *A. fumigatus*, *N. fischeri* and *A. clavatus* genes are species specific. Interestingly, 46% of *A. fumigatus*-specific genes with paralogues have been found to be telomere proximal, suggesting that they may have been duplicated recently and translocated to these regions (Fedorova *et al.*, 2008). In keeping with this observation, the most intriguing finding was the existence of genomic islands, conserved among the Affc lineage species, wherein recently acquired genes (relative to other sequenced members of the genus *Aspergillus*) are enriched. The position of the islands was biased towards the telomere proximal regions of the chromosomes, a finding that gains still more significance once gene expression in response to the mammalian host is considered (McDonagh *et al.*, 2008). Telomeric bias is emerging as a common theme in terms of genomic sequestration of genes enriched in fungal pathogens. In the case of *A. fumigatus*, such genes are significantly smaller in size than core conserved genes and contain fewer exons (Fedorova *et al.*, 2008). Gene clustering is another phenomenon where genomic context appears to be relevant. Obvious examples of such clusters include those directing secondary metabolite biosynthesis. Similarly, clustered lineage-specific genes simultaneously induced in infected tissue and predominantly encoding proteins destined for secretion have been observed in the ubiquitous maize pathogen *Ustilago maydis* (Howlett *et al.*, 2007).

17.3 Functional Genomics

To date, functional genomics analyses have informed us about fungal factors required for virulence to a much greater extent than host factors. Loss of fungal gene function can lead to either heightened susceptibility or resistance in the host. While the former category of gene functions (constituting genes conferring hypervirulence) are informative with respect to understanding the nature of the host–pathogen interaction, genes whose function are required for virulence are likely to be the best targets for novel antifungal therapeutics (Fig. 17.2).

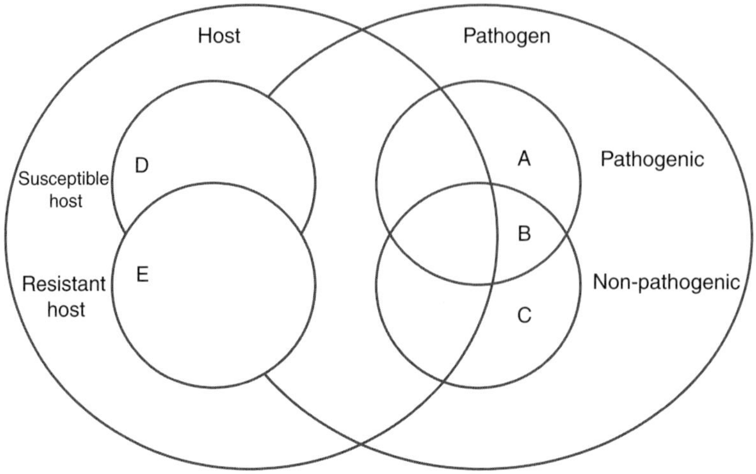

Fig. 17.2. Analysis of host and pathogen gene function can inform target discovery on multiple levels. Loss of fungal gene function can lead to heightened resistance (hypovirulence) or susceptibility (hypervirulence) in the host. Fungal gene functions that are essential for fungal survival are attractive candidates for novel therapy. These need not be restricted to pathogenic fungi but are most often limited to those that are absent or not highly conserved in mammalian hosts (A, B and C). Mouse knockout mutants can lead to heightened susceptibility (D) or resistance (E) to infection with non-mutated pathogenic fungi, thereby identifying important mechanisms of natural defence against fungal infections and novel avenues for immunotherapy.

17.3.1 Target-based drug discovery: essential genes

To a great extent, the traditional approach to drug discovery has involved whole-cell screening against small molecules and natural products to identify those that cause cell death. Such approaches are now being superseded by advances in target identification and assay development. It has long been accepted that a good target should be essential for microbial survival and should be broadly represented among target organisms but not homologous to any eukaryotic component, and should be 'druggable'. For fungal pathogens, several approaches have been used to identify essential genes. Among these, efforts have been most advanced for *C. albicans*.

As *C. albicans* exists predominantly in a diploid genetic state, loss of one functional copy of a gene can often result in a measurable phenotype. Uhl *et al.* (2003) used transposon-mediated mutagenesis to construct and screen 18,000 *C. albicans* mutants for morphogenetic phenotypes. The switch from blastospore to filamentous growth is a recognized virulence trait in this organism, and the authors relied on haploinsufficiency to identify functions crucial for filamentation in response to serum or nutrient starvation. Among 146 genes identified in this study, approximately one-third lacked homologues in *S. cerevisiae* and other model organisms and might therefore constitute drug targets.

de Backer *et al.* (2001) constructed an integrative vector for conditional expression of antisense RNA under the control of the *GAL1* promoter and exploited the regulatory consequences of two possible modes of vector integration into genomic DNA. The authors reasoned that galactose-inducible expression of antisense RNA would be achievable regardless of vector integration site; however, if the vector integrated at the genomic locus of the cloned cDNA insert, promoter interference would additionally result, due to convergent orientation of the vector-borne and native gene promoters. This approach thus specifically relies on lowering the level of specific *C. albicans* mRNAs by either of the above mechanisms, thereby decreasing the expression level of the corresponding protein. If this *C. albicans* protein is critical for growth, the cell will grow more slowly or die. Having used the vector to clone a library of cDNA inserts, the *C. albicans* strain CAI-4 was transformed and more than 2000 transformants were screened for reduced growth upon activation of the *GAL1* promoter. The screen was performed in lithium acetate-containing medium to prolong the G_1 phase of the life cycle during which antisense RNA is presumed to act most strongly. Parallel measurement of growth in non-inducing and inducing media was performed for all of the transformants, and cDNA inserts from the integrated antisense library were isolated from the disruptants by polymerase chain reaction (PCR). Many of the identified genes were already known to be essential in *S. cerevisiae* or in other organisms and included, for example, ribosomal proteins and translation elongation factors. Genes involved in carbon source metabolism and nutrient uptake (for example, the galactose permease *HXT6*), were also identified. Based on observations in bacteria and in yeast, which demonstrated that the underexpression of any component of a process leads to increased sensitivity to an inhibitor of a relevant step in that process, the mutant *C. albicans* strains were used in high-throughput screening for antifungal drugs in order to identify deficient growth of mutants relative to a wild-type strain. If lowering the dosage of a specific gene in *C. albicans* resulted in a heterozygote that was sensitized to a drug, an indication of the site or pathway at which compounds exert their effect could be derived.

A large-scale gene-replacement and conditional expression (GRACE™) approach was adopted by Becker *et al.* (2010) to identify a drug target gene set for *C. albicans*. By means of a number of strategic design features, this particular study was entirely geared towards producing tools that would be useful for drug discovery whereby the use of a tetracycline-regulatable promoter provided the basis for repressing gene expression *in vitro* and also in an animal host. In general terms, the system employs two components: (i) a chimeric transactivator protein (consisting of the *Escherichia coli* TetR DNA-binding domain fused to a transcriptional activator domain; and (ii) a promoter rendered tetracycline responsive by virtue of insertion of multiple Tet operator elements. Conditional repression is achieved by provision of tetracycline (or analogues) in the growth medium, which prevents the stable association between the transactivator and the Tet-responsive promoter. The GRACE approach involves the precise deletion of one gene copy and controllable expression of the remaining allele by promoter replacement with the Tet-responsive promoter, thereby placing the remaining gene copy under Tet promoter control. A further independent means of repressing conditionally regulated genes was built into the platform whereby expression of a *URA3*-marked plasmid, stably integrated as a tandem duplication at one of the two native *LEU2* loci, provided a means by which to effect the forced loss of the transactivator plasmid by 5-fluoroorotic acid counterselection. The system therefore provided two independent means of achieving transcriptional repression. Using this approach, the authors were able to construct promoter-replacement alleles for 1152 genes. Among these, 567 genes were identified as essential in *C. albicans*. Tetracycline-mediated repression of gene promoters among this cohort, coupled with analysis of terminal phenotypes, provided the means by which to distinguish between cidal versus static terminal phenotypes. Effectively, this distinguishes mutants lacking gene functions essential for growth and cell division from those where loss of gene function leads to cell death (as defined by an inability to further produce colony forming units following a 20 min exposure to tetracycline *in vitro*). The capacity to repress gene function during animal disease is also provided via supplementation of the animals' drinking water with tetracycline, which represses gene expression *in vivo*. Finally, the promoter-replacement strains were also used as whole-cell screening reagents whereby the activity of a drug targeting the repressed gene function would be expected to have heightened activity against an organism that lacks the ability to express that function. In *C. albicans*, such manipulations can be achieved relatively easily using a PCR-based methodology, due to the high rates of homologous recombination in *C. albicans* and minimal requirements for flanking homologous sequences.

A later study assessed 177 selected conditionally essential tetracycline-regulatable alleles for virulence testing in a murine model of systemic candidiasis (Becker *et al.* 2010) and found 102 of these to be required for early- and late-stage diseases, as tested by stage-specific, doxycycline-mediated repression of the genes of interest. This approach permitted the interrogation of potential targets within the context of either prophylaxis or severe disease. Several interesting findings, having direct relevance to drug discovery strategies, were highlighted by the study. Certain gene functions were found to be essential for growth *in vitro* but dispensable in the murine host, late-pathway ergosterol biosynthetic genes being a case in point. *ERG9* and *ERG11* were found to be non-essential in a murine model of disease, which might be due to the fact that *C. albicans* is able to scavenge cholesterol in the mammalian host when fungal ergosterol biosynthesis is not possible. Beyond those involved in ergosterol biosynthesis, a further 17 gene functions were demonstrated to be similarly relevant to host, but not *in vitro*, growth. It therefore seems likely that inhibitors of such functions would have therapeutic utility.

Although *A. fumigatus* has the benefit (from a molecular geneticist's perspective) of existing solely in the haploid genetic state, it exhibits a comparatively low frequency of homologous recombination such that PCR-mediated approaches must tackle large gene-replacement constructs because significant regions of flanking homology are required to achieve targeted integration. These shortcomings can be overridden by the use of non-homologous end-rejoining mutants (da Silva Ferreira *et al.*, 2006). However, there are serious concerns regarding genome stability in such genetic backgrounds. The prolonged retention of such mutations in isolates destined for virulence analyses or, indeed, large-scale phenotypic or drug discovery investigations, is unacceptably risky. An exemplar drug-discovery gene set for *A. fumigatus* identified by the use of a conditional promoter-replacement strategy and employing the nitrogen-responsive promoter p*NiiA* has been reported (Hu *et al.*, 2007). Repression of the p*NiiA* promoter is achieved in the presence of ammonium, regardless of the presence of other nitrogen sources. From the outset, the study was streamlined by identifying *A. fumigatus* genes homologous to those whose products were already known to be essential for survival in *S. cerevisiae* and *C. albicans*. A conditional *A. fumigatus* promoter-replacement approach was applied to 54 genes of diverse biological functions having orthologues essential for growth in *S. cerevisiae* and *C. albicans*. Among them, 35 were found also to be essential for growth in *A. fumigatus*. These included genes directing amino acid biosynthesis ($n = 6$), cell-wall biosynthesis ($n = 5$), metabolism ($n = 6$), ergosterol biosynthesis ($n = 4$), protein modification, translation or transport ($n = 12$) and ribosome biogenesis ($n = 8$). Similar to the GRACE approach described above, the experimental strategy permits analysis of cidal versus static phenotypes, and the use of conditional promoter-replacement strains as whole-cell screening reagents. Although in a number of instances mutants having terminal phenotypes in murine diseases were identifiable, the repression of the promoter during disease was fortuitously effected by nitrogen availability in the host tissue, not by regulated means.

A further point of interest is the fact that the functional relevance of many gene products is reliant upon environmental conditions. Given that microbes face a multiplicity of external stresses in the host environment, it is only to be expected that certain gene functions dispensable for growth *in vitro* are essential in the murine host. It is also feasible that distinct members of multigene families are preferentially required in the host environment, and for both of the aforementioned reasons, a precedent is set for testing mutant alleles in whole animals. By considering conservation in *A. fumigatus* and human genomes, the rarity of potential targets having broad-spectrum relevance becomes apparent, and this is further restricted when fungal selectivity is further imposed on the generally accepted definition of a good drug target. It therefore seems likely that relaxation of the previously held views on target prioritization will need to be exercised on a case-by-case basis in future rational approaches to antifungal drug discovery. The caveat still exists that human orthologues for such genes do exist, and the success of target-driven approaches remains to be proven.

17.3.2 Chemical genetics

Once access to large collections of repressible or mutant alleles can be secured, the opportunity to perform mode-of-action studies for existing and novel small molecules or novel compounds will arise. As yet, no such investigations have been reported for any fungal pathogen. In this context, the phenotype resulting from deletion of an essential gene would resemble that of the same (but wild-type) organism treated with a drug that inactivates the product of that gene. None the less, proof of principal has been more than adequately demonstrated by systematic analyses of collections of *S. cerevisiae* non-essential gene deletions (Hughes *et al.*, 2000; Parsons *et al.*, 2003, 2004, 2006). Several studies of chemical–genetic interactions have been reported for this model yeast. The most extensive study (Hillenmeyer *et al.*, 2010) analysed the effects of more than 4000 small molecules on more than 6000 *S. cerevisiae* gene-deletion mutants, amounting to more than 6 million single gene measurements. The aim of the study was to assign a phenotype to as many gene deletion mutants as possible, combining a chemical genomic approach with analysis of growth in response to environmental stress. Further compendiums of chemical–genetic profiles have been contributed by Parsons *et al.* (2006) and Hughes *et al.* (2000) wherein targeted analyses of the effects of exposure to 82 and 12 compounds, respectively, revealed new information on modes of action of existing drugs.

Recognizing that, for compounds having highly specific modes of action, compound specific gene sets buffer the cell from drug activity, Parsons *et al.* (2004) studied drug hypersensitivity on a global scale using *S. cerevisiae* gene deletions. Testing the viable gene-deletion mutants for drug-sensitive phenotypes provided a chemical–genetic interaction profile for each of the 12 compounds studied. As a loss-of-function mutation in a gene that is the target of a compound phenocopies the effect of the compound on the wild-type organism, the authors theorized that crossing such a mutation into the genetic background of viable *S. cerevisiae* gene-deletion strains would provide a genetic interaction profile for the target gene that should resemble the chemical–genetic interaction profile of its inhibitory compound. This prediction was well borne out by the subsequent experimentation. For example, of 27 genes identified as synthetic lethal or sick with the ergosterol biosynthetic gene *ERG11*, 13 were also fluconazole sensitive. Similarly Hughes *et al.* (2000) identified novel modes of action for existing therapeutic drugs, including the breast cancer therapeutic tamoxifen, which was found to disrupt calcium homeostasis.

17.3.3 Host genetics and susceptibility to infection

In 1996, Le Maitre *et al.* (1996) reported that Toll signalling was essential for resistance to *A. fumigatus* in the fruit fly *Drosophila melanogaster*. Subsequent to these seminal observations, the field of mammalian TLRs and innate fungal immunity has rapidly progressed to completely redefine the way we think about interactions between innate and adaptive immunity. It has subsequently been demonstrated that TLR4 polymorphisms are a critical determinant of susceptibility to invasive aspergillosis in human transplant patients (Bochud *et al.*, 2008). These observations demonstrate the power of animal models to fundamentally advance our understanding of human disease states. There is now growing interest in the use of high-throughput screening in model animal systems, such as *D. melanogaster* and *Caenorhabditis elegans*, both in terms of therapeutic drug screening and identification of host genetic susceptibility to disease (Lionakis and Kontoyiannis, 2010). Recent studies in *C. elegans* led to the eventual identification of the scavenger receptors SCARF1 and CD36 as key innate receptors for *C. albicans* and *Cryptococcus neoformans* (Means *et al.*, 2009). The future promises a growing resource of animal models with wide-scale genetic deletions for the high-throughput identification of susceptibility to IFI. Understanding the critical components of immunity that govern disease susceptibility will enable us to identify targeted immunotherapies when disease is established.

17.4 Transcriptomics

While whole-genome collections of gene-deletion mutants are currently unavailable for most pathogenic fungi, whole-genome transcription data is increasingly accessible. In particular, studies documenting transcription in the infected host deliver insight regarding the primary stresses experienced by host-colonizing organisms and, increasingly, concomitant documentation of the host response (Fig. 17.3). In a recent review of studies documenting the host-infecting fungal transcriptome, we assessed transcriptional data sets within the context of several disease models, thereby comparatively analysing transcriptome behaviour for several actively infecting animal and plant fungal pathogens (Cairns *et al.*, 2010). It was possible to draw broad conclusions on, for example, disease-relevant carbon metabolism and iron limitation. The commentary provides a highly detailed overview of the various methods adopted thus far for scrutinization of host-infecting fungal transcriptomes, including ways to circumvent the technical limitations associated with such analyses. Interestingly, the highest concordance between host-infecting transcriptomes (based on best-hit bidirectional blast analysis) was found between data sets obtained by analyses of fungal RNA extracted from the bronchoalveolar lavage fluid of *A. fumigatus*- and *C. neoformans*-infected mice (Hu *et al.*,

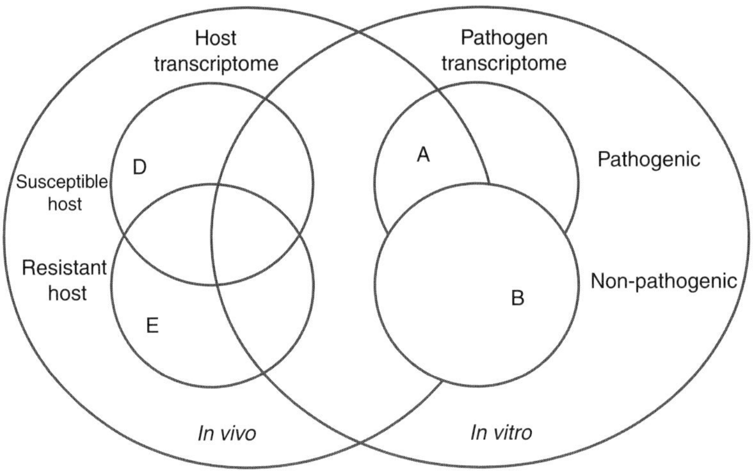

Fig. 17.3. Utility of host and pathogen transcriptomics for informing target discovery. Genes that are differentially expressed *in vivo* relative to *in vitro* growth may encode protein functions that are employed preferentially during host colonization, in particular those where orthologues are limited to pathogenic species (A), which may represent important virulence factors and/or pathways, but also those directing normal growth, cellular homeostasis and stress adaptation (B) that are present in both pathogenic and non-pathogenic species. Genes whose expression is specifically regulated in response to stress can be identified from controlled *in vitro* experimentation and identified among those identified as significant *in vivo*. This can aid the identification of signalling and adaptation mechanisms having likely therapeutic value. Among all of these genes and pathways, those that do not have human homologues, e.g. secondary metabolite biosynthesizing genes, are potential targets. Profiling of host-gene expression in resistant (E), non-immunocompromised hosts versus those suffering chemically or genetically induced immune deficits (D) will provide information about appropriate control of inflammation and tissue damage during normal sterilizing immune responses and how damage is mediated in invasive aspergillosis.

2008; McDonagh *et al.*, 2008), both of which initiate infection in the mammalian lung, albeit in hosts of disparate immune status. This would indicate that the nutritional and physiological constraints imposed by the lung are dominant as drivers of pathogen gene expression, independent of host immune status. Ultimately, from comparative analyses, it would be useful to identify those genes that are actively transcribed during infection, and among them the genes that are not present or active in non-pathogenic species. Such an approach has already generated significant insight in studies of *Aspergillus* spp. (Fedorova *et al.*, 2008; McDonagh *et al.*, 2008).

17.4.1 The fungal transcriptome during infection in whole-animal models of disease

A number of studies have analysed fungal gene expression during infection of whole mammal hosts (for a review, see Cairns *et al.*, 2010). In the case of *A. fumigatus*, there is currently a single published study in this realm (McDonagh *et al.*, 2008). None the less, significant insight has already been derived and a number of further studies from our laboratories will be forthcoming. McDonagh *et al.* (2008) established a methodology for measuring fungal transcript abundance during initiation of neutropenic murine infection point by selectively harvesting fungal germlings at 14 h post-infection. The application of linear mRNA amplification produced sufficient amplified RNA for microarray experiments, and a first snapshot of the *A. fumigatus* transcriptome during initiation of infection in the mammalian lung was obtained. A number of extremely insightful observations were derived from this first analysis. First, by incorporating a comparative analysis of all sequenced *Aspergillus* genomes, the authors were able to identify gene functions that have been acquired recently in the closely related but differently virulent *A. fumigatus* lineage (Affc) species, namely *A. fumigatus*, *A. clavatus* and *N. fischeri*. By plotting gene expression as a function of genetic locus, overlaid upon the eight *A. fumigatus* chromosomes, it was possible to visualize concordance between loci exhibiting higher transcript abundances and those where lineage-specific genes were preferentially located. This was strongly suggestive of a recent acquisition of gene functions employed during host colonization and highlighted regions of the genome in which to search more carefully for virulence attributes and therefore novel therapeutic targets. A further fascinating insight relates to the biased chromosomal distribution of genes whose transcripts are in higher transcript abundance during early infection, relative to laboratory culture. Genes having higher transcript abundance in the host relative to laboratory culture were found to form a significantly increased proportion of differentially regulated functions in intermediate and subtelomeric regions of the chromosomes (defined as regions spanning 300–600 and 0–300 kb from the telomeres, respectively). While only 16% of the predicted *A. fumigatus* gene repertoire is housed within 300 kb of the telomeres, 29% of transcripts having increased abundance, relative to laboratory culture, in the murine lung could be located to such subtelomeric areas, compared with just 11% of downregulated transcripts. Moreover, 28% of the entire subtelomeric gene repertoire was found to be represented in the induced data set compared with only 8% of subtelomeric genes represented among downregulated functions. Furthermore, a large number of upregulated gene functions were found to cluster into regions of five or more contiguous, co-regulated genes. More than 70 such gene clusters were identified by a study in neutropenic mice (McDonagh *et al.*, 2008). Of these, more than half are also upregulated during colonization of corticosteroid-treated hosts (L. Alcazar-Fuoli and E. Bignell, unpublished data). Functions are assignable only to a fraction of these gene clusters, predominantly those involved in secondary metabolite biosynthesis, for example gliotoxin, or siderophore biosynthesis (Gardiner and Howlett, 2005; Schrettl *et al.*, 2008). Based on the presence of genes encoding putative signal peptides, and unlike gene clusters identified in the *U. maydis* plant-infecting transcriptome (Howlett *et al.*, 2007), there is no obvious sequestration of classical protein effectors among the gene clusters identified in *A. fumigatus*. Studies are under way in our laboratories to identify those gene clusters having novel roles in virulence.

17.4.2 Defining responses to host-imposed stress

By comparing the behaviour of fungal transcriptomes exposed to defined *in vitro* stresses, it is possible to extract similar transcription signatures from genes upregulated during host disease. This can either be achieved by mining available published data or in a focused, controlled study, as described by McDonagh *et al.* (2008), who identified multiple genes involved in alkaline adaptation, iron acquisition and nutrient starvation among those induced during host disease. If one can identify adaptation mechanisms that are crucial for host disease such as pH or siderophore biosynthesis, more focused studies of regulatory circuits and possible synergistic interactions with existing drugs become possible. For example, pH adaptation in *S. cerevisiae* and *C. albicans* requires calcium signalling via the FK506 target phosphatase, calcineurin, and the transcription factor Crz1p. Given that multiple, licensed, non-antifungal drugs target calcium homeostasis (Afeltra and Verweij, 2003) and specifically calcineurin activity, molecules that target pH adaptation in the host might have synergistic activities with existing drugs. Thus, the hierarchical organization of such regulatory pathways, rather than components of the individual pathways themselves become open to investigation as potential therapeutic targets. Importantly, transcriptional rewiring of regulatory circuitry is often observed when comparing the behaviour of diverse species of fungal pathogens, and the insight afforded by transcriptional studies will therefore be important for deciphering network inhibitors having broad-spectrum inhibitory potential. With respect to defining targets having therapeutic significance in mammalian hosts, a crucial realization is that the host environment itself determines the growth rate and morphological development of the infecting fungus. It is therefore imperative that we understand the stage-specific regulation of transcription in multiple relevant infection models to accurately identify *A. fumigatus* virulence factors relevant to the broadest possible spectrum of related disease.

17.4.3 Transcript profiling of immune responses and aspergillosis

In order to better understand the molecular events that govern the early host response to invasive aspergillosis, we have adopted a transcriptomic approach to gain a greater understanding of how immune responses to aspergillosis are regulated (Armstrong-James *et al.*, 2009). Such an approach has given us a far greater understanding of how tissue damage is controlled during normal sterilizing immune responses in *A. fumigatus* exposure and how tissue damage is mediated in invasive aspergillosis. Understanding these processes at a molecular level has provided a rational framework for the development of novel drugs that augment host immunity or reduce host-mediated tissue damage.

In order to better understand the key mechanisms that mediate normal clearance of *A. fumigatus* disease, we inoculated immunocompetent mice with an intranasal *A. fumigatus* challenge and characterized the early host transcriptional events that occur during normal clearance of disease by whole-lung microarray analysis. This approach enabled us to identify the key transcriptional events that control normal clearance of disease. Two key groups of genes were identified as being upregulated at 24 h after inoculation. The first group contained a set of genes that all had roles in control of cellular proliferation and apoptosis and in regulation of lung tissue injury. These findings strongly suggested that, during normal control of *Aspergillus* disease, a primary function of the host response is to limit excessive immune responses that may cause tissue damage and inflammation, and that this occurs partly through apoptotic pathways. The second group of genes identified as upregulated during normal control of *Aspergillus* disease encode proteins involved in activation and regulation of innate immune responses and phagocytic clearance. Taken together, these observations indicate that sterilizing host immunity to *A. fumigatus* is mediated by a highly controlled and innate immune response characterized by phagocytosis, control of neutrophil influx, host-cell apoptosis and control of macrophage and T-cell differentiation. Developing a greater understanding of how the host normally clears *Aspergillus* disease has provided us with insights into those biological processes that may need to be harnessed in order to develop novel host-based therapies to enable efficient clearance of disease.

We have also used transcript profiling to characterize the early host response to disease in the neutropenic murine model of invasive aspergillosis. In this model, mice die rapidly from angioinvasive aspergillosis. Our studies demonstrated a major increase in the expression of genes encoding proteins involved in TNF-α expression and signal transduction at 24 h after disease. In addition, there was transcriptional evidence of activation of early pathways associated with Th17 T-cell differentiation. These observations suggest that neutropenic angioinvasive aspergillosis is associated with TNF-α-mediated tissue inflammation, failure to develop a controlled Th1 response, and an aberrant and pro-inflammatory Th17 response. This raises the possibility that immunotherapies that either block TNF-α production, such as monoclonal anti-TNF-α antibodies, or that drive aberrant adaptive immune responses back to Th1 polarization, may have therapeutic benefit in invasive *Aspergillus* syndromes.

In this respect, the identification of fungal virulence factors and secreted effectors that modulate the human immune system, such as exotoxins, small molecules or extracellular enzymes, is another important goal.

17.5 Proteomics: Global Host–Pathogen Interaction Screens

Global analyses of host–pathogen protein interactions have not yet been described for fungal pathogens. However, the feasibility of such approaches, at least in terms of *in vitro* and *ex vivo* infection models, is almost certain given recent publications in the fields of viral and bacterial pathogenesis. It is less obvious how such experimentation might be performed in the whole animal, although from a technical perspective, the use of split-marker technology has seen success with visualizing protein–protein interactions in living mice (Paulmurugan *et al.*, 2002). Genome-wide small interfering RNA (siRNA) studies have been used to identify host factors that might influence disease progression. For example, König *et al.* (2008) used a luciferase-expressing HIV-1 reporter virus and an arrayed genome-wide siRNA library to study the effect of neutralizing 20,000 human gene functions in infected 293T cells. The authors used a yeast two-hybrid protein–protein interaction database to derive an extended interactome network of 2458 host proteins affecting HIV infection and integrated the HIV–human protein interactions obtained by testing each of the HIV-encoded proteins against a library of human proteins. Additionally, the authors imported mRNA expression data on host genes of interest from publicly accessible gene expression databases to specifically identify genes having patterns of expression coincident with that of the viral receptors CD41 and the co-receptors CXCR4 and CD4/CCR5. The various lines of evidence were combined to create a decision matrix for prioritization of host factors most likely to impact on HIV-1 replication and approximately 800 genes were identified as strongly supported in regulating HIV-1 replication in host cells. Over 40 new factors were identified as influencing the initiation and/or kinetics of HIV-1 DNA synthesis, nuclear import or viral DNA integration.

17.6 From Bench to Bedside: Translation of Insights Derived from Pathosystematic Studies into Therapeutic Benefit

17.6.1 Recombinant interferon-γ immunotherapy

Recent evidence suggests that invasive fungal diseases are associated with inadequate Th1 host immune responses (Walsh *et al.*, 1994;

Jorgensen *et al.*, 2003; Allison and Eugui, 2005). This has been compounded by the move to T-cell-based immunosuppressive drug regimens for transplantation, because these drugs also target Th1 host immune responses (Jorgensen *et al.*, 2003). This results in a cumulative failure to produce adequate interferon (IFN)-γ-driven responses to invasive fungal diseases. On this basis, recombinant IFN-γ therapy has been explored as a potential adjunctive therapy for invasive fungal diseases in a number of different clinical settings. Pilot studies in the context of HIV-associated cryptococcal meningitis have demonstrated increase cerebrospinal fluid sterilization. These studies were recently reported as having been validated in large-scale randomized controlled studies in South Africa (Tom Harrison, Immunology of Fungal Infections, Gordon Research Conference, 2011, unpublished data). In addition recombinant IFN-γ immunotherapy is now used as standard prophylaxis against fungal disease in individuals with chronic granulomatous disorder.

Our studies in a neutropenic murine model of invasive pulmonary aspergillosis showed that clearance of the disease in immunocompetent mice required an effective host Th1-orientated transcriptional programme (Armstrong-James *et al.*, 2009). Mortality in immunosuppressed mice was associated with a disordered transcriptional programme that was characterized by the increased expression of genes encoding TNF-related proteins, TNF signalling and proteins responsible for the activation and expansion of Th2/Th17 $CD4^+$ T cells (Armstrong-James *et al.*, 2009). These mice also showed a deficiency of IFN-γ production in the infected lung. In addition, our studies in solid-organ transplant patients have demonstrated that invasive fungal diseases are associated with impaired IFN-γ response and excessive IL-10 responses. On this basis, we have been using recombinant human IFN-γ therapy as an adjunctive therapy in solid-organ transplant patients with refractory or disseminated invasive fungal diseases. Our studies demonstrate that such an approach appears safe and is associated with rapid sterilization of disease (Armstrong-James *et al.*, 2010). In addition, IFN-γ therapy did not lead to deterioration of graft function and was associated with augmentation of endogenous IFN-γ production, a burst in the pro-inflammatory cytokine response and reversal of excessive IL-10 production. Clearly, multicentre studies will be required to further validate these observations.

17.6.2 Adoptive immunotherapy

Over the past two decades, it has become increasingly clear that Th1 lymphocytes play an important role in immunity to invasive fungal diseases (Romani, 2011). In the context of HSCT, major advances have been made in the identification, isolation and clinical-scale generation of antifungal T cells. Adoptive transfer of such cells either in patients with invasive aspergillosis and impaired T-cell immunity or as prophylaxis after HSCT, is a potentially attractive option that may complement antifungal therapies. In particular, invasive *Aspergillus* has become a major problem in patients with T-cell immunodeficiencies, such as patients on T-cell-based immunosuppressive regimens for solid-organ transplantation or graft-versus-host disease. There is clear evidence emerging that patients who develop invasive fungal diseases have impaired Th1 responses. Furthermore, studies in stem-cell transplant patients indicate that these patients have significantly reduced anti-*Aspergillus* T cells when compared with normal individuals (Beck *et al.*, 2008). These observations provide a clear therapeutic rationale for the targeted use of adoptive immunotherapy with Th1 IFN-γ-producing fungal-specific T-cell-adoptive therapy. Such an approach has already gained popularity in the context of post-transplant cytomegalovirus disease with clear therapeutic benefit (Cobbold *et al.*, 2005). Therefore, extending such approaches in the stem-cell laboratory to address aspergillosis and other invasive mycoses has been relatively straightforward due to the prior establishment of clinical methodologies for cytomegalovirus.

One of the key challenges in adoptive immunotherapy is identification of the appropriate fungal T-cell antigenic stimuli in order to enable the comprehensive identification of the complete antifungal T-cell repertoire through stimulation assays. In the context of *Aspergillus* spp., this is further complicated by the complex relationship that exists between fungal morphogenesis (condial–hyphal transmission) and host immunological responses (conidia induce Th1 responses, while hyphae Th2 responses). One hypothesis is that the identification of 'globally expressed antigens' that are expressed throughout hyphal transition would be ideal. While superficially it would be reasonable to assume that conidial antigens would be ideal, as conidia induce Th1 responses, this may not reflect the true mechanisms underlying disease establishment, where control of hyphal transition may be a critical determinant of outcome.

Ideally, for clinical good medical practice-grade applications, recombinant antigens are preferable, as these can be easily and reproducibly synthesized, whereas considerable variation may occur in fungal cultures, which in addition may cause contamination of cell cultures. Current approaches that have been tested include live conidial stimulation, fungal extracts and specific recombinant antigens or proteins, or even carbohydrates. Subsequent identification and physical isolation of antifungal T cells is based on commercially available IFN-γ capture assays. This approach usually yields in the range of 10^7 antifungal T cells, which can be further amplified in culture. Therefore, it is possible to isolate these cells prior to transplantation, for subsequent use after cryopreservation, should disease occur post-transplantation. In landmark studies in haploidentical stem-cell transplant patients with probable aspergillosis, infusion of anti-*Aspergillus* T cells had a clear therapeutic benefit, with a significant reduction in serum galactomannan concentrations when compared with controls at 6 weeks. In complementary studies, the utility of dendritic cell vaccination for protection against fungal disease has also been explored. In key animal studies, adoptive transfer of *Aspergillus*-pulsed dendritic cells led to T-cell priming and enhanced resistance to invasive aspergillosis (Perruccio *et al*., 2004). Other immunotherapeutic modalities with promise for the treatment of IFIs currently being explored in mice include the collection of Pentraxin 3 (Gaziano *et al*., 2004).

In conclusion, both cytokine-based and adoptive cellular immunotherapy show great potential for treating patients with invasive mycoses. Future multicentre studies will be required to validate such approaches.

17.6.3 Monoclonal antibodies

Monoclonal antibodies have become a major novel class of biological pharmaceuticals over the last decade, with a number of novel monoclonals licensed for the treatment of neoplastic and autoimmune diseases. The relative lack of direct drug toxicities associated with this class of drugs, as well as established protocols for production, make monoclonals an attractive approach for therapy of infectious diseases. The first monoclonal demonstrated to have antifungal activity was efungumab. Efungumab is a monoclonal antibody specific for fungal heat-shock protein 90 (HSP90). HSP90 is a molecular chaperone that is key to stress responses in many organisms. In fungi, it has been shown to be involved in pathogen drug resistance mechanisms in response to exposure to azoles and echinocandins. Therefore, from a hypothetical perspective, blockade of HSP90 may potentiate the antifungal effects of these compounds. Furthermore, HSP90 itself is expressed at the cell wall in fungi, and has been demonstrated to generate production of natural antibodies in patients with invasive candidiasis. Indeed, efungumab was initially derived from a human-generated antibody. In terms of structure, the pharmacological agent is composed of heavy and light chains but does not contain the Fc component. *In vitro* studies of efungumab therapy, either on its own or in combination with azoles, echinocandins or polyenes, indicate that efungumab has synergy with fluconazole for *C. albicans*, reducing the minimum inhibitory concentration fourfold. Very similar synergistic properties were identified when efungumab was combined with amphotericin B or echinocandins. In animal models of invasive candidiasis, further studies indicate that combination therapy with efungumab and either amphotericin B or caspofungin was superior in terms of reduction of fungal burden, when compared with either monotherapy.

A major breakthrough for efungumab was a randomized, double-blind trial that investigated the efficacy of efungumab in combination with liposomal amphotericin B in patients with invasive candidiasis (Pachi *et al.*, 2006) For this study, the primary outcome measure was overall treatment response at 10 days. Notably, both primary and secondary outcomes were shown to be superior in the efungumab arm of the trial, with a complete clinical response rate of 84% compared with 48% in the placebo arm. However, Herbrecht *et al.* (2006) called into question the validity of the study design and analysis. Subsequently, the European Committee for Medicinal Products for Human Use turned down licensing for this agent on the basis of a lack of clear data on clinical efficacy and the observation of a cytokine release syndrome in some patients, most worryingly manifesting as changes in blood pressure in some patients. Despite these issues, the efungumab story has demonstrated an important proof of principle for the development of monoclonal antibodies with antifungal activity.

17.6.4 Natural antifungals

Genomics is transforming our view of the fungal kingdom. Queries of fungal genomic sequence databases show that large numbers of genes encoding proteins involved in the biosynthesis of so far unknown metabolites are present, underlining the potential for novel active substances. Fungal secondary metabolites exhibit a huge diversity of chemical structure and are thought to function in reproductive and pathogenic development, intercellular or interorganism communication, and defence against natural predators. Although genome sequencing identifies genetic loci that have putative roles in secondary metabolite biosynthesis, the conditions under which transcriptional expression of many such genes becomes active are not known, and many potentially priceless biosynthetic loci are subject to silencing mechanisms of currently unknown molecular basis.

Two of the major classes of antifungal drugs currently used for invasive mycoses are natural products. Polyenes such as amphotericin B or nystatin, which disrupt fungal ergosterol in the cell wall, are macrocyclic lactones first isolated in *Streptomyces* species (Donovick *et al.*, 1955; Medoff and Kobayashi, 1980). In addition, the echinocandins, which are commonly used for *Candida* spp. diseases, are fungal secondary metabolites, such as anidulafungin, first isolated from *A. nidulans* (Denning *et al.*, 2003). A number of other echinocandins have either been brought to market, such as caspofungin or mycafungin, or are in development for use as antifungals in man. Other natural peptides under investigation are aerothricin-related cyclic peptides isolated from Deuteromycotina (Kohchi *et al.*, 2001). These drugs have promising *in vitro* antifungal activity but have not been tested in man.

A large number of other naturally occurring compounds have shown potential as antifungal agents that could be developed for human use. Cispentacin is a novel amino acid antibiotic that is naturally produced by *Bacillus cereus* in broth culture and has been found to have antifungal activity against *C. albicans* and other fungi (Konishi *et al.*, 1989). Structure–activity relationship studies for cispentacin led to the subsequent development of the related compound icofungipen, which has shown potential as an oral agent in animal models of invasive candidiasis (Mittendorf *et al.*, 2003). An antifungal metabolite, sordarin, isolated from *Sordaria araneosa*, has also been identified with broad antifungal activity, and a number of other sordarin derivatives are being investigated. High-throughput screening identified a sordarin analogue, GR135402, that was shown to be a strong and selective inhibitor of protein synthesis in *C. albicans* (Domínguez and Martín, 1998). A semi-synthetic sordarin derivative, currently known as FR290581, has been shown to have enhanced *in vitro* activity against *Candida* spp. and showed efficacy in animal models of invasive candidiasis (Hanadate *et al.*, 2009). Novel macrolides such as rustmicin, produced by *Streptomyces galbus*, have been shown to exhibit good antifungal activity against yeasts, and are also currently being investigated (Mandala *et al.*, 1998).

17.6.5 Iron-chelation therapy for mucormycosis

Zygomycetes are lower fungi from the order Mucorales and are opportunistic pathogens. Diseases primarily occur in patients who are immunocompromised, and particularly those with diabetic ketoacidosis. There is a clear historical association between the use of the iron chelator deferoxamine and risk of development of mucormycosis (Boelaert *et al.*, 1994). Notably, while deferoxamine acts as an iron chelator for the host, it has the opposite effect for *Rhizopus oryzae*, instead acting as a siderophore, thereby supplying iron to the fungus (Boelaert *et al.*, 1994). In contrast, it has been demonstrated that the alternative iron chelator deferasirox also has iron-chelating activity for *R. oryzae*. Furthermore, this agent improved survival in murine models of zygomycosis, in synergy with liposomal amphotericin B (Ibrahim-Granet *et al.*, 2003). Subsequent to these observations, a Phase II study of adjuvant deferasirox for the treatment of mucormycosis is under way (the DEFEAT Mucor study).

17.7 Conclusion

In this chapter, we have delineated and examined progress in areas of pathosystematic study, which will inform future therapeutic strategy. As the research community embraces these approaches and recognizes more fully the value and timeliness of integrative biology in deciphering the origin and physiological basis of fungal virulence, the capacity of basic fungal biological research to inform rationalized anti-infective development, and natural product mining, will increase exponentially. Future efforts must retain a focus on the extent to which mycological research can be exploited for novel therapeutic advantage and, given the pace at which technological advances occur, the challenge for research scientists will be in harnessing these new tools in order to maximize the translational potential of their research.

References

Afeltra, J. and Verweij, P.E. (2003) Antifungal activity of nonantifungal drugs. *European Journal of Clinical Microbiology and Infectious Diseases* 22, 397–407.

Allison, A.C. and Eugui, E.M. (2005) *Mechanisms of action of mycophenolate mofetil in preventing acute and chronic allograft rejection.* Transplantation 80 (Suppl. 2), S181–S190.

Armstrong-James, D.P., Turnbull, S.A., Teo, I., Stark, J., Rogers, N.J., Rogers, T.R., Bignell, E. and Haynes, K. (2009) Impaired interferon-γ responses, increased interleukin-17 expression, and a tumor necrosis factor-α transcriptional program in invasive aspergillosis. *Journal of Infectious Diseases* 200, 1341–1351.

Armstrong-James, D., Teo, I.A., Shrivistava, S., Petrou, M.A., Taube, D., Dorling, A. and Shaunak, S. (2010) Exogenous interferon-γ immunotherapy for invasive fungal infections in kidney transplant patients. *American Journal of Transplantation* 10, 1796–1803.

Babovic-Vuksanovic D., Snow, K. and Ten, R.M. (1999) Mannose-binding lectin (MBL) deficiency. Variant alleles in a midwestern population of the United States. *Annals of Allergy, Asthma and Immunology* 82, 134–143.

Becker, J.M., Kauffman, S.J., Hauser, M., Huang, L., Lin, M., Sillaots, S., Jiang, B., Xu, D. and Roemer, T. (2010) Pathway analysis of *Candida albicans* survival and virulence determinants in a murine infection model. *Proceedings of the National Academy of Sciences USA* 107, 22044–22049.

Babula, O., Lazdane, G., Kroica, J., Ledger, W.J. and Witkin, S.S. (2003) Relation between recurrent vulvovaginal candidiasis, vaginal concentrations of mannose-binding lectin, and a mannose-binding lectin gene polymorphism in Latvian women. *Clinical Infectious Diseases* 37, 733–737.

Balloy, V., Si-Tahar M., Takeuchi, O., Philippe, B., Nahori, M.A., Tanguy, M., Huerre, M., Akira, S., Latgé, J.P. and Chignard, M. (2005) Involvement of Toll-like receptor 2 in experimental invasive pulmonary aspergillosis. *Infection and Immunity* 73, 5420–5425.

Beck, O., Koehl, U., Tramsen, L., Mousset, S., Latgé, J.P., Müller, K., Schwabe, D., Bader, P., Klingebiel, T. and Lehrnbecher, T. (2008) Enumeration of functionally active anti-*Aspergillus* T-cells in human peripheral blood. *Journal of Immunological Methods* 335, 41–45.

Ben-Ami R., Lewis, R.E., Leventakos, K. and Kontoyiannis, D.P. (2009) *Aspergillus fumigatus* inhibits angiogenesis through the production of gliotoxin and other secondary metabolites. *Blood* 114, 5393–5399.

Bignell, E., Negrete-Urtasun, S., Calcagno, A.M., Haynes, K., Arst, H.N. Jr and Rogers, T. (2005) The *Aspergillus* pH-responsive transcription factor PacC regulates virulence. *Molecular Microbiology* 55, 1072–1084.

Bochud, P.-Y., Chien, J.W., Marr, K.A., Leisenring, W.M., Upton, A., Janer, M., Rodrigues, S.D., Li, S., Hansen, J.A., Zhao, L.P., Aderem, A. and Boeckh, M. (2008) Toll-like receptor 4 polymorphisms and aspergillosis in stem-cell transplantation. *New England Journal of Medicine* 359, 1766–1777.

Boelaert, J.R., de Locht, M. and Schneider, Y.J. (1994) The effect of deferoxamine on different zygomycetes. *Journal of Infectious Diseases* 169, 231–232.

Braun, B.R., van Het, H.M., d'Enfert, C., Martchenko, M., Dungan, J., Kuo, A., Inglis, D.O., Uhl, M.A., Hogues, H., Berriman, M., Lorenz, M., Levitin, A., Oberholzer, U., Bachewich, C., Harcus, D., Marcil, A., Dignard, D., Iouk, T., Zito, R., Frangeul, L., Tekaia, F., Rutherford, K., Wang, E., Munro, C.A., Bates, S., Gow, N.A., Hoyer, L.L., Kohler, G., Morschhauser, J., Newport, G., Znaidi, S., Raymond, M., Turcotte, B., Sherlock, G., Costanzo, M., Ihmels, J., Berman, J., Sanglard, D., Agabian, N., Mitchell, A.P., Johnson, A.D., Whiteway, M. and Nantel, A. (2005) A human-curated annotation of the *Candida albicans* genome. *PLoS Genetics* 1, 36–57.

Bruns, S., Kniemeyer, O., Hasenberg, M., Aimanianda, V., Nietzsche, S., Thywißen, A., Jeron, A., Latgé, J.-P., Brakhage, A.A. and Gunzer, M. (2010) Production of extracellular traps against *Aspergillus fumigatus in vitro* and in infected lung tissue is dependent on invading neutrophils and influenced by hydrophobin RodA. *PLoS Pathogens* 6, e1000873.

Butler, G., Rasmussen, M.D., Lin, M.F., Santos, M.A., Sakthikumar, S., Munro, C.A., Rheinbay, E., Grabherr, M., Forche, A., Reedy, J.L., Agrafioti, I., Arnaud, M.B., Bates, S., Brown, A.J., Brunke, S., Costanzo, M.C., Fitzpatrick, D.A., de Groot, P.W., Harris, D., Hoyer, L.L., Hube, B., Klis, F.M., Kodira, C., Lennard, N., Logue, M.E., Martin, R., Neiman, A.M., Nikolaou, E., Quail, M.A., Quinn, J., Santos, M.C., Schmitzberger, F.F., Sherlock, G., Shah, P., Silverstein, K.A., Skrzypek, M.S., Soll, D., Staggs, R., Stansfield, I., Stumpf, M.P., Sudbery, P.E., Srikantha, T., Zeng, Q., Berman, J., Berriman, M., Heitman, J., Gow, N.A., Lorenz, M.C., Birren, B.W., Kellis, M. and Cuomo, C.A. (2009) Evolution of pathogenicity and sexual reproduction in eight *Candida* genomes. *Nature* 459, 657–662.

Cairns, T., Minuzzi, F. and Bignell, E. (2010) The host-infecting fungal transcriptome. *FEMS Microbiology Letters* 307, 1–11.

Capilla, J., Clemons, K.V. and Stevens, D.A. (2007) Animal models: an important tool in mycology. *Medical Mycology* 45, 657–684.

Carvalho, A., Cunha, C., Pasqualotto, A.C., Pitzurra, L., Denning, D.W. and Romani, L. (2010) Genetic variability of innate immunity impacts human susceptibility to fungal diseases. *International Journal of Infectious Diseases* 14, e460–e468.

Casadevall, A. and Pirofski, L.A. (2003) The damage-response framework of microbial pathogenesis. *Nature Reviews Microbiology* 1, 17–24.

Casadevall, A. and Pirofski, L.A. (2009) Virulence factors and their mechanisms of action: the view from a damage-response framework. *Journal of Water Health* 7 (Suppl. 1), S2–S18.

Clemons, K.V. and Stevens, D.A. (2005) The contribution of animal models of aspergillosis to understanding pathogenesis, therapy and virulence. *Medical Mycology* 43 (Suppl. 1), S101–S110.

Cobbold, M., Khan, N., Pourgheysari, B., Tauro, S., McDonald, D., Osman, H., Assenmacher, M., Billingham, L., Steward, C., Crawley, C., Olavarria, E., Goldman, J., Chakraverty, R., Mahendra, P., Craddock, C. and Moss, P.A.H. (2005) Adoptive transfer of cytomegalovirus-specific CTL to stem cell transplant patients after selection by HLA-peptide tetramers. *Journal of Experimental Medicine* 202, 379–396.

Cross, C.E. and Bancroft, G.J. (1995) Ingestion of acapsular *Cryptococcus neoformans* occurs via mannose and β-glucan receptors, resulting in cytokine production and increased phagocytosis of the encapsulated form. *Infection and Immunity* 63, 2604–2611.

Cunha, C., Di, I.M., Bozza, S., Giovannini, G., Zagarella, S., Zelante, T., D'Angelo, C., Pierini, A., Pitzurra, L., Falzetti, F., Carotti, A., Perruccio, K., Latge, J.P., Rodrigues, F., Velardi, A., Aversa, F., Romani, L. and Carvalho, A. (2010) Dectin-1 Y238X polymorphism associates with susceptibility to invasive aspergillosis in hematopoietic transplantation through impairment of both recipient- and donor-dependent mechanisms of antifungal immunity. *Blood* 116, 5394–5402.

da Silva Ferreira, M.E., Kress, M.R., Savoldi, M., Goldman, M.H., Hartl, A., Heinekamp, T.,

Brakhage, A.A. and Goldman, G.H. (2006) The *akuB*^{KU80} mutant deficient for nonhomologous end joining is a powerful tool for analyzing pathogenicity in *Aspergillus fumigatus*. *Eukaryotic Cell* 5, 207–211.

Davis, D., Edwards, J.E. Jr, Mitchell, A.P. and Ibrahim, A.S. (2000) *Candida albicans* RIM101 pH response pathway is required for host–pathogen interactions. *Infection and Immunity* 68, 5953–5959.

de Backer, M.D., Nelissen, B., Logghe, M., Viaene, J., Loonen, I., Vandoninck, S., de, H.R., Dewaele, S., Simons, F.A., Verhasselt, P., Vanhoof, G., Contreras, R. and Luyten, W.H. (2001) An antisense-based functional genomics approach for identification of genes critical for growth of *Candida albicans*. *Nature Biotechnology* 19, 235–241.

de Repentigny, R.L. (2004) Animal models in the analysis of *Candida* host–pathogen interactions. *Current Opinion in Microbiology* 7, 324–329.

Dennehy, K.M., Ferwerda, G., Faro-Trindade I., Pyz, E., Willment, J.A., Taylor, P.R., Kerrigan, A., Tsoni, S.V., Gordon, S. and Meyer-Wentrup, F. (2008) Syk kinase is required for collaborative cytokine production induced through Dectin-1 and Toll-like receptors. *European Journal of Immunology* 38, 500–506.

Denning, D.W., Riniotis, K., Dobrashian, R. and Sambatakou, H. (2003) Chronic cavitary and fibrosing pulmonary and pleural aspergillosis: case series, proposed nomenclature change, and review. *Clinical Infectious Diseases* 37 (Suppl. 3), S265–S280.

Domínguez, J.M. and Martín, J.J. (1998) Identification of elongation factor 2 as the essential protein targeted by sordarins in *Candida albicans*. *Antimicrobial Agents and Chemotherapy* 42, 2279–2283.

Donders, G.G., Babula, O., Bellen, G., Linhares, I.M. and Witkin, S.S. (2008) Mannose-binding lectin gene polymorphism and resistance to therapy in women with recurrent vulvovaginal candidiasis. *BJOG* 115, 1225–1231

Donovick, R., Gold, W., Pagano, J.F. and Stout, H.A. (1955) Amphotericins A and B antifungal antibiotics produced by a streptomycete. I. *In vitro* studies. *Antibiotics Annual* 3, 579–586.

Fedorova, N.D., Khaldi, N., Joardar, V.S., Maiti, R., Amedeo, P., Anderson, M.J., Crabtree, J., Silva, J.C., Badger, J.H., Albarraq, A., Angiuoli, S., Bussey, H., Bowyer, P., Cotty, P.J., Dyer, P.S., Egan, A., Galens, K., Fraser-Liggett, C.M., Haas, B.J., Inman, J.M., Kent, R., Lemieux, S., Malavazi, I., Orvis, J., Roemer, T., Ronning, C.M., Sundaram, J.P., Sutton, G., Turner, G., Venter, J.C., White, O.R., Whitty, B.R., Youngman, P., Wolfe, K.H., Goldman, G.H., Wortman, J.R., Jiang, B., Denning, D.W. and Nierman, W.C. (2008) Genomic islands in the pathogenic filamentous fungus *Aspergillus fumigatus*. *PLoS Genetics* 4, e1000046.

Ferwerda, B., Ferwerda, G., Plantinga, T.S., Willment, J.A., van Spriel, A.B., Venselaar, H., Elbers, C.C., Johnson, M.D., Cambi, A., Huysamen, C., Jacobs, L., Jansen, T., Verheijen, K., Masthoff, L., Morré, S.A., Vriend, G., Williams, D.L., Perfect, J.R., Joosten, L.A., Wijmenga, C., van der Meer, J.W., Adema, G.J., Kullberg, B.J., Brown, G.D. and Netea, M.G. (2009) Human dectin-1 deficiency and mucocutaneous fungal infections. *New England Journal of Medicine* 361, 1760–1767.

Gardiner, D.M. and Howlett, B.J. (2005) Bioinformatic and expression analysis of the putative gliotoxin biosynthetic gene cluster of *Aspergillus fumigatus*. *FEMS Microbiology Letters* 248, 241–248.

Garred, P., Nielsen, M.A., Kurtzhals, J.A., Malhotra, R., Madsen, H.O., Goka, B.Q., Akanmori, B.D., Sim, R.B. and Hviid, L. (2003) Mannose-binding lectin is a disease modifier in clinical malaria and may function as opsonin for *Plasmodium falciparum*-infected erythrocytes. *Infection and Immunity* 71, 5245–5253.

Gaziano, R., Bozza, S., Bellocchio, S., Perruccio, K., Montagnoli, C., Pitzurra, L., Salvatori, G., De Santis, R., Carminati, P., Mantovani, A. and Romani, L. (2004) Anti-*Aspergillus* fumigatus efficacy of pentraxin 3 alone and in combination with antifungals. *Antimicrobial Agents and Chemotherapy* 48, 4414–4421.

Giraldo, A.M., Lynn, J.W., Purpera, M.N., Godke, R.A. and Bondioli, K.R. (2007) DNA methylation and histone acetylation patterns in cultured bovine fibroblasts for nuclear transfer. *Molecular Reproduction and Development* 74, 1514–1524.

Glocker, E.O., Hennigs, A., Nabavi, M., Schäffer, A.A., Woellner, C., Salzer, U., Pfeifer, D., Veelken, H., Warnatz, K., Tahami, F., Jamal, S., Manguiat, A., Rezaei, N., Amirzargar, A.A., Plebani, A., Hannesschläger, N., Gross, O., Ruland, J. and Grimbacher, B. (2009) A homozygous CARD9 mutation in a family with susceptibility to fungal infections. *New England Journal of Medicine* 361, 1727–1735.

Granell, M., Urbano-Ispizua, A., Suarez, B., Rovira, M., Fernández-Avilés, F., Martínez, C., Ortega, M., Uriburu, C., Gaya, A., Roncero, J.M., Navarro, A., Carreras, E., Mensa, J., Vives, J., Rozman, C., Montserrat, E. and Lozano, F. (2006) Mannan-binding lectin pathway deficiencies and invasive fungal infections following allogeneic stem cell transplantation. *Experimental Hematology* 34, 1435–1441.

Gross, O., Gewies, A., Finger, K., Schäfer, M., Sparwasser, T., Peschel, C., Förster, I. and Ruland, J. (2006) Card9 controls a non-TLR signalling pathway for innate anti-fungal immunity. *Nature* 442, 651–656

Hanadate, T., Tomishima, M., Shiraishi, N., Tanabe, D., Morikawa, H., Barrett, D., Matsumoto, S., Ohtomo, K. and Maki, K. (2009) FR290581, a novel sordarin derivative: synthesis and antifungal activity. *Bioorganic and Medicinal Chemistry Letters* 19, 1465–1468.

Herbrecht, R., Fohrer, C. and Nivoix, Y. (2006) Mycograb for the treatment of invasive candidiasis. *Clinical Infectious Diseases* 43, 1083; author reply 1083–1084.

Hillenmeyer, M.E., Ericson, E., Davis, R.W., Nislow, C., Koller, D. and Giaever, G. (2010) Systematic analysis of genome-wide fitness data in yeast reveals novel gene function and drug action. *Genome Biology* 11, R30.

Howlett, B.J., Idnurm, A. and Heitman, J. (2007) Fungal pathogenesis: gene clusters unveiled as secrets within the *Ustilago maydis* code. *Current Biology* 17, R87–R90.

Hu, G., Cheng, P.Y., Sham, A., Perfect, J.R. and Kronstad, J.W. (2008) Metabolic adaptation in *Cryptococcus neoformans* during early murine pulmonary infection. *Molecular Microbiology* 69, 1456–1475.

Hu, W., Sillaots, S., Lemieux, S., Davison, J., Kauffman, S., Breton, A., Linteau, A., Xin, C., Bowman, J., Becker, J., Jiang, B. and Roemer, T.(2007) Essential gene identification and drug target prioritization in *Aspergillus fumigatus*. *PLoS Pathogens* 3, e24.

Hughes, T.R., Marton, M.J., Jones, A.R., Roberts, C.J., Stoughton, R., Armour, C.D., Bennett, H.A., Coffey, E., Dai, H., He, Y.D., Kidd, M.J., King, A.M., Meyer, M.R., Slade, D., Lum, P.Y., Stepaniants, S.B., Shoemaker, D.D., Gachotte, D., Chakraburtty, K., Simon, J., Bard, M. and Friend, S.H. (2000) Functional discovery via a compendium of expression profiles. *Cell* 102, 109–126.

Ibrahim-Granet, O., Philippe, B., Boleti, H., Boisvieux-Ulrich, E., Grenet, D., Stern, M. and Latge, J.P. (2003) Phagocytosis and intracellular fate of *Aspergillus fumigatus* conidia in alveolar macrophages. *Infection and Immunity* 71, 891–903.

Jack, D.L., Read, R.C., Tenner, A.J., Frosch, M., Turner, M.W. and Klein, N.J. (2001) Mannose-binding lectin regulates the inflammatory response of human professional phagocytes to *Neisseria meningitidis* serogroup B. *Journal of Infectious Diseases* 1184, 1152–1162.

Jorgensen, K.A., Koefoed-Nielsen, P.B. and Karamperis, N. (2003) Calcineurin phosphatase activity and immunosuppression. A review on the role of calcineurin phosphatase activity and the immunosuppressive effect of cyclosporin A and tacrolimus. *Scandinavian Journal of Immunology* 57, 93–98.

Jurevic, R.J., Bai, M., Chadwick, R.B., White, T.C. and Dale, B.A. (2003) Single-nucleotide polymorphisms (SNPs) in human β-defensin 1: high-throughput SNP assays and association with *Candida* carriage in type I diabetics and nondiabetic controls. *Journal of Clinical Microbiology* 41, 90–96.

Kirkpatrick, C.H. (2001) Chronic mucocutaneous candidiasis. *Pediatric Infectious Disease Journal* 20, 197–206.

Kohchi, M., Masubuchi, K., Murata, T., Okada, T. and Shimma, N. (2001) Aerothricin derivatives. *World Patents* 53, 322.

König, R., Zhou, Y., Elleder, D., Diamond, T.L., Bonamy, G.M., Irelan, J.T., Chiang, C.Y., Tu B.P., De Jesus, P.D., Lilley, C.E., Seidel, S., Opaluch, A.M., Caldwell, J.S., Weitzman, M.D., Kuhen, K.L., Bandyopadhyay, S., Ideker, T., Orth, A.P., Miraglia, L.J., Bushman, F.D., Young, J.A. and Chanda, S.K. (2008) Global analysis of host–pathogen interactions that regulate early-stage HIV-1 replication. *Cell* 135, 49–60.

Konishi, M., Nishio, M., Saitoh, K., Miyaki, T., Oki, T. and Kawaguchi, H. (1989) Cispentacin, a new antifungal antibiotic. I. Production, isolation, physico-chemical properties and structure. *Journal of Antibiotics (Tokyo)* 42, 1749–1755.

Kwon-Chung, K.J. and Sugui, J.A. (2009) What do we know about the role of gliotoxin in the pathobiology of *Aspergillus fumigatus*? Medical Mycology 47 (Suppl. 1), S97–S103.

Lambourne, J., Agranoff, D., Herbrecht, R., Troke, P.F., Buchbinder, A., Willis, F., Letscher-Bru, V., Agrawal, S., Doffman, S., Johnson, E., White, P.L., Barnes, R.A., Griffin, G., Lindsay, J.A. and Harrison, T.S. (2009) Association of mannose-binding lectin deficiency with acute invasive aspergillosis in immunocompromised patients. *Clinical Infectious Diseases* 49, 1486–1491.

Latge, J.P. (1999) *Aspergillus fumigatus* and aspergillosis. *Clinical Microbiology Reviews* 12, 310–350.

Lavoie, H., Hogues, H., Mallick, J., Sellam, A., Nantel, A. and Whiteway, M. (2010) Evolutionary tinkering with conserved components of a transcriptional regulatory network. *PLoS Biology* 8, e1000329.

Le Maitre, B., Nicolas, E., Michaut, L., Reichhart, J.M. and Hoffmann, J.A. (1996) The dorsoventral regulatory gene cassette spatzle/Toll/cactus controls the potent antifungal response in *Drosophila* adults. *Cell* 86, 973–983.

Lewis, R.E. and Wiederhold, N.P. (2005) Murine model of invasive aspergillosis. *Methods in Molecular Medicine* 118, 129–142.

Lewis, R.E., Wiederhold, N.P., Lionakis, M.S., Prince, R.A. and Kontoyiannis, D.P. (2005) Frequency and species distribution of gliotoxin-producing *Aspergillus* isolates recovered from patients at a tertiary-care cancer center. *Journal of Clinical Microbiology* 43, 6120–6122.

Lionakis, M.S. and Kontoyiannis, D.P. (2010) The growing promise of *Toll*-deficient *Drosophila melanogaster* as a model for studying *Aspergillus* pathogenesis and treatment. *Virulence* 1, 488–499.

Ma, L.J., van der Does, H.C., Borkovich, K.A., Coleman, J.J., Daboussi, M.J., Di, P.A., Dufresne, M., Freitag, M., Grabherr, M., Henrissat, B., Houterman, P.M., Kang, S., Shim, W.B., Woloshuk, C., Xie, X., Xu, J.R., Antoniw, J., Baker, S.E., Bluhm, B.H., Breakspear, A., Brown, D.W., Butchko, R.A., Chapman, S., Coulson, R., Coutinho, P.M., Danchin, E.G., Diener, A., Gale, L.R., Gardiner, D.M., Goff, S., Hammond-Kosack, K.E., Hilburn, K., Hua-Van, A., Jonkers, W., Kazan, K., Kodira, C.D., Koehrsen, M., Kumar, L., Lee, Y.H., Li, L., Manners, J.M., Miranda-Saavedra, D., Mukherjee, M., Park, G., Park, J., Park, S.Y., Proctor, R.H., Regev, A., Ruiz-Roldan, M.C., Sain, D., Sakthikumar, S., Sykes, S., Schwartz, D.C., Turgeon, B.G., Wapinski, I., Yoder, O., Young, S., Zeng, Q., Zhou, S., Galagan, J., Cuomo, C.A., Kistler, H.C. and Rep, M. (2010) Comparative genomics reveals mobile pathogenicity chromosomes in *Fusarium. Nature* 464, 367–373.

Mandala, S.M., Thornton, R.A., Milligan, M., Rosenbach, M., Garcia-Calvo, M., Bull, H.G., Harris, G.K., Abruzzo, K., Flattery, A.M., Gill, C.J., Bartizal, S., Dreikorn, S. and Kurtz, M.B. (1998) Rustmicin, a potent antifungal agent, inhibits sphingolipid synthesis at inositol phosphoceramide synthase. *Journal of Biological Chemistry* 273, 19492–19494.

McDonagh, A., Fedorova, N.D., Crabtree, J., Yu, Y., Kim, S., Chen, D., Loss, O., Cairns, T., Goldman, G., Armstrong-James, D., Haynes, K., Haas, H., Schrettl, M., May, G., Nierman, W.C. and Bignell, E. (2008) Sub-telomere directed gene expression during initiation of invasive aspergillosis. *PLoS Pathogens* 4, e1000154.

Means, T.K., Mylonakis, E., Tampakakis, E., Colvin, R.A., Seung, E., Puckett, L., Tai, M.F., Stewart, C.R., Pukkila-Worley, R., Hickman, S.E., Moore, K.J., Calderwood, S.B., Hacohen, N., Luster, A.D. and El Khoury, J. (2009) Evolutionarily conserved recognition and innate immunity to fungal pathogens by the scavenger receptors SCARF1 and CD36. *Journal of Experimental Medicine* 206, 637–653.

Medoff, G. and Kobayashi, G.S. (1980) Strategies in the treatment of systemic fungal infections. *New England Journal of Medicine* 302, 145–155.

Mencacci, A., Perruccio, K., Bacci, A., Cenci, E., Benedetti, R., Martelli, M.F., Bistoni, F., Coffman, R., Velardi, A. and Romani, L. (2001) Defective antifungal T-helper 1 (TH1) immunity in a murine model of allogeneic T-cell-depleted bone marrow transplantation and its restoration by treatment with TH2 cytokine antagonists. *Blood* 97, 1483–1490.

Mezger, M., Einsele, H. and Loeffler, J. (2010) Genetic susceptibility to infections with *Aspergillus fumigatus. Critical Reviews in Microbiology* 36, 168–177.

Mittendorf, J., Kunisch, F., Matzke, M., Militzer, H.C., Schmidt, A. and Schönfeld, W. (2003) Novel antifungal β-amino acids: synthesis and activity against *Candida albicans. Bioorganic and Medicinal Chemistry Letters* 13, 433–436.

Moran, G.P., Coleman, D.C. and Sullivan, D.J. (2011) Comparative genomics and the evolution of pathogenicity in human pathogenic fungi. *Eukaryotic Cell* 10, 34–42.

Morrison, B.E., Park, S.J., Mooney, J.M. and Mehrad, B. (2003) Chemokine-mediated recruitment of NK cells is a critical host defense mechanism in invasive aspergillosis. *Journal of Clinical Investigation* 112, 1862–1870.

Moss, R.B. (2010) Allergic bronchopulmonary aspergillosis and *Aspergillus* infection in cystic fibrosis. *Current Opinion in Pulmonary Medicine* 16, 598–603.

Neth, O., Jack, D.L., Dodds, A.W., Holzel, H., Klein, N.J. and Turner, M.W. (2000) Mannose-binding lectin binds to a range of clinically relevant microorganisms and promotes complement deposition. *Infection and Immunity* 68, 688–693.

Odds, F.C., Gow, N.A. and Brown, A.J. (2001) Fungal virulence studies come of age. *Genome Biology* 2, reviews1009-reviews1009.4.

Orciuolo, E., Stanzani, M., Canestraro, M., Galimberti, S., Carulli, G., Lewis, R., Petrini, M. and Komanduri, K.V. (2007) Effects of *Aspergillus fumigatus* gliotoxin and methylprednisolone on human neutrophils: implications for the pathogenesis of invasive aspergillosis. *Journal of Leukocyte Biology* 82, 839–848.

Pachi, J., Svoboda, P., Jacobs, F., Vandewoude, K., van der Hoven, B., Spronk, P., Masterson, G., Malbrain, M., Aoun, M., Garbino, J., Takala, J., Drgona, L., Burnie, J., Matthews R and the Mycograb Invasive Candidiasis Study Group (2006) A randomized, blinded, multicenter trial of lipid-associated amphotericin B alone versus in combination with an antibody-based inhibitor of heat shock protein 90 in patients with invasive candidiasis. *Clinical Infectious Diseases* 42, 1404–1413.

Pardo, J., Urban, C., Galvez, E.M., Ekert, P.G., Müller, U., Kwon-Chung, J., Lobigs, M., Müllbacher, A., Wallich, R., Borner, C. and Simon, M.M. (2006) The mitochondrial protein Bak is pivotal for gliotoxin-induced apoptosis and a critical host factor of *Aspergillus fumigatus* virulence in mice. *Journal of Cell Biology* 174, 509–519.

Parsons, A.B., Brost, R.L., Ding, H., Li, Z., Zhang, C., Sheikh, B., Brown, G.W., Kane, P.M., Hughes, T.R. and Boone, C. (2004) Integration of chemical-genetic and genetic interaction data links bioactive compounds to cellular target pathways. *Nature Biotechnology* 22, 62–69.

Parsons, A.B., Geyer, R., Hughes, T.R. and Boone, C. (2003) Yeast genomics and proteomics in drug discovery and target validation. *Progress in Cell Cycle Research* 5, 159–166.

Parsons, A.B., Lopez, A., Givoni, I.E., Williams, D.E., Gray, C.A., Porter, J., Chua, G., Sopko, R., Brost, R.L., Ho, C.H., Wang, J., Ketela, T., Brenner, C., Brill, J.A., Fernandez, G.E., Lorenz, T.C., Payne, G.S., Ishihara, S., Ohya, Y., Andrews, B., Hughes, T.R., Frey, B.J., Graham, T.R., Andersen, R.J. and Boone, C. (2006) Exploring the mode-of-action of bioactive compounds by chemical-genetic profiling in yeast. *Cell* 126, 611–625.

Paulmurugan, R., Umezawa, Y., and Gambhir, S.S. (2002) Noninvasive imaging of protein–protein interactions in living subjects using reporter protein complementation and reconstitution strategies. *Proceedings of the National Academy of Sciences* USA 99, 15608–15613.

Perruccio, K., Bozza, S., Montagnoli, C., Bellocchio, S., Aversa, F., Martelli, M., Bistoni, F., Velardi, A. and Romani, L. (2004) Prospects for dendritic cell vaccination against fungal infections in hematopoietic transplantation. *Blood Cells, Molecules, and Diseases* 33, 248–255.

Plantinga, T.S., Hamza, O.J., Willment, J.A., Ferwerda, B., van de Geer, N.M., Verweij, P.E., Matee, M.I., Banahan, K., O'Neill L.A., Kullberg, B.J., Brown, G.D., van der Ven, A.J. and Netea, M.G. (2010) Genetic variation of innate immune genes in HIV-infected African patients with or without oropharyngeal candidiasis. *Journal of Acquired Immune Deficiency Syndromes* 55, 87–94.

Pollock, J.D., Williams, D.A., Gifford, M.A.C., Li L.L., Du, X., Fisherman, J., Orkin, S.J., Doerschuk, C.M., Dinauer, M. (1995) Mouse model of X-linked chronic granulomatous disease, an inherited defect in phagocyte superoxide production. *Nature Genetics* 9, 202–209.

Romani, L. (2011) Immunity to fungal infections. *Nature Reviews Immunology* 11, 275–288.

Romani, L., Bistoni, F., Perruccio, K., Montagnoli, C., Gaziano, R., Bozza, S., Bonifazi, P., Bistoni, G., Rasi, G., Velardi, A., Fallarino, F., Garaci, E. and Puccetti, P. (2006) Thymosin $\alpha 1$ activates dendritic cell tryptophan catabolism and establishes a regulatory environment for balance of inflammation and tolerance. *Blood* 108, 2265–2274.

Sambatakou, H., Pravica, V., Hutchinson, I.V. and Denning, D.W. (2006) Cytokine profiling of pulmonary aspergillosis. *International Journal of Immunogenetics* 33, 297–302.

Schrettl, M., Bignell, E., Kragl, C., Joechl, C., Rogers, T., Arst, H.N. Jr, Haynes, K. and Haas, H. (2004) Siderophore biosynthesis but not reductive iron assimilation is essential for *Aspergillus fumigatus* virulence. *Journal of Experimental Medicine* 200, 1213–1219.

Schrettl, M., Bignell, E., Kragl, C., Sabiha, Y., Loss, O., Eisendle, M., Wallner, A., Arst, H.N. Jr, Haynes, K. and Haas, H. (2007) Distinct roles for intra- and extracellular siderophores during *Aspergillus fumigatus* infection. *PLoS Pathogens* 3, 1195–1207.

Schrettl, M., Kim, H.S., Eisendle, M., Kragl, C., Nierman, W.C., Heinekamp, T., Werner, E.R., Jacobsen, I., Illmer, P., Yi, H., Brakhage, A.A. and Haas, H. (2008) SreA-mediated iron regulation in *Aspergillus fumigatus. Molecular Microbiology* 70, 27–43.

Steffensen, R., Thiel, S., Varming, K., Jersild, C. and Jensenius, J.C. (2000) Detection of structural gene mutations and promoter polymorphisms in the mannan-binding lectin (MBL) gene by polymerase chain reaction with sequence-specific primers. *Journal of Immunological Methods* 241, 33–42

Sugui, J.A., Pardo, J., Chang, Y.C., Zarember, K.A., Nardone, G., Galvez, E.M., Mullbacher, A., Gallin, J.I., Simon, M.M. and Kwon-Chung, K.J. (2007) Gliotoxin is a virulence factor of *Aspergillus fumigatus*: gliP deletion attenuates virulence in mice immunosuppressed with hydrocortisone. *Eukaryotic Cell* 6, 1562–1569.

Szabo, E.K. and MacCallum. D.M. (2011) The contribution of mouse models to our understanding of systemic candidiasis. *FEMS Microbiology Letters* 320, 1–8.

Tekaia, F. and Latge, J.P. (2005) *Aspergillus fumigatus*: saprophyte or pathogen? *Current Opinion in Microbiology* 8, 385–392.

Uhl, M.A., Biery, M., Craig, N. and Johnson, A.D. (2003) Haploinsufficiency-based large-scale forward genetic analysis of filamentous growth in the diploid human fungal pathogen *C. albicans. EMBO Journal* 22, 2668–2678.

Vaid, M., Kaur, S., Sambatakou, H., Madan, T., Denning, D.W. and Sarma, P.U. (2007) Distinct alleles of mannose-binding lectin (MBL) and surfactant proteins A (SP-A) in patients with chronic cavitary pulmonary aspergillosis and allergic bronchopulmonary aspergillosis. *Clinical Chemistry and Laboratory Medicine* 45, 183–186.

van der Meer, J.W., van der Veerdonk, F.L., Joosten, L.A., Kullberg, B.J. and Netea, M.G. (2010) Severe *Candida* spp. infections: new insights into natural immunity. *International Journal of Antimicrobial Agents* 36 (Suppl. 2), S58–S62.

van Het, H.M., Rast, T.J., Martchenko, M., Grindle, S., Dignard, D., Hogues, H., Cuomo, C., Berriman, M., Scherer, S., Magee, B.B., Whiteway, M., Chibana, H., Nantel, A. and Magee, P.T. (2007) Assembly of the *Candida albicans* genome into sixteen supercontigs aligned on the eight chromosomes. *Genome Biology* 8, R52.

Walsh, T.J., Hiemenz, J. and Pizzo, P.A. (1994) Evolving risk factors for invasive fungal infections – all neutropenic patients are not the same. Clinical Infectious Diseases 18, 793–798.

Zaas, A.K., Liao, G., Chien, J.W., Weinberg, C., Shore, D., Giles, S.S., Marr, K.A., Usuka, J., Burch, L.H., Perera, L., Perfect, J.R., Peltz, G. and Schwartz, D.A. (2008) Plasminogen alleles influence susceptibility to invasive aspergillosis. *PLoS Genetics* 4, e1000101.

Zak, D.E. and Aderem, A. (2009) Systems biology of innate immunity. *Immunology Reviews* 227, 264–282.

Zmeili, O.S. and Soubani, A.O. (2007) Pulmonary aspergillosis: a clinical update. *Quarterly Journal Of Medicine* 100, 317–334.

18 *In Vivo* High-throughput Antimicrobial Discovery Screens Utilizing *Caenorhabditis elegans* as an Alternative Host

Jeffrey J. Coleman and Eleftherios Mylonakis
Division of Infectious Diseases, Massachusetts General Hospital, Harvard Medical School, Boston, Massachusetts, USA

18.1 Introduction

The identification and development of compounds with antimicrobial activity remains of paramount importance to circumvent the increasing frequency of infection from antibiotic-resistant microbial pathogens. Traditionally, antimicrobial compounds have been screened and identified by their ability to directly inhibit microbial growth (microbiostatic) or kill the microbe (microbicidal). While this drug-discovery method has provided many useful antibiotics, shortcomings exist such as a limited number of potential target sites, and therefore antibiotic discovery has been unable to keep pace with the acquired antimicrobial resistance to these compounds (Walsh, 2003; Bush, 2004; Wright, 2007; Miller and Waldrop, 2010). Additionally, many of the compounds identified as having antimicrobial properties are toxic to mammalian cells, creating the potential for harmful side effects. Another shortfall to conventional antimicrobial assays includes an inability to assess physiochemical properties (e.g. solubility, tissue penetration/permeability) of the compound. To circumvent these issues, *in vivo* screening of potential antimicrobial compounds allows simultaneous assessment of antimicrobial activity and toxicity and other physiochemical properties.

18.2 *Caenorhabditis elegans* as a Host for *In Vivo* Studies

A number of metazoan alternative hosts have been developed to study microbial infection, including the fruit fly (*Drosophila melanogaster*), larvae of the greater wax moth (*Galleria mellonella*) and zebrafish (*Danio rerio*), all of which have been reviewed previously (Fuchs and Mylonakis, 2006; Mylonakis *et al.*, 2007; Mylonakis, 2008; O'Callaghan and Vergunst, 2010). However, *C. elegans*, a transparent, free-living nematode from soil, has been used extensively as an alternative host for a number of bacterial and fungal pathogens for studies on both the immune response of the nematode and virulence of the pathogen.

The attractiveness of *C. elegans* as a model host has arisen for several reasons. Adult nematodes are hermaphroditic and so self-fertilize, creating numerous genetically identical progeny within their short reproductive cycle. The small size and transparent body of the nematode enables numerous worms to be placed within a single microtitre plate well, which then can be monitored by microscopy. Furthermore, numerous molecular techniques have been developed for use on *C. elegans*, in particular RNA interference for each gene of the nematode (Kamath *et al.*, 2003), where the mRNA of specific genes of interest is selectively degraded, essentially drastically reducing the amount of gene product that is translated into active protein. Previous research using the nematode has mapped the cell linage of the adult nematode, and the animal's genome has been sequenced and annotated.

Portions of the innate immune system of the nematode are evolutionarily conserved with humans (Irazoqui *et al.*, 2010). The *C. elegans* p38 mitogen-activated protein (MAP) kinase signalling pathway, composed of NSY-1/SEK-1/PMK-1, is involved in the immune response to a number of microbial pathogens (Kim *et al.*, 2002). Additionally, *C. elegans* possesses several other cellular immune response pathways that appear to function in parallel with the p38 MAP kinase cascade. The insulin/insulin growth factor receptor pathway composed of DAF-2 and DAF-16 is able to confer a phenotype suggestive of being involved in the immune response to both Gram-positive and Gram-negative bacterial pathogens; however, during pathogen infection of the nematode, DAF-16 does not appear to be activated (Garsin *et al.*, 2002). Nevertheless, a number of alternative pathways involving various immune response patterns have been identified, including a transforming growth factor-β pathway, a programmed cell death/unfolded protein response, a pathway with FSHR-1 as a receptor and a pathway involving β-catenin (Aballay and Ausubel, 2001; Haskins *et al.*, 2008; Irazoqui *et al.*, 2008; Powell *et al.*, 2009).

Many microbial pathogens form a lethal persistent infection, usually colonizing the intestinal tract of the nematode (Sifri *et al.*, 2005). These pathogens rely on some of the same virulence factors to establish and maintain these infections in *C. elegans* as they do in mammals. These factors include secreted proteins and toxins, type III secretion systems and their associated effectors, traits of the microbial cell wall involved in virulence and the regulatory proteins involved in cellular signalling during infection (Sifri *et al.*, 2005).

C. elegans has been used previously as a whole organism amendable to high-throughput or semi-high-throughput compound screens (Kwok *et al.*, 2006; Gosai *et al.*, 2010). Besides conservation of the innate immune response in the nematode, the organism has several additional attributes that have made it ideal for use in high-throughput antimicrobial compound screens. The facile infection procedure for the nematode requires replacing the normal *Escherichia coli* food source with the pathogen of interest and allowing sufficient time for the nematode to feed on the pathogenic microbe. In addition to circumventing the aforementioned toxicity and permeability issues, the *in vivo* nature of the antimicrobial screens permits detection of compounds that may otherwise be overlooked in traditional antimicrobial assays. As some microbial virulence factors are only expressing during the infection process, compounds that inhibit these virulence factors and confer an increase in nematode survival can only be identified during *in vivo* assays. Alternatively, compounds that are capable of favourably altering the immune response to the pathogen will only be identified using a suitable host. As antimicrobial assays using *C. elegans* as a heterologous host allow identification of compounds that have these characteristics, although not necessarily direct antimicrobial activity, a more precise term for compounds able to increase nematode survival are 'anti-infective' compounds (Moy *et al.*, 2006).

18.3 Antibacterial Drug Discovery

The feasibility of infecting *C. elegans* with bacterial pathogens has aided its utility as a heterologous host for numerous clinically important pathogens including *Acinetobacter baumannii*, *Burkholderia cepacia*, pathogenic *E. coli*, *Enterococcus faecalis*, *Pseudomonas aeruginosa*, *Salmonella enterica*, *Serratia marcescens*, *Staphylococcus aureus*, *Streptococcus pneumoniae*, *Streptococcus pyogenes* and *Yersinia pestis* (Sifri *et al.*, 2005). The enterococci, commensal bacteria that inhabit the intestine of many metazoans, are collectively the third most common cause of bacteraemia, causing enterococcal sepsis leading to death in up to 50% of cases (Jett *et al.*, 1994). Of the enterococci, the isolated causative organism in approximately 80% of the cases is *E. faecalis* (Jett *et al.*, 1994). Although *E. faecalis* is frequently found in the gastrointestinal tract, several virulence factors have been identified that allow the bacterium to adhere to and invade host tissues (Jett *et al.*, 1994). *E. faecalis* is intrinsically resistant to a number of clinically used antibiotics, and plasmid- or transposon-acquired resistance has emerged for several other antibiotics including vancomycin (Huycke *et al.*, 1998), which is usually viewed as the antibiotic of 'last resort'. The prevalence and resistance profile to antibiotics has generated a renewed interest in developing alternative antibiotics for additional treatment options (Huycke *et al.*, 1998).

The first anti-infective compound screen utilizing *C. elegans* was carried out to identify compounds active against *E. faecalis* (Moy *et al.*, 2006). This study developed the assay for screening in a liquid medium, which ultimately enabled the procedure to be adapted for use with instrumentation. A screen of 7136 compounds (6000 synthesized small-molecule compounds and 1136 natural-product extracts) identified 18 synthesized compounds (0.3% hit rate) and nine natural-product extracts (0.8% hit rate) responsible for increased survival of *E. faecalis*-infected nematodes (Moy *et al.*, 2006). Sixteen of the small-molecule compounds were evaluated further, and five were capable of increasing nematode survival threefold or more, while another eight increased nematode survival at least twofold (Moy *et al.*, 2006). Seven of these compounds had a low minimum inhibitory concentration (MIC); however, six of the small-molecule compounds (and two of the natural-product extracts) had an MIC higher than the concentration required to confer an increase in nematode survival *in vivo*, suggesting that their activity may be derived from something other than direct inhibition of bacterial growth (Moy *et al.*, 2006). None of the 16 small-molecule compounds demonstrated cytotoxicity to *C. elegans* or was able to cause haemolysis of sheep erythrocytes (Moy *et al.*, 2006).

Advancements made to the *E. faecalis/C. elegans* 'curing' assay enabled an increase in accuracy and the number of compounds that could be screened at a single time. This was accomplished by use of the nematodes in a 384-well microtitre plate, instrumentation to dispense the correct number of nematodes within the wells and an imaging system/procedure/software to facilitate scoring the results of the screen (Moy *et al.*, 2009). A total of 37,214 small molecules and natural-product extracts were screened using this procedure, identifying 92 compounds and extracts (0.25% hit rate) able to increase *E. faecalis*-infected nematode survival (Moy *et al.*, 2009). Of these 92 compounds, 65 were compounds with previously known antimicrobial activity or with a chemical structure similar to a known antimicrobial agent (Moy *et al.*, 2009). Twenty-one of the remaining 27 compounds were subjected to further analysis, and nine of the compounds were capable of curing *C. elegans* of the *E. faecalis* infection at a significantly lower concentration than the MIC, suggesting that the compounds acted by either inhibiting virulence factors or by promoting the immune response (Moy *et al.*, 2009). In total, six structural classes of small molecules were identified as anti-infectives that may act in a novel fashion to overcome the bacterial infection (Moy *et al.*, 2009).

One of the most time-consuming steps in the antimicrobial compound discovery screens is scoring the nematodes at the conclusion of the assay. Previously, in order to determine whether nematodes were alive or dead, the shape of the nematodes was assessed, as dead worms frequently take on a rod shape while those that are alive have a sinusoidal shape (Moy *et al.*, 2006). In lieu of this subjective scoring method, staining the worms with SYTOX® Orange allowed rapid assessment of *C. elegans* survival, as the dye is readily taken up by cells with damaged membranes and therefore specifically stains dead nematodes (Fig. 18.1) (Gill *et al.*, 2003). A series of several steps using the image analysis software CellProfiler further facilitated the scoring of the nematodes by calculating the ratio between the fluorescent area within a well and the total area of the well (Moy *et al.*, 2006). Several developments of the software CellProfiler and CellProfiler Analyst allow image-based data from high-throughput screens to be quickly analysed enabling scoring without visual confirmation by microscopy (Carpenter *et al.*, 2006; Lamprecht *et al.*, 2007; Jones *et al.*, 2008).

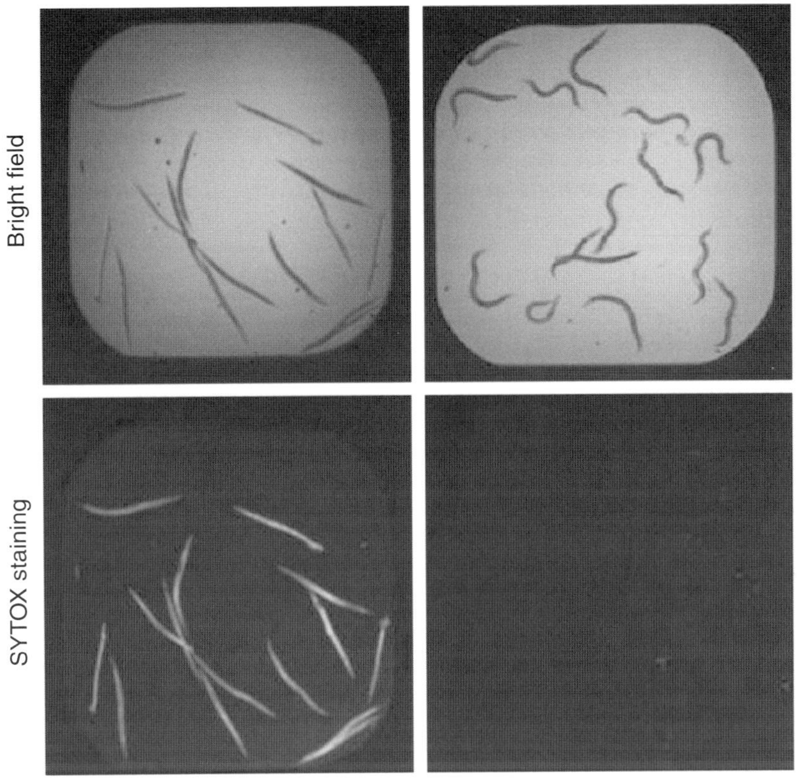

Fig. 18.1. Representative wells at the conclusion of the drug discovery screen utilizing SYTOX Orange for scoring. The top images are of two wells visualized by bright-field microscopy, while the bottom images are the same wells after staining with SYTOX Orange. The left panels are representative of a compound unable to 'cure' the worms of the bacterial infection, while the right panels are of a compound able to confer an increase in nematode survival. Dead nematodes have a characteristic rod shape, whereas live nematodes retain their sinusoidal shape.

18.4 Antifungal Drug Discovery

C. elegans has served as an alternative host for several medically important fungi such as *Candida albicans*, *Candida glabrata*, *Cryptococcus neoformans* and *Histoplasma capsulatum* (Mylonakis *et al.*, 2002; Breger *et al.*, 2007; Thakur *et al.*, 2008; Johnson *et al.*, 2009). *Candida* spp. are the fourth most common pathogen isolated from the bloodstream, and nosocomial bloodstream infections may reach a mortality rate of approximately 40% (Pfaller and Diekema, 2007; Pukkila-Worley *et al.*, 2009a). The prevalence of *Candida* spp. in patients, the ability of the fungus to form a biofilm on medical devices and the incidence of resistance to clinically used antifungal agents has created a need for either improved antifungal compounds or new classes of compounds capable of inhibiting the progression of *Candida* spp. (d'Enfert, 2006; Spanakis *et al.*, 2006).

Candida spp., including *C. albicans*, have been shown to be able to form a persistent lethal infection in *C. elegans* (Breger *et al.*, 2007). The switch from yeast morphology to hyphal growth has been shown to be a key virulence factor in mammalian systems (Calderone and Fonzi, 2001; Kumamoto and Vinces, 2005). *C. albicans* hyphal formation is also a virulence factor for *C. elegans*, as mutations of key components involved in this morphological transition render the fungus less virulent (Breger *et al.*, 2007; Pukkila-Worley *et al.*, 2009b). Several transcription factors involved in either hyphal formation or fungal cell-wall integrity are virulence factors for both mammals and *C. elegans* (Pukkila-Worley *et al.*, 2009b), further supporting the use of *C. elegans* as an suitable alternative host for fungi, including *in vivo* antifungal compound screens.

A screen of 1266 compounds for antifungal activity utilizing *C. elegans* as a heterologous host initially identified 15 compounds (1.18% hit rate) that were able to significantly prolong the life of *C. albicans*-infected nematodes and were able to inhibit fungal filamentation (Breger *et al.*, 2007). Three of the compounds identified were subsequently tested in a murine model for treatment of candidiasis, and caffeic acid phenethyl ester (CAPE) and enoxacin displayed efficacy in this mammalian system. Furthermore, CAPE was capable of inhibiting biofilm formation of *C. albicans*. This initial screen worked by feeding the nematodes *C. albicans* prior to placing the nematodes into the microtitre plate containing the compound, thereby making the screening process labour-intensive. Subsequently, modifications to the procedure demonstrated that the screen could be conducted without prior infection of *C. elegans* with *C. albicans*, reducing the time necessary to carry out the assay (Tampakakis *et al.*, 2008; Okoli *et al.*, 2009).

These modifications allowed a second screen of 3228 compounds to be carried out for antifungal activity (Okoli *et al.*, 2009). Nineteen compounds were identified (0.59% hit rate) that were able to prolong nematode survival, including seven clinically used antifungal agents and three immunosuppressants (Fig. 18.2; Okoli *et al.*, 2009). Importantly, both antifungal screens were able to successfully identify all known compounds with antifungal activity (Breger *et al.*, 2007; Okoli *et al.*, 2009). Moreover, this screen was able to demonstrate that the *C. elegans*/*C. albicans* antifungal assay is able to determine if a compound is toxic at higher concentrations. Malachite green carbinol base was able to confer an increase in nematode survival; however, as the concentration of compound increased, *C. elegans* survival rapidly decreased, despite no apparent growth of *C. albicans* in the well, suggesting that higher concentrations of the compound is toxic to *C. elegans* (Okoli *et al.*, 2009). In agreement with this data, malachite green was previously shown to be cytotoxic to mammalian cells (Fessard *et al.*, 1999).

The *C. elegans*/*C. albicans* antifungal compound screen was able to identify several natural products with efficacy against the fungal pathogen. Twelve compounds from plants, termed saponins, were able to significantly prolong nematode survival when challenged with *C. albicans* (Coleman *et al.*, 2010). Based on dose–response curves, some of the saponins were able to confer nematode survival to

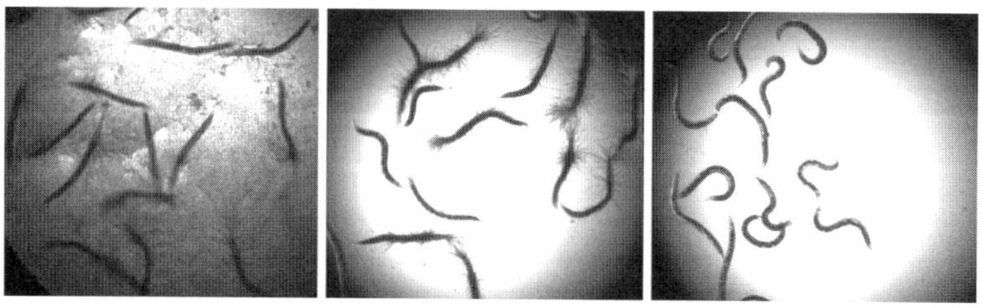

Fig. 18.2. Depiction of *C. albicans*-infected nematodes at the conclusion of an antifungal compound assay. The left panel shows a microtitre plate well containing a compound with no antifungal activity. Note the rod shape of the dead *C. elegans* and growth of *C. albicans* in the medium in the well. The middle panel shows a well containing a compound able to inhibit *C. albicans* growth *in vitro*, although not able to confer an increase in nematode survival, as hyphal filaments are visible extending from the body of the nematode. The right panel shows a microtitre plate well containing a compound with *in vivo* antifungal activity conferring nematode survival. The sinusoidal shape of the nematodes suggest that they are still alive. (Modified from Okoli *et al.*, 2009.)

a similar degree as amphotericin B, an antifungal agent in clinical use (Coleman *et al.*, 2010). Two saponins were selected for further evaluation and were able to impede biofilm formation and displayed no haemolytic activity, a trait normally associated with saponins (Coleman *et al.*, 2010). The saponins were able to facilitate photodynamic inactivation of the fungus by increasing membrane permeability, enabling the photosensitizer to enter the fungal cell more efficiently. The identification of many compounds within the saponin class of natural products using the *C. elegan/C. albicans* antifungal assay validates the ability of this system to detect structure–activity relationships that could be exploited for further development of antifungal agents for future use.

18.5 Conclusions

Several characteristics of *C. elegans* are advantageous for amenability to high-throughput screening assays for antimicrobial compounds. The evolutionarily conserved pathways of the innate immune response between the nematode and mammals and the overlap of virulence factors required for infection of the host allow an *in vivo* screening method to identify novel compounds that can be exploited for further development. These compounds may not only directly inhibit the growth of the microbe but may also impede the virulence of the pathogen and/or alter the immune response, and are therefore referred to as anti-infectives. High-throughput drug-discovery screening assays have been developed using *E. faecalis* and *C. albicans* as pathogens, yielding numerous compounds that have not previously been identified or explored as potential antibiotics. The success of these few screens have indicated that additional compounds are yet to be discovered by taking advantage of *C. elegans* in whole-animal *in vivo* antimicrobial discovery assays.

Acknowledgements

We would like to thank Younghoon Kim for providing the images used in Fig. 18.1. This work was supported by a National Institutes of Health R01 award (AI075286), a P01 award (AI083214) and an R21 award (AI079569) to E.M. and a T32 award (AI007061) to J.J.C.

References

Aballay, A. and Ausubel, F.M. (2001) Programmed cell death mediated by *ced-3* and *ced-4* protects *Caenorhabditis elegans* from *Salmonella typhimurium*-mediated killing. *Proceedings of the National Academy of Sciences USA* 98, 2735–2739.

Breger, J., Fuchs, B.B., Aperis, G., Moy, T.I., Ausubel, F.M. and Mylonakis, E. (2007) Antifungal chemical compounds identified using a *C. elegans* pathogenicity assay. *PLoS Pathogens* 3, e18.

Bush, K. (2004) Antibacterial drug discovery in the 21st century. *Clinical Microbiology and Infection* 10 (Suppl. 4), 10–17.

Calderone, R.A. and Fonzi, W.A. (2001) Virulence factors of *Candida albicans. Trends in Microbiology* 9, 327–335.

Carpenter, A., Jones, T., Lamprecht, M., Clarke, C., Kang, I., Friman, O., Guertin, D., Chang, J., Lindquist, R., Moffat, J., Golland, P. and Sabatini, D. (2006) CellProfiler: image analysis software for identifying and quantifying cell phenotypes. *Genome Biology* 7, R100.

Coleman, J.J., Okoli, I., Tegos, G.P., Holson, E.B., Wagner, F.F., Hamblin, M.R. and Mylonakis, E. (2010) Characterization of plant-derived saponin natural products against *Candida albicans. ACS Chemical Biology* 5, 321–332.

d'Enfert, C. (2006) Biofilms and their role in the resistance of pathogenic *Candida* to antifungal agents. *Current Drug Targets* 7, 465–470.

Fessard, V., Godard, T., Huet, S., Mourot, A. and Poul, J.M. (1999) Mutagenicity of malachite green and leucomalachite green in *in vitro* tests. *Journal of Applied Toxicology* 19, 421–430.

Fuchs, B.B. and Mylonakis, E. (2006) Using non-mammalian hosts to study fungal virulence and host defense. *Current Opinion in Microbiology* 9, 346–351.

Garsin, D.A., Villanueva, J.M., Begun, J., Kim, D.H., Sifri, C.D., Calderwood, S.B., Ruvkun, G. and Ausubel, F.M. (2002) Long-lived *C. elegans daf-2* mutants are resistant to bacterial pathogens. *Science* 300, 1921.

Gill, M.S., Olsen, A., Sampayo, J.N. and Lithgow, G.J. (2003) An automated high-throughput assay for survival of the nematode *Caenorhabditis elegans. Free Radical Biology and Medicine* 35, 558–565.

Gosai, S.J., Kwak, J.H., Luke, C.J., Long, O.S., King, D.E., Kovatch, K.J., Johnston, P.A., Shun, T.Y., Lazo, J.S., Perlmutter, D.H., Silverman, G.A. and Pak, S.C. (2010) Automated high-content live animal drug screening using *C. elegans* expressing the aggregation prone serpin α1-antitrypsin Z. *PLoS ONE,* 5, e15460.

Haskins, K.A., Russell, J.F., Gaddis, N., Dressman, H.K. and Aballay, A. (2008) Unfolded protein response genes regulated by CED-1 are required for *Caenorhabditis elegans* innate immunity. *Developmental Cell* 15, 87–97.

Huycke, M.M., Sahm, D.F. and Gilmore, M.S. (1998) Multiple-drug resistant enterococci: the nature of the problem and an agenda for the future. *Emerging Infectious Diseases* 4, 239–249.

Irazoqui, J.E., Ng, A., Xavier, R.J. and Ausubel, F.M. (2008) Role for β-catenin and HOX transcription factors in *Caenorhabditis elegans* and mammalian host epithelial–pathogen interactions. *Proceedings of the National Academy of Sciences USA* 105, 17469–17474.

Irazoqui, J.E., Urbach, J.M. and Ausubel, F.M. (2010) Evolution of host innate defence: insights from *Caenorhabditis elegans* and primitive invertebrates. *Nature Reviews Immunology* 10, 47–58.

Jett, B.D., Huycke, M.M. and Gilmore, M.S. (1994) Virulence of enterococci. *Clinical Microbiology Reviews* 7, 462–478.

Johnson, C.H., Ayyadevara, S., McEwen, J.E. and Reis, R.J.S. (2009) *Histoplasma capsulatum* and *Caenorhabditis elegans*: a simple nematode model for an innate immune response to fungal infection. *Medical Mycology* 47, 808–813.

Jones, T., Kang, I., Wheeler, D., Lindquist, R., Papallo, A., Sabatini, D., Golland, P. and Carpenter, A. (2008) CellProfiler Analyst: data exploration and analysis software for complex image-based screens. *BMC Bioinformatics* 9, 482.

Kamath, R.S., Fraser, A.G., Dong, Y., Poulin, G., Durbin, R., Gotta, M., Kanapin, A., Le Bot, N., Moreno, S., Sohrmann, M., Welchman, D.P., Zipperlen, P. and Ahringer, J. (2003) Systematic functional analysis of the *Caenorhabditis elegans* genome using RNAi. *Nature* 421, 231–237.

Kim, D.H., Feinbaum, R., Alloing, G., Emerson, F.E., Garsin, D.A., Inoue, H., Tanaka-Hino, M., Hisamoto, N., Matsumoto, K., Tan, M.-W. and Ausubel, F.M. (2002) A conserved p38 MAP kinase pathway in *Caenorhabditis elegans* innate immunity. *Science* 297, 623–626.

Kumamoto, C.A. and Vinces, M.D. (2005) Contributions of hyphae and hypha-co-regulated genes to *Candida albicans* virulence. *Cellular Microbiology* 7, 1546–1554.

Kwok, T.C., Ricker, N., Fraser, R., Chan, A.W., Burns, A., Stanley, E.F., McCourt, P., Cutler, S.R. and Roy, P.J. (2006) A small-molecule screen in *C. elegans* yields a new calcium channel antagonist. *Nature* 441, 91–95.

Lamprecht, M.R., Sabatini, D.M. and Carpenter, A.E. (2007) CellProfiler: free versatile software for automated biological image analysis. *Biotechniques* 42, 71–75.

Miller, J.R. and Waldrop, G.L. (2010) Discovery of novel antibacterials. *Expert Opinion on Drug Discovery* 5, 145–154.

Moy, T.I., Ball, A.R., Anklesaria, Z., Casadei, G., Lewis, K. and Ausubel, F.M. (2006) Identification of novel antimicrobials using a live-animal infection model. *Proceedings of the National Academy of Sciences USA* 103, 10414–10419.

Moy, T.I., Conery, A.L., Larkins-Ford, J., Wu, G., Mazitschek, R., Casadei, G., Lewis, K., Carpenter, A.E. and Ausubel, F.M. (2009) High-throughput screen for novel antimicrobials using a whole animal infection model. *ACS Chemical Biology* 4, 527–533.

Mylonakis, E. (2008) *Galleria mellonella* and the study of fungal pathogenesis: making the case for another genetically tractable model host. *Mycopathologia* 165, 1–3.

Mylonakis, E., Ausubel, F.M., Perfect, J.R., Heitman, J. and Calderwood, S.B. (2002) Killing of *Caenorhabditis elegans* by *Cryptococcus neoformans* as a model of yeast pathogenesis. *Proceedings of the National Academy of Sciences USA* 99, 15675–15680.

Mylonakis, E., Casadevall, A. and Ausubel, F.M. (2007) Exploiting amoeboid and non-vertebrate animal model systems to study the virulence of human pathogenic fungi. *PLoS Pathogens* 3, e101.

O'Callaghan, D. and Vergunst, A. (2010) Non-mammalian animal models to study infectious disease: worms or fly fishing? *Current Opinion in Microbiology* 13, 79–85.

Okoli, I., Coleman, J.J., Tampakakis, E., An, W.F., Holson, E., Wagner, F., Conery, A.L., Larkins-Ford, J., Wu, G., Stern, A., Ausubel, F.M. and Mylonakis, E. (2009) Identification of antifungal compounds active against *Candida albicans* using an improved high-throughput *Caenorhabditis elegans* assay. *PLoS ONE* 4, e7025.

Pfaller, M.A. and Diekema, D.J. (2007) Epidemiology of invasive candidiasis: a persistent public health problem. *Clinical Microbiology Reviews* 20, 133–163.

Powell, J.R., Kim, D.H. and Ausubel, F.M. (2009) The G protein-coupled receptor FSHR-1 is required for the *Caenorhabditis elegans* innate

immune response. *Proceedings of the National Academy of Sciences USA* 106, 2782–2787.
Pukkila-Worley, R., Holson, E., Wagner, F. and Mylonakis, E. (2009a) Antifungal drug discovery through the study of invertebrate model hosts. *Current Medicinal Chemistry* 16, 1588–1595.
Pukkila-Worley, R., Peleg, A.Y., Tampakakis, E. and Mylonakis, E. (2009b) *Candida albicans* hyphal formation and virulence assessed using a *Caenorhabditis elegans* infection model. *Eukaryotic Cell* 8, 1750–1758.
Sifri, C.D., Begun, J. and Ausubel, F.M. (2005) The worm has turned – microbial virulence modeled in *Caenorhabditis elegans. Trends in Microbiology* 13, 119–127.
Spanakis, E., Aperis, G. and Mylonakis, E. (2006) New agents for the treatment of fungal infections: clinical efficacy and gaps in coverage. *Clinical Infectious Diseases* 43, 1060–1068.
Tampakakis, E., Okoli, I. and Mylonakis, E. (2008) A *C. elegans*-based, whole animal, *in vivo* screen for the identification of antifungal compounds. *Nature Protocols* 3, 1925–1931.
Thakur, J., Arthanari, H., Yang, F., Pan, S.-J., Fan, X., Breger, J., Frueh, D., Gulshan, K., Li, D., Mylonakis, E., Struhl, K., Moye-Rowley, S., Cormack, B., Wagner, G. and Naar, A. (2008) A nuclear receptor-like pathway regulating multidrug resistance in fungi. *Nature* 452, 604–609.
Walsh, C. (2003) Where will new antibiotics come from? *Nature Reviews Microbiology* 1, 65–70.
Wright, G.D. (2007) The antibiotic resistome: the nexus of chemical and genetic diversity. *Nature Reviews Microbiology* 5, 175–186.

19 *Drosophila melanogaster* as a Versatile Model for the Discovery of Drugs Effective Against Human Microbe-induced Infection and Pathology

Yiorgos Apidianakis[1] and Dimitrios P. Kontoyiannis[2]
[1]*Department of Biological Sciences, University of Cyprus, Nicosia, Cyprus;*
[2]*Department of Infectious Diseases, Infection Control and Employee Health, The University of Texas: MD Anderson Cancer Center, Houston, Texas, USA*

19.1 Introduction

Antimicrobial drug discovery has focused mainly on the identification of microbicidal and microbiostatic drugs that kill and stop the growth of microbes, respectively. Indeed, many *in vitro* high-throughput drug screens have been employed, and many antibiotics that target microbial survival and growth outside hosts have been developed. Yet this approach comes with significant caveats. First, the rate of identification of new antibiotics has dropped over the last two decades, and secondly, microbes have exhibited remarkable efficiency in becoming resistant to existing antibiotics (Gould, 2010).

Microbes are infectious because of their interaction with the host. This means that using chemicals that either inhibit pathogen virulence or alter host defence (e.g. by boosting the immune response to increase resistance to infection) is an open area of drug development (Martinez and Silley, 2010). Therefore, a reasonable procedure is to assess the antimicrobial efficiency of drugs in mammalian hosts that mimic human disease. However, using mammalian models of infectious disease is costly, laborious and time-consuming; thus, these models are inappropriate for high-throughput or large-scale drug screening. Simpler model organisms can be used as bridges between *in vitro* and mammalian model-based screening (Kurz and Ewbank, 2007; Giacomotto and Ségalat, 2010). Among these simpler models, *Drosophila melanogaster* has unique benefits.

In this chapter, we will describe the benefits and limitations of using *Drosophila* as a model for identification of anti-infective drugs, i.e. drugs that modulate microbial virulence or host defence. We will also describe the efforts to model human bacterial and fungal infections in flies. We will not discuss studies of microbial infections that affect flies but not humans, because they are not directly applicable to human infectious diseases or antimicrobial drug discovery, even though they are very important in terms of basic biology. Finally, we will discuss the potential of large-scale toxicity analysis and anti-infective drug screening using *Drosophila*.

19.2 *D. melanogaster* as a Simple Host for Studying Infections

19.2.1 Biology of the fly

Flies are facile and cost-effective models. They can be cultured in small (20–100 ml) vials or bottles on a cornmeal medium supplemented with yeast, sucrose and agar. At 25°C, the generation time from egg to adult ranges from 10 to 12 days. The fly life cycle has four stages: embryo, larva, pupa and adult. Embryogenesis is completed in about 24 h at 25°C. The larval stage lasts for 4 days, during which time the larval body size increases 30-fold. This is followed by the pupal stage, which lasts for 5–6 days and is when metamorphosis, a dramatic period of tissue reorganization culminating in the development of the adult structures from the precursor imaginal disc tissues, takes place. A newly hatched adult fly can feed on the same medium on which it is cultured, mate and proceed through the *Drosophila* life cycle (Miller, 1994).

19.2.2 Innate immunity, blood cells and the fat body

The value of flies in studying infectious disease was established over the past two decades mainly because of seminal work on the identification of conserved innate immune pathways, the tissues in which they are activated and their specificity against different microbes (Lemaitre *et al.*, 1996, Lemaitre and Hoffmann, 2007). Indeed, *Drosophila* elicits a highly conserved response to bacteria, fungi and viruses mainly via the activation of Imd, Toll, Jak/Stat and Jnk pathways, leading to the expression of antimicrobial peptides and many other genes (de Gregorio *et al.*, 2001). In addition, flies have haemocytes, which are types of blood cells that are equivalent to human macrophages, and the fat body, which is equivalent to adipose tissue and the liver in humans (Lemaitre and Hoffmann, 2007). Haemocyte-like cell lines are available, allowing the study of antiphagocytic and signalling properties of haemocytes. To date, many screens of haemocyte-derived cells have been performed at various institutions, including the *Drosophila* RNAi Screening Center at Harvard Medical School (http://www.flyrnai.org), providing the possibility of combined gene knockdown and high-throughput small-molecule screening (Perrimon *et al.*, 2007; Mohr *et al.*, 2010). Haemocytes, the fat body and *Drosophila* epithelial immune responses activate antimicrobial peptides, which are conserved in humans. However, flies lack adaptive immunity, a closed circulatory system and specialized cells that bridge mammalian innate and adaptive immunity (e.g. dendritic cells and mast cells). Thus, notwithstanding the anatomical and immunological differences between flies and mammals, research focusing on the conserved aspects of host–microbe interaction in *D. melanogaster* can reveal novel mechanistic insights that can shift current paradigms regarding pathogenesis and provide ample opportunity for drug screening assay development.

19.2.3 Muscle and intestinal infections

Human wound, systemic and intestinal infections can be easily mimicked in *Drosophila* after pricking, injecting and feeding flies, respectively, with pathogens (Apidianakis and Rahme, 2009). For example, studies of wound infections in flies have highlighted the role of muscle tissue homeostasis in the infection process. Specifically, wound infection proceeds more rapidly if *Drosophila* muscle gene expression is impaired (Apidianakis *et al.*, 2007). Importantly, the fly musculature has significant similarities with the mammalian musculature in terms of cell biology and metabolism (Daczewska *et al.*, 2010). Thus, muscle regeneration and wasting following wounding and infection can be studied in flies.

In addition, the fly gut and mammalian gut are strikingly similar (Apidianakis and Rahme, 2011). Fly intestines have epithelial monolayers that contain stem cells and mature enterocytes, some of which, similarly to mammals, have subcellular extensions on the apical side called microvilli that face the gut lumen (Gartner, 1970; Baumann, 2001; Shanbhag and Tripathi, 2009). In addition, a layer of mucus protects both mammals and flies from infection by intestinal microbes, whereas the *Drosophila* gut is also lined by a chitin layer that helps protect it from direct contact with microbes (Vodovar *et al.*, 2005). The epithelial monolayer resides on an extracellular collagenous matrix called the basement membrane. Attached to the basement membrane longitudinal and circular muscles are innervated and oxygenated by the trachea to drive the peristaltic movements of the *Drosophila* gut (Jiang and Edgar, 2009). A similar arrangement of intestinal external musculature is found in the outer layers of the mammalian intestine, which is also innervated and oxygenated via a vasculature plexus (Kvietys and Granger, 1986; Rhee *et al.*, 2009). Noticeably, the space between the outer musculature and the basement membrane is filled, particularly in mammals, by three additional layers: the submucosa, the muscularis mucosae muscle and the lamina propria layer. Thus, interaction of microbes with human intestinal epithelium but not with the lamina propria or submucosa layers can be effectively modelled in *Drosophila*.

19.3 Human Bacterial Infections in *D. melanogaster*

The Gram-negative bacteria *Vibrio cholerae*, *Serratia marcescens* and *Pseudomonas aeruginosa*, the Gram-positive bacteria *Enterococcus faecalis*, *Staphylococcus aureus* and *Listeria monocytogenes*, and the fungi *Cryptococcus neoformans*, *Candida albicans*, *Aspergillus fumigatus* and Zygomycetes are the most common human pathogens that can be studied effectively in flies (Mansfield *et al.*, 2003; Cox and Gilmore, 2007; Nehme *et al.*, 2007; Apidianakis *et al.*, 2009; Apidianakis and Rahme, 2009). Fly models of human bacterial infections allow assessment of the virulence of various pathogens' genes and the mechanisms that the pathogens use to infect hosts.

19.3.1 *P. aeruginosa*

P. aeruginosa is a common clinical pathogen that can cause severe infections, most notably in patients with cystic fibrosis or in those in intensive care units (Lyczak *et al.*, 2000). A recent increase in the incidence of infection with multidrug-resistant isolates of *P. aeruginosa* has raised serious concerns (Hirsch and Tam, 2010). *P. aeruginosa* is the most studied human bacterial pathogen in *Drosophila*. Researchers have shown that a very low number of bacteria can kill flies very efficiently in a matter of hours (D'argenio *et al.*, 2001; Lau *et al.*, 2003). Moreover, studies using *Drosophila* have revealed the anti-innate immunity action of this pathogen. Indeed, *P. aeruginosa* can suppress antimicrobial peptide induction and local tissue responses via prominent virulence factors (Apidianakis *et al.*, 2005). Thus, investigators have employed large-scale virulence screens to discover many new virulence factors (D'argenio *et al.*, 2001; Kim *et al.*, 2008). In addition, intestinal *P. aeruginosa* infection exhibits compensatory proliferation, which benefits a wild-type host but is detrimental to a host genetically predisposed to tumour development (Apidianakis *et al.*, 2009).

19.3.2 *V. cholerae*

Cholera, the pandemic diarrhoeal disease caused by the Gram-negative bacterium *V. cholerae*, remains a major public health concern in the developing world (Ritchie and Waldor, 2009). The cholera toxin, which is responsible for the voluminous stools that accompany cholera, constitutively activates adenylyl cyclase in the host, resulting in the export of ions from enterocytes to the intestinal lumen (Vanden Broeck *et al.*, 2007). Researchers have developed models of this disease in *Drosophila* (Blow *et al.*, 2005) and found that, similarly to *P. aeruginosa*, *V. cholerae* induces intestinal cell apoptosis, which in turn acts as a host defence response (Berkey *et al.*, 2009). In addition, as with the genes for *P. aeruginosa* and *Yersinia pseudotuberculosis*, the *V. cholerae* gene *kerV* is an important virulence factor in flies as well as in mammals (An *et al.*, 2009). Another similarity with *P. aeruginosa* is that researchers have proposed that *V. colerae* virulence factors inhibit innate immunity in *Drosophila* (Park *et al.*, 2005).

19.3.3 *S. marcescens*

S. marcescens is an important cause of hospital-acquired infections, especially in neonatal intensive care units (Dessi *et al.*, 2009). Work with *S. marcescens* has shown that this pathogen can cause intestinal infections that may become systemic (Flyg *et al.*, 1980; Nehme *et al.*, 2007). In addition, intestinal infections with *S. marcescens* activate the Jak/Stat pathway, which plays an important role in intestinal regeneration and the defence response (Cronin *et al.*, 2009; Kallio *et al.*, 2010). Interestingly, a whole-genome screen using the *Drosophila/S. marcescens* model of infection revealed multiple host genes that either increase or decrease virulence (Cronin *et al.*, 2009).

19.3.4 *E. faecalis*

E. faecalis is a normal commensal in the intestinal tract but can also cause serious, life-threatening, hospital-borne infections (Sava *et al.*, 2010). This is a result of the emergence of multidrug-resistant *E faecalis* strains and the virulence factors that they bear (Palmer *et al.*, 2010). Although sequencing of *E. faecalis* has provided much insight into its genetic makeup, drugs that are effective against the pathogenic stains of this species are lacking. Studies in *Drosophila* have shown that *E. faecalis* can colonize the intestine, and strains that express the virulence factor cytolysin are significantly more virulent than non-cytolysin-expressing strains. This is similar to what is observed in mammalian models of infection (Cox and Gilmore, 2007).

19.3.5 *S. aureus*

S. aureus is an important pathogen in humans, causing a range of superficial and potentially life-threatening diseases (Cataldo *et al.*, 2010). In *Drosophila*, this pathogen causes lethal systemic infections with similarities to infections in mammalian models. For example, *Drosophila* flies infected with reporter gene fusion strains of *S. aureus* exhibited expression of virulence factors and microcolony formation during infection. In this disease model, antibiotics typically used in the clinic proved to be efficient in clearing the bacteria. In addition, screening of specific *S. aureus* mutants for virulence identified genes important for pathogenesis (Needham *et al.*, 2004).

19.3.6 *L. monocytogenes*

L. monocytogenes, a facultative anaerobic intracellular bacterium, causes listeriosis and is one of the most virulent food-borne pathogens (Ramaswamy *et al.*, 2007). It is capable of replicating in a broad range of host-cell types and species. *L. monocytogenes* can also grow extensively and cause lethal infections in *Drosophila* adults and larvae. This bacterium can be found in the cytosol of *Drosophila* phagocytes and is capable of directing polymerization of the host-cell actin. *L. monocytogenes* gene products necessary for intracellular replication and cell-to-cell spread in mammalian cells behave similarly in fly cells. A previous study suggested that *L. monocytogenes* virulence gene expression requires temperatures higher than 30°C. Nevertheless, in insect cells, this bacterium can express virulence determinants at 25°C (Mansfield *et al.*, 2003).

19.4 Human Fungal Infections in *D. melanogaster*

The incidence of fungal infections has increased over the last three decades, making the identification of new antifungal drug targets more important than ever. The mediocre clinical efficacy of antifungals and our incomplete understanding of fungal pathogenesis contribute to an overall poor prognosis for fungal infections (Richardson and Lass-Florl, 2008). Although logistically difficult to use on a large scale, conventional animal models of fungal infections provide valuable information about both antifungal drug efficacy and fungal virulence. Existing *in vivo* mammalian models can be complemented by studies using *D. melanogaster* because the most clinically important fungal infections are effectively modelled in this species (Lionakis and Kontoyiannis, 2005; Chamilos *et al.*, 2006).

19.4.1 *C. neoformans*

C. neoformans is a facultative intracellular pathogen in macrophages that is unique among medically important fungi because it is covered by a polysaccharide capsule. Although primarily a pathogen in patients infected with human immunodeficiency virus (HIV), it can also cause severe forms of meningitis and meningoencephalitis in immunocompetent individuals (Olszewski *et al.*, 2010). Modelling of *C. neoformans* infections in flies has shown that different innate immunity pathways are used against this pathogen depending on the route of infection. Specifically, systemic infection can be cleared when the Toll innate immunity pathway is active, but the same pathway is not necessary for host defence against lethal intestinal infections (Apidianakis *et al.*, 2004).

19.4.2 *A. fumigatus* and *C. albicans*

C. albicans is the predominant fungal pathogen in humans and is an important cause of death in immunocompromised patients (Moudgal and Sobel, 2010). Similarly, invasive aspergillosis is a significant cause of morbidity and death in severely immunocompromised patients (Ben-Ami *et al.*, 2010). Modelling infections with *Aspergillus* and *Candida* spp. is possible in immunocompromised but not wild-type *Drosophila* flies, as the fly Toll pathway can clear the infection (Lionakis and Kontoyiannis, 2005; Chamilos *et al.*, 2006). Interestingly, a number of studies using *Drosophila* and mouse models of these mycoses showed qualitatively similar results regarding the role of various virulence factors and drugs (Lionakis and Kontoyiannis, 2005, 2010; Lionakis *et al.*, 2005; Chamilos *et al.*, 2006, 2009, 2010; Spikes *et al.*, 2008).

19.4.3 Zygomycetes

Zygomycosis (formerly called mucormycosis) is a fungal infection with *Mucor*, *Rhizopus* or other fungal species having common morphologies. Zygomycosis is an increasing threat to patients with HIV infection (Severo *et al.*, 2010). Treatment of zygomycosis is different from that of the more common mycoses such as candidiasis and aspergillosis. Indeed, Zygomycetes are emerging opportunistic moulds that are resistant to most conventional antifungals (Alastruey-Izquierdo *et al.*, 2009). Therefore, studying zygomycosis in flies would result in a significant contribution to biomedical research. These fungi are highly virulent in wild-type flies, and infections with them respond similarly to pharmacological treatments in both fly and mammalian model hosts (Chamilos *et al.*, 2008; Lamaris *et al.*, 2009).

19.5 The Promise of Large-scale Drug Screens

Benefits of the *Drosophila* model include genetic amenability, low cost and culture conditions compatible with large-scale drug screening. The main advantage of flies over *in vitro* models is that screening is feasible using the entire animal. Although neuropharmacological studies have employed large-scale drug screens using *Drosophila* (Stilwell *et al.*, 2006; Chang *et al.*, 2008), such screening has yet to be established for anti-infective compounds. Anti-infective high-throughput screening would be possible *in vivo* using *Drosophila* embryos and larvae that can be dispensed into fly food mixed with microbes and chemicals obtained from a library of compounds (Fig. 19.1a). This approach has several benefits. First, the small size of the *Drosophila* embryo ($150 \times 500\,\mu m$) allows the rearing of many embryos in 96-well or even 384-well plates. Also, similarly staged embryos are easily obtained via timed egg laying and controlled incubation methods. For example, the COPAS™ Select Large-particle Sorter (Union Biometrica, Holliston, Massachusetts) is capable of automated embryo sorting based on embryo size, shape and fluorescence intensity and can distribute embryos in multiwell plates. In addition, the BD Pathway™ High-content Bioimager (BD Biosciences, Franklin Lakes, New Jersey) is capable of high-resolution image capture and analysis in a multiwell format. Given the availability of transgenic fluorescent reporter genes, automatic assessment of live versus dead *Drosophila* larvae feeding on a microbe/drug mixture is possible because *Drosophila* larvae are transparent. Indeed, larvae can carry ubiquitously expressed markers such as green fluorescent protein, which allows automatic scoring of fluorescence in these larvae (Fig. 19.1b).

Larval high-throughput screens would allow the identification of new active compounds that may eventually be validated in mammals. In addition, this approach is unbiased because it is not dependent on prior identification of a target for *in vitro* activity, i.e. a drug can boost host defence or decrease the virulence of a pathogen independently of its effect on microbe growth arrest and/or killing. Lastly, establishing a database containing information linking drug efficacy and toxicological data with their chemical structures is possible. This approach has two main benefits. First, toxicological assessment and survival of infection can be assessed simultaneously. Secondly, more than 80,000 commercially available chemicals are currently in use for screening, and approximately 2000 new chemicals are introduced each year, for which little or no toxicological data are available (National Toxicology programme: http://ntp.niehs.nih.gov/).

A caveat regarding this approach is that only a larval feeding model appears to be feasible for high-throughput screening using *D. melanogaster* models. This is because current drug screening requires analysis of 10,000–100,000 chemicals over periods ranging from 1 day to 1 week (http://www.pharmainfo.net/akshat0026/high-throughput-screening-high-speed-drug-discovery). This is logistically challenging when manual scoring is required.

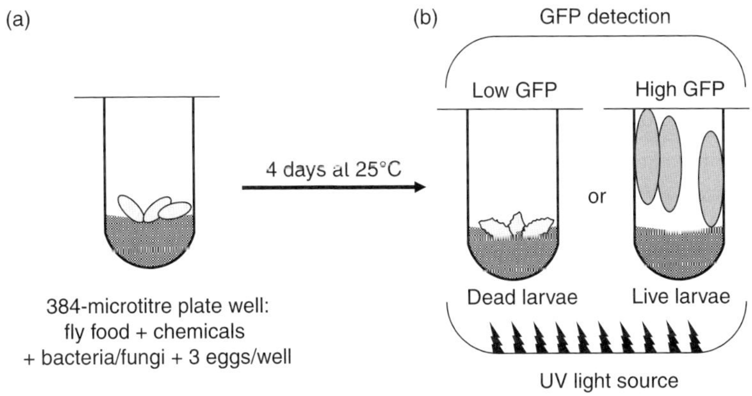

Fig. 19.1. Illustration of a proposed high-throughput drug screen in *D. melanogaster* in a 384-well plate. (a) A few microlitres of fly food, a bacterial or fungal solution, and chemicals obtained from a library of compounds can be mixed and aliquotted at the bottom of each well using robotic systems. Three *Drosophila* eggs per well can then be dispensed automatically, and the plates can be sealed with UV light-transparent wrap and incubated at 25°C for 4 days. (b) Genetically modified *Drosophila* eggs with ubiquitous expression of green fluorescent protein (GFP), which can easily be detected in young hatching larvae, are able to survive placement in microbially contaminated food mixed with the chemical and increase in size (normally about 30-fold), thus emitting a strong detectable signal. A fluorescent plate reader can be used to illuminate the larvae beneath each plate with UV light and detect GFP in each well.

Thus, high-throughput drug screening via pricking, feeding or injecting adult flies with a library of chemicals is not currently feasible. Nevertheless, following primary selection of drugs from a larval high-throughput screen, medium-scale toxicological and inflammatory screens can be performed in adult flies. In this respect, injection or feeding of drugs in adult flies can be followed by antimicrobial peptide expression and enterocyte damage and stress assessments in order to evaluate further the cytotoxicity and inflammatory potential of selected drugs.

19.6 Conclusions

Use of *Drosophila* models has contributed to many of the fundamental genetic, molecular and developmental biology advances over the past century. The ability to infect *D. melanogaster* at different stages of development via feeding, pricking or injecting microbes and the fly's high innate immunity and tissue physiology conservation have made this model organism suitable for biomedical research focused on identifying the biological activity of anti-infective drugs. *Drosophila* models of infection have certain shortcomings, such as the inability to use adult flies, different modes of infection and various types of readout in high-throughput screening. None the less, the ability to use different *Drosophila* infection models depending on the desired scale of drug screening (Table 19.1) warrants a more central role for *Drosophila* in anti-infective drug screening and toxicity analysis.

Table 19.1. Advantages of performing drug screens in *Drosophila*.

Conservation in innate immune response and tissue physiology
Availability of disparate models of infection
Feasibility for high-throughput screens using *Drosophila* larvae
Drugs are selected not only when microbiocidal or microbiostatic, but also when inhibiting virulence factors or boosting the host defence
Toxicological (i.e. fly mortality) data can be obtained in parallel
Facile follow-up of inflammatory and cytotoxicity/cell-stress assessments

References

Alastruey-Izquierdo, A., Castelli, M.V., Cuesta, I., Zaragoza, O., Monzon, A., Mellado, E. and Rodriguez-Tudela, J.L. (2009) *In vitro* activity of antifungals against Zygomycetes. *Clinical Microbiology and Infection* 15 (Suppl. 5), 71–76.

An, D., Apidianakis, Y., Boechat, A.L., Baldini, R.L., Goumnerov, B.C. and Rahme, L.G. (2009) The pathogenic properties of a novel and conserved gene product, KerV, in proteobacteria. *PLoS One* 4, e7167.

Apidianakis, Y. and Rahme, L.G. (2009) *Drosophila melanogaster* as a model host for studying *Pseudomonas aeruginosa* infection. *Nature Protocols* 4, 1285–1294.

Apidianakis, Y. and Rahme, L.G. (2011) *Drosophila melanogaster* as a model for human intestinal infection and pathology. *Disease Models and Mechanisms* 4, 21–30.

Apidianakis, Y., Rahme, L.G., Heitman, J., Ausubel, F.M., Calderwood, S.B. and Mylonakis, E. (2004) Challenge of *Drosophila melanogaster* with *Cryptococcus neoformans* and role of the innate immune response. *Eukaryotic Cell* 3, 413–419.

Apidianakis, Y., Mindrinos, M.N., Xiao, W., Lau, G.W., Baldini, R.L., Davis, R.W. and Rahme, L.G. (2005) Profiling early infection responses: *Pseudomonas aeruginosa* eludes host defenses by suppressing antimicrobial peptide gene expression. *Proceedings of the National Academy of Sciences USA* 102, 2573–2578.

Apidianakis, Y., Mindrinos, M.N., Xiao, W., Tegos, G.P., Papisov, M.I., Hamblin, M.R., Davis, R.W., Tompkins, R.G. and Rahme, L.G. (2007) Involvement of skeletal muscle gene regulatory network in susceptibility to wound infection following trauma. *PLoS One* 2, e1356.

Apidianakis, Y., Pitsouli, C., Perrimon, N. and Rahme, L. (2009) Synergy between bacterial infection and genetic predisposition in intestinal dysplasia. *Proceedings of the National Academy of Sciences USA* 106, 20883–20888

Baumann, O. (2001) Posterior midgut epithelial cells differ in their organization of the membrane skeleton from other *Drosophila* epithelia. *Experimental Cell Research* 270, 176–187.

Ben-Ami, R., Lewis, R.E. and Kontoyiannis, D.P. (2010) Enemy of the (immunosuppressed) state: an update on the pathogenesis of *Aspergillus fumigatus* infection. *British Journal of Haematology* 150, 406–417.

Berkey, C.D., Blow, N. and Watnick, P.I. (2009) Genetic analysis of *Drosophila melanogaster* susceptibility to intestinal *Vibrio cholerae* infection. *Cellular Microbiology* 11, 461–474.

Blow, N.S., Salomon, R.N., Garrity, K., Reveillaud, I., Kopin, A., Jackson, F.R. and Watnick, P.I. (2005) *Vibrio cholerae* infection of *Drosophila melanogaster* mimics the human disease cholera. *PLoS Pathogens* 1, e8.

Cataldo, M.A., Taglietti, F. and Petrosillo, N. (2010) Methicillin-resistant *Staphylococcus aureus*: a community health threat. *Postgraduation Medicine* 122, 16–23.

Chamilos, G., Lionakis, M.S., Lewis, R.E., Lopez-Ribot, J.L., Saville, S.P., Albert, N.D., Halder, G. and Kontoyiannis, D.P. (2006) *Drosophila melanogaster* as a facile model for large-scale studies of virulence mechanisms and antifungal drug efficacy in *Candida* species. *Journal of Infectious Diseases* 193, 1014–1022.

Chamilos, G., Lewis, R.E., Hu, J., Xiao, L., Zal, T., Gilliet, M., Halder, G. and Kontoyiannis, D.P. (2008) *Drosophila melanogaster* as a model host to dissect the immunopathogenesis of zygomycosis. *Proceedings of the National Academy of Sciences USA* 105, 9367–9372.

Chamilos, G., Nobile, C.J., Bruno, V.M., Lewis, R.E., Mitchell, A.P. and Kontoyiannis, D.P. (2009) *Candida albicans* Cas5, a regulator of cell wall integrity, is required for virulence in murine and Toll mutant fly models. *Journal of Infectious Diseases* 200, 152–157.

Chamilos, G., Bignell, E.M., Schrettl, M., Lewis, R.E., Leventakos, K., May, G.S., Haas, H. and Kontoyiannis, D.P. (2010) Exploring the concordance of *Aspergillus fumigatus* pathogenicity in mice and *Toll*-deficient flies. *Medical Mycology* 48, 506–510.

Chang, S., Bray, S.M., Li, Z., Zarnescu, D.C., He, C., Jin, P. and Warren, S.T. (2008) Identification of small molecules rescuing fragile X syndrome phenotypes in *Drosophila*. *Nature Chemical Biology* 4, 256–263.

Cox, C.R. and Gilmore, M.S. (2007) Native microbial colonization of *Drosophila melanogaster* and its use as a model of *Enterococcus faecalis* pathogenesis. *Infection and Immunity* 75, 1565–1576.

Cronin, S.J., Nehme, N.T., Limmer, S., Liegeois, S., Pospisilik, J.A., Schramek, D., Leibbrandt, A., Simoes R. de M., Gruber, S., Puc, U., Ebersberger, I., Zoranovic, T., Neely, G.G., Von Haeseler, A., Ferrandon, D. and Penninger, J.M. (2009) Genome-wide RNAi screen identifies genes involved in intestinal pathogenic bacterial infection. *Science* 325, 340–343.

Daczewska, M., Picchio, L., Jagla, T., Figeac, N. and Jagla, K. (2010) Muscle development and regeneration in normal and pathological conditions: learning from *Drosophila*. *Current Pharmaceutical Design* 16, 929–941.

D'argenio, D.A., Gallagher, L.A., Berg, C.A. and Manoil, C. (2001) *Drosophila* as a model host for *Pseudomonas aeruginosa* infection. *Journal of Bacteriology* 183, 1466–1471.

de Gregorio, E., Spellman, P.T., Rubin, G.M. and Lemaitre, B. (2001) Genome-wide analysis of the *Drosophila* immune response by using oligonucleotide microarrays. *Proceedings of the National Academy of Sciences USA* 98, 12590–5.

Dessi, A., Puddu, M., Testa, M., Marcialis, M.A., Pintus, M.C. and Fanos, V. (2009) *Serratia marcescens* infections and outbreaks in neonatal intensive care units. *Journal of Chemotherapy* 21, 493–499.

Flyg, C., Kenne, K. and Boman, H.G. (1980) Insect pathogenic properties of *Serratia marcescens*: phage-resistant mutants with a decreased resistance to *Cecropia* immunity and a decreased virulence to *Drosophila*. *Journal of General Microbiology* 120, 173–181.

Gartner, L.P. (1970) Submicroscopic morphology of the adult *Drosophila* midgut. *Journal of the Baltimore College of Dental Surgery* 25, 64–76.

Giacomotto, J. and Ségalat, L. (2010) High-throughput screening and small animal models, where are we? *British Journal of Pharmacology* 160, 204–216.

Gould, I.M. (2010) Coping with antibiotic resistance: the impending crisis. *International Journal of Antimicrobial Agents* 36 (Suppl. 3), S1–S2.

Hirsch, E.B. and Tam, V.H. (2010) Impact of multidrug-resistant *Pseudomonas aeruginosa* infection on patient outcomes. *Expert Review of Pharmacoeconomics and Outcomes Research* 10, 441–451.

Jiang, H. and Edgar, B.A. (2009) EGFR signaling regulates the proliferation of *Drosophila* adult midgut progenitors. *Development* 136, 483–493.

Kallio, J., Myllymaki, H., Gronholm, J., Armstrong, M., Vanha-Aho, L.M., Makinen, L., Silvennoinen, O., Valanne, S. and Ramet, M. (2010) Eye transformer is a negative regulator of *Drosophila* JAK/STAT signaling. *FASEB Journal* 24, 4467–4479.

Kim, S.H., Park, S.Y., Heo, Y.J. and Cho, Y.H. (2008) *Drosophila melanogaster*-based screening for multihost virulence factors of *Pseudomonas aeruginosa* PA14 and identification of a virulence-attenuating factor, HudA. *Infection and Immunity* 76, 4152–4162.

Kurz, C.L. and Ewbank, J.J. (2007) Infection in a dish: high-throughput analyses of bacterial pathogenesis. *Current Opinions in Microbiology* 10, 10–16.

Kvietys, P.R. and Granger, D.N. (1986) Physiology and pathophysiology of the colonic circulation. *Clinical Gastroenterology* 15, 967–983.

Lamaris, G.A., Ben-Ami, R., Lewis, R.E., Chamilos, G., Samonis, G. and Kontoyiannis, D.P. (2009) Increased virulence of Zygomycetes organisms following exposure to voriconazole: a study involving fly and murine models of zygomycosis. *Journal of Infectious Diseases* 199, 1399–1406.

Lau, G.W., Goumnerov, B.C., Walendziewicz, C.L., Hewitson, J., Xiao, W., Mahajan-Miklos, S., Tompkins, R.G., Perkins, L.A. and Rahme, L.G. (2003) The *Drosophila melanogaster* Toll pathway participates in resistance to infection by the Gram-negative human pathogen *Pseudomonas aeruginosa. Infection and Immunity* 71, 4059–4066.

Lemaitre, B. and Hoffmann, J. (2007) The host defense of *Drosophila melanogaster. Annual Review of Immunology* 25, 697–743.

Lemaitre, B., Nicolas, E., Michaut, L., Reichhart, J.M. and Hoffmann, J.A. (1996) The dorsoventral regulatory gene cassette *spätzle/Toll/cactus* controls the potent antifungal response in *Drosophila* adults. *Cell* 86, 973–983.

Lionakis, M.S. and Kontoyiannis, D.P. (2005) Fruit flies as a minihost model for studying drug activity and virulence in *Aspergillus. Medical Mycology* 43 (Suppl. 1), S111–S114.

Lionakis, M.S. and Kontoyiannis, D.P. (2010) The growing promise of Toll-deficient *Drosophila melanogaster* as a model for studying *Aspergillus* pathogenesis and treatment. *Virulence* 1, 488–499.

Lionakis, M.S., Lewis, R.E., May, G.S., Wiederhold, N.P., Albert, N.D., Halder, G. and Kontoyiannis, D.P. (2005) Toll-deficient *Drosophila* flies as a fast, high-throughput model for the study of antifungal drug efficacy against invasive aspergillosis and *Aspergillus* virulence. *Journal of Infectious Diseases* 191, 1188–1195.

Lyczak, J.B., Cannon, C.L. and Pier, G.B. (2000) Establishment of *Pseudomonas aeruginosa* infection: lessons from a versatile opportunist. *Microbes and Infection* 2, 1051–1060.

Mansfield, B.E., Dionne, M.S., Schneider, D.S. and Freitag, N.E. (2003) Exploration of host–pathogen interactions using *Listeria monocytogenes* and *Drosophila melanogaster. Cellular Microbiology* 5, 901–911.

Martinez, M. and Silley, P. (2010) Antimicrobial drug resistance. *Handbook of Experimental Pharmacology* 227–264.

Miller, A. (1994) The internal anatomy and histology of the imago of *Drosophila melanogaster.* In: Demerec, M. (ed.) *Biology of* Drosophila. Cold Spring Harbor Press, Cold Spring Harbor, New York, pp. 420–534.

Mohr, S., Bakal, C. and Perrimon, N. (2010) Genomic screening with RNAi: results and challenges. *Annual Reviews in Biochemistry* 79, 37–64.

Moudgal, V. and Sobel, J. (2010) Antifungals to treat *Candida albicans. Expert Opinions in Pharmacotherapy* 11, 2037–2048.

Needham, A.J., Kibart, M., Crossley, H., Ingham, P.W. and Foster, S.J. (2004) *Drosophila melanogaster* as a model host for *Staphylococcus aureus* infection. *Microbiology* 150, 2347–2355.

Nehme, N.T., Liegeois, S., Kele, B., Giammarinaro, P., Pradel, E., Hoffmann, J.A., Ewbank, J.J. and Ferrandon, D. (2007) A model of bacterial intestinal infections in *Drosophila melanogaster. PLoS Pathogens* 3, e173.

Olszewski, M.A., Zhang, Y. and Huffnagle, G.B. (2010) Mechanisms of cryptococcal virulence and persistence. *Future Microbiology* 5, 1269–1288.

Palmer, K.L., Kos, V.N. and Gilmore, M.S. (2010) Horizontal gene transfer and the genomics of enterococcal antibiotic resistance. *Current Opinions in Microbiology* 13, 632–639.

Park, S.Y., Heo, Y.J., Kim, K.S. and Cho, Y.H. (2005) *Drosophila melanogaster* is susceptible to *Vibrio cholerae* infection. *Molecules to Cells* 20, 409–415.

Perrimon, N., Friedman, A., Mathey-Prevot, B. and Eggert, U.S. (2007) Drug-target identification in *Drosophila* cells: combining high-throughout RNAi and small-molecule screens. *Drug Discovery Today* 12, 28–33.

Ramaswamy, V., Cresence, V.M., Rejitha, J.S., Lekshmi, M.U., Dharsana, K.S., Prasad, S.P. and Vijila, H.M. (2007) Listeria – review of epidemiology and pathogenesis. *Journal of Microbiology Immunology and Infection* 40, 4–13.

Rhee, S.H., Pothoulakis, C. and Mayer, E.A. (2009) Principles and clinical implications of the brain–gut–enteric microbiota axis. *Nature Reviews in Gastroenterology and Hepatology* 6, 306–314.

Richardson, M. and Lass-Florl, C. (2008) Changing epidemiology of systemic fungal infections. *Clinical Microbiology and Infection* 14 (Suppl. 4), 5–24.

Ritchie, J.M. and Waldor, M.K. (2009) *Vibrio cholerae* interactions with the gastrointestinal tract: lessons from animal studies. *Current Topics in Microbiology and Immunology* 337, 37–59.

Sava, I.G., Heikens, E. and Huebner, J. (2010) Pathogenesis and immunity in enterococcal infections. *Clinical Microbiology and Infection* 16, 533–540.

Severo, C.B., Guazzelli, L.S. and Severo, L.C. (2010) Zygomycosis. *Jornal Brasileiro de Pneumologia* 36, 134–141.

Shanbhag, S. and Tripathi, S. (2009) Epithelial ultrastructure and cellular mechanisms of acid and base transport in the *Drosophila* midgut. *Journal of Experimental Biology* 212, 1731–1744.

Spikes, S., Xu, R., Nguyen, C.K., Chamilos, G., Kontoyiannis, D.P., Jacobson, R.H., Ejzykowicz, D.E., Chiang, L.Y., Filler, S.G. and May, G.S. (2008) Gliotoxin production in *Aspergillus fumigatus* contributes to host-specific differences in virulence. *Journal of Infectious Diseases* 197, 479–486.

Stilwell, G.E., Saraswati, S., Littleton, J.T. and Chouinard, S.W. (2006) Development of a *Drosophila* seizure model for *in vivo* high-throughput drug screening. *European Journal of Neuroscience* 24, 2211–2222.

Vanden Broeck, D., Horvath, C. and de Wolf, M.J. (2007) *Vibrio cholerae*: cholera toxin. *International Journal of Biochemistry and Cellular Biology* 39, 1771–1775.

Vodovar, N., Vinals, M., Liehl, P., Basset, A., Degrouard, J., Spellman, P., Boccard, F. and Lemaitre, B. (2005) *Drosophila* host defense after oral infection by an entomopathogenic *Pseudomonas* species. *Proceedings of the National Academy of Sciences USA* 102, 11414–11419.

20 Antimicrobial Photosensitizers: Harnessing the Power of Light to Treat Infections

Sulbha K. Sharma, Tianhong Dai and Michael R. Hamblin
Wellman Center for Photomedicine, Massachusetts General Hospital, Boston, Massachusetts, USA

20.1 Introduction

Photodynamic therapy (PDT) is a successful and clinically approved therapeutic modality for the treatment of cancer, which is currently available in several countries (Dougherty, 2002; Brown *et al.*, 2004). It is based on the use of a photosensitive drug or photosensitizer (PS) in combination with light of suitable wavelength (600–900nm) in the presence of oxygen to generate cytotoxic reactive oxygen species (ROS). The basic principle in PDT is that the excited state of the PS, in the presence of oxygen, transfers energy or electrons to ground-state molecular oxygen producing ROS, such as singlet oxygens and hydroxyl radicals, which are responsible for the killing of cells (Ochsner, 1997). This therapy has now also been proposed for the treatment of infectious diseases (Levy and Obochi, 1996) and has become more relevant as antibiotic-resistant bacterial infections represent an important and rising public health threat. When the cells to be killed are pathogenic microorganisms, the procedure is termed photodynamic inactivation (PDI) or antimicrobial PDT (aPDT). A diversity of different antimicrobial PSs are used in research for testing the efficacy of aPDT for infections. Before discussing these antimicrobial PSs, a brief history and overview of aPDT will be discussed.

Over the last 60 years, the use of antimicrobial drugs in medicine has prompted bacteria to develop highly efficient biochemical and genetic mechanisms that enable them to live safely in the antibiotic environment. Thus, the emergence of multidrug-resistant pathogens is leading to increased morbidity. The methods adopted by these bacteria include the thickening of their outer wall, encoding of new proteins that prevent the penetration of drugs or that mediate the active efflux of antibiotics and the generation of mutants deficient in porin channels, which permit the entry of externally added chemicals. When considering these highly protective mechanism adopted by the microorganism, it becomes difficult to visualize a broadly applicable approach to fight all the problems simultaneously (Smith *et al.*, 1999). PDT may therefore become one therapy that adds to the armamentarium of effective antimicrobial therapy.

The first evidence for this came when, in 1900, Raab noticed the killing of paramecia with acridine orange in the presence of light (Raab, 1900). However, early results demonstrated that the common PSs used for cancer were not adequately effective for the PDT killing of some well-known pathogens (Wainwright, 2004b). More recently, in the 1990s, there were reports showing that cationic PSs such as phenothiaziniums (Wilson *et al.*, 1995), porphyrins (Merchat *et al.*, 1996) and phthalocyanines (Minnock *et al.*, 1996) induced a rapid and extensive light-mediated killing of Gram-negative bacteria such as *Escherichia coli* and *Pseudomonas aeruginosa*, as well as killing fungi and Gram-positive bacteria. Besides being a broad-spectrum antimicrobial therapy, aPDT has several other advantages:

1. It is broad spectrum and can kill a wide range of microbes such as Gram-positive and Gram-negative bacteria, yeasts, fungi and parasitic protozoa, as well as inactivating viruses.
2. There is thought to be no (or little) possibility of developing photoresistant species, even after multiple treatments.
3. PS and drug–light intervals can be designed that exhibit selectivity for microbes over host cells and tissue.
4. There is a low risk of inducing mutagenic effects.
5. aPDT kills microbial cells rapidly (in minutes), while antibiotics can take days to work.
6. Because PSs are delivered topically into infected areas, aPDT can be effective in traumatic infections where the blood supply is compromised, preventing systemically administered antibiotics reaching the microbes.
7. It has been demonstrated that aPDT can be effective in biofilm infections that are resistant to antibiotics.
8. Last but not the least, it can be a less expensive therapy compared with other known therapies.

20.1.1 The general features of microbial cells for PDI

Different microorganisms are found to be differentially susceptible to aPDT; the reason for this is the difference in size and configuration of the cell wall of different microorganisms. Gram-positive and Gram-negative bacteria differ in susceptibility due to differences in morphology: Gram-positive bacteria are surrounded by a layer of only peptidoglycan and lipoteichoic acid, which is comparatively porous, while Gram-negative bacteria have a somewhat more complex, non-porous cell-wall structure consisting of an inner cytoplasmic membrane and an outer membrane, which are separated by the peptidoglycan-containing periplasm (Fig. 20.1). Fungal cells have intermediate permeability between Gram-positive and Gram-negative bacteria. In addition, the cysts formed by protozoa also represent difficult targets. Therefore, the method for the treatment of infections should focus on microbial pathogens with very diverse characteristics.

20.1.2 Photobiological processes

The PS in its excited state can follow two different types of pathway known as type I and type II. When the ground-state PS absorbs a photon, it is converted into its long-lived triplet state via a short-lived singlet state. This triplet state is the reactive intermediate. In the type I mechanism, the triplet state PS transfers an electron to ground-state molecular oxygen to produce ROS such as superoxide, hydroxyl radicals and peroxides, while in the type II mechanism, the triplet state of the PS undergoes energy transfer to the ground state of oxygen, which is also in the triplet state, to give another ROS, i.e. a singlet oxygen (Fig. 20.2). The lifetime of the singlet oxygen is very small and this singlet oxygen then reacts further with the surrounding biomolecules. The main molecules targeted by both the mechanisms (types I and II) are certain amino acids (tryptophan, histidine, tyrosine, cysteine and methionine), pyrimidine and purine bases of DNA/RNA and unsaturated lipids. The wide range of biomolecules damaged by ROS means that the spectrum of microbial targets of PDT is very broad.

Some of the properties considered to be favourable for ideal antimicrobial PSs are as follows:

1. The PS should have long-lived, excited triplet state and a high quantum yield for the generation of ROS on excitation with visible light.
2. It should have a high extinction coefficient mainly in the red and far-red region where

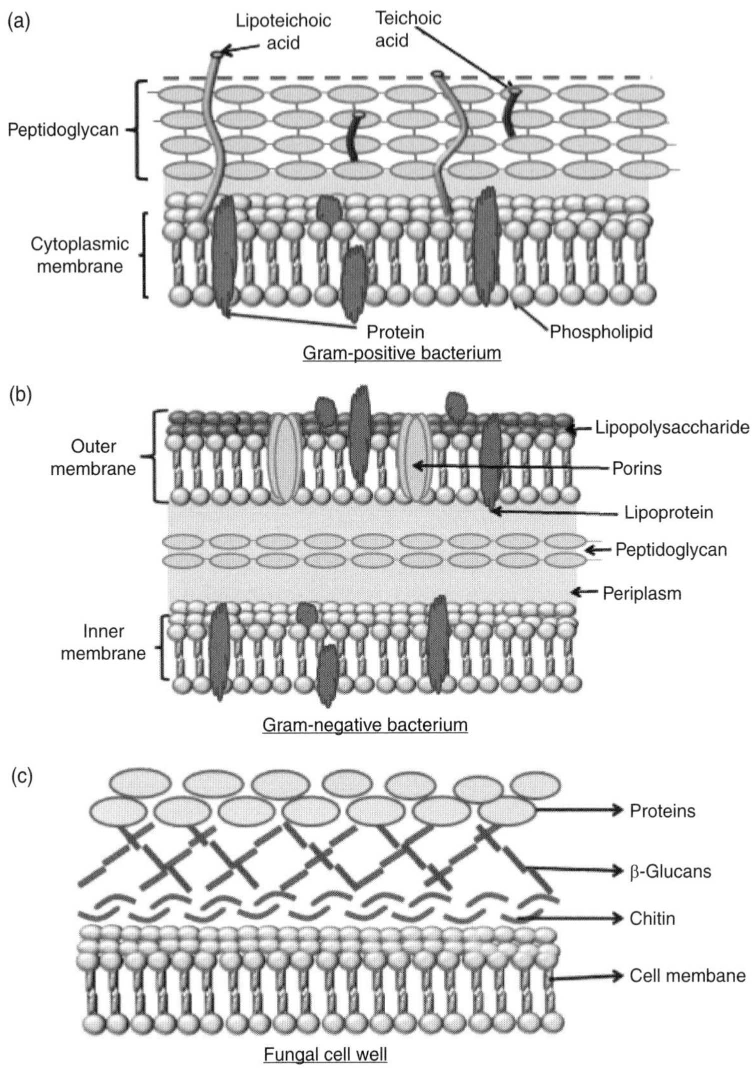

Fig. 20.1. Structures of cell walls of representative pathogenic microbial cells. (a) A Gram-positive bacterium; (b) a Gram-negative bacterium; (c) a fungal yeast.

light transmission through tissue is maximal, although for the treatment of superficial infections, the intensely absorbed blue light (400–420 nm) is also useful.
3. It should have high affinity for the broadest possible range of microbial cells.
4. The PS should bind selectively to the cytoplasmic membrane; as a result, cell death will mainly be due to damage of the membrane rather than of the genetic material.
5. The mechanisms involved in PDI should have no mutagenic effect.
6. It should have a broad spectrum of action against bacteria, fungi, yeasts and parasites to help the treatment of infectious diseases that are considered to be the result of the presence of a varied flora of pathogens.
7. The cell-selective binding conferred by the molecular structure should be such that there is maximum damage to the microbes with minimal damage to the host tissue.

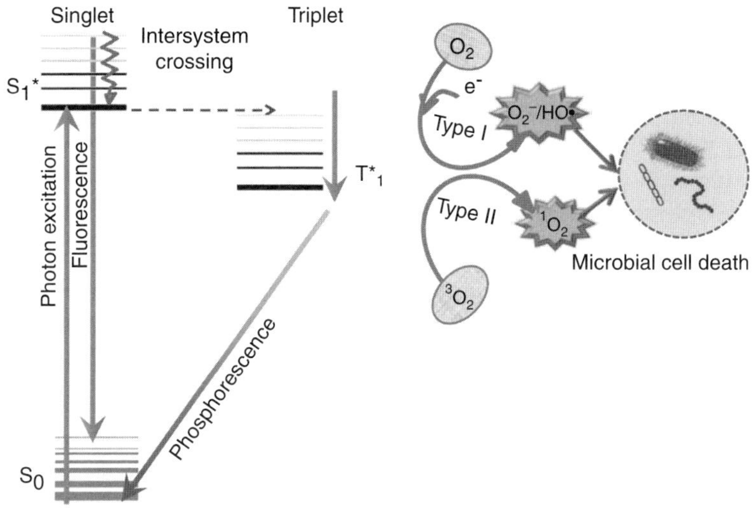

Fig. 20.2. Jablonski diagram of the mechanism of antimicrobial photodynamic therapy. Light absorbed by the photosensitizer (PS) in the ground state (S_0) excites the PS to a short-lived first excited state (S_1), which can lose energy by fluorescence or undergo intersystem crossing to a long-lived triplet state (T^*_1). The triplet PS can carry out energy transfer to a ground-state triplet oxygen ($^3O_2$) to produce a reactive singlet oxygen ($^1O_2$). Alternatively, the triplet PS can carry out electron transfer to oxygen to produce the superoxide O_2^-, which goes on to form hydroxyl radicals ($HO^•$). Both $^1O_2$ and $HO^•$ can efficiently kill microbial cells.

The advantage of the broad-spectrum of activity exhibited by PDT means that it could be used to treat a localized infection before the clinical microbiology laboratory identifies the culprit microbe and the appropriate antibiotic is selected. Moreover, a more limited range of antimicrobial PSs could be stocked up in pharmacies compared with the wide range of antibiotics currently needed.

20.2 Drug Discovery and aPDT

It has been known for many decades that Gram-positive bacteria are highly susceptible to killing by traditional PSs with the same molecular features as those PSs that were used to kill cancer cells (such as porphyrins), but later it was realized that they were not well suited for antimicrobial application (Malik *et al.*, 1990). In the 1990s, it was discovered that PSs with a cationic charge could kill Gram-negative bacteria, which had previously been thought to be resistant to many aPDT procedures (Malik *et al.*, 1992; Merchat *et al.*, 1996; Minnock *et al.*, 1996). Other classes of pathogen such as viruses (both enveloped and non-enveloped) (Wainwright, 2004a), yeasts (Bliss *et al.*, 2004; Fuchs *et al.*, 2007), filamentous fungi (Gonzales *et al.*, 2010), protozoa (Kassab *et al.*, 2003) and parasites (Gottlieb *et al.*, 1995; Akilov *et al.*, 2006) have been reported to be susceptible to aPDT mediated by cationic PSs. We will discuss some examples of compounds that have been investigated as antimicrobial PSs, and a selection of chemical structures are given in Fig. 20.3.

20.2.1 Cationic porphyrins

Porphyrins can be changed into cationic PSs by the insertion of positively charged substituents (quaternary amino groups) in the peripheral positions of the tetrapyrrole macrocycle. Insertion of the cationic group affects the kinetics and increases the binding with microbial cells. This is often done by altering phenyl groups substituted in the *meso*-position of the porphyrin macrocycle. It was

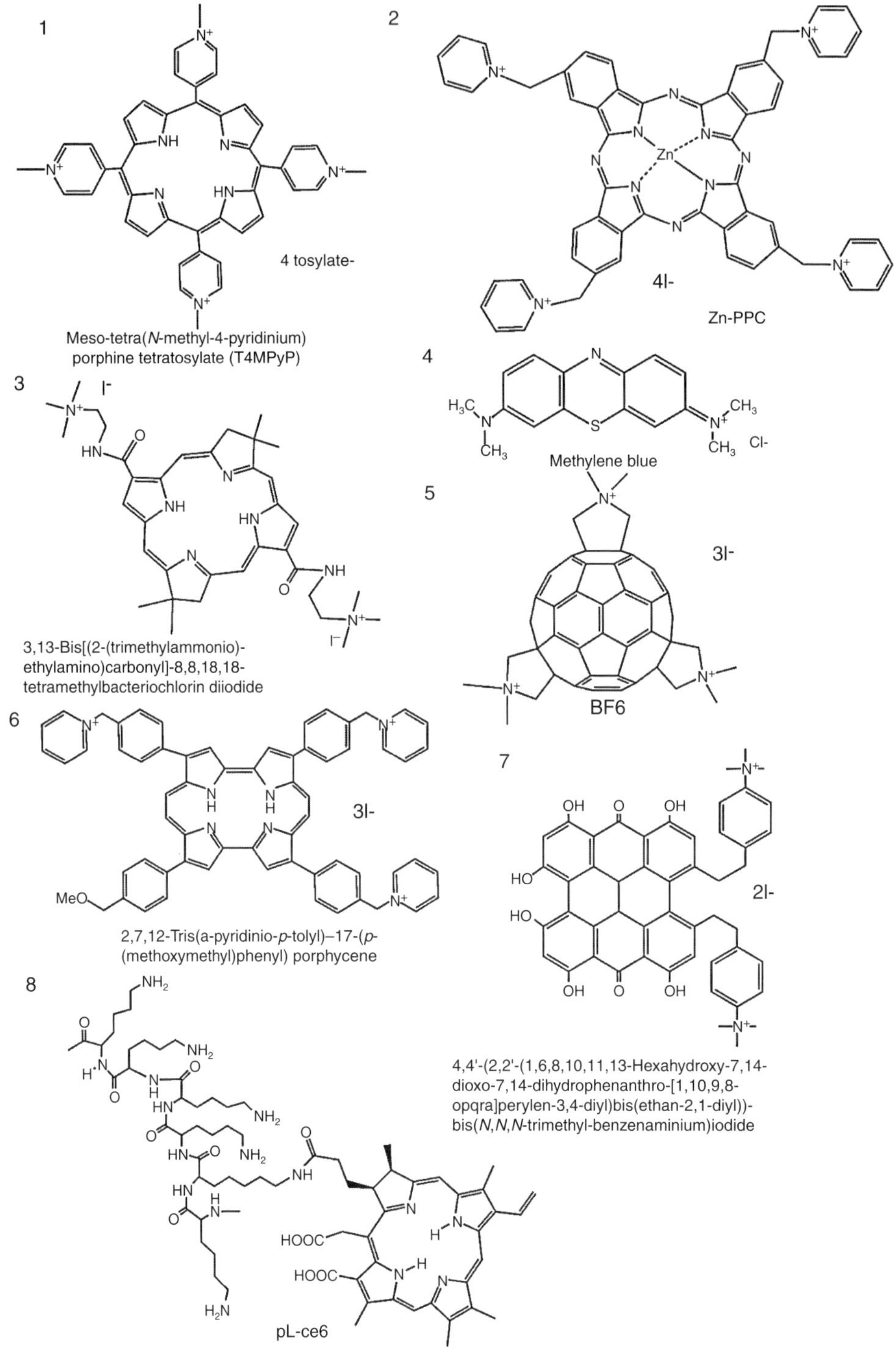

Fig. 20.3. Chemical structures of a selection of different classes of antimicrobial PSa. 1, Tetracationic porphyrin; 2, tetracationic zinc phthalocyanine; 3, bis-cationic bacteriochlorin; 4, phenothiazinium dye; 5, tris-cationic fullerene; 6, tris-cationic porphycene; 7, bis-cationic hypericin derivative; 8, conjugate between chlorin(e6) and poly-L-lysine.

demonstrated by Merchat *et al.* (1996) that cationic *meso*-substituted porphyrins, namely tetra(4*N*-methyl-pyridyl) porphine tetraiodide (T4MPyP) (Fig. 20.3, compound 1) and tetra(4*N*,*N*,*N*-trimethylanilinium) porphine tetraiodide (T4MAP), effectively mediated aPDT of Gram-negative bacteria. Another cationic porphyrin, 5-phenyl-10,15,20-tris(*N*-methyl-4-pyridyl)-porphyrin chloride (PTMPP) or Sylsens B, demonstrated effective killing of bacteria, *Candida* and the dermatophyte *Trichophyton rubrum* (Lambrechts *et al.*, 2004, 2005a; Smijs *et al.*, 2009). Maisch *et al.* (2005) showed that bis-cationic porphyrins such as XF70 were broad-spectrum antimicrobial PSs, giving good photokilling of methicillin-resistant (MRSA) and methicillin-sensitive *Staphylococcus aureus* strains, methicillin-resistant *Staphylococcus epidermidis* and *E. coli*. Other reports have used a wide range of substituted cationic porphyrins to mediate aPDT of diverse species of pathogens (Banfi *et al.*, 2006; Carvalho *et al.*, 2007; Grinholc *et al.*, 2008; Alves *et al.*, 2009; Costa *et al.*, 2010). Sylsens B has been tested for mediating PDT of burn wound infections in mice. The burns were illuminated directly after the application of the PTMPP with red light and periodic imaging of the mice using a sensitive camera to detect the bioluminescence signal. More than 98% of the bacteria were eradicated after a light dose of 210 J/cm^2 in the presence of PTMPP. However, bacterial regrowth was observed. Collectively, these data suggested that PDT has the potential to rapidly reduce the bacterial load in infected burns but treatment needs to be optimized to reduce wound damage and prevent recurrence (Lambrechts *et al.*, 2005b).

20.2.2 Cationic phthalocyanines

Phthalocyanines can also be turned into suitable antimicrobial PSs by attaching cationic substituents. Phthalocyanines are usually arranged with central coordinated metal atoms to avoid aggregation and improve photochemical properties. The diamagnetic metal ions such as zinc (II), when centrally coordinated, impart a high fluorescence quantum yield, long triplet lifetimes and high triplet quantum yields, which lead to a high probability of energy or electron transfer. Minnock *et al.* (1996) evaluated phthalocyanine zinc (II) molecules with different charges to kill bacteria and demonstrated that the Gram-negative bacteria could be photoinactivated when illuminated in the presence of a tetracationic water-soluble zinc pyridinium phthalocyanine, Zn-PPC (Fig. 20.3, compound 2). Mantareva *et al.* (2007) showed that one cationic phthalocyanine with four cationic groups was able to photoinactivate Gram-positive *S. aureus*, the Gram-negative *P. aeruginosa* and the fungal species *Candida albicans*. A recent paper (Mantareva *et al.*, 2010) from the same group described a Ga (III)-substituted phthalocyanine with eight cationic groups that was able to mediate photoinactivation of Gram-positive and Gram-negative bacteria and *Candida* spp. in planktonic form, an in biofilms. Giuliani *et al.* (2010) showed that another tetracationic zinc phthalocyanine designated RLP068 (Kassab *et al.*, 2003) could photoinactivate *S. aureus*, *P. aeruginosa* and *C. albicans* and moreover did not generate any resistance, even after 20 successive cycles of sublethal PDT and regrowth.

20.2.3 Cationic bacteriochlorins

Bacteriochlorins possess an intense absorption band in the near-infrared spectrum (>700 nm) due to the two opposed reduced pyrrole rings in the macrocycle. In a similar manner to porphyrins, they can be synthesized with peripheral cationic groups to give antimicrobial PSs. Compounds such as bis-cationic (Fig. 20.3, compound 3), tetrakis cationic and hexakis cationic bacteriochlorins are efficient in killing Gram-positive and Gram-negative bacteria and fungi. Moreover, they show good selectivity for microbial cells over host cells. These are prepared using entirely synthetic methods, which renders them stable by introduction of gem-dimethyl groups that prevent adventitious reoxidation of the reduced rings (Huang *et al.*, 2010).

20.2.4 Phenothiazinium dyes

The members of this class include compounds with a single cationic charge that is delocalized over the three-ring structure. Some of the most widely used members of this class are methylene blue (MB; Fig. 20.3, compound 4) and toluidine blue O (TBO) (Wainwright *et al.*, 1997a; Wainwright and Crossley, 2002; Phoenix *et al.*, 2003). These compounds have an added advantage over others and because of this MB has been clinically approved as an injectable intravenous therapy for methaemoglobinaemia (Wainwright and Crossley, 2002). Both of these compounds are considered safe for topical application (Wainwright, 2010). There are some other PSs in this class that have been tested for their antimicrobial activity including new methylene blue (NMB) (Ragàs *et al.*, 2010) and dimethyl-methylene blue (O'Neill *et al.*, 2003) and these have proved to be more potent antimicrobial PSs compared with MB and TBO (Wainwright *et al.*, 1997b). Studies performed *in vivo* in our group (Ragàs *et al.*, 2010) investigated PDT mediated by NMB in mouse burn infections. NMB was applied 30 min after infection followed by illumination with red light at 635 nm. PDT of *Acinetobacter baumannii* led to a 3.2 $\log_{10}$ reduction of the bacterial luminescence after 360 J/cm^2 was delivered. We have also tested aPDT in a mouse model of localized *C. albicans* infection (Dai *et al.*, 2011). After 24 h, topical application of NMB solution followed by illumination with red light produced a light-dose-dependent reduction in bioluminescence.

20.2.5 Cationic fullerenes

Fullerenes, commonly called buckyballs, are closed cage compounds made up only of carbon atoms. The buckminsterfullerene (C_{60}) is the most widely used member among these. These molecules absorb in the visible and UV region due to the presence of an extended system of conjugated double bonds. Furthermore, they have a triplet yield approaching unity and hence no fluorescence. The long-lived triplet state can undergo either energy transfer to produce a singlet oxygen or electron transfer to produce a superoxide and subsequently hydroxyl radical. Although C_{60} is highly insoluble, these molecules can be developed as efficient antimicrobial PSs by functionalization of the periphery with the appropriate cationic groups. The tris-cationic fullerene (Fig. 20.3, compound 5) was shown by our laboratory (Tegos *et al.*, 2005) to be a broad-spectrum PS able to mediate photoinactivation of Gram-positive and Gram-negative bacteria and fungi. Another study by our group (Huang *et al.*, 2010) showed that cationic fullerenes with six cationic groups were also highly effective. Other laboratories (Spesia *et al.*, 2008) have shown that cationic fullerenes with two cationic groups are also effective against Gram-negative bacteria.

20.2.6 Miscellaneous cationic PSs

Porphycenes are structural isomers of the porphyrin backbone (Stockert *et al.*, 2007). These authors synthesized a cationic PS by attaching three quaternary pyridinium groups to the porphycene (Fig. 20.3, compound 6), which proved to be an efficient broad-spectrum antimicrobial PS, demonstrating the ability to kill Gram-positive and Gram-negative bacteria, as well as a fungal yeast. Moreover, this cationic porphycene was also able to effectively treat an *in vivo* mouse infection model using aPDT. In a model comprising mouse third-degree burns infected with a bioluminescent MRSA strain there was a 2.6 log reduction ($P < 0.001$) of the bacterial bioluminescence for the PDT-treated group after irradiation with 180 J/cm^2 of red light (Ragàs *et al.*, 2010).

Hypericin is a natural produce isolated from St John's Wort and has been widely used as a PS for PDT of cancer. Hager *et al.* (2009) synthesized bis-cationic derivatives of hypericin such as compound 7 (Fig. 20.3) and demonstrated these PSs could be used for PDI of *Propionibacterium acnes*.

20.2.7 Conjugates between PS and cationic polymers

Our laboratory prepared a microbial-targeted PS by covalently attaching a non-cationic PS, chlorin(e6) (ce6) to amino groups present on a cationic polymer such as poly-L-lysine (pL) to form a pL–ce6 conjugate (Fig. 20.3, compound 8) (Soukos *et al.*, 1997). Various forms of the cationic pL–ce6 conjugate proved to be effective in killing Gram-positive and Gram-negative bacteria (Soukos *et al.*, 1998; Hamblin *et al.*, 2002b).

Hamblin *et al.* (2002a) developed a mouse model of excisional wound infections for performing aPDT. A rapid light-dose-dependent effect was observed after PDT with the pL–ce6 conjugate. Topical application of pL–ce6 followed by laser illumination at 665 nm led to a 99% reduction in bacterial luminescence. The mouse model was also used by the same group (Hamblin *et al.*, 2003) to test the efficacy of aPDT with pL–ce6 conjugate against infections induced by a more invasive species, *P. aeruginosa*. To allow the conjugate to bind to and penetrate the bacteria, illumination at 665 nm was commenced at 30 min after the inoculation of bacteria. It was seen from a set of luminescence images that PDT produced a light-dose-dependent loss of luminescence, until only a trace remained, after 240 J/cm^2 had been delivered. Nine out of ten (90%) of the PDT-treated mice survived; in contrast, all of the non-treated control mice (n=10) died within 5 days. In addition, the wounds treated with PDT healed better than wounds that were treated with an alternative topical antimicrobial (silver nitrate). This improvement in healing was attributed to the fact that PDT can also destroy protease enzymes responsible for slowing down wound healing.

A similar synthetic approach using polyethylenimine (PEI) allowed the formation of a PEI–ce6 conjugate that had the additional advantages of being protease stable and more cost effective (Tegos *et al.*, 2006). PDT of *A. baumannii* in a burn wound infection was studied by Dai *et al.* (2009) using the PEI–ce6 conjugate and non-coherent red light at 660 nm. The burn wounds were created as described by Lambrechts *et al.* (2005b). Antimicrobial PDT was performed and induced approximately a 1.8 log reduction in bacterial luminescence from the mouse burn. Bacterial regrowth in the treated burn was observed but was generally modest. In addition, PDT did not lead to inhibition of wound healing. These data suggest that PDT may be an effective new treatment for multidrug-resistant localized *A. baumannii* infections.

A mouse model of a skin abrasion wound infected with MRSA was developed by Dai *et al.* (2010) and treated with PEI–ce6 PDT. In six of the ten PDT-treated mice, complete wound healing was achieved within 4 days post-infection. The reason for the large advantage of wound healing in the PDT group probably reflects the fact that an abrasion has unbroken skin between the scratches that can form a nucleus for wound healing. However, this normal skin can be destroyed by the bacteria if the infection is untreated, leading to a uniform large wound that takes much longer to heal. Findings from this study demonstrated that PDT significantly reduced the bioburden of MRSA in the mouse wounds, which would otherwise develop severe infections. In addition, wound healing and morbidity (body weight loss) were greatly benefited by the eradication of MRSA from the wounds. PDT may represent an alternative approach for the treatment of MRSA skin infections.

The concept of polycationic PS conjugates to mediate PDT of infections has proved to be fruitful and has been studied extensively both in our laboratory (Hamblin *et al.*, 2002a, 2003; Gad *et al.*, 2004a,b; Demidova and Hamblin, 2005; Garcez *et al.*, 2007, 2008; Dai *et al.*, 2009, 2010) and by others (Polo *et al.*, 2000; Rovaldi *et al.*, 2000; Lauro *et al.*, 2002).

20.2.8 PSs encapsulated into cationic liposomes and nanoparticles

It has been shown that, by encapsulation of PSs in cationic liposomes rather than the more usual liposomes composed of anionic or neutral lipids, the ability of non-cationic PSs such as *m*-tetrahydroxyphenylchlorin (mTHPC) to kill microbial cells can be enhanced (Bombelli *et al.*, 2008). A similar report (Ferro *et al.*, 2006) used cationic liposomes composed with *N*-(1-(2,3-dioleoyloxy)propyl)-*N*,*N*,*N*-trimethylammonium methylsulfate (DOTAP) and containing either haematoporphyrin or chlorophyll a to mediate aPDT of MRSA.

Similarly, the attention in nanoparticles has led researchers to prepare nanoparticles containing both PSs and cationic charges for antimicrobial photoinactivation. Schwiertz *et al.* (2009) found that calcium phosphate nanoparticles containing a PS and bearing cationic charges were superior PS delivery vehicles, especially for the Gram-negative *P. aeruginosa*. Ferro *et al.* (2009) compared a monocationic porphyrin, 5-(4-(1-dodecanoylpyridinium))-10,15,20-triphenyl-porphine (TDPyP) complexed into supramolecular aggregates of cationic amphiphilic β-cyclodextrin with the same porphyrin encapsulated in cationic liposomes (Ferro *et al.*, 2007). The cationic cyclodextrin porphyrin was more effective in mediating photoinactivation of both Gram-positive and Gram-negative bacteria than the cationic liposome formulation.

20.2.9 Conjugates between PSs and antibodies

The use of monoclonal antibodies (mAbs) conjugated to PSs appears to be one exception to the rule that cationic groups are mandatory to produce a PS that can efficiently photoinactivate Gram-negative bacteria. A conjugate between mAb NO76 and Sn-ce6 (Lu *et al.*, 1992) was used by Yarmush and co-workers to kill the resistant Gram-negative species *Pseudomonas aeruginosa* both *in vitro* (Friedberg *et al.*, 1991) and *in vivo* (Berthiaume *et al.*, 1994). The conjugate did not kill *S. aureus* to which the mAb did not bind. This finding (effectiveness despite the lack of cationic charge) may be explained by the tight binding between the antibody and the bacterial cell.

20.3 Conclusion

In recent years, the use of aPDT in clinical infections has become increasingly common. PDT is becoming the treatment of choice for periodontitis where PS and light from a laser fibre is inserted into the dental pocket (Andersen *et al.*, 2007; Pinheiro *et al.*, 2010; Novaes *et al.*, 2011). MB (Periowave™, Ondine Biomedical; Ge *et al.*, 2011) and TBO (HELBO Photodynamic Systems; Neugebauer *et al.*, 2004) are frequently employed PSs. Other dental applications have been reported such as from Denfotex in the UK using PDT to sterilize dental cavities. We (with our collaborators in Brazil) have published a study (Garcez *et al.*, 2007) in which the PEI–ce6 conjugate invented in our laboratory was used to combat endodontic infection in patient root canals in conjunction with a red fibre-optic laser. Other studies on endodontic infection have been reported (Garcez *et al.*, 2008, 2010). Ondine Biomedical recently embarked on a large clinical trial (6000 patients) of PDT for nasal decontamination of MRSA in the anterior nares prior to surgery (http://www.ondinebio.com/wp-content/uploads/2011/04/OBP-NR-041511-Final.pdf). As mupirocin resistance is spreading, leading to discouragement of mupirocin use, and PDT can readily destroy the bacterial contamination for the crucial 48 h period during and after surgery, this would appear to be an ideal application for aPDT. Clinical trials are also planned using PDT for *in situ* microbial photodisinfection of endotracheal tubes as a means to prevent ventilator-associated pneumonia (http://www.ondinebio.com/wp-content/uploads/2011/05/OBP-NR-051011-Final.pdf) and a related company, Sinuwave, is exploring the use of MB PDT to combat chronic sinusitis (http://www.sinuwave.com/). Our laboratory (Ganz *et al.*, 2005; Lembo *et al.*, 2009) and one other (Wilder-Smith *et al.*, 2002) have published clinical studies on PDT for *Helicobacter pylori* infection in the human stomach. Photopharmica in Leeds in the UK has carried out a clinical trial of PDT for infected leg ulcers, Other reports have used PDT with 5-aminolevulinic acid for various localized superficial infections such as cutaneous leishmaniasis (El-On *et al.*, 2004; Asilian and Davami, 2006;), athlete's foot (Calzavara-Pinton *et al.*, 2004) and viral warts (Mizuki *et al.*, 2003; Chen *et al.*, 2004; Herzinger *et al.*, 2006).

Acknowledgements

This work was supported by the NIH (grant RO1 AI050875 to M.R.H.) and US Air Force MFEL Program (FA9550-04-1-0079).

References

Akilov, O.E., Kosaka, S., O'Riordan, K., Song, X., Sherwood, M., Flotte, T.J., Foley, J.W. and Hasan, T. (2006) The role of photosensitizer molecular charge and structure on the efficacy of photodynamic therapy against *Leishmania* parasites. *Chemistry and Biology* 13, 839–847.

Alves, E., Costa, L., Carvalho, C.M., Tome, J.P., Faustino, M.A., Neves, M.G., Tome, A.C., Cavaleiro, J.A., Cunha, A. and Almeida, A. (2009) Charge effect on the photoinactivation of Gram-negative and Gram-positive bacteria by cationic meso-substituted porphyrins. *BMC Microbiology* 9, 70.

Andersen, R., Loebel, N., Hammond, D. and Wilson, M. (2007) Treatment of periodontal disease by photodisinfection compared to scaling and root planing. *Journal of Clinical Dentistry* 18, 34–38.

Asilian, A. and Davami, M. (2006) Comparison between the efficacy of photodynamic therapy and topical paromomycin in the treatment of Old World cutaneous leishmaniasis: a placebo-controlled, randomized clinical trial. *Clinical and Experimental Dermatology* 31, 634–637.

Banfi, S., Caruso, E., Buccafurni, L., Battini, V., Zazzaron, S., Barbieri, P. and Orlandi, V. (2006) Antibacterial activity of tetraaryl-porphyrin photosensitizers: an *in vitro* study on Gram negative and Gram positive bacteria. *Journal of Photochemistry and Photobiology B* 85, 28–38.

Berthiaume, F., Reiken, S.R., Toner, M., Tompkins, R.G. and Yarmush, M.L. (1994) Antibody-targeted photolysis of bacteria *in vivo*. *Biotechnology (New York)* 12, 703–706.

Bliss, J.M., Bigelow, C.E., Foster, T.H. and Haidaris, C.G. (2004) Susceptibility of *Candida* species to photodynamic effects of photofrin. *Antimicrobial Agents and Chemotherapy* 48, 2000–2006.

Bombelli, C., Bordi, F., Ferro, S., Giansanti, L., Jori, G., Mancini, G., Mazzuca, C., Monti, D., Ricchelli, F., Sennato, S. and Venanzi, M. (2008) New cationic liposomes as vehicles of *m*-tetrahydroxyphenylchlorin in photodynamic therapy of infectious diseases. *Molecular Pharmacology* 5, 672–679.

Brown, S.B., Brown, E.A. and Walker, I. (2004) The present and future role of photodynamic therapy in cancer treatment. *Lancet Oncology* 5, 497–508.

Calzavara-Pinton, P.G., Venturini, M., Capezzera, R., Sala, R. and Zane, C. (2004) Photodynamic therapy of interdigital mycoses of the feet with topical application of 5-aminolevulinic acid. *Photodermatology, Photoimmunology and Photomedicine* 20, 144–147.

Carvalho, C.M., Gomes, A.T., Fernandes, S.C., Prata, A.C., Almeida, M.A., Cunha, M.A., Tome, J.P., Faustino, M.A., Neves, M.G., Tome, A.C., Cavaleiro, J.A., Lin, Z., Rainho, J.P. and Rocha, J. (2007) Photoinactivation of bacteria in wastewater by porphyrins: bacterial β-galactosidase activity and leucine-uptake as methods to monitor the process. *Journal of Photochemistry and Photobiology B* 88, 112–118.

Chen, H.M., Chen, C.T., Yang, H., Kuo, M.Y., Kuo, Y.S., Lan, W.H., Wang, Y.P., Tsai, T. and Chiang, C.P. (2004) Successful treatment of oral verrucous hyperplasia with topical 5-aminolevulinic acid-mediated photodynamic therapy. *Oral Oncology* 40, 630–637.

Costa, L., Carvalho, C.M., Faustino, M.A., Neves, M.G., Tome, J.P., Tome, A.C., Cavaleiro, J.A., Cunha, A. and Almeida, A. (2010) Sewage bacteriophage inactivation by cationic porphyrins: influence of light parameters. *Photochemical and Photobiological Sciences* 9, 1126–1133.

Dai, T., Tegos, G.P., Lu, Z., Huang, L., Zhiyentayev, T., Franklin, M.J., Baer, D.G. and Hamblin, M.R. (2009) Photodynamic therapy for *Acinetobacter baumannii* burn infections in mice. *Antimicrobial Agents and Chemotherapy* 53, 3929–3934.

Dai, T., Tegos, G.P., Zhiyentayev, T., Mylonakis, E. and Hamblin, M.R. (2010) Photodynamic therapy for methicillin-resistant *Staphylococcus aureus* infection in a mouse skin abrasion model. *Lasers in Surgery and Medicine* 42, 38–44.

Demidova, T.N. and Hamblin, M.R. (2005) Effect of cell-photosensitizer binding and cell density on microbial photoinactivation. *Antimicrobial Agents and Chemotherapy* 49, 2329–2335.

Dougherty, T.J. (2002) An update on photodynamic therapy applications. *Journal of Clinical Laser Medicine and Surgery* 20, 3–7.

El-On, J., Katz, M. and Weinrauch, L. (2004) Treatment of cutaneous leishmaniasis by photodynamic therapy. *Journal of the American Academy of Dermatology* 50, e12; author reply e13.

Ferro, S., Ricchelli, F., Mancini, G., Tognon, G. and Jori, G. (2006) Inactivation of methicillin-resistant *Staphylococcus aureus* (MRSA) by liposome-delivered photosensitising agents. *Journal of Photochemistry and Photobiology B* 83, 98–104.

Ferro, S., Ricchelli, F., Monti, D., Mancini, G. and Jori, G. (2007) Efficient photoinactivation of methicillin-resistant *Staphylococcus aureus* by a novel porphyrin incorporated into a poly-cationic liposome. *International Journal of Biochemistry and Cell Biology* 39, 1026–1034.

Ferro, S., Jori, G., Sortino, S., Stancanelli, R., Nikolov, P., Tognon, G., Ricchelli, F.

and Mazzaglia, A. (2009) Inclusion of 5-[4-(1-dodecanoylpyridinium)]-10,15,20-triphenylporphine in supramolecular aggregates of cationic amphiphilic cyclodextrins: physicochemical characterization of the complexes and strengthening of the antimicrobial photosensitizing activity. *Biomacromolecules* 10, 2592–2600.

Friedberg, J.S., Tompkins, R.G., Rakestraw, S.L., Warren, S.W., Fischman, A.J. and Yarmush, M.L. (1991) Antibody-targeted photolysis. Bacteriocidal effects of Sn (IV) chlorin e6–dextran–monoclonal antibody conjugates. *Annals of the New York Academy of Sciences* 618, 383–393.

Fuchs, B.B., Tegos, G.P., Hamblin, M.R. and Mylonakis, E. (2007) Susceptibility of *Cryptococcus neoformans* to photodynamic inactivation is associated with cell wall integrity. *Antimicrobial Agents and Chemotherapy* 51, 2929–2936.

Gad, F., Zahra, T., Francis, K.P., Hasan, T. and Hamblin, M.R. (2004a) Targeted photodynamic therapy of established soft-tissue infections in mice. *Photochemical and Photobiological Sciences* 3, 451–458.

Gad, F., Zahra, T., Hasan, T. and Hamblin, M.R. (2004b) Effects of growth phase and extracellular slime on photodynamic inactivation of Gram-positive pathogenic bacteria. *Antimicrobial Agents and Chemotherapy* 48, 2173–2178.

Ganz, R.A., Viveiros, J., Ahmad, A., Ahmadi, A., Khalil, A., Tolkoff, M.J., Nishioka, N.S. and Hamblin, M.R. (2005) *Helicobacter pylori* in patients can be killed by visible light. *Lasers in Surgery and Medicine* 36, 260–265.

Garcez, A.S., Ribeiro, M.S., Tegos, G.P., Nunez, S.C., Jorge, A.O. and Hamblin, M.R. (2007) Antimicrobial photodynamic therapy combined with conventional endodontic treatment to eliminate root canal biofilm infection. *Lasers in Surgery and Medicine* 39, 59–66.

Garcez, A.S., Nunez, S.C., Hamblin, M.R. and Ribeiro, M.S. (2008) Antimicrobial effects of photodynamic therapy on patients with necrotic pulps and periapical lesion. *Journal of Endodontics* 34, 138–142.

Garcez, A.S., Nunez, S.C., Hamblin, M.R., Suzuki, H. and Ribeiro, M.S. (2010) Photodynamic therapy associated with conventional endodontic treatment in patients with antibiotic-resistant microflora: a preliminary report. *Journal of Endodontics* 36, 1463–1466.

Ge, L., Shu, R., Li, Y., Li, C., Luo, L., Song, Z., Xie, Y. and Liu, D. (2011) Adjunctive effect of photodynamic therapy to scaling and root planing in the treatment of chronic periodontitis. *Photomedicine and Laser Surgery* 29, 33–37.

Giuliani, F., Martinelli, M., Cocchi, A., Arbia, D., Fantetti, L. and Roncucci, G. (2010) *In vitro* resistance selection studies of RLP068/Cl, a new Zn(II) phthalocyanine suitable for antimicrobial photodynamic therapy. *Antimicrobial Agents and Chemotherapy* 54, 637–642.

Gonzales, F.P., da Silva, S.H., Roberts, D.W. and Braga, G.U. (2010) Photodynamic inactivation of conidia of the fungi *Metarhizium anisopliae* and *Aspergillus nidulans* with methylene blue and toluidine blue. *Photochemistry and Photobiology* 86, 653–661.

Gottlieb, P., Shen, L.G., Chimezie, E., Bahng, S., Kenney, M.E., Horowitz, B. and Ben-Hur, E. (1995) Inactivation of *Trypanosoma cruzi* trypomastigote forms in blood components by photodynamic treatment with phthalocyanines. *Photochemistry and Photobiology* 62, 869–874.

Grinholc, M., Kawiak, A., Kurlenda, J., Graczyk, A. and Bielawski, K.P. (2008) Photodynamic effect of protoporphyrin diarginate (PPArg2) on methicillin-resistant *Staphylococcus aureus* and human dermal fibroblasts. *Acta Biochimica Polonica* 55, 85–90.

Hager, B., Strauss, W.S. and Falk, H. (2009) Cationic hypericin derivatives as novel agents with photobactericidal activity: synthesis and photodynamic inactivation of *Propionibacterium acnes*. *Photochemistry and Photobiology* 85, 1201–1206.

Hamblin, M.R., O'Donnell, D.A., Murthy, N., Contag, C.H. and Hasan, T. (2002a) Rapid control of wound infections by targeted photodynamic therapy monitored by *in vivo* bioluminescence imaging. *Photochemistry and Photobiology* 75, 51–57.

Hamblin, M.R., O'Donnell, D.A., Murthy, N., Rajagopalan, K., Michaud, N., Sherwood, M.E. and Hasan, T. (2002b) Polycationic photosensitizer conjugates: effects of chain length and Gram classification on the photodynamic inactivation of bacteria. *Journal of Antimicrobial Chemotherapy* 49, 941–951.

Hamblin, M.R., Zahra, T., Contag, C.H., McManus, A.T. and Hasan, T. (2003) Optical monitoring and treatment of potentially lethal wound infections *in vivo*. *International Journal of Infectious Diseases* 187, 1717–1725.

Herzinger, T., Wienecke, R., Weisenseel, P., Borelli, C., Berking, C. and Degitz, K. (2006) Photodynamic therapy of genital condylomata in men. *Clinical and Experimental Dermatology* 31, 51–53.

Huang, L., Huang, Y.Y., Mroz, P., Tegos, G.P., Zhiyentayev, T., Sharma, S.K., Lu, Z., Balasubramanian, T., Krayer, M., Ruzie, C., Yang, E., Kee, H.L., Kirmaier, C., Diers, J.R., Bocian, D.F., Holten, D., Lindsey, J.S. and Hamblin, M.R.

(2010) Stable synthetic cationic bacteriochlorins as selective antimicrobial photosensitizers. *Antimicrobial Agents and Chemotherapy* 54, 3834–3841.

Kassab, K., Dei, D., Roncucci, G., Jori, G. and Coppellotti, O. (2003) Phthalocyanine-photosensitized inactivation of a pathogenic protozoan, *Acanthamoeba palestinensis*. *Photochemical and Photobiological Sciences* 2, 668–672.

Lambrechts, S.A., Aalders, M.C., Langeveld-Klerks, D.H., Khayali, Y. and Lagerberg, J.W. (2004) Effect of monovalent and divalent cations on the photoinactivation of bacteria with meso-substituted cationic porphyrins. *Photochemistry and Photobiology* 79, 297–302.

Lambrechts, S.A., Aalders, M.C. and van Marle, J. (2005a) Mechanistic study of the photodynamic inactivation of *Candida albicans* by a cationic porphyrin. *Antimicrobial Agents and Chemotherapy* 49, 2026–2034.

Lambrechts, S.A., Demidova, T.N., Aalders, M.C., Hasan, T. and Hamblin, M.R. (2005b) Photodynamic therapy for *Staphylococcus aureus* infected burn wounds in mice. *Photochemical and Photobiological Sciences* 4, 503–509.

Lauro, F.M., Pretto, P., Covolo, L., Jori, G. and Bertoloni, G. (2002) Photoinactivation of bacterial strains involved in periodontal diseases sensitized by porphycene–polylysine conjugates. *Photochemical and Photobiological Sciences* 1, 468–470.

Lembo, A.J., Ganz, R.A., Sheth, S., Cave, D., Kelly, C., Levin, P., Kazlas, P.T., Baldwin, P.C. III, Lindmark, W.R., McGrath, J.R. and Hamblin, M.R. (2009) Treatment of *Helicobacter pylori* infection with intra-gastric violet light phototherapy: a pilot clinical trial. *Lasers in Surgery and Medicine* 41, 337–344.

Levy, J.G. and Obochi, M. (1996) New applications in photodynamic therapy. Introduction. *Photochemistry and Photobiology* 64, 737–739.

Lu, X.M., Fischman, A.J., Stevens, E., Lee, T.T., Strong, L., Tompkins, R.G. and Yarmush, M.L. (1992) Sn-chlorin e6 antibacterial immunoconjugates. An *in vitro* and *in vivo* analysis. *Journal of Immunological Methods* 156, 85–99.

Maisch, T., Bosl, C., Szeimies, R.M., Lehn, N. and Abels, C. (2005) Photodynamic effects of novel XF porphyrin derivatives on prokaryotic and eukaryotic cells. *Antimicrobial Agents and Chemotherapy* 49, 1542–1552.

Malik, Z., Hanania, J. and Nitzan, Y. (1990) Bactericidal effects of photoactivated porphyrins – an alternative approach to antimicrobial drugs. *Journal of Photochemistry and Photobiology B* 5, 281–293.

Malik, Z., Ladan, H. and Nitzan, Y. (1992) Photodynamic inactivation of Gram-negative bacteria: problems and possible solutions. *Journal of Photochemistry and Photobiology B* 14, 262–266.

Mantareva, V., Kussovski, V., Angelov, I., Borisova, E., Avramov, L., Schnurpfeil, G. and Wohrle, D. (2007) Photodynamic activity of water-soluble phthalocyanine zinc(II) complexes against pathogenic microorganisms. *Bioorganic and Medicinal Chemistry* 15, 4829–4835.

Mantareva, V., Kussovski, V., Angelov, I., Wohrle, D., Dimitrov, R., Popova, E. and Dimitrov, S. (2010) Non-aggregated Ga(III)-phthalocyanines in the photodynamic inactivation of planktonic and biofilm cultures of pathogenic microorganisms. *Photochemical and Photobiological Sciences* 2011, 10, 91–102.

Merchat, M., Bertolini, G., Giacomini, P., Villanueva, A. and Jori, G. (1996) Meso-substituted cationic porphyrins as efficient photosensitizers of Gram-positive and Gram-negative bacteria. *Journal of Photochemistry and Photobiology B* 32, 153–157.

Minnock, A., Vernon, D.I., Schofield, J., Griffiths, J., Parish, J.H. and Brown, S.T. (1996) Photoinactivation of bacteria. Use of a cationic water-soluble zinc phthalocyanine to photoinactivate both Gram-negative and Gram-positive bacteria. *Journal of Photochemistry and Photobiology B* 32, 159–164.

Mizuki, D., Kaneko, T. and Hanada, K. (2003) Successful treatment of topical photodynamic therapy using 5-aminolevulinic acid for plane warts. *British Journal of Dermatology* 149, 1087–1088.

Neugebauer, J., Jozsa, M. and Kubler, A. (2004) Antimicrobial photodynamic therapy for prevention of alveolar ostitis and post-extraction pain. *Mund-, Kiefer- und Gesichtschirurgie* 8, 350–355.

Novaes, A.B. Jr., Schwartz-Filho, H.O., de Oliveira, R.R., Feres, M., Sato, S. and Figueiredo, L.C. (2011) Antimicrobial photodynamic therapy in the non-surgical treatment of aggressive periodontitis: microbiological profile. *Lasers in medical science* doi:10.1007/s10103-011-0901-6 (Epub ahead of print).

O'Neill, J., Wilson, M. and Wainwright, M. (2003) Comparative antistreptococcal activity of photobactericidal agents. *Journal of Chemotherapy* 15, 329–334.

Ochsner, M. (1997) Photophysical and photobiological processes in the photodynamic therapy of tumours. *Journal of Photochemistry and Photobiology B* 39, 1–18.

Phoenix, D.A., Sayed, Z., Hussain, S., Harris, F. and Wainwright, M. (2003) The phototoxicity of phenothiazinium derivatives against *Escherichia coli* and *Staphylococcus aureus*. *FEMS Immunology and Medical Microbiology* 39, 17–22.

Pinheiro, S.L., Donega, J.M., Seabra, L.M., Adabo, M.D., Lopes, T., do Carmo, T.H., Ribeiro, M.C. and Bertolini, P.F. (2010) Capacity of photodynamic therapy for microbial reduction in periodontal pockets. *Lasers in Medical Science* 25, 87–91.

Polo, L., Segalla, A., Bertoloni, G., Jori, G., Schaffner, K. and Reddi, E. (2000) Polylysine–porphycene conjugates as efficient photosensitizers for the inactivation of microbial pathogens. *Journal of Photochemistry and Photobiology B* 59, 152–158.

Raab, O. (1900) Über die Wirkung fluoresceinder Stoffe and Infusorien. *Zeit für Biology* 39, 524–546.

Ragàs, X., Dai, T., Tegos, G.P., Agut, M., Nonell, S. and Hamblin, M.R. (2010) Photodynamic inactivation of *Acinetobacter baumannii* using phenothiazinium dyes: *in vitro* and *in vivo* studies. *Lasers in Surgery and Medicine* 42, 384–390.

Rovaldi, C.R., Pievsky, A., Sole, N.A., Friden, P.M., Rothstein, D.M. and Spacciapoli, P. (2000) Photoactive porphyrin derivative with broad-spectrum activity against oral pathogens *in vitro*. *Antimicrobial Agents and Chemotherapy* 44, 3364–3367.

Schwiertz, J., Wiehe, A., Grafe, S., Gitter, B. and Epple, M. (2009) Calcium phosphate nanoparticles as efficient carriers for photodynamic therapy against cells and bacteria. *Biomaterials* 30, 3324–3331.

Smijs, T.G., Pavel, S., Talebi, M. and Bouwstra, J.A. (2009) Preclinical studies with 5,10,15-Tris(4-methylpyridinium)-20-phenyl-[21H,23H]-porphine trichloride for the photodynamic treatment of superficial mycoses caused by *Trichophyton rubrum*. *Photochemistry and Photobiology* 85, 733–739.

Smith, T.L., Pearson, M.L., Wilcox, K.R., Cruz, C., Lancaster, M.V., Robinson-Dunn, B., Tenover, F.C., Zervos, M.J., Band, J.D., White, E. and Jarvis, W.R. (1999) Emergence of vancomycin resistance in *Staphylococcus aureus*. Glycopeptide-Intermediate *Staphylococcus aureus* Working Group. *New England Journal of Medicine* 340, 493–501.

Soukos, N.S., Hamblin, M.R. and Hasan, T. (1997) The effect of charge on cellular uptake and phototoxicity of polylysine chlorin(e6) conjugates. *Photochemistry and Photobiology* 65, 723–729.

Soukos, N.S., Ximenez-Fyvie, L.A., Hamblin, M.R., Socransky, S.S. and Hasan, T. (1998) Targeted antimicrobial photochemotherapy. *Antimicrobial Agents and Chemotherapy* 42, 2595–2601.

Spesia, M.B., Milanesio, M.E. and Durantini, E.N. (2008) Synthesis, properties and photodynamic inactivation of *Escherichia coli* by novel cationic fullerene C60 derivatives. *European Journal of Medicinal Chemistry* 43, 853–861.

Stockert, J.C., Canete, M., Juarranz, A., Villanueva, A., Horobin, R.W., Borrell, J.I., Teixido, J. and Nonell, S. (2007) Porphycenes: facts and prospects in photodynamic therapy of cancer. *Current Medicinal Chemistry* 14, 997–1026.

Tegos, G.P., Demidova, T.N., Arcila-Lopez, D., Lee, H., Wharton, T., Gali, H. and Hamblin, M.R. (2005) Cationic fullerenes are effective and selective antimicrobial photosensitizers. *Chemistry and Biology* 12, 1127–1135.

Tegos, G.P., Anbe, M., Yang, C., Demidova, T.N., Satti, M., Mroz, P., Janjua, S., Gad, F. and Hamblin, M.R. (2006) Protease-stable polycationic photosensitizer conjugates between polyethyleneimine and chlorin(e6) for broad-spectrum antimicrobial photoinactivation. *Antimicrobial Agents and Chemotherapy* 50, 1402–1410.

Wainwright, M. (2004a) Photoinactivation of viruses. *Photochemical and Photobiological Sciences* 3, 406–411.

Wainwright, W. (2004b) Photoantimicrobials – a PACT against resistance and infection. *Drug Future* 29, 85–93.

Wainwright, M. (2010) 'Safe' photoantimicrobials for skin and soft-tissue infections. *International Journal of Antimicrobial Agents* 36, 14–18.

Wainwright, M. and Crossley, K.B. (2002) Methylene Blue – a therapeutic dye for all seasons? *Journal of Chemotherapy* 14, 431–443.

Wainwright, M., Phoenix, D.A., Marland, J., Wareing, D.R. and Bolton, F.J. (1997a) A study of photobactericidal activity in the phenothiazinium series. *FEMS Immunology and Medical Microbiology* 19, 75–80.

Wainwright, M., Phoenix, D.A., Rice, L., Burrow, S.M. and Waring, J. (1997b) Increased cytotoxicity and phototoxicity in the methylene blue series via chromophore methylation. *Journal of Photochemistry and Photobiology B* 40, 233–239.

Wilder-Smith, C.H., Wilder-Smith, P., Grosjean, P., van den Bergh, H., Woodtli, A., Monnier, P., Dorta, G., Meister, F. and Wagnieres, G. (2002) Photoeradication of *Helicobacter pylori* using 5-aminolevulinic acid: preliminary human studies. *Lasers in Surgery and Medicine* 31, 18–22.

Wilson, M., Burns, T., Pratten, J. and Pearson, G.J. (1995) Bacteria in supragingival plaque samples can be killed by low-power laser light in the presence of a photosensitizer. *Journal of Applied Bacteriology* 78, 569–574.

21 Nanoparticle Platforms for Antimicrobial Therapy

David Trofa and Joshua D. Nosanchuk
Departments of Medicine (Division of Infectious Diseases) and Microbiology and Immunology, Albert Einstein College of Medicine, New York, USA

21.1 Introduction

Nanoparticles have unique characteristics that make them ideal drug-delivery vehicles capable of targeting virtually any anatomical site within the human body. They are in the size range of 1–100 nm, have a high surface-area-to-volume ratio and are individually designed with the capacity to interact with cells and tissues at the molecular level (Zhang *et al.*, 2008). The fate of nanoparticles within the human body is determined by the interactions of the nanoparticles with their local environment, which can be influenced by their composition, size and surface properties. Charges, for example, that are slightly negative or positive usually have minimal self–self and self–non-self interactions, while larger charges increase macrophage scavenging and clearance by the reticuloendothelial system. A particularly important area of nanotechnology application is the development of nanoparticles that can target difficult-to-reach areas of the body such as bone marrow and the central nervous system.

Nanoparticle applications include antimicrobial therapeutics, cancer therapy, *in vivo* imaging, *in vitro* diagnostics, biomaterial formulations and active implants (Wagner *et al.*, 2006). Further developments in nanoparticle technology may allow detection of the molecular changes responsible for disease pathogenesis, better diagnostic imaging and improved drug therapeutics, with more vehicle delivery options capable of combined drug therapies, thus enabling technologies to accelerate scientific and medical discoveries. Currently, the most common nanotech platforms include polymeric nanoparticles, nanoshells, micelles, liposomes, dendrimers, nucleic acid-based nanoconstructs, engineered viral nanoparticles, magnetic nanoparticles, silicon oxide nanoparticles and quantum dots (Farokhzad and Langer, 2006).

Certain antimicrobial drugs are difficult to administer due to low water solubility, cytotoxicity to host tissues, rapid clearance from the bloodstream and poor membrane transport ability. Nanoparticles facilitate antimicrobial delivery to infection sites by increasing drug serum solubility, prolonging systemic circulation and allowing controlled delivery and drug release in targeted tissues and cells, with the option of delivering multiple therapeutic agents for combination therapy (Davis *et al.*, 2008; Zhang *et al.*, 2008). Furthermore, nanoparticles have two mechanisms of drug delivery, fusion with the pathogen or binding to the cell wall or membrane and subsequent deposition of drug. Nanoparticles can also enter host cells via endocytosis and release drug payloads to treat intracellular infections, an important mechanism as pathogenic microorganisms have developed multiple ways to avoid intracellular killing including phagosome escape, inhibition of phagosome–lysosome fusion, and lysosomal enzyme or oxidative and non-oxidative killing mechanism resistance (Zhang *et al.*, 2010). Hence, nanoparticles have been designed to specifically target some of the resistance mechanisms that microbes have evolved in response to the use of antimicrobial drugs of recent decades.

In this chapter, we summarize the use of nanoparticles as antimicrobial agents and detail the most common vehicles used for antimicrobial delivery; including liposomes, polymeric nanoparticles, solid lipid nanoparticles, dendrimers and silver nanoparticles (Zhang *et al.*, 2010). We also discuss nanoparticles in the context of some important infectious diseases, including tuberculosis (TB), malaria and human immunodeficiency virus/acquired immunodeficiency syndrome (HIV/AIDS). While most nanoparticle-based drug-delivery systems are currently in pre-clinical development, a few have been used clinically (Table 21.1), and with the promising ongoing research discussed here, such platforms may be instrumental in treating life-threatening infectious diseases in the future.

21.2 Antimicrobial Platforms

21.2.1 Liposomes

Liposomes were first described in 1965 (Bangham *et al.*, 1965) and proposed as a drug-delivery platform in the 1970s. They are currently the most widely used antimicrobial drug-delivery system. Liposomes form nanoparticles through the non-spontaneous assembly of a spherical amphiphilic bilayer membrane composed of natural or synthetic lipids, the surface of which can be customized

Table 21.1. US Food and Drug Administration (FDA)-approved antimicrobial nanomedicines.

Product	Composition and nanotech component	Delivery route[a]	FDA-approved indications	FDA approval date	Company
Abelcet	Amphotericin B–lipid complex	IV	Fungal infections	1995	Enzon (Bridgewater, New Jersey, USA)
Amphotec	Amphotericin B colloidal dispersion	SC	Fungal infections	1996	InterMune (Brisbane, California, USA)
Ambisome	Amphotericin B liposomes	IV	Fungal infections	1997	Gilead Sciences (Foster City, California, USA)
PEGIntron	PEG–α-interferon 2b	SC	Chronic hepatitis C in patients with compensated liver disease	2001	Enzon Schering-Plough (Kenilworth, New Jersey, USA)
Pegasys	PEG–α-interferon 2a	SC	Chronic hepatitis C	2002	Nektar (San Carlos, California, USA)
			Chronic hepatitis B	2005	Hoffmann-La Roche (Basel)
Acticoat	Silver nanoparticles	Topical	Antimicrobial wound care	1998	Nucryst (Wakefield, Massachusetts, USA)
SilvaGard	Silver nanoparticles	Topical	Antimicrobial wound care	2005	AcryMed Inc. (Beaverton, Oregon, USA)

[a]IV, intravenous; SC, subcutaneous.

with various functional groups to enhance *in vivo* stability or target specific ligands, such as alveolar macrophages (see section 21.3.2) (Farokhzad and Langer, 2006; Zhang *et al.*, 2008). The most commonly used lipid in liposome preparation is phosphatidylcholine, an electrically neutral phospholipid containing fatty acyl chains of varying degrees of saturation and length. The liposomal lipid bilayers mimic pathogen cell membranes, facilitating their fusion with microbes and resulting in the intracellular release of concentrated drug payloads that improve drug efficacy by potentially overcoming certain microbial drug-resistant pathways, such as antibiotic reflux where protein pumps in pathogen membranes efflux antibiotics out of the cell (Fischbach and Walsh, 2009). This property is not selective for liposomes and also occurs in other nanoparticle vehicles.

Clinically, liposomes have been especially instrumental in treating invasive fungal infections. Amphotericin B (AmB) deoxycholate is a broad-range antifungal drug limited by two safety concerns. First, it is associated with various drug toxicities such as chills, fever, anaphylaxis and other serious adverse effects that may require drug cessation. Secondly, its nephrotoxicity has a cumulative effect with progressive dosing that limits the maximum daily dose (Kelsey *et al.*, 1999). AmBisome® (NeXstar Pharmaceuticals; California, USA) has AmB intercalated into the phospholipid bilayer of liposomes consisting of hydrogenated soy phosphatidylcholine, cholesterol and distearoyl phosphatidylglycerol (Hiemenz and Walsh, 1996). Compared with standard AmB, AmBisome has a longer systemic circulation half-life, reduced plasma toxicity and enhanced therapeutic efficacy (Walsh *et al.*, 2001).

AmBisome delivers its payload via an absorption mechanism, releasing the drug following fusion of the liposome with the fungal cell. For example, AmBisome has been shown to attach to the outer wall of *Candida glabrata*, resulting in disruption of the liposome, accumulation of AmB in the cytoplasm and fungal death (Adler-Moore and Proffitt, 2002). The localization of AmBisome to the site of fungal infection is quite remarkable, as shown by the localization of fluorescently labelled AmBisome to the site of infection in *Candida*-infected mice (Adler-Moore, 1994). Two other US Food and Drug Administration (FDA)-approved nanomedicine products on the market that deliver an AmB payload include Abelcet® (Enzon; New Jersey, USA), which uses an AmB–lipid complex, and Amphotec® (InterMune; California, USA), which uses a lipid colloidal dispersion (Wagner *et al.*, 2006). Fungisome™, liposomal AmB and Ampholip™, an AmB–lipid complex, have been approved in India (Table 21.2).

Several antibacterial agents have been packaged as liposomes for experimental use with excellent results. Improved activity relative to standard drug formulations has been demonstrated *in vitro* and/or *in vivo* with liposomes loaded with AmB against *Salmonella typhimurium* (Fattal *et al.*, 1991; Schumacher and Margalit, 1997), benzyl penicillin against *Staphylococcus aureus* (Kim and Jones, 2004), ciprofloxacin against *Salmonella* Dublin (Magallanes *et al.*, 1993), gentamicin and streptomycin against *Brucella* spp. (Fountain

Table 21.2. Other antimicrobial nanomedicines in clinical use.

Product	Composition and nanotech component	Indication	Company
Epaxal	Virosomal hepatitis A vaccine	Hepatitis A vaccine	Berna Biotech (Switzerland)
Inflexal V	Virosomal influenza vaccine	Influenza	Berna Biotech (Switzerland)
Fungisome	Liposomal amphotericin B	Fungal infections	Lifecare Innovations (India)
Ampholip	Amphotericin B–lipid complex	Fungal infections	Bharat Serums and Vaccines Ltd (India)

et al., 1985), and vancomycin and teicoplanin against methicillin-resistant *S. aureus* (MRSA) (Onyeji *et al.*, 1994). Polymyxin B is a potent drug for multidrug-resistant Gram-negative bacteria, but its use is limited by toxicities, including nephrotoxicity, ototoxicity and neuromuscular blockade. However, liposomal encapsulation of polymyxin B reduces toxicity while improving the microbial activity against *Pseudomonas aeruginosa* (Alipour *et al.*, 2008).

21.2.2 Polymeric nanoparticles

Polymeric nanoparticles have unique characteristics that make them another ideal platform for antimicrobial drug delivery. Besides being structurally stable and having the capacity to load high concentrations of hydrophilic and hydrophobic drugs, particle properties such as size, zeta potentials and drug-release profiles can be customized during synthesis. Moreover, the surface of polymeric nanoparticles can be chemically modified with functional groups, drug moieties or targeting ligands. For instance, conjugation of lectin, a protein that binds to simple or complex carbohydrates on most bacterial cell walls, allows nanoparticles to bind *Helicobacter pylori* cell-wall carbohydrate receptors (Umamaheshwari and Jain, 2003). Hence, polymeric nanoparticles are being extensively studied to increase drug solubility, enhance *in vivo* stability and improve targeting (Soppimath *et al.*, 2001; Delie and Blanco-Prieto, 2005).

There are two main types of polymeric nanoparticles for antimicrobial drug delivery. The nanosphere is a self-assembled diblock copolymer consisting of a hydrophobic polymeric core containing the drugs and a hydrophilic shielding section to prevent osponization and degradation of the core. The length of the hydrophobic chain can vary the rate of drug release, allowing increased control and customization of the nanoparticle. Furthermore, the hydrophobic nature of the nanoparticle core allows polymeric nanoparticles to carry and deliver poorly water-soluble drugs (Cheng *et al.*, 2007; Gu *et al.*, 2008). Examples of biodegradable polymers used to form the hydrophobic polymeric core include poly(lactic acid) (PLA), poly(glycolic acid) (PGA), poly(lactide-co-glycolide) (PLGA), poly (ε-caprolactone) (PCL) and poly(cyano-acrylate) (PCA). Polyethylene glycol (PEG) has been commonly used as a hydrophilic segment to help prolong nanoparticle circulation times in the bloodstream by preventing host immune system recognition (Sosnik *et al.*, 2010).

The second type of polymeric nanoparticles is nanocapsules, formed through an emulsification polymerization of linear polymers such as polyalkyl acrylates and polymethyl methacrylate. Hydrophobic drugs can be absorbed to the nanocapsules during the polymerization process, while hydrophilic drugs are normally attached to the particle via covalent conjugation. Interestingly, antimicrobials can be inactivated by covalent attachment, as noted in a study on staphylococcal infections where β-lactam and ciprofloxacin retained their potency while penicillin was inactivated following attachment (Abeylath *et al.*, 2008).

Polymeric nanoparticles have recently become a mainstay in the treatment of chronic hepatitis B and C virus infection. Standard therapy for hepatitis C consists of a combination of pegylated interferon (IFN) combined with ribavirin, a nucleoside analogue (Foster, 2010). As a result of the increased half-life of IFN after pegylation, sustained virological response rates climbed to over 60% in patients treated with pegylated IFN plus ribavirin compared with 40% with standard IFN with ribavirin (Manns *et al.*, 2001; Fried *et al.*, 2002; Hadziyannis *et al.*, 2004). There are two FDA-approved pegIFNs currently available, PEG–α-IFN-2b (PegIntron™) and PEG–α-IFN-2a (Pegasys™), which differ in the IFN-α modified, the size and nature of pegylation, and the covalent attachment of the PEG (Foster, 2010). A recent report indicates that PEG–α-IFN-2a plus ribavirin achieved a higher sustained virological response rate than PEG–α-IFN-2b plus ribavirin (68.8 versus 54.4%; Ascione *et al.*, 2010).

PEG–α-IFN-2a is the only pegylated form of IFN approved for the treatment of hepatitis B in the USA (Lok and McMahon,

2009). In clinical trials, pegylated IFN-α has also shown equal or greater efficacy compared with standard IFN in the treatment of chronic hepatitis B (Lok and McMahon, 2009). Additionally, pegylated IFN-α achieved a higher rate of seroconversion in hepatitis B virus e antigen (HBeAg)-positive patients versus standard IFN-α (Cooksley *et al.*, 2003). In the same patient population, PEG–α-IFN-2a was more successful than lamivudine in inducing sustained HBeAg seroconversion, while also achieving similar results to combination therapy of pegIFN-2a and lamivudine (Lau *et al.*, 2005). PegIFN-2a also showed efficacy in HBeAg-negative patients (Marcellin *et al.*, 2004).

Additional experimental polymeric nanoparticles for infectious diseases include AmB-loaded PCL nanospheres, which have enhanced *in vitro* efficacy against *Leishmania donovani* (Espuelas *et al.*, 2002), while rifampicin-loaded polybutylcyanoacrylate nanoparticles have increased antibacterial activity both *in vitro* and *in vivo* against *S. aureus* and *Mycobacterium avium* (Skidan *et al.*, 2003).

21.2.3 Solid lipid nanoparticles

Solid lipid nanoparticles (SLNs) are particulate systems with mean diameters ranging from 50 to 1000 nm and composed of lipids (e.g. fatty acids, triglycerides, steroids, partial glycerides and waxes) and surfactants (e.g. soybean lecithin, phosphatidylcholine, poloxamer 188, sodium cholate and sodium glycocholate) (zur Mühlen *et al.*, 1998).

SLNs have an occlusive property so that they form a thin film when applied topically, which retains skin moisture and promotes molecule penetration into the skin. This enhances drug penetration and decreases the rate of drug clearance, as seen in a comparison of retinol and retinyl palmitate SNLs versus free drug (Müller *et al.*, 2002). Furthermore, because SLNs are stable in water and dermal cream, they are prime candidates for use in skin-care products (Wissing and Müller, 2003). SLNs have been developed to treat superficial fungal infections with the water-insoluble azole drugs, such as clotrimazole, miconazole, exonazole, oxiconazole and tioconazole (Gupta and Cooper, 2008). The advantages of using SLNs as a means to deliver antifungal agents to treat superficial infections include an increase in drug diffusion to deeper skin layers, higher drug loading, sustained drug release profiles and physiochemical stability (Sanna, Gavini *et al.*, 2007; Yang *et al.*, 2008). Compared with other nanoparticles, SLNs have improved stability and better encapsulation efficiency than liposomes, and require fewer organic solvents during production than polymeric nanoparticles (Sosnik *et al.*, 2010).

SLN formulations have also been used for the oral administration of drugs. For example, tobramycin is an antibacterial drug that is particularly used against *P. aeruginosa* infections in cystic fibrosis patients (Gilligan, 1991). Although tobramycin is typically administered via aerosolization or intravenous infusion, SNL preparations of tobramycin achieve systemic drug levels by bypassing P-glycoprotein, an ATP-dependent drug-efflux pump, on the brush border of the small intestine that actively removes diffused drugs from the cells. As tobramycin-loaded SLNs penetrate the intestinal linings through endocytosis as opposed to passive diffusion, the activity of the efflux pump is drastically reduced (Bargoni *et al.*, 2001). SLNs have also been investigated for the treatment of TB (see Section 21.3.2).

21.2.4 Dendrimer delivery

Dendrimers are highly ordered and regularly branched globular macromolecules consisting of three distinct architectural regions: a focal moiety or a core, layers of branched repeat units emerging from the core and functional end groups on the outer layer of repeat units (Grayson and Fréchet, 2001). This allows hydrophobic drugs to be stored in the hydrophobic core, while hydrophilic drugs can be attached to the surface by covalent conjugation or electrostatic interactions (Gillies and Frechet, 2005).

Certain qualities of dendrimers make them appropriate vehicles for antimicrobial delivery. First, dendrimers are highly branched, providing an enormous surface-area-to-size ratio, allowing increased interaction with pathogens. Additionally, antimicrobials can be used as building blocks in the synthesis of dendrimers. For example, dendrimers can contain quaternary ammonium salts, which disrupt bacterial membranes, as functional end groups. Furthermore, electrostatic interactions between the polycationic structure of dendrimer biocides and the negatively charged bacteria facilitates adsorption and allows more dendrimers to enter the bacterium, leading to eventual disintegration of the bacterial membrane (Chen and Cooper, 2002).

One of the most studied types of antimicrobial dendrimers is polyamidoamine (PAMAM), which has a high density of functional groups making it hydrophilic and more capable of conjugating to antimicrobial compounds. PAMAM dendrimers loaded with silver salts have demonstrated significant antimicrobial activity against *S. aureus*, *P. aeruginosa* and *Escherichia coli* (Balogh *et al.*, 2001), while sulfamethoxazole-loaded PAMAM dendrimers increase the drug's aqueous solubility and have higher antibacterial activity against *E. coli* (Ma *et al.*, 2007).

21.2.5 Silver nanoparticles

Long before the advent of antibiotics, silver in various forms was used to treat burns, wounds and a number of bacterial infections (Rai *et al.*, 2009). Silver possesses broad-spectrum antimicrobial activity against Gram-positive and Gram-negative bacteria, fungi, protozoa and some viruses (see Section 21.3.4) (Monteiro *et al.*, 2009). The ability to manipulate silver into nanoparticles, as well as the increase in antibiotic-resistant pathogens, has led to a recent resurgence in its use to treat and protect against antimicrobial infections. Silver is also non-toxic to humans in minute concentrations, and most studies suggest that silver nanoparticles are non-toxic as well.

The bactericidal activity of silver nanoparticles involves interaction with sulfur-containing proteins in the bacterial membrane and phosphorous-containing compounds, such as DNA, within cells, as well as interruption of the respiratory chain leading to cell death (Feng *et al.*, 2000; Sondi and Salopek-Sondi, 2004; Morones *et al.*, 2005; Rai *et al.*, 2009). Applications for silver nanoparticles (Rai *et al.*, 2009), include dressings, creams and gels that effectively reduce bacterial infections in chronic wounds (Rupp *et al.*, 2004; Taylor *et al.*, 2005; Ip *et al.*, 2006; Leaper, 2006; Jun *et al.*, 2007), silver-impregnated implantable medical devices for antimicrobial activity (Furno *et al.*, 2004) and antibacterial water filters (Jain and Pradeep, 2005). Additionally, antimicrobial polymeric films containing silver nanoparticles may find clinical use for coating prosthetic devices in orthopaedics and dentistry (Travan *et al.*, 2011). Currently, one of the most significant uses for silver nanoparticles is as medical device liners that protect the surface from the attachment and subsequent biofilm formation of microbes.

21.3 Recent Nanoparticle Development for Specific Diseases

21.3.1 *S. aureus*

S. aureus is a major cause of superficial and invasive infections in community and hospital settings and is a leading pathogen that has evolved resistance to standard antibiotics. Recent investigations demonstrating the efficacy of silane-based nanoparticles that release sustained concentrations of nitric oxide (NO) (Friedman *et al.*, 2008) for the treatment of skin and soft tissue infections due to drug-resistant *S. aureus* provide promising data that illustrates the therapeutic potential of compounds that are unlikely to be resisted by bacteria (Han *et al.*, 2009; Martinez *et al.*, 2009). NO is an important component of the host defence mechanism, but its efficacy as a therapeutic has been limited by poor delivery options. In addition to the antimicrobial potency, the NO nanoparticles significantly improved wound healing. These data suggest that NO-releasing nanoparticles could serve as a novel class of topically applied antimicrobials to treat cutaneous infections and wounds. Notably, the NO-releasing nanoparticles were also therapeutic in a murine wound infection model with multidrug-resistant *Acinetobacter baumannii* (Mihu *et al.*, 2010). Applications of this NO nanoparticle platform are extensive and multidisciplinary because of the important role NO plays in immunity and the wound-healing process. NO-based therapeutics can aid in wound healing complicated by common co-morbidities such as obesity, diabetes, atopic dermatitis and peripheral vascular disease.

21.3.2 TB

Nanotechnology use in TB has been reviewed recently (Griffiths *et al.*, 2010; Sosnik *et al.*, 2010). Currently, the most effective pharmacotherapy for susceptible TB is a multidrug combination of isoniazid, pyrazinamide and rifampicin, taken with ethambutol for the first 2 months of treatment (the initial intensive stage), followed by a 4-month regimen of rifampicin and isoniazid (Onyebujoh *et al.*, 2005). This prolonged length of treatment and the extensive pill burden results in low patient compliance and decreased cure rates, which contributes to the development of microbial resistance. Treatment of multidrug-resistant TB consists of the use of second- or third-line drugs that are more toxic, more expensive, less active and require longer treatment periods (Sosnik *et al.*, 2010). It is hoped that nano-based drugs for TB will provide an effective treatment that will increase compliance while overcoming multidrug-resistant organisms. A number of nanoplatforms have been used in various *in vitro* and *in vivo* investigations of TB therapeutics, usually encapsulated forms of first-line TB drugs (Sosnik *et al.*, 2010), including liposomes (Deol and Khuller, 1997; Deol *et al.*, 1997), polymeric nanoparticles (Pandey *et al.*, 2003a; Pandey and Khuller, 2004), SLNs (Sharma *et al.*, 2004; Pandey *et al.*, 2005), dendrimers (Lenaerts *et al.*, 2005; Kumar *et al.*, 2007) and nanodispersions (Jain and Vyas, 1995; Mullaicharam and Murthy, 2004).

As TB largely manifests as a respiratory infection, it is desirable to enhance local delivery of drugs to the lungs, particularly to the alveolar macrophages harbouring the mycobacterium reservoir (Gill *et al.*, 2007; Azarmi *et al.*, 2008; Sosnik *et al.*, 2010). SLNs are attractive, as their delivery to the lungs is followed by phagocytosis by alveolar macrophages and subsequent delivery of drug payloads (Gelperina *et al.*, 2005; Pandey and Khuller, 2005). This translocation and biodistribution through pulmonary delivery has been studied using radiolabelled aerosol SLNs in rats with effective uptake of SLNs in lungs and subsequent accumulation of particles in the periaortic, axillary and inguinal lymph nodes. Another mechanism used to target alveolar macrophages is through the attachment of mannose to liposomes. Mannose is recognized by lectin receptors on macrophages, and mannose-coated liposomes have *in vitro* and *in vivo* preferential uptake by alveolar macrophages compared with non-coated liposomes (Lane *et al.*, 1998; Irache *et al.*, 2008; Wijagkanalan *et al.*, 2008).

Polymeric nanoparticles have been investigated for the targeted delivery to the lungs (Azarmi *et al.*, 2008). In one study, rifampicin, isoniazid and pyrazinamide were encapsulated in PLGA nebulizable nanoparticles and aerosolized particles could be detected at therapeutic concentrations in guinea pig lungs for 11 days (Pandey *et al.*, 2003b). Additionally, five such treatments administered every 10 days were as effective against TB as 46 oral daily doses. In another study, the uptake of encapsulated rifampicin PLGA nanoparticles into alveolar macrophages was enhanced through conjugation with mannitol (Ohashi *et al.*, 2009). Aerosolized rifampicin-loaded liposomes have been shown to increase drug concentrations in lungs compared with nebulized rifampicin alone (Vyas *et al.*, 2004). Liposomes coated with *O*-stearoyl amylopectin, in particular, were effective at targeting alveolar macrophages.

21.3.3 Malaria

The application of nanotechnology to treat malaria was reviewed recently (Santos-Magalhaes and Mosqueira, 2010). Historically, the most important drug used in malaria treatment is chloroquine (CQ), although widespread resistance to CQ has developed (Price *et al.*, 2007; Fidock *et al.*, 2008). Important qualities of nanoparticles for targeting malaria include long circulating times to increase interactions with infected red blood cells (Mosqueira *et al.*, 2004), protection of unstable drugs, surface modifications with ligands to improve binding (Kayser and Kiderlen, 2003; Date *et al.*, 2007) and enhanced intracellular drug delivery to overcome drug resistance mechanisms. In support of nanoparticle approaches, CQ encapsulation in fluid-state (Peeters *et al.*, 1989a) or gel-state liposomes increased therapeutic and prophylactic efficacy in animal malaria models (Peeters *et al.*, 1989b).

CQ liposomes have also been coated with polysaccharides (phosphatidylcholine and phosphatidylglycerol), chitosan (Henriksen *et al.*, 1997) and antibodies targeting erythrocytes (Singhal and Gupta, 1986; Agrawal *et al.*, 1987). In a mouse model, CQ-loaded liposomes coated with such antibodies effectively treated CQ-susceptible and -resistant *Plasmodium berghei* infections (Owais *et al.*, 1995). Cure rates for CQ-resistant *P. berghei* at 4 and 6 days post-infection were 75 and 90%, respectively. Interestingly, transferring-conjugated SLNs can increase the concentration of quinine in the brain for the treatment of cerebral malaria (Gupta *et al.*, 2007). CQ PEGylated dendrimers, both uncoated and coated with chondroitin sulfate, can prolong serum CQ concentrations in an intravenous rat model (Bhadra *et al.*, 2006). Finally, quinine encapsulation in a polymeric nanocapsule improved the survival of malaria-infected rats by 30% compared with free quinine (Haas *et al.*, 2009).

Other malarial drugs in early-stage investigation as nanoparticle platforms include primaquine liposomes, nanospheres, dendrimers, artemether dendrimers and halofantrine nanocapsules (Santos-Magalhaes and Mosqueira, 2010).

21.3.4 HIV

Issues with current antiretroviral therapy for HIV include non-adherence, drug–drug interactions, and adverse side effects, as well as a failure to eradicate the virus (Kim and Read, 2010). Nanoparticles can potentially impact on all of these issues, and although the research is in its early stages, the outlook is promising. One area of particular focus has been the development of nanosuspensions that significantly extend the release and/or increase the solubility of loviride, rilpivirine, lopinavir, ritonavir and efavirenz (van Eerdenbrugh *et al.*, 2007; Destache *et al.*, 2008; van't Klooster *et al.*, 2010). Sharma and Garg (2010) reviewed the polymeric micelles, polymeric nanoparticles and dendrimers that have been developed for *in vitro* and small-animal *in vivo* studies, which have provided evidence that nanoparticles can address the above-stated issues with current HIV antiretroviral therapy (Sharma and Garg, 2010).

Silver nanoparticles have also shown promising protective activity against free and cell-associated HIV-1, including drug-resistant strains (Elechiguerra *et al.*, 2005; Sun *et al.*, 2005; Lara *et al.*, 2010). The silver nanoparticles bind to gp120 on the viral surface to prevent CD4-dependent virion binding and fusion with the host cells.

21.4 Nanoparticle Vaccines

The application of nanotechnology for the development of vaccines is a promising option for the prevention of many infectious diseases. Currently, there are two non-FDA-approved nanoparticle vaccines on the market, both of which are virosomes. Virosomes are unilamellar phospholipid bilayer vesicles that can present virus antigens. They are biodegradable, non-toxic and do not induce antibodies against themselves (Cryz *et al.*, 1996) but are capable of inducing both T- and B-cell responses (Arkema *et al.*, 2000; Bungener *et al.*, 2002; Cusi, 2006; Moser *et al.*, 2007). Epaxal® and Inflexal® V are two virosome vaccines manufactured by Berna Biotech (Table 21.2). Epaxal is a virosomal, aluminium-free vaccine for hepatitis A that contains reconstituted influenza virosomes (Glück *et al.*, 2004; Moser *et al.*, 2007). Studies show that patients remain protected for 10–12 years post-immunization (van Herck *et al.*, 2004; Hammitt *et al.*, 2008).

Inflexal V was introduced in 1997 and has been shown to be highly efficacious at delivering influenza antigens to illicit a strong immune response in patients of all ages (Herzog *et al.*, 2009).

Mucosal nanoparticle formulations, in particular, are a promising option that can serve important roles in developing nations where devastating infectious diseases pose significant risks (Chadwick *et al.*, 2010). Accordingly, an intranasal vaccine has been developed with liposomes complexed with DNA for *Mycobacterium tuberculosis* heat-shock protein 65 antigen and immunostimulatory CpG motifs (Rosada *et al.*, 2008). In mice, this vaccine can induce a cellular immune response that significantly reduces the number of bacilli in the lungs after a single intranasal immunization. Additional options for TB vaccination include nanoparticle-based DNA vaccines capable of strong T-cell responses after aerosol delivery, as well as nanoparticles loaded with genes of interest, which are then attached to attenuated bacteria for delivery (Bivas-Benita *et al.*, 2004; Akin *et al.*, 2007). These options for nanoparticle-based TB vaccination and other promising options have been reviewed recently (Griffiths *et al.*, 2010). A nanoemulsion formulation for use as an intranasal hepatitis B vaccine containing a viral surface antigen can induce significant levels of mucosal IgA levels and T-helper 1 (Th1)-associated cellular immunity responses in murine models, which facilitates the control of infection (Makidon *et al.*, 2008). An experimental intranasal HIV vaccine comprising liposomes containing haemagglutinating virus of Japan fusion proteins, which are taken up by nasal epithelium-associated cells and antigen-presenting cells, and HIV glycoprotein gp160 has been shown to induce antibody and Th1/Th2 T-cell responses that are encouraging for prophylactic and therapeutic applications against HIV (Sakaue *et al.*, 2003).

21.5 Conclusion

Nanoparticles possess unique qualities that make them ideal vehicles for the treatment of many infectious diseases. These compounds have the capacity to improve antimicrobial solubility, reduce cytotoxicity to the host, achieve higher intracellular concentrations and provide combination drug therapy. Additionally, the ability to customize nanomedicines for specific pathogen targeting ensures that nanoparticles will play an increasingly significant role against resistance microbes such as *S. aureus*. Given the recent boom in publications, funding and patents over the last few years, the continued development of novel nanoparticle antimicrobials should be expected in the future (Wagner *et al.*, 2006).

References

Abeylath, S.C., Turos, E., Dickey, S. and Lim, D.V. (2008) Glyconanobiotics: novel carbohydrated nanoparticle antibiotics for MRSA and *Bacillus anthracis*. *Bioorganic and Medicinal Chemistry* 16, 2412–2418.

Adler-Moore, J. (1994) AmBisome targeting to fungal infections. *Bone Marrow Transplant* 14 (Suppl. 5), S3–S7.

Adler-Moore, J. and Proffitt, R.T. (2002) AmBisome: liposomal formulation, structure, mechanism of action and pre-clinical experience. *Journal of Antimicrobial Chemothery* 49 (Suppl. 1), 21–30.

Agrawal, A.K., Singhal, A. and Gupta, C.M. (1987) Functional drug targeting to erythrocytes *in vivo* using antibody bearing liposomes as drug vehicles. *Biochemical and Biophysical Research Communications* 148, 357–361.

Akin, D., Sturgis, J., Ragheb, K., Sherman, D., Burkholder, K., Robinson, J.P., Bhunia, A.K., Mohammed, S. and Bashir, R. (2007) Bacteria-mediated delivery of nanoparticles and cargo into cells. *Nature Nanotechnology* 2, 441–449.

Alipour, M., Halwani, M., Omri, A. and Suntres, Z.E. (2008) Antimicrobial effectiveness of liposomal polymyxin B against resistant Gram-negative bacterial strains. *International Journal of Pharmaceutics* 355, 293–298.

Arkema, A., Huckriede, A., Schoen, P., Wilschut, J. and Daemen, T. (2000) Induction of cytotoxic T lymphocyte activity by fusion-active peptide-containing virosomes. *Vaccine* 18, 1327–1333.

Ascione, A., de Luca, M., Tartaglione, M.T., Lampasi, F., di Costanzo, G.G., Lanza, A.G., Picciotto, F.P., Marino-Marsilia G., Fontanella, L. and Leandro, G. (2010) Peginterferon alfa-2a plus ribavirin is more effective than peginterferon alfa-2b plus ribavirin for treating chronic hepatitis C virus infection. *Gastroenterology* 138, 116–122.

Azarmi, S., Roa, W.H. and Löbenberg, R. (2008) Targeted delivery of nanoparticles for the treatment of lung diseases. *Advanced Drug Delivery Reviews* 60, 863–875.

Balogh, L., Swanson, D.R, Tomalia, D.A., Hagnauer, G.L. and McManus, A.T. (2001) Dendrimer–silver complexes and nanocomposites as antimicrobial agents. *Nano Letters* 1, 18–21.

Bangham, A.D., Standish, M.M. and Watkins, J.C. (1965) Diffusion of univalent ions across the lamellae of swollen phospholipids. *Journal of Molecular Biology* 13, 238–252.

Bargoni, A., Cavalli, R., Zara, G.P., Fundarò, A., Caputo, O. and Gasco, M.R. (2001) Transmucosal transport of tobramycin incorporated in solid lipid nanoparticles (SLN) after duodenal administration to rats. Part II – tissue distribution. *Pharmacological Research* 43, 497–502.

Bhadra, D., Bhadra, S. and Jain, N.K. (2006) PEGylated peptide dendrimeric carriers for the delivery of antimalarial drug chloroquine phosphate. *Pharmacological Research* 23, 623–633.

Bivas-Benita, M., van Meijgaarden, K.E., Franken, K.L., Junginger, H.E., Borchard, G., Ottenhoff, T.H. and Geluk, A. (2004) Pulmonary delivery of chitosan–DNA nanoparticles enhances the immunogenicity of a DNA vaccine encoding HLA-A*0201-restricted T-cell epitopes of *Mycobacterium tuberculosis. Vaccine* 22, 1609–1615.

Bungener, L., Serre, K., Bijl, L., Leserman, L., Wilschut, J., Daemen, T. and Machy, P. (2002) Virosome-mediated delivery of protein antigens to dendritic cells. *Vaccine* 20, 2287–2295.

Chadwick, S., Kriegel, C. and Amiji, M. (2010) Nanotechnology solutions for mucosal immunization. *Advanced Drug Delivery Reviews* 62, 394–407.

Chen, C.Z. and Cooper, S.L. (2002) Interactions between dendrimer biocides and bacterial membranes. *Biomaterials* 23, 3359–3368.

Cheng, J., Teply, B.A., Sherifi, I., Sung, J., Luther, G., Gu, F.X., Levy-Nissenbaum, E., Radovic-Moreno, A.F., Langer, R. and Farokhzad, O.C. (2007) Formulation of functionalized PLGA-PEG nanoparticles for *in vivo* targeted drug delivery. *Biomaterials* 28, 869–876.

Cooksley, W.G., Piratvisuth, T., Lee, S.D., Mahachai, V., Chao, Y.C., Tanwandee, T., Chutaputti, A., Chang, W.Y., Zahm, F.E. and Pluck, N. (2003) Peginterferon α-2a (40 kDa): an advance in the treatment of hepatitis B e antigen-positive chronic hepatitis B. *Journal of Viral Hepatitis* 10, 298–305.

Cryz, S.J., Que, J.U. and Glück, R. (1996) A virosome vaccine antigen delivery system does not stimulate an antiphospholipid antibody response in humans. *Vaccine* 14, 1381–1383.

Cusi, M.G. (2006) Applications of influenza virosomes as a delivery system. *Human Vaccine* 2, 1–7.

Date, A.A., Joshi, M.D. and Patravale, V.B. (2007) Parasitic diseases: liposomes and polymeric nanoparticles versus lipid nanoparticles. *Advanced Drug Delivery Reviews* 59, 505–521.

Davis, M.E., Chen, Z.G. and Shin, D.M. (2008) Nanoparticle therapeutics: an emerging treatment modality for cancer. *Nature Reviews Drug Discovery* 7, 771–782.

Delie, F. and Blanco-Prieto, M.J. (2005) Polymeric particulates to improve oral bioavailability of peptide drugs. *Molecules* 10, 65–80.

Deol, P. and Khuller, G.K. (1997) Lung specific stealth liposomes: stability, biodistribution and toxicity of liposomal antitubercular drugs in mice. *Biochimica et Biophysica Acta* 1334, 161–172.

Deol, P., Khuller, G.K. and Joshi, K. (1997) Therapeutic efficacies of isoniazid and rifampin encapsulated in lung-specific stealth liposomes against *Mycobacterium tuberculosis* infection induced in mice. *Antimicrobial Agents and Chemother* 41, 1211–1214.

Destache, C., Belgum, T., Elsasser, G., Christensen, K. and Shibata, A. (2008) Ritonavir-, lopinavir-, and efavirenz-containing nanoparticles: *in vitro* release of ART. In: *15th Conference on Retroviruses and Opportunistic Infections*, Boston, Massachusetts, 3–6 February. Abstract 743.

Elechiguerra, J.L., Burt, J.L., Morones, J.R., Camacho-Bragado, A., Gao, X., Lara, H.H., Yacaman, M.J. (2005) Interaction of silver nanoparticles with HIV-1. *Journal of Nanobiotechnology* 3, 6.

Espuelas, M.S., Legrand, P., Loiseau, P.M., Bories, C., Barratt, G. and Irache, J.M. (2002) *In vitro* antileishmanial activity of amphotericin B loaded in poly(epsilon-caprolactone) nanospheres. *Journal of Drug Targeting* 10, 593–599.

Farokhzad, O.C. and Langer, R. (2006) Nanomedicine: developing smarter therapeutic and diagnostic modalities. *Advanced Drug Delivery Reviews* 58, 1456–1459.

Fattal, E., Rojas, J., Youssef, M., Couvreur, P. and Andremont, A. (1991) Liposome-entrapped ampicillin in the treatment of experimental murine listeriosis and salmonellosis. *Antimicrobial Agents and Chemotherapy* 35, 770–772.

Feng, Q.L., Wu J., Chen, G.Q., Cui, F.Z., Kim, T.N. and Kim, J.O. (2000) A mechanistic study of the antibacterial effect of silver ions on *Escherichia coli* and *Staphylococcus aureus*. *Journal of Biomedical Materials Research* 52, 662–668.

Fidock, D.A., Eastman, R.T., Ward, S.A. and Meshnick, S.R. (2008) Recent highlights in antimalarial drug resistance and chemotherapy research. *Trends in Parasitology* 24, 537–544.

Fischbach, M.A. and Walsh, C.T. (2009) Antibiotics for emerging pathogens. *Science* 325, 1089–1093.

Foster, G.R. (2010) Pegylated interferons for the treatment of chronic hepatitis C: pharmacological and clinical differences between peginterferon-α-2a and peginterferon-α-2b. *Drugs* 70, 147–165.

Fountain, M.W., Weiss, S.J., Fountain, A.G., Shen, A. and Lenk, R.P. (1985) Treatment of *Brucella canis* and *Brucella abortus in vitro* and *in vivo* by stable plurilamellar vesicle-encapsulated aminoglycosides. *Journal of Infectious Disease* 152, 529–535.

Fried, M.W., Shiffman, M.L., Reddy, K.R., Smith, C., Marinos, G., Gonçales, F.L. Jr, Häussinger, D., Diago, M., Carosi, G., Dhumeaux, D., Craxi, A., Lin, A., Hoffman, J., Yu J. (2002) Peginterferon alfa-2a plus ribavirin for chronic hepatitis C virus infection. *New England Journal of Medicine* 347, 975–982.

Friedman, A.J., Han, G., Navati, M.S., Chacko, M., Gunther, L., Alfieri, A. and Friedman, J.M. (2008) Sustained release nitric oxide releasing nanoparticles: characterization of a novel delivery platform based on nitrite containing hydrogel/glass composites. *Nitric Oxide* 19, 12–20.

Furno, F., Morley, K.S., Wong, B., Sharp, B.L., Arnold, P.L., Howdle, S.M., Bayston, R., Brown, P.D., Winship, P.D. and Reid, H.J. (2004) Silver nanoparticles and polymeric medical devices: a new approach to prevention of infection? *Journal of Antimicrobial Chemotherapy* 54, 1019–1024.

Gelperina, S., Kisich, K., Iseman, M.D. and Heifets, L. (2005) The potential advantages of nanoparticle drug delivery systems in chemotherapy of tuberculosis. *American Journal of Respiratory and Critical Care Medicine* 172, 1487–1490.

Gill, S., Löbenberg, R., Ku, T., Azarmi, S., Roa, W. and Prenner, E.J. (2007) Nanoparticles: characteristics, mechanisms of action, and toxicity in pulmonary drug delivery – a review. *Journal of Biomedical Nanotechnology* 3, 107–119.

Gillies, E.R. and Frechet, J.M. (2005) Dendrimers and dendritic polymers in drug delivery. *Drug Discovery Today* 10, 35–43.

Gilligan, P.H. (1991) Microbiology of airway disease in patients with cystic fibrosis. *Clinical Microbiology Reviews* 4, 35–51.

Glück, R., Moser, C. and Metcalfe, I.C. (2004) Influenza virosomes as an efficient system for adjuvanted vaccine delivery. *Expert Opinion on Biological Therapy* 4, 1139–1145.

Grayson, S.M. and Fréchet, J.M. (2001) Convergent dendrons and dendrimers: from synthesis to applications. *Chemical Reviews* 101, 3819–3868.

Griffiths, G., Nyström, B., Sable, S.B. and Khuller, G.K. (2010) Nanobead-based interventions for the treatment and prevention of tuberculosis. *Nature Reviews Microbiology* 8, 827–834.

Gu, F., Zhang, L., Teply, B.A., Mann, N., Wang, A., Radovic-Moreno A.F., Langer, R. and Farokhzad, O.C. (2008) Precise engineering of targeted nanoparticles by using self-assembled biointegrated block copolymers. *Proceedings of the National Academy of Sciences USA* 105, 2586–2591.

Gupta, A.K. and Cooper, E.A. (2008) Update in antifungal therapy of dermatophytosis. *Mycopathologia* 166, 353–367.

Gupta, Y., Jain, A. and Jain, S.K. (2007) Transferrin-conjugated solid lipid nanoparticles for enhanced delivery of quinine dihydrochloride to the brain. *Journal of Pharmacy and Pharmacology* 59, 935–940.

Haas, S.E., Bettoni, C.C., de Oliveira, L.K., Guterres, S.S. and Dalla Costa, T. (2009) Nanoencapsulation increases quinine antimalarial efficacy against *Plasmodium berghei in vivo*. *International Journal of Antimicrobial Agents* 34, 156–161.

Hadziyannis, S.J., Sette, H. Jr, Morgan, T.R., Balan, V., Diago, M., Marcellin, P., Ramadori, G., Bodenheimer H. Jr, Bernstein, D., Rizzetto, M., Zeuzem, S., Pockros, P.J., Lin, A., Ackrill, A.M. and the PEGASYS International Study Group (2004) Peginterferon-α2a and ribavirin combination therapy in chronic hepatitis C: a randomized study of treatment duration and ribavirin dose. *Annals of Internal Medicine* 140, 346–355.

Hammitt, L.L., Bulkow, L., Hennessy, T.W., Zanis, C., Snowball, M., Williams, J.L., Bell, B.P. and McMahon, B.J. (2008) Persistence of antibody to hepatitis A virus 10 years after vaccination among children and adults. *Journal of Infectious Disease* 198, 1776–1782.

Han, G., Martinez, L.R., Mihu, M.R., Friedman, A.J., Friedman, J.M. and Nosanchuk, J.D. (2009) Nitric oxide releasing nanoparticles are therapeutic for *Staphylococcus aureus* abscesses in a murine model of infection. *PLoS One* 4, e7804.

Henriksen, I., S.R. Våagen, Sande, S.A., Smistad, G. and Karlsen, J. (1997) Interactions between liposomes and chitosan II: Effect of selected parameters on aggregation and leakage. *International Journal of Pharmaceutics* 146, 193–203.

Herzog, C., Hartmann, K., Künzi, V., Kürsteiner, O., Mischler, R., Lazar, H. and Glück, R. (2009) Eleven years of Inflexal V – a virosomal adjuvanted influenza vaccine. *Vaccine* 27, 4381–4387.

Hiemenz, J.W. and Walsh, T.J. (1996) Lipid formulations of amphotericin B: recent progress and future directions. *Clinical Infectious Diseases* 22 (Suppl. 2), S133–S144.

Ip, M., Lui, S.L., Poon, V.K., Lung, I. and Burd, A. (2006) Antimicrobial activities of silver dressings: an *in vitro* comparison. *Journal of Medical Microbiology* 55, 59–63.

Irache, J.M., Salman, H.H., Gamazo, C. and Espuelas, S. (2008) Mannose-targeted systems for the delivery of therapeutics. *Expert Opinion on Drug Delivery* 5, 703–724.

Jain, C.P. and Vyas, S.P. (1995) Preparation and characterization of niosomes containing rifampicin for lung targeting. *Journal of Microencapsulation* 12, 401–407.

Jain, P. and Pradeep, T. (2005) Potential of silver nanoparticle-coated polyurethane foam as an antibacterial water filter. *Biotechnology and Bioengineering* 90, 59–63.

Jun, J., Yuan, D.Y., Shao, W.H., Shao, Z.F. and Zhong, W.Y. (2007) Preparation and characterization of antibacterial silver-containing nanofibers for wound dressing applications. *Journal of US–China Medical Science* 4, 52–54.

Kayser, O. and Kiderlen, A.F. (2003) Delivery strategies for antiparasitics. *Expert Opinion on Investigational Drugs* 12, 197–207.

Kelsey, S.M., Goldman, J.M., McCann S., Newland, A.C., Scarffe, J.H., Oppenheim, B.A. and Mufti, G.J. (1999) Liposomal amphotericin (AmBisome) in the prophylaxis of fungal infections in neutropenic patients: a randomised, double-blind, placebo-controlled study. *Bone Marrow Transplant* 23, 163–168.

Kim, H.J. and Jones, M.N. (2004) The delivery of benzyl penicillin to *Staphylococcus aureus* biofilms by use of liposomes. *Journal of Liposome Research* 14, 123–139.

Kim, P.S. and Read, S.W. (2010) Nanotechnology and HIV: potential applications for treatment and prevention. *Wiley Interdisciplinary Reviews: Nanomedicine and Nanobiotechnology* 2, 693–702.

Kumar, P.V., Agashe, H., Dutta, T. and Jain, N.K. (2007) PEGylated dendritic architecture for development of a prolonged drug delivery system for an antitubercular drug. *Current Drug Delivery* 4, 11–19.

Lane, K.B., Egan, B., Vick, S., Abdolrasulnia, R. and Shepherd, V.L. (1998) Characterization of a rat alveolar macrophage cell line that expresses a functional mannose receptor. *Journal of Leukocyte Biology* 64, 345–350.

Lara, H.H., Ayala-Nuñez, N.V., Ixtepan-Turrent, L. and Rodriguez-Padilla C. (2010) Mode of antiviral action of silver nanoparticles against HIV-1. *Journal of Nanobiotechnology* 8, 1.

Lau, G.K., Piratvisuth, T., Luo, K.X., Marcellin, P., Thongsawat, S., Cooksley, G., Gane, E., Fried, M.W., Chow, W.C., Paik, S.W., Chang, W.Y., Berg, T., Flisiak, R., McCloud P., Pluck, N. and the Peginterferon Alfa-2a HBeAg-Positive Chronic Hepatitis B Study Group (2005) Peginterferon Alfa-2a, lamivudine, and the combination for HBeAg-positive chronic hepatitis B. *New England Journal of Medicine* 352, 2682–2695.

Leaper, D.J. (2006) Silver dressings: their role in wound management. *International Wound Journal* 3, 282–294.

Lenaerts, A.J., Gruppo, V., Marietta, K.S., Johnson, C.M., Driscoll, D.K., Tompkins, N.M., Rose, J.D., Reynolds, R.C. and Orme, I.M. (2005) Preclinical testing of the nitroimidazopyran PA-824 for activity against *Mycobacterium tuberculosis* in a series of *in vitro* and *in vivo* models. *Antimicrobial Agents and Chemotherapy* 49, 2294–2301.

Lok, A.S.F. and McMahon, B.J. (2009) Chronic hepatitis B: update 2009. *Hepatology* 50, 661–662.

Ma, M., Cheng, Y., Xu Z., Xu P., Qu H., Fang, Y., Xu T. and Wen, L. (2007) Evaluation of polyamidoamine (PAMAM) dendrimers as drug carriers of anti-bacterial drugs using sulfamethoxazole (SMZ) as a model drug. *European Journal of Medicinal Chemistry* 42, 93–98.

Magallanes, M., Dijkstra, J. and Fierer, J. (1993) Liposome-incorporated ciprofloxacin in treatment of murine salmonellosis. *Antimicrobial Agents and Chemothery* 37, 2293–2297.

Makidon, P.E., Bielinska, A.U., Nigavekar, S.S., Janczak, K.W., Knowlton, J., Scott, A.J., Mank, N., Cao, Z., Rathinavelu, S., Beer, M.R., Wilkinson, J.E., Blanco, L.P., Landers, J.J. and Baker, J.R. Jr (2008) Pre-clinical evaluation of a novel nanoemulsion-based hepatitis B mucosal vaccine. *PLoS One* 3, e2954.

Manns, M.P., McHutchison, J.G., Gordon, S.C., Rustgi, V.K., Shiffman, M., Reindollar, R., Goodman, Z.D., Koury, K., Ling, M. and Albrecht, J.K. (2001) Peginterferon alfa-2b plus ribavirin compared with interferon alfa-2b plus ribavirin for initial treatment of chronic hepatitis C: a randomised trial. *Lancet* 358, 958–965.

Marcellin, P., Lau, G.K., Bonino, F., Farci, P., Hadziyannis, S., Jin, R., Lu Z.M., Piratvisuth, T.,

Germanidis, G., Yurdaydin, C., Diago, M., Gurel, S., Lai, M.Y., Button, P., Pluck, N. and the Peginterferon Alfa-2a HBeAg-Negative Chronic Hepatitis B Study Group (2004) Peginterferon alfa-2a alone, lamivudine alone, and the two in combination in patients with HBeAg-negative chronic hepatitis B. *New England Journal of Medicine* 351, 1206–1217.

Martinez, L.R., Han, G., Chacko, M., Mihu, M.R., Jacobson, M., Gialanella, P., Friedman, A.J., Nosanchuk, J.D. and Friedman, J.M. (2009) Antimicrobial and healing efficacy of sustained release nitric oxide nanoparticles against *Staphylococcus aureus* skin infection. *Journal of Investigative Dermatology* 129, 2463–2469.

Mihu, M.R., Sandkovsky, U., Han, G., Friedman, J.M., Nosanchuk, J.D. and Martinez, L.R. (2010) The use of nitric oxide releasing nanoparticles as a treatment against *Acinetobacter baumannii* in wound infections. *Virulence* 1, 62–67.

Monteiro, D.R., Gorup, L.F., Takamiya, A.S., Ruvollo-Filho A.C., de Camargo, E.R. and Barbosa, D.B. (2009) The growing importance of materials that prevent microbial adhesion: antimicrobial effect of medical devices containing silver. *International J ournal of Antimicrobial Agents* 34, 103–110.

Morones, J.R., Elechiguerra, J.L., Camacho, A., Holt, K., Kouri, J.B., Ramírez, J.T. and Yacaman, M.J. (2005) The bactericidal effect of silver nanoparticles. *Nanotechnology* 16, 2346–2353.

Moser, C., Amacker, M., Kammer, A.R., Rasi, S., Westerfeld, N. and Zurbriggen, R. (2007) Influenza virosomes as a combined vaccine carrier and adjuvant system for prophylactic and therapeutic immunizations. *Expert Reviews of Vaccines* 6, 711–721.

Mosqueira, V.C., Loiseau, P.M., Bories, C., Legrand, P., Devissaguet, J.P. and Barratt, G. (2004) Efficacy and pharmacokinetics of intravenous nanocapsule formulations of halofantrine in *Plasmodium berghei*-infected mice. *Antimicrobial Agents and Chemotherapy* 48, 1222–1228.

Mullaicharam, A.R. and Murthy, R.S.R. (2004) Lung accumulation of niosome-entrapped rifampicin following intravenous and intratracheal administration in the rat. *Journal of Drug Delivery Science and Technology* 14, 99–104.

Müller, R.H., Radtke, M. and Wissing, S.A. (2002) Solid lipid nanoparticles (SLN) and nanostructured lipid carriers (NLC) in cosmetic and dermatological preparations. *Advanced Drug Delivery Reviews* 54 (Suppl. 1), S131–S155.

Ohashi, K., Kabasawa, T., Ozeki, T. and Okada, H. (2009) One-step preparation of rifampicin/poly(lactic-co-glycolic acid) nanoparticle-containing mannitol microspheres using a four-fluid nozzle spray drier for inhalation therapy of tuberculosis. *Journal of Controlled Release* 135, 19–24.

Onyebujoh, P., Zumla, A., Ribeiro, I., Rustomjee, R., Mwaba, P., Gomes, M. and Grange, J.M. (2005) Treatment of tuberculosis: present status and future prospects. *Bulletin World Health Organization* 83, 857–865.

Onyeji, C.O., Nightingale, C.H. and Marangos, M.N. (1994) Enhanced killing of methicillin-resistant *Staphylococcus aureus* in human macrophages by liposome-entrapped vancomycin and teicoplanin. *Infection* 22, 338–342.

Owais, M., Varshney, G.C., Choudhury, A., Chandra, S. and Gupta, C.M. (1995) Chloroquine encapsulated in malaria-infected erythrocyte-specific antibody-bearing liposomes effectively controls chloroquine-resistant *Plasmodium berghei* infections in mice. *Antimicrobial Agents and Chemotherapy* 39, 180–184.

Pandey, R. and Khuller, G.K. (2004) Subcutaneous nanoparticle-based antitubercular chemotherapy in an experimental model. *Journal of Antimicrobial Chemotherapy* 54, 266–268.

Pandey, R. and Khuller, G.K. (2005) Solid lipid particle-based inhalable sustained drug delivery system against experimental tuberculosis. *Tuberculosis (Edinburgh, Scotland)* 85, 227–234.

Pandey, R., Zahoor, A., Sharma, S. and Khuller, G.K. (2003a) Nanoparticle encapsulated antitubercular drugs as a potential oral drug delivery system against murine tuberculosis. *Tuberculosis (Edinburgh, Scotland)* 83, 373–378.

Pandey, R., Sharma, A., Zahoor, A., Sharma, S., Khuller, G.K. and Prasad, B. (2003b) Poly (DL-lactide-co-glycolide) nanoparticle-based inhalable sustained drug delivery system for experimental tuberculosis. *Journal of Antimicrobial Chemotherapy* 52, 981–986.

Pandey, R., Sharma, S. and Khuller, G.K. (2005) Oral solid lipid nanoparticle-based antitubercular chemotherapy. *Tuberculosis (Edinburgh, Scotland)* 85, 415–420.

Peeters, P.A., Brunink, B.G., Eling, W.M. and Crommelin, D.J. (1989a) Therapeutic effect of chloroquine(CQ)-containing immunoliposomes in rats infected with *Plasmodium berghei* parasitized mouse red blood cells: comparison with combinations of antibodies and CQ or liposomal CQ. *Biochimica et Biophysica Acta* 981, 269–276.

Peeters, P.A., de Leest, K., Eling, W.M. and Crommelin, D.J. (1989b) Chloroquine blood levels after administration of the liposome-encapsulated drug in relation to therapy of murine malaria. *Pharmaceutical Research* 6, 787–793.

Price, R.N., Dorsey, G., Ashley, E.A., Barnes, K.I., Baird, J.K., d'Alessandro U., Guerin, P.J., Laufer, M.K., Naidoo, I., Nosten, F., Olliaro, P., Plowe, C.V., Ringwald, P., Sibley, C.H., Stepniewska, K. and White, N.J. (2007) World Antimalarial Resistance Network I: clinical efficacy of antimalarial drugs. *Malaria Jouranl* 6, 119.

Rai, M., Yadav, A. and Gade, A. (2009) Silver nanoparticles as a new generation of antimicrobials. *Biotechnology Advances* 27, 76–83.

Rosada, R.S., de la Torre, L.G., Frantz, F.G., Trombone, A.P., Zárate-Bladés C.R., Fonseca, D.M., Souza, P.R., Brandão, I.T., Masson, A.P., Soares, E.G., Ramos, S.G., Faccioli, L.H., Silva, C.L., Santana, M.H. and Coelho-Castelo, A.A. (2008) Protection against tuberculosis by a single intranasal administration of DNA-hsp65 vaccine complexed with cationic liposomes. *BMC Immunology* 9, 38.

Rupp, M.E., T Fitzgerald, T., Marion, N., Helget, V., Puumala, S., Anderson, J.R. and Fey, P.D. (2004) Effect of silver-coated urinary catheters: efficacy, cost-effectiveness, and antimicrobial resistance. *American Journal of Infection Control* 32, 445–450.

Sakaue, G., Hiroi, T., Nakagawa, Y., Someya, K., Iwatani, K., Sawa, Y., Takahashi, H., Honda, M., Kunisawa, J. and Kiyono, H. (2003) HIV mucosal vaccine: nasal immunization with gp160-encapsulated hemagglutinating virus of Japan-liposome induces antigen-specific CTLs and neutralizing antibody responses. *Jouranl of Immunology* 170, 495–502.

Sanna, V., Gavini, E., Cossu, M., Rassu, G. and Giunchedi, P. (2007) Solid lipid nanoparticles (SLN) as carriers for the topical delivery of econazole nitrate: in-vitro characterization, ex-vivo and in-vivo studies. *Journal of Pharmacy and Pharmacology* 59, 1057–1064.

Santos-Magalhaes, N.S. and Mosqueira, V.C. (2010) Nanotechnology applied to the treatment of malaria. *Advanced Drug Delivery Reviews* 62, 560–575.

Schumacher, I. and Margalit, R. (1997) Liposome-encapsulated ampicillin: physicochemical and antibacterial properties. *Journal of Pharmaceutical Sciences* 86, 635–641.

Sharma, A., Sharma, S. and Khuller, G.K. (2004) Lectin-functionalized poly (lactide-co-glycolide) nanoparticles as oral/aerosolized antitubercular drug carriers for treatment of tuberculosis. *Jouranl of Antimicrobial Chemotherapy* 54, 761–766.

Sharma, P. and Garg, S. (2010) Pure drug and polymer based nanotechnologies for the improved solubility, stability, bioavailability and targeting of anti-HIV drugs. *Advanced Drug Delivery Reviews* 62, 491–502.

Singhal, A. and Gupta, C.M. (1986) Antibody-mediated targeting of liposomes to red cells in vivo. *FEBS Letters* 201, 321–326.

Skidan, I.N., Gel'perina, S.E., Severin, S.E. and Guliaev, A.E. (2003) [Enhanced activity of rifampicin loaded with polybutyl cyanoacrylate nanoparticles in relation to intracellularly localized bacteria]. *Antibiotiki I Khimioterapiia* 48, 23–26 (in Russian).

Sondi, I. and Salopek-Sondi, B. (2004) Silver nanoparticles as antimicrobial agent: a case study on *E. coli* as a model for Gram-negative bacteria. *Journal of Colloid and Interface Science* 275, 177–182.

Soppimath, K.S., Aminabhavi, T.M., Kulkarni, A.R. and Rudzinski, W.E. (2001) Biodegradable polymeric nanoparticles as drug delivery devices. *Journal of Controlled Release* 70, 1–20.

Sosnik, A., Carcaboso, A.M., Glisoni, R.J., Moretton, M.A. and Chiappetta, D.A. (2010) New old challenges in tuberculosis: potentially effective nanotechnologies in drug delivery. *Advanced Drug Delivery Reviews* 62, 547–559.

Sun, R.W., Chen, R., Chung, N.P., Ho, C.M., Lin, C.L. and Che, C.M. (2005) Silver nanoparticles fabricated in Hepes buffer exhibit cytoprotective activities toward HIV-1 infected cells. *Chemical Communications* 5059–5061.

Taylor, P.L., Ussher, A.L. and Burrell, R.E. (2005) Impact of heat on nanocrystalline silver dressings. Part I: Chemical and biological properties. *Biomaterials* 26, 7221–7229.

Travan, A., Marsich, E., Donati, I., Benincasa, M., Giazzon, M., Felisari, L. and Paoletti, S. (2011) Silver-polysaccharide nanocomposite antimicrobial coatings for methacrylic thermosets. *Acta Biomaterialia* 7, 337–346.

Umamaheshwari, R.B. and Jain, N.K. (2003) Receptor mediated targeting of lectin conjugated gliadin nanoparticles in the treatment of *Helicobacter pylori. Journal of Drug Targeting* 11, 415–423; discussion 423–414.

van't Klooster, G., Hoeben, E., Borghys, H., Looszova, A., Bouche, M.P., van Velsen, F. and Baert, L. (2010) Pharmacokinetics and disposition of rilpivirine (TMC278) nanosuspension as a long-acting injectable antiretroviral formulation. *Antimicrobial Agents and Chemotherapy* 54, 2042–2050.

van Eerdenbrugh, B., Froyen, L., Martens, J.A., Blaton, N., Augustijns, P., Brewster, M., van den Mooter, G. (2007) Characterization of physico-chemical properties and pharmaceutical performance of sucrose co-freeze-dried solid nanoparticulate powders of the anti-HIV agent loviride prepared by media milling. *International Journal of Pharmaceutics* 338, 198–206.

van Herck, K., van Damme, P., Lievens, M. and Stoffel, M. (2004) Hepatitis A vaccine: indirect evidence of immune memory 12 years after the primary course. *Journal of Medical Virology* 72, 194–196.

Vyas, S.P., Kannan, M.E., Jain, S., Mishra, V. and Singh, P. (2004) Design of liposomal aerosols for improved delivery of rifampicin to alveolar macrophages. *International Journal of Pharmaceutics* 269, 37–49.

Wagner, V., Dullaart, A., Bock, A.K. and Zweck, A. (2006) The emerging nanomedicine landscape. *Nature Biotechnology* 24, 1211–1217.

Walsh, T.J., Goodman, J.L., Pappas, P., Bekersky, I., Buell, D.N., Roden, M., Barrett, J. and Anaissie, E.J. (2001) Safety, tolerance, and pharmacokinetics of high-dose liposomal amphotericin B (AmBisome) in patients infected with *Aspergillus* species and other filamentous fungi: maximum tolerated dose study. *Antimicrobial Agents and Chemotherapy* 45, 3487–3496.

Wijagkanalan, W., Kawakami, S., Takenaga, M., Igarashi, R., Yamashita, F. and Hashida, M. (2008) Efficient targeting to alveolar macrophages by intratracheal administration of mannosylated liposomes in rats. *Journal of Controlled Release* 125, 121–130.

Wissing, S.A. and Müller, R.H. (2003) Cosmetic applications for solid lipid nanoparticles (SLN). *International Journal of Pharmaceutics* 254, 65–68.

Yang, W., Wiederhold, N.P., Williams, R.O. III (2008) Drug delivery strategies for improved azole antifungal action. *Expert Opinion on Drug Delivery* 5, 1199–1216.

Zhang, L., Gu, F.X., Chan, J.M., Wang, A.Z., Langer, R.S. and Farokhzad, O.C. (2008) Nanoparticles in medicine: therapeutic applications and developments. *Clinical Pharmacology and Therapeutics* 83, 761–769.

Zhang, L., Pornpattananangku, D., Hu, C.M. and Huang, C.M. (2010) Development of nanoparticles for antimicrobial drug delivery. *Current Medicinal Chemistry* 17, 585–594.

zur Mühlen, A., Schwarz, C. and Mehnert, W. (1998) Solid lipid nanoparticles (SLN) for controlled drug delivery – drug release and release mechanism. *European Journal of Pharmaceutics and Biopharmaceutics* 45, 149–155.

22 Antimicrobial Activity of Carbon Nanotubes

Shaobin Liu and Yuan Chen*
School of Chemical and Biomedical Engineering, Nanyang Technological University, Singapore

22.1 Introduction

Carbon nanotubes (CNTs) are hollow cylinders rolled up from a single or several layers of one-atom-thick hexagonal carbon sheets. They are referred to as single-walled CNTs (SWCNTs), double-walled CNTs (DWCNTs) or multiwalled CNTs (MWCNTs) according to the number of carbon walls (Fig. 22.1a). CNTs are synthetic materials. SWCNTs were first synthesized in 1993 (Bethune *et al.*, 1993; Iijima and Ichihashi, 1993), while the finding of MWCNTs has been traced back much earlier (Iijima 1991; Monthioux and Kuznetsov 2006). Common CNT synthesis methods (Iijima and Ichihashi, 1993; Guo *et al.*, 1995; Dai *et al.*, 1996) share the same principle. Atomic carbon species derived either from solid carbon sources or from carbon-bearing gases organize into thermodynamically stable nanoscale CNTs on catalyst nanoparticles at high temperatures (normally 700–1000°C). CNTs have diameters ranging from 0.4nm to a few hundred nanometres (typically 1nm for SWCNTs and tens of nanometres for MWCNTs) with high length-to-diameter ratios, and their lengths range from hundreds of nanometres to centimetres (Zheng *et al.*, 2004). Most earlier studies focused on their extraordinary electronic, thermal and mechanical properties, resulting from their unique one-dimensional nanostructures (Endo *et al.*, 2008). Soon, their potential biomedical applications started to be extensively explored because on the one hand, they can be easily internalized by cells (Porter *et al.*, 2007) and therefore can act as delivery vehicles of various molecules (Bhirde *et al.*, 2009), while on the other hand, their electronic and spectroscopic properties offer opportunities in detection and treatment of diseases (Kostarelos *et al.*, 2009; Z. Liu *et al.*, 2009). However, most biomedical studies have focused on the impact of CNTs on mammalian cells.

A few early studies showed that functionalized CNTs have antimicrobial activity (Gu *et al.*, 2005; Wang *et al.*, 2006). The first direct evidence that pristine CNTs show strong antimicrobial activity appeared in 2007 (Kang *et al.*, 2007). The results showed that direct contact between CNTs and *Escherichia coli* caused severe membrane damage and subsequent cell inactivation. A number of other studies on the antimicrobial activity of CNTs appeared over the next 3 years (Upadhyayula *et al.*, 2009a; Upadhyayula and Gadhamshetty, 2010). Most of these studies have been conducted with regard to understanding the environmental impacts of CNTs, using CNTs for removal of contaminants in drinking water and developing antimicrobial surface coatings containing CNTs.

* Corresponding author (chenyuan@ntu.edu.sg).

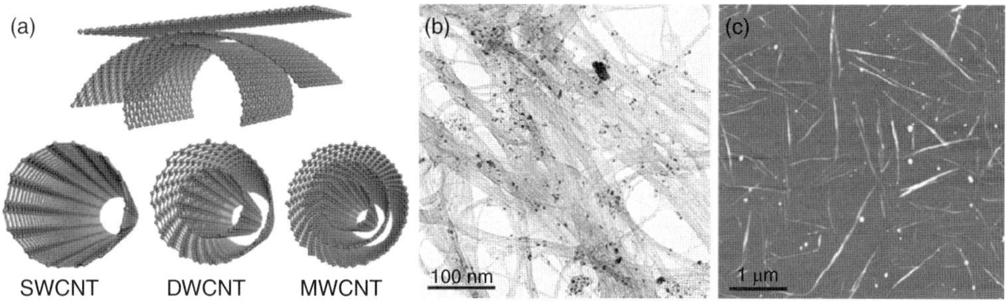

Fig. 22.1. (a) Schematic illustration of CNTs. (b) TEM image of CNT samples containing various impurities. (c) AFM image of CNT bundles with different diameters and lengths. (From Wei *et al.*, 2008.)

In this chapter, we will focus on the common problems faced in investigation of the antimicrobial activity of CNTs. The heterogeneous nature of common CNT samples is introduced first. The findings on the correlation between antimicrobial activity and specific structural features of CNTs are then discussed in details, followed by some proposed antimicrobial mechanisms. Lastly, potential applications suggested by the current studies are summarized.

22.2 Heterogeneous Nature of CNT Samples

Unlike regular chemical agents, which have a well-defined size, molecular structure, properties and purity, commonly available CNT samples are a mixture of many chemical species. They include non-carbon impurities, such as transition metal residues and nanosized catalyst supports; carbon impurities, such as amorphous carbon, carbon particles, graphite and carbon fibres; and CNTs. As shown in the transmission electron microscope (TEM) image in Fig. 22.1b, CNTs are also different in diameter, length, chirality (the direction in which a carbon layer rolls up to form a nanotube; Ouyang *et al.*, 2002a,b), morphology, surface functional groups and defects. In addition, because of the strong van der Waals forces among CNTs, they often aggregate together to form CNT bundles of different sizes (Fig. 22.1c) (Girifalco *et al.*, 2000; Wang *et al.*, 2005). Thus, it is essential to determine reliable correlations between specific CNT structural and chemical characteristics and the antimicrobial activity of CNT samples, so we can increase the potential of CNTs in antimicrobial applications, while at the same time reducing any risks. To get such reliable correlations, the properties of CNTs, such as concentration, dispersion and surface functional group, all need to be well managed in antimicrobial assays.

The exact composition and properties of CNT samples depend on how they are synthesized, purified and functionalized. Various purification strategies have been developed to improve the purity of CNT samples. Haddon *et al.* (2004) summarized the common strategies. Most purification methods rely on one or more of these steps: gas- or vapour-phase oxidation, wet chemical oxidation/treatment, centrifugation and filtration (including chromatographic methods). Pristine CNTs are not soluble in water because of their hydrophobic graphitic surfaces. Functionalization is needed to obtain a homogeneous CNT aqueous dispersion. Both covalent (e.g. introducing carboxyl groups, amino groups or other functional groups) and non-covalent (surfactant or polymer wrapping) functionalization methods are available for achieving CNT solubilization (Tasis *et al.*, 2006; Karousis *et al.*, 2010). In the last few years, significant efforts have also been devoted to obtaining monodispersed CNT samples through both selective synthesis and post-synthetic approaches. For instance, SWCNTs with controlled chirality, such as (9,8)- (Wang *et al.*, 2010), (6,5)- (Ghorannevis *et al.*, 2010; He *et al.*, 2010) and (7,5)-CNTs (Chen *et al.*, 2004a,b; Ciuparu *et al.*, 2004) can be produced by chirality selective synthesis. SWCNTs with different lengths can also be selectively synthesized (Du *et al.*, 2006; Lopez *et al.*, 2009; Moon *et al.*, 2009). Post-synthetic enrichment approaches include selective chemistry, electrical breakdown, dielectrophoresis, chromatography and ultra-centrifugation (Banerjee *et al.*, 2005; Hersam, 2008; Liu and Hersam, 2010). CNT samples with controlled diameter, length and/or chirality to some extent are already available commercially. These efforts have already been and are likely to further speed up our understanding, eventually realizing the applications of the antimicrobial activity of CNTs. However, it is worth mentioning that the evaluation of CNT properties relies on many analytical techniques, such as optical absorbance, photoluminescence, Raman spectroscopy, scanning probe microscopy, scanning electron microscopy (SEM) and TEM, atomic force microscopy (AFM), thermogravimetric analysis (TGA), X-ray photoelectron spectroscopy (XPS) and inductively coupled plasma (ICP) analysis. Until now, widely accepted evaluation standards for establishing CNT purity levels are still not available. Thus, it should be noted that the property data provided by some CNT producers may not be reliable. Careful evaluation of CNT sample properties is necessary for their antimicrobial applications.

22.3 Antimicrobial Activity of CNTs

Physiochemical properties affect the antimicrobial activity of nanomaterials (Rivera Gil *et al.*, 2010). CNT is a perfect example of this claim. In the last 3 years, many physiochemical properties of CNTs have been studied, such as size, electronic properties, concentration, impurities, functionalization, solution chemistry and incubation time. Various antimicrobial activity assays have been adopted, including live/dead bacterial viability assays (Brady-Estevez *et al.*, 2008; Kang *et al.*, 2008a), metabolic activity assays (Creach *et al.*, 2003; Kang *et al.*, 2008a; Hu *et al.*, 2010), the plate counting method (Wang *et al.*, 2006; S. Liu *et al.*, 2009) and turbidity measurement (Arias and Yang, 2009; Yang *et al.*, 2010).

22.3.1 CNT size: diameter, length and dispersion/aggregation

Physiochemical properties of CNTs vary as a function of their sizes. This size dependence has been clearly observed in their antimicrobial activity. Among two different types of CNTs (SWCNTs and MWCNTs), the smaller-diameter SWCNTs have stronger antimicrobial activity than the large-diameter MWCNTs (Kang *et al.*, 2008a). Yang *et al.* (2010) compared three SWCNT samples with different lengths (<1, 1–5 and >5 μm), and found that longer SWCNTs displayed stronger antimicrobial activity towards *Salmonella typhimurium* than shorter SWCNTs at the same nanotube weigh concentration. However, the length effect is not universal. Aslan *et al.* (2010) reported that shorter SWCNTs showed stronger antimicrobial activity towards both *E. coli* and *Staphylococcus epidermidis*. Because of the strong interaction among CNTs, the aggregation of CNTs results in nanotube bundles in different sizes. This also affects their antimicrobial activity. S. Liu *et al.* (2009) found that well-dispersed individual SWCNTs assisted by the biocompatible surfactant Tween 20 display much stronger antimicrobial activity than larger SWCNT bundles in 0.9% NaCl solution.

22.3.2 CNT metallicity

Depending on the chirality of SWCNTs (the rolling direction of the carbon sheet), an unsorted SWCNT sample usually contains two-thirds semi-conducting nanotubes and one-third metallic nanotubes (Dresselhaus *et al.*, 1992; Saito *et al.*, 1992). This electronic structure difference also has a strong impact on the antimicrobial activity of SWCNTs. Metallic SWCNTs showed much stronger antimicrobial activity than semi-conducting SWCNTs under the same evaluation condition (Vecitis *et al.*, 2010).

22.3.3 CNT concentration

CNTs also show a clear concentration-dependent antimicrobial activity (Arias and Yang, 2009; S. Liu *et al.*, 2009). A higher concentration of CNTs usually results in a higher death rate of bacteria. For example, the death rate of *E. coli* increases with an increase in SWCNT concentration from 5 to 80 μg/ml (S. Liu *et al.*, 2009). Arias and Yang (2009) reported that the antimicrobial activity of SWNTs with surface groups of –OH and –COOH both increased with an increase in SWCNT concentration (Arias and Yang, 2009).

22.3.4 CNT functionalization

CNTs can be functionalized with different surface groups, which may change the antimicrobial activity of CNTs. For instance, the antimicrobial activity of three different functionalized SWCNTs (SWCNT–OH, SWCNT–COOH and SWCNT–NH_2) on *S. typhimurium* were compared (Arias and Yang, 2009). The results showed that SWCNT–OH and SWCNT–COOH had antimicrobial activity at approximately 50 mg/ml, while SWCNT–NH_2 only showed antimicrobial activity at much higher concentrations. In addition, MWCNTs functionalized with –OH, –COOH and –NH_2 did not show antimicrobial activity to any of the tested bacterial cells up to s concentration of 500–875 mg/ml (Arias and Yang, 2009). However, another study reported that functionalized MWCNTs (produced by sonication in a mixture of H_2SO_4 and HNO_3 and thus containing –OH and –COOH) presented stronger antimicrobial activity than pristine MWCNTs (Kang *et al.*, 2008b). Furthermore, SWCNTs have also been functionalized with sugars, such as mannose or galactose (Gu *et al.*, 2005; Wang *et al.*, 2006; Luo *et al.*, 2009), and these materials were efficient in capturing *E. coli* (Gu *et al.*, 2005) and *Bacillus anthracis* spores (Luo *et al.*, 2009), resulting in a significant decline in the number of bacterial spores.

22.3.5 Impurities in CNT samples

Metal residues resulting from catalysts used for CNT synthesis are one of the major concerns in terms of CNT toxicity towards mammalian cells (Guo *et al.*, 2007; X.Y. Liu *et al.*, 2007). However, studies on SWCNTs (with Co residues; S. Liu *et al.*, 2009) and MWCNTs (with Fe residues; Kang *et al.*, 2008b) have suggested that small amount of metal residues have little influence on the antimicrobial activity of CNTs. S. Liu *et al.* (2009) compared SWCNT samples containing different amount of Co ranging from 19.28 to 0.17 atom %, and no significant differences among these samples were found. Other than metal residues, Kang *et al.* (2008b) demonstrated that amorphous carbon had no noticeable effects on the antimicrobial activity of CNTs.

22.3.6 Solution chemistry

In CNT antimicrobial activity studies, solution chemistry refers to the physiochemical properties of the culture solutions used. It includes the type of culture media, ionic strength, pH and its dissolved natural organic matters. Arias and Yang (2009) investigated the behaviour of functionalized SWNCTs in various media, including deionized water, 0.9% NaCl, PBS buffer and brain–heart infusion broth. They found that SWCNTs had strong antimicrobial activity in deionized water and 0.9% NaCl. However, SWCNTs displayed no antimicrobial activity in PBS buffer and brain–heart infusion broth. Ionic strength is an important factor influencing the performance of CNT-based water filters (Brady-Estevez *et al.*, 2010a,b,c). CNT filters could remove more viruses at higher ionic strengths (NaCl), and the authors claimed that this was because of the suppression of repulsive electrostatic interactions between viruses and CNTs. Different salts have diverse effects, for example adding $CaCl_2$ improves virus removal by CNT filters, whereas adding $MgCl_2$ reduces virus removal (Brady-Estevez *et al.*, 2010a,c). The pH of the solution also influences virus removal using CNT filters. Using a solution with pH 3.9, CNT filters showed a higher virus removal rate than using a solution with pH 9.0 (Brady-Estevez *et al.*, 2010a,c). These researchers predicted that natural organic matter may alter the surface charge, aggregation behaviour and mobility of CNTs in solution, thus modifying the interactions between CNTs and bacteria. Conversely, a recent antimicrobial assay showed no significant differences when natural organic matter from a river was present (Kang *et al.*, 2009). This may have been because of the low concentration of natural river organic matter present in the study.

22.3.7 Incubation time

Studies from different research groups have shown that the antimicrobial activity of CNTs is time dependent. A longer incubation time can increase the antimicrobial effect of CNTs. Vecitis *et al.* (2010) reported that most of the SWCNT antimicrobial action toward *E. coli* occurs shortly after contact between the bacteria and the SWCNTs, while Kang *et al.* (2009) found that the inactivation rate of *Bacillus subtilis* increased with an increase of incubation time from 1 to 4 h. SWCNT–COOH and SWCNT–OH also showed a time-dependent antimicrobial effect towards *S. typhimurium* in deionized water (Arias and Yang, 2009).

22.4 Antimicrobial Mechanisms of CNTs

It is important to elucidate the antimicrobial mechanism of CNTs so that their potential application can be realized without causing problems to humans and the environment. Unfortunately, it still not clear exactly how CNTs kill microbes. Some possible mechanisms have been studied by researchers, as illustrated in Fig. 22.2(a).

Kang *et al.* (2007) hypothesized that the antimicrobial activity of SWCNTs was induced by direct physical contact between bacterial cell membranes and SWCNT aggregates. According to their observation, most *E. coli* cells (79.9 ± 9.8 %) adhering to SWCNT aggregates were inactivated, while only a few of the free-swimming cells (7.6 ± 2.1%) were inactivated. When cell membranes are damaged after contact with CNTs, cell cytoplasmic constituents such as RNA and DNA can be detected in cell cultures. The concentration of RNA and DNA is significantly higher after incubation with SWCNTs, compared with cell cultures without SWCNTs (Kang *et al.*, 2008a,b; S. Liu *et al.*, 2009). Damage of bacterial membranes has also been observed by SEM (Wang *et al.*, 2006; Kang *et al.*, 2007, 2008a,b; S. Liu *et al.*, 2009; Vecitis *et al.*, 2010) (Fig. 22.2d,e). AFM images also reveal dynamic changes of bacterial morphology when cells are incubated with SWCNTs (Obraztsova *et al.*, 2009; S. Liu *et al.*, 2009) (Fig. 22.2b,c). S. Liu *et al.* (2009) proposed that individually dispersed

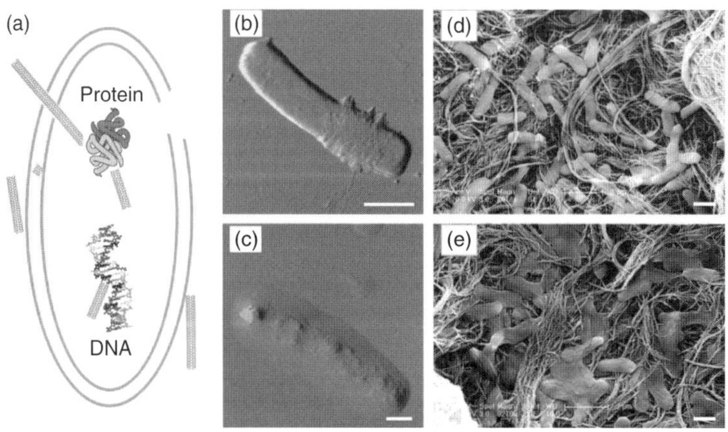

Fig. 22.2. (a) Schematic illustration of the antimicrobial mechanism of CNTs. (b) AFM image showing SWCNT networks covering one part of the surface of an *E. coli* cell. (From Liu *et al.*, 2009.) (c) AFM image showing the morphology changes in *E. coli* after incubation with SWCNTs. (From Liu *et al.*, 2009.) (d, e) SEM images showing damaged bacterial cells after contact with a CNT network. (From Kang *et al.*, 2008a.)

SWCNTs may be visualized as numerous moving 'nano darts' in solution, constantly attacking bacterial cells, thereby degrading bacterial cell integrity and causing cell death. Molecular dynamic simulation supported the observation that CNTs can penetrate the lipid bilayer of bacterial membranes (Lopez *et al.*, 2004). Liu *et al.* (2010) further mimicked the interaction between SWCNTs and bacterial cells using a sharp AFM tip to puncture bacterial cells. However, this AFM study indicated that a single collision by a nanotube is unlikely to introduce direct physical damages to a bacterial cell. SWCNT networks were found on *E. coli* cells after 2 h incubation (Fig. 22.2b), suggesting that bacterial death related to the accumulation effect of a large amount of nanotubes. CNTs can direct adsorb to bacterial cells through collisions (Deng *et al.*, 2008; Upadhyayula *et al.*, 2008; Akasaka and Watari, 2009; Upadhyayula *et al.*, 2009b). It has also been reported that bacteria in contact with SWCNT networks have much less biofilm growth (Rodrigues and Elimelech, 2010), suggesting that multiple contacts between CNTs and bacteria are necessary for the bacterial death.

As well as the physical damage induced by CNTs, the 'chemical' effects of CNTs on bacteria may also be important. Oxidative stress induced by CNTs could be a major cause of the antimicrobial activity of CNTs. DNA microarray analysis was applied to study gene expression in *E. coli* after exposure to SWCNTs and MWCNTs (Kang *et al.*, 2008a), and it was found that *E. coli* expresses a high level of stress-related σ-factor mRNA and other stress-related gene products after incubation with CNTs. Several expressed genes are part of the *soxRS* and *oxyR* systems, which are linked to the bacterial oxidative stress response (Kang *et al.*, 2008a). The oxidative stress of SWCNTs is dependent on their metallicity (Vecitis *et al.*, 2010). Glutathione was employed as an indicator of the cell oxidative stress. The extent of glutathione oxidation is higher when it reacts with metallic SWCNTs. Correspondingly, the death rate of *E. coli* is higher when they are exposed to metallic SWCNTs compared with incubation with semi-conducting SWCNTs. However, it should be noted that an oxidation–reduction potential analysis indicates that SWCNT is not a strong oxidant (Lopez *et al.*, 2004; S. Liu *et al.*, 2009). A thiol and sulfide quantization kit test also indicated that a free protein (bovine serum albumin) was not oxidized by SWCNTs (S. Liu *et al.*, 2009). On the other hand, although metal residue-induced oxidative stress has been considered as one of the major CNT toxicity mechanisms in mammalian cells (Guo *et al.*, 2007; X.Y. Liu *et al.*, 2007), metal residues play a minor role in the antimicrobial activity of CNTs, especially when high-purity CNT samples were used (Kang *et al.*, 2008b; S. Liu *et al.*, 2009).

Current observations suggest that the antimicrobial activity of CNTs is a synergistic effect of both 'physical' and 'chemical' effects (Vecitis *et al.*, 2010). When bacteria are incubated with CNTs, intensive collisions between CNTs and bacterial cells may cause physical damages on cell membranes as observed by researchers (Kang *et al.*, 2008a; Vecitis *et al.*, 2010). At the same time, some 'small' CNTs could be internalized by bacterial cells, while other 'larger' CNT aggregates may stick on the surface of bacterial cells (Wang *et al.*, 2006; Kang *et al.*, 2007; S. Liu *et al.*, 2010). Oxidative stress induced by CNTs on cell surfaces or inside cells may damage glutathione, lipids or proteins in the cytoplasm and membrane components (Kang *et al.*, 2008a; Vecitis *et al.*, 2010). The details of CNT antimicrobial mechanisms require further study.

22.5 Potential Applications

The strong antimicrobial activity of CNTs has motivated researchers to study their various potential applications. The general strategy is to use CNTs as active building blocks to form nanocomposites with various desired morphologies and functions, which may be suitable for specific purposes.

22.5.1 Antifouling surfaces and CNT filters

Many studies have focused on applying CNTs to water disinfection. When CNTs enter an aquatic environment, they may inactivate bacteria (Kang *et al.*, 2009). Surfaces deposited with SWCNT layers were found to be able to inhibit the formation of bacterial biofilms (Rodrigues and Elimelech, 2010). Bacteria and viruses can also be removed effectively by membrane filters containing SWCNTs or MWCNTs (Brady-Estevez *et al.*, 2008; Brady-Estevez *et al.*, 2010a,b,c). SWCNT filters were fabricated by depositing a thin layer of SWCNTs on a polyvinylidene fluoride or polytetrafluoroethylene (PTFE)-based microporous membrane (5 mm pore size) (Brady-Estevez *et al.*, 2008, 2010a), while MWCNT filters were made by depositing MWCNTs on a 5 mm pore-size PTFE membrane (Brady-Estevez *et al.*, 2010b). MWCNT filters removed more bacteriophage MS2 viruses than SWCNT filters under similar CNT loadings. The better performance of MWCNT filters was credited to the better uniformity of MWCNT layers (Brady-Estevez *et al.*, 2010b). A dual-layer SWCNT/MWCNT hybrid filter was then produced to improve its performance further. The hybrid filter was composed of a thin SWCNT layer (0.05 mg/cm^2) on top of a thicker MWCNT layer (0.27 mg/cm^2) supported on a 5 mm pore-size PTFE membrane (Brady-Estevez *et al.*, 2010b). This filter showed significantly higher virus removal efficiency compared with an SWCNT or MWCNT filter alone. Furthermore, Schoen *et al.* (2010) fabricated a water filter composed of silver nanowires, CNTs and cotton. This composite filter was able to kill concentrated bacteria in a high-throughput gravity-fed device under a moderate voltage bias at 20 V.

22.5.2 Antimicrobial CNT–polymer nanocomposites

Various CNT–polymer composites have been studied for their potential antimicrobial biomedical applications. A microporous film composed of SWCNTs and polyvinylpyrrolidone-iodine (PVPI) was prepared as antiseptic bands (Simmons *et al.*, 2009). The antiseptic iodine was available on the surface of SWCNTs wrapped together in polymer, and this film showed high antimicrobial activity towards *E. coli*. Aslan *et al.* (2010) dispersed SWCNTs in a biomedical polymer, poly(lactic-co-glycolic acid) (PLGA), to form thin films. This SWCNT–PLGA film were coated on cover glasses with the weight ratio of SWCNTs to PLGA ranging from 1:7000 to 1:70, and could effectively decrease the viability of *E. coli* and *S. epidermidis*. Schiffman and Elimelech (2011) incorporated SWCNTs into electrospun polysulfone mats and applied them as a conformal coating. The freestanding polymer mats with a low weight percentage of incorporated SWCNTs showed strong antimicrobial activity towards *E. coli*. The death rate of bacteria increased from 18 to 76% when the SWCNT content increased from 0.1 to 1.0 weight percentage. A CNT–agar composite also has been investigated for potential photothermal antimicrobial therapy (Akasaka *et al.*, 2010). Acrylic acid-grafted poly (butylene adipate-co-terephthalate) (PBAT-g-AA) and multihydroxyl-functionalized MWCNTs (MWCNT-OH) were used to prepare a hybrid material (PBAT-g-AA–MWCNT-OH), also exhibiting high antimicrobial activity (Wu 2009). Nepal *et al.* (2008) fabricated a multifunctional biomimetic film composed of SWCNT, DNA and lysozyme, using a layer-by-layer assembly method. This composite film with a high Young's modulus and controlled morphology showed excellent long-term antimicrobial activity. CNTs coated with silver particles have attracted interest from several research groups (T. Liu *et al.*, 2007; Yuan *et al.*, 2008; Kosaka *et al.*, 2009). Silver nanoparticles were grafted on to MWCNTs with the assistance of dendritic poly(amidoamine) (d-MWCNTs–Ag) and the composite showed strong antimicrobial activity against various bacteria (Yuan *et al.*, 2008). Similarly, silver-coated SWCNTs were prepared by attaching silver nanoparticles on the surface of amino-functionalized SWCNTs, and exhibited strong antimicrobial activity against *E. coli* and *S. aureus* (Kosaka *et al.*, 2009). Silver-coated CNTs with high antimicrobial activity can also be prepared by ion beam-assisted deposition (T. Liu *et al.*, 2007). Nanocomposites containing CNTs and titanium dioxide are another class of promising antimicrobial materials, especially under light irradiation. MWCNT–TiO_2 composites were synthesized using oxidized MWCNTs with different titanium alkoxide precursors in a benzene solvent and effectively inhibited the growth of bacteria when exposed to sunlight (Oh *et al.*, 2009).

22.5.3 Targeted antimicrobial activity

In potential antimicrobial drug applications, it is desirable that CNTs can recognize harmful microbes and do not show toxic effects to other cells or organisms. CNTs have often been studied as a tool for transport and cellular translocation of therapeutic molecules (Bianco *et al.*, 2005; Kostarelos *et al.*, 2009). For instance, CNTs have been studied intensively in tumour targeted drug delivery (Z. Liu *et al.*, 2007; McDevitt *et al.*, 2007; Bhirde *et al.*, 2009). However, few studies have investigated the targeted and specified antimicrobial activity of either pristine or functionalized CNTs in the presence of microbial and other kinds of cells. A recent study showed that a conjugate of functionalized CNT and amphotericin B exhibited strong antifungal activity without significant toxic effects on Jurkat cells (Wu *et al.*, 2005; Benincasa *et al.*, 2011). In this study, functionalized CNTs were used as a carrier of amphotericin B, rather than the active antimicrobial agent. We expect that more research will be carried out on the targeted and specified antimicrobial activity of CNTs in the near future. Various novel functionalization methods will play essential roles in producing and controlling the targeted antimicrobial activity of CNTs.

22.6 Summary and Perspectives

The antimicrobial activity of CNTs depends on their diameter, length, dispersion, electronic structure, surface functionalization and solution chemistry, as well as concentration and incubation time. Currently, a priority in this area is to establish reliable correlations between antimicrobial activity and specific CNT characteristics. Novel methods are needed for synthesis, purification, functionalization and enrichment of CNT samples, so that CNT samples with well-defined properties can be evaluated. New functionalization methods are also important to create and then manipulate the targeted antimicrobial activity of CNTs. Innovative fabrication methods are useful to fabricate CNT nanocomposites with desired composition and functions. These efforts would eventually realize their potential antimicrobial applications. Moreover, efficacy and toxicology studies are required to provide the necessary risk-to-benefit assessments. From a broader aspect, the antimicrobial activity of CNTs can be also combined with their unique electrical, thermal and spectroscopic properties for the development of innovative environmental and biomedical applications.

References

Akasaka, T. and Watari, F. (2009) Capture of bacteria by flexible carbon nanotubes. *Acta Biomaterialia* 5, 607–612.

Akasaka, T., Matsuoka, M., Hashimoto, T., Abe, S., Uo, M. and Watari, F. (2010) The bactericidal effect of carbon nanotube/agar composites irradiated with near-infrared light on *Streptococcus mutans. Materials Science and Engineering B – Advanced Functional Solid-state Materials* 173, 187–190.

Arias, L.R. and Yang, L.J. (2009) Inactivation of bacterial pathogens by carbon nanotubes in suspensions. *Langmuir* 25, 3003–3012.

Aslan, S., Loebick, C.Z., Kang, S., Elimelech, M., Pfefferle, L.D. and Van Tassel, P.R. (2010) Antimicrobial biomaterials based on carbon nanotubes dispersed in poly(lactic-co-glycolic acid). *Nanoscale* 2, 1789–1794.

Banerjee, S., Hemraj-Benny, T. and Wong, S.S. (2005) Routes towards separating metallic and semiconducting nanotubes. *Journal for Nanoscience and Nanotechnology* 5, 841–855.

Benincasa, M., Pacor, S., Wu, W., Prato, M., Bianco, A. and Gennaro, R. (2011) Antifungal activity of amphotericin B conjugated to carbon nanotubes. *ACS Nano* 5, 199–208.

Bethune, D.S., Kiang, C.H., Devries, M.S., Gorman, G., Savoy, R., Vazquez, J. and Beyers, R. (1993) Cobalt-catalyzed growth of carbon nanotubes with single-atomic-layer walls. *Nature* 363, 605–607.

Bhirde, A.A., Patel, V., Gavard, J., Zhang, G.F., Sousa, A.A., Masedunskas, A., Leapman, R.D.,

Weigert, R., Gutkind, J.S. and Rusling, J.F. (2009) Targeted killing of cancer cells *in vivo* and *in vitro* with EGF-directed carbon nanotube-based drug delivery. *ACS Nano* 3, 307–316.

Bianco, A., Kostarelos, K. and Prato, M. (2005) Applications of carbon nanotubes in drug delivery. *Current Opinion in Chemical Biology* 9, 674–679.

Brady-Estevez, A.S., Kang, S. and Elimelech, M. (2008) A single-walled-carbon-nanotube filter for removal of viral and bacterial pathogens. *Small* 4, 481–484.

Brady-Estevez, A.S., Nguyen, T.H., Gutierrez, L. and Elimelech, M. (2010a) Impact of solution chemistry on viral removal by a single-walled carbon nanotube filter. *Water Research* 44, 3773–3780.

Brady-Estevez, A.S., Schnoor, M.H., Kang, S. and Elimelech, M. (2010b) SWNT–MWNT hybrid filter attains high viral removal and bacterial inactivation. *Langmuir* 26, 19153–19158.

Brady-Estevez, A.S., Schnoor, M.H., Vecitis, C.D., Saleh, N.B. and Ehmelech, M. (2010c) Multiwalled carbon nanotube filter: improving viral removal at low pressure. *Langmuir* 26, 14975–14982.

Chen, Y., Ciuparu, D., Lim, S., Yang, Y.H., Haller, G.L. and Pfefferle, L. (2004a) Synthesis of uniform diameter single wall carbon nanotubes in co-mcm-41: effects of co pressure and reaction time. *Journal of Catalysis* 226, 351–362.

Chen, Y., Ciuparu, D., Lim, S.Y., Yang, Y.H., Haller, G.L. and Pfefferle, L. (2004b) Synthesis of uniform diameter single-wall carbon nanotubes in Co-MCM-41: effects of the catalyst prereduction and nanotube growth temperatures. *Journal of Catalysis* 225, 453–465.

Ciuparu, D., Chen, Y., Lim, S., Haller, G.L. and Pfefferle, L. (2004) Uniform-diameter single-walled carbon nanotubes catalytically grown in cobalt-incorporated mcm-41. *Journal of Physical Chemistry B* 108, 503–507.

Creach, V., Baudoux, A.C., Bertru, G. and Le Rouzic, B. (2003) Direct estimate of active bacteria: CTC use and limitations. *Journal of Microbiological Methods* 52, 19–28.

Dai, H.J., Rinzler, A.G., Nikolaev, P., Thess, A., Colbert, D.T. and Smalley, R.E. (1996) Single-wall nanotubes produced by metal-catalyzed disproportionation of carbon monoxide. *Chemical Physics Letters* 260, 471–475.

Deng, S.G., Upadhyayula, V.K.K., Smith, G.B. and Mitchell, M.C. (2008) Adsorption equilibrium and kinetics of microorganisms on single-wall carbon nanotubes. *IEEE Sensors Journal* 8, 954–962.

Dresselhaus, M.S., Dresselhaus, G. and Saito, R. (1992) Carbon-fibers based on c-60 and their symmetry. *Physical Review B: Condensed Matter and Materials Physics* 45, 6234–6242.

Du, F., Ma, Y.F., Lv, X., Huang, Y., Li, F.F. and Chen, Y.S. (2006) The synthesis of single-walled carbon nanotubes with controlled length and bundle, size using the electric arc method. *Carbon* 44, 1327–1330.

Endo, M., Strano, M.S. and Ajayan, P.M. (2008) Potential applications of carbon nanotubes. In: Ado, J., Dresselhaus, G. and Dresselhaus, M.S. (eds) *Carbon Nanotubes. Advanced Topics in the Synthesis, Structure, Properties and Applications.* Springer, Berlin/Heidelberg/New York, pp. 13–61.

Ghorannevis, Z., Kato, T., Kaneko, T. and Hatakeyama, R. (2010) Narrow-chirality distributed single-walled carbon nanotube growth from nonmagnetic catalyst. *Journal of the American Chemical Society* 132, 9570–9572.

Girifalco, L.A., Hodak, M. and Lee, R.S. (2000) Carbon nanotubes, buckyballs, ropes, and a universal graphitic potential. *Physical Review B: Condensed Matter and Materials Physics* 62, 13104–13110.

Gu, L.R., Elkin, T., Jiang, X.P., Li, H.P., Lin, Y., Qu, L.W., Tzeng, T.R.J., Joseph, R. and Sun, Y.P. (2005) Single-walled carbon nanotubes displaying multivalent ligands for capturing pathogens. *Chemical Communications* 874–876.

Guo, L., Morris, D.G., Liu, X.Y., Vaslet, C., Hurt, R.H. and Kane, A.B. (2007) Iron bioavailability and redox activity in diverse carbon nanotube samples. *Chemistry of Materials* 19, 3472–3478.

Guo, T., Nikolaev, P., Thess, A., Colbert, D.T. and Smalley, R.E. (1995) Catalytic growth of single-walled nanotubes by laser vaporization. *Chemical Physics Letters* 243, 49–54.

Haddon, R.C., Sippel, J., Rinzler, A.G. and Papadimitrakopoulos, F. (2004) Purification and separation of carbon nanotubes. *MRS Bulletin* 29, 252–259.

He, M., Chernov, A.I., Fedotov, P.V., Obraztsova, E.D., Sainio, J., Rikkinen, E., Jiang, H., Zhu, Z., Tian, Y., Kauppinen, E.I., Niemelä, M. and Krause, A.O.I. (2010) Predominant (6,5) single-walled carbon nanotube growth on a copper-promoted iron catalyst. *Journal of the American Chemical Society* 132, 13994–13996.

Hersam, M.C. (2008) Progress towards monodisperse single-walled carbon nanotubes. *Nature Nanotechnology* 3, 387–394.

Hu, W.B., Peng, C., Luo, W.J., Lv, M., Li, X.M., Li, D., Huang, Q. and Fan, C.H. (2010) Graphene-based antibacterial paper. *ACS Nano* 4, 4317–4323.

Iijima, S. (1991) Helical microtubules of graphitic carbon. *Nature* 354, 56–58.

Iijima, S. and Ichihashi, T. (1993) Single-shell carbon nanotubes of 1-nm diameter. *Nature* 363, 603–605.

Kang, S., Pinault, M., Pfefferle, L.D. and Elimelech, M. (2007) Single-walled carbon nanotubes exhibit strong antimicrobial activity. *Langmuir* 23, 8670–8673.

Kang, S., Herzberg, M., Rodrigues, D.F. and Elimelech, M. (2008a) Antibacterial effects of carbon nanotubes: size does matter. *Langmuir* 24, 6409–6413.

Kang, S., Mauter, M.S. and Elimelech, M. (2008b) Physicochemical determinants of multiwalled carbon nanotube bacterial cytotoxicity. *Environmental Science and Technology* 42, 7528–7534.

Kang, S., Mauter, M.S. and Elimelech, M. (2009) Microbial cytotoxicity of carbon-based nanomaterials: implications for river water and wastewater effluent. *Environmental Science and Technology* 43, 2648–2653.

Karousis, N., Tagmatarchis, N. and Tasis, D. (2010) Current progress on the chemical modification of carbon nanotubes. *Chemical Reviews* 110, 5366–5397.

Kosaka, T., Ohgami, A., Nakamura, T., Ohana, T. and Ishihara, M. (2009) The preparation of Ag nanoparticle-modified single-walled carbon nanotubes and their antibacterial activity. *Biocontrol Science* 14, 133–138.

Kostarelos, K., Bianco, A. and Prato, M. (2009) Promises, facts and challenges for carbon nanotubes in imaging and therapeutics. *Nature Nanotechnology* 4, 627–633.

Liu, J. and Hersam, M.C. (2010) Recent developments in carbon nanotube sorting and selective growth. *MRS Bulletin* 35, 315–321.

Liu, S., Wei, L., Hao, L., Fang, N., Chang, M.W., Xu, R., Yang, Y.H. and Chen, Y. (2009) Sharper and faster "nano darts" kill more bacteria: a study of antibacterial activity of individually dispersed pristine single-walled carbon nanotube. *ACS Nano* 3, 3891–3902.

Liu, S., Ng, A.K., Xu, R., Wei, J., Tan, C.M., Yang, Y. and Chen, Y. (2010) Antibacterial action of dispersed single-walled carbon nanotubes on *Escherichia coli* and *Bacillus subtilis* investigated by atomic force microscopy. *Nanoscale* 2, 2744–2750.

Liu, T., Tang, H.Q., Cai, X.M., Zhao, J., Li, D.J., Li, R. and Sun, X.L. (2007) A study on bactericidal properties of Ag coated carbon nanotubes. *Nuclear Instruments and Methods in Physics Research Section B – Beam Interactions with Materials and Atoms* 264, 282–286.

Liu, X.Y., Gurel, V., Morris, D., Murray, D.W., Zhitkovich, A., Kane, A.B. and Hurt, R.H. (2007) Bioavailability of nickel in single-wall carbon nanotubes. *Advanced Materials* 19, 2790–2796.

Liu, Z., Cai, W.B., He, L.N., Nakayama, N., Chen, K., Sun, X.M., Chen, X.Y. and Dai, H.J. (2007) *In vivo* biodistribution and highly efficient tumour targeting of carbon nanotubes in mice. *Nature Nanotechnology* 2, 47–52.

Liu, Z., Tabakman, S., Welsher, K. and Dai, H.J. (2009) Carbon nanotubes in biology and medicine: *in vitro* and *in vivo* detection, imaging and drug delivery. *Nano Research* 2, 85–120.

Lopez, C.F., Nielsen, S.O., Moore, P.B. and Klein, M.L. (2004) Understanding nature's design for a nanosyringe. *Proceedings of the National Academy of Sciences USA* 101, 4431–4434.

Lopez, V., Welte, L., Fernandez, M.A., Moreno-Moreno, M., Gomez-Herrero, J., De Pablo, P.J. and Zamora, F. (2009) Dependence of the single walled carbon nanotube length with growth temperature and catalyst density by chemical vapor deposition. *Journal of Nanoscience and Nanotechnology* 9, 2830–2835.

Luo, P.J.G., Wang, H.F., Gu, L.R., Lu, F.S., Lin, Y., Christensen, K.A., Yang, S.T. and Sun, Y.P. (2009) Selective interactions of sugar-functionalized single-walled carbon nanotubes with *Bacillus* spores. *ACS Nano* 3, 3909–3916.

McDevitt, M.R., Chattopadhyay, D., Kappel, B.J., Jaggi, J.S., Schiffman, S.R., Antczak, C., Njardarson, J.T., Brentjens, R. and Scheinberg, D.A. (2007) Tumor targeting with antibody-functionalized, radiolabeled carbon nanotubes. *Journal of Nuclear Medicine* 48, 1180–1189.

Monthioux, M. and Kuznetsov, V.L. (2006) Who should be given the credit for the discovery of carbon nanotubes? *Carbon* 44, 1621–1623.

Moon, Y.K., Lee, J., Lee, J.K., Kim, T.K. and Kim, S.H. (2009) Synthesis of length-controlled aerosol carbon nanotubes and their dispersion stability in aqueous solution. *Langmuir* 25, 1739–1743.

Nepal, D., Balasubramanian, S., Simonian, A.L. and Davis, V.A. (2008) Strong antimicrobial coatings: single-walled carbon nanotubes armored with biopolymers. *Nano Letters* 8, 1896–1901.

Obraztsova, E.A., Lukashev, E.P., Zarubina, A.P., Parkhomenko, I.M. and Yaminsky, I.V. (2009) Bactericidal action of single-walled carbon nanotubes. *Moscow University Physics Bulletin* 64, 320–323.

Oh, W.C., Zhang, F.J. and Chen, M.L. (2009) Preparation of MWCNT/TiO2 composites by using MWCNTs and titanium(IV) alkoxide precursors in benzene and their photocatalytic effect and bactericidal activity. *Bulletin of the Korean Chemical Society* 30, 2637–2642.

Ouyang, M., Huang, J.L. and Lieber, C.M. (2002a) Fundamental electronic properties and applications of single-walled carbon nanotubes. *Accounts of Chemical Research* 35, 1018–1025.

Ouyang, M., Huang, J.L. and Lieber, C.M. (2002b) Scanning tunneling microscopy studies of the one-dimensional electronic properties of single-walled carbon nanotubes. *Annual Review of Physical Chemistry* 53, 201–220.

Porter, A.E., Gass, M., Muller, K., Skepper, J.N., Midgley, P.A. and Welland, M. (2007) Direct imaging of single-walled carbon nanotubes in cells. *Nature Nanotechnology* 2, 713–717.

Rivera Gil, P., Oberdörster, G.N., Elder, A., Puntes, V.C. and Parak, W.J. (2010) Correlating physico-chemical with toxicological properties of nanoparticles: the present and the future. *ACS Nano* 4, 5527–5531.

Rodrigues, D.F. and Elimelech, M. (2010) Toxic effects of single-walled carbon nanotubes in the development of *E. coli* biofilm. *Environmental Science and Technology* 44, 4583–4589.

Saito, R., Fujita, M., Dresselhaus, G. and Dresselhaus, M.S. (1992) Electronic-structure of graphene tubules based on C60. *Physical Review B: Condensed Matter and Materials Physics* 46, 1804–1811.

Schiffman, J.D. and Elimelech, M. (2011) Antibacterial activity of electrospun polymer mats with incorporated narrow diameter single-walled carbon nanotubes. *ACS Applied Materials and Interfaces* 3, 462–468.

Schoen, D.T., Schoen, A.P., Hu, L., Kim, H.S., Heilshorn, S.C. and Cui, Y. (2010) High speed water sterilization using one-dimensional nanostructures. *Nano Letters* 10, 3628–3632.

Simmons, T.J., Lee, S.H., Park, T.J., Hashim, D.P., Ajayan, P.M. and Linhardt, R.J. (2009) Antiseptic single wall carbon nanotube bandages. *Carbon* 47, 1561–1564.

Tasis, D., Tagmatarchis, N., Bianco, A. and Prato, M. (2006) Chemistry of carbon nanotubes. *Chemical Reviews* 106, 1105–1136.

Upadhyayula, V.K.K. and Gadhamshetty, V. (2010) Appreciating the role of carbon nanotube composites in preventing biofouling and promoting biofilms on material surfaces in environmental engineering: a review. *Biotechnology Advances* 28, 802–816.

Upadhyayula, V.K.K., Deng, S.G., Mitchell, M.C., Smith, G.B., Nair, V.K. and Ghoshroy, S. (2008) Adsorption kinetics of *Escherichia coli* and *Staphylococcus aureus* on single-walled carbon nanotube aggregates. *Water Science and Technology* 58, 179–184.

Upadhyayula, V.K.K., Deng, S.G., Mitchell, M.C. and Smith, G.B. (2009a) Application of carbon nanotube technology for removal of contaminants in drinking water: a review. *Science of the Total Environment* 408, 1–13.

Upadhyayula, V.K.K., Deng, S.G., Smith, G.B. and Mitchell, M.C. (2009b) Adsorption of *Bacillus subtilis* on single-walled carbon nanotube aggregates, activated carbon and NanoCeram™. *Water Research* 43, 148–156.

Vecitis, C.D., Zodrow, K.R., Kang, S. and Elimelech, M. (2010) Electronic-structure-dependent bacterial cytotoxicity of single-walled carbon nanotubes. *ACS Nano* 4, 5471–5479.

Wang, F., Dukovic, G., Brus, L.E. and Heinz, T.F. (2005) The optical resonances in carbon nanotubes arise from excitons. *Science* 308, 838–841.

Wang, H., Wang, B., Quek, X.Y., Wei, L., Zhao, J.W., Li, L.J., Chan-Park, M.B., Yang, Y.H. and Chen, Y.A. (2010) Selective synthesis of (9,8) single walled carbon nanotubes on cobalt incorporated TUD-1 catalysts. *Journal of the American Chemical Society* 132, 16747–16749.

Wang, H.F., Gu, L.R., Lin, Y., Lu, F.S., Meziani, M.J., Luo, P.G.J., Wang, W., Cao, L. and Sun, Y.P. (2006) Unique aggregation of anthrax (*Bacillus anthracis*) spores by sugar-coated single-walled carbon nanotubes. *Journal of the American Chemical Society* 128, 13364–13365.

Wei, L., Wang, B., Wang, Q., Li, L.J., Yang, Y.H. and Chen, Y. (2008) Effect of centrifugation on the purity of single-walled carbon nanotubes from MCM-41 containing cobalt. *Journal of Physical Chemistry C* 112, 17567–17575.

Wu, C.S. (2009) Antibacterial and static dissipating composites of poly(butylene adipate-co-terephthalate) and multi-walled carbon nanotubes. *Carbon* 47, 3091–3098.

Wu, W., Wieckowski, S., Pastorin, G., Benincasa, M., Klumpp, C., Briand, J.P., Gennaro, R., Prato, M. and Bianco, A. (2005) Targeted delivery of amphotericin B to cells by using functionalized carbon nanotubes. *Angewandte Chemie International Edition* 44, 6358–6362.

Yang, C.N., Mamouni, J., Tang, Y.A. and Yang, L.J. (2010) Antimicrobial activity of single-walled carbon nanotubes: length effect. *Langmuir* 26, 16013–16019.

Yuan, W., Jiang, G.H., Che, J.F., Qi, X.B., Xu, R., Chang, M.W., Chen, Y., Lim, S.Y., Dai, J. and Chan-Park, M.B. (2008) Deposition of silver nanoparticles on multiwalled carbon nanotubes grafted with hyperbranched poly(amidoamine) and their antimicrobial effects. *Journal of Physical Chemistry C* 112, 18754–18759.

Zheng, L.X., O'Connell, M.J., Doorn, S.K., Liao, X.Z., Zhao, Y.H., Akhadov, E.A., Hoffbauer, M.A., Roop, B.J., Jia, Q.X. and Dye, R.C. (2004) Ultralong single-wall carbon nanotubes. *Nature Materials* 3, 673–676.

Index